WORLD *of* MICROBIOLOGY AND IMMUNOLOGY

WORLD *of*

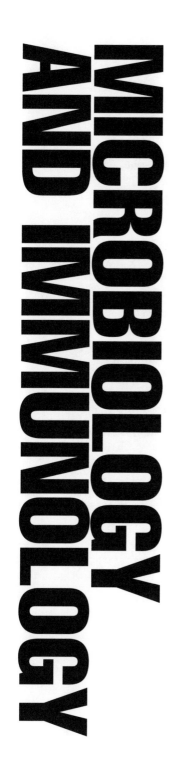

K. Lee Lerner and Brenda Wilmoth Lerner, *Editors*

Volume 1
A-L

GALE®

THOMSON

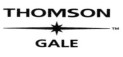

GALE

Detroit • New York • San Diego • San Francisco • Cleveland • New Haven, Conn. • Waterville, Maine • London • Munich

THOMSON
— ★ —
™
GALE

World of Microbiology and Immunology

K. Lee Lerner and Brenda Wilmoth Lerner, *Editors*

Project Editor
Brigham Narins

Editorial
Mark Springer

Permissions
Margaret Chamberlain, Jackie Jones

Imaging and Multimedia
Leitha Etheridge-Sims, Mary K. Grimes, Lezlie
Light, Dan Newell, David G. Oblender,
Christine O'Bryan, Robyn V. Young

Product Design
Michael Logusz

Manufacturing
Rhonda Williams

LIBRARY OF CONGRESS CATALOGING-IN-PUBLICATION DATA

World of microbiology and immunology / K. Lee Lerner and Brenda Wilmoth
Lerner, editors.
    p. ; cm.
        Includes bibliographical references and index.
        ISBN 0-7876-6540-1 (set : alk. paper)—
        ISBN 0-7876-6541-X (v. 1 : alk. paper)—
        ISBN 0-7876-6542-8 (v. 2 : alk. paper)
        1. Microbiology—Encyclopedias. 2. Immunology—Encyclopedias.
        [DNLM: 1. Allergy and Immunology—Encyclopedias—English.
        2. Microbiology—Encyclopedias—English. QW 13 W927 2003]
        I. Lerner, K. Lee. II. Lerner, Brenda Wilmoth.
QR9 .W675 2003
579'.03—dc21   2002010181
ISBN: 0-7876-6541-X

Printed in the United States of America
10 9 8 7 6 5 4 3 2 1

CONTENTS

INTRODUCTION vii

HOW TO USE THIS BOOK ix

ACKNOWLEDGMENTS xiii

ENTRIES
    Volume 1: A-L 1
    Volume 2: M-Z 359

SOURCES CONSULTED 619

HISTORICAL CHRONOLOGY 643

GENERAL INDEX 661

INTRODUCTION

Although microbiology and immunology are fundamentally separate areas of biology and medicine, they combine to provide a powerful understanding of human health and disease—especially with regard to infectious disease, disease prevention, and tragically, of the growing awareness that bioterrorism is a real and present worldwide danger.

World of Microbiology and Immunology is a collection of 600 entries on topics covering a range of interests—from biographies of the pioneers of microbiology and immunology to explanations of the fundamental scientific concepts and latest research developments. In many universities, students in the biological sciences are not exposed to microbiology or immunology courses until the later half of their undergraduate studies. In fact, many medical students do not receive their first formal training in these subjects until medical school. Despite the complexities of terminology and advanced knowledge of biochemistry and genetics needed to fully explore some of the topics in microbiology and immunology, every effort has been made to set forth entries in everyday language and to provide accurate and generous explanations of the most important terms. The editors intend *World of Microbiology and Immunology* for a wide range of readers. Accordingly, the articles are designed to instruct, challenge, and excite less experienced students, while providing a solid foundation and reference for more advanced students. The editors also intend that *World of Microbiology and Immunology* be a valuable resource to the general reader seeking information fundamental to understanding current events.

Throughout history, microorganisms have spread deadly diseases and caused widespread epidemics that threatened and altered human civilization. In the modern era, civic sanitation, water purification, immunization, and antibiotics have dramatically reduced the overall morbidity and the mortality of disease in advanced nations. Yet much of the world is still ravaged by disease and epidemics, and new threats constantly appear to challenge the most advanced medical and public health systems. For all our science and technology, we are far from mastering the microbial world.

During the early part of the twentieth century, the science of microbiology developed somewhat independently of other biological disciplines. Although for many years it did not exist as a separate discipline at all—being an "off-shoot" of chemistry (fermentation science) or medicine—with advances in techniques such as microscopy and pure culturing methodologies, as well as with the establishment of the germ theory of disease and the rudiments of vaccination, microbiology suddenly exploded as a separate discipline. Whereas other biological disciplines were concerned with such topics as cell structure and function, the ecology of plants and animals, the reproduction and development of organisms, the nature of heredity and the mechanisms of evolution, microbiology had a very different focus. It was concerned primarily with the agents of infectious disease, the immune response, the search for chemotherapeutic agents and bacterial metabolism. Thus, from the very beginning, microbiology as a science had social applications. A more detailed historical perspective of the development of the field may be found in the article "History of Microbiology" in this volume.

Microbiology established a closer relationship with other biological disciplines in the 1940s because of its association with genetics and biochemistry. This association also laid the foundations for the subsequent and still rapidly developing field of genetic engineering, which holds promise of profound impact on science and medicine.

Microorganisms are extremely useful experimental subjects because they are relatively simple, grow rapidly, and can be cultured in large quantities. George W. Beadle and Edward L. Tatum studied the relationship between genes and enzymes in 1941 using mutants of the bread mold *Neurospora*. In 1943 Salvador Luria and Max Delbrück used bacterial mutants to show that gene mutations were apparently spontaneous and not directed by the environment. Subsequently, Oswald Avery, Colin M. MacLeod, and Maclyn McCarty provided strong evidence that DNA was the genetic material and carried genetic information during transformation. The interactions between microbiology, genetics, and biochemistry soon led to the development of modern, molecularly oriented genetics.

Recently microbiology has been a major contributor to the rise of molecular biology, the branch of biology dealing with the physical and chemical bases of living matter and its function. Microbiologists have been deeply involved in studies of the genetic code and the mechanisms of DNA, RNA, and protein synthesis. Microorganisms were used in many of the early studies on the regulation of gene expression and the control of enzyme activity. In the 1970s new discoveries in microbiology led to the development of recombinant gene technology and genetic engineering. One indication of the importance of microbiology today is the number of Nobel Prizes awarded for work in physiology and medicine during the twentieth century; about a third of these were awarded to scientists working on microbiological problems.

Microorganisms are exceptionally diverse, are found almost everywhere, and affect human society in countless ways. The modern study of microbiology is very different from the chemically and medically oriented discipline pioneered by Louis Pasteur and Robert Koch. Today it is a large discipline with many specialities. It has impact on medicine, agricultural and food sciences, ecology, genetics, biochemistry, and many other fields. Today it clearly has both basic and applied aspects.

Many microbiologists are interested in the biology of the microorganisms themselves. They may focus on a specific group of microorganisms and be called virologists (scientists who study viruses), bacteriologists (scientists who study bacteria), phycologists or algologists (scientists who study algae), mycologists (scientists who study fungi), or protozoologists (scientists who study protozoa). Others may be interested in microbial morphology or particular functional processes and work in fields such as microbial cytology, physiology, ecology, genetics, taxonomy, and molecular biology. Some microbiologists may have a more applied orientation and work on problems in fields such as medical microbiology, food and dairy microbiology, or public health. Because the various fields of microbiology are interrelated, an applied microbiologist must always be familiar with basic microbiology. For example, a medical microbiologist must have a good understanding of microbial taxonomy, genetics, immunology, and physiology to identify and properly respond to the pathogen of concern.

It is clear that scientists study the microbial world in much the same way as they studied the world of multicellular organisms at the beginning of the twentieth century, when microbiology was a young discipline. This is in part due to the huge developments and refinements of techniques, which now allow scientists to more closely and fully investigate the world of bacteria and viruses.

One of the focuses of this book is the field of medical microbiology and its connection with immunology. Medical microbiology developed between the years 1875 and 1918, during which time many disease-causing bacteria were identified and the early work on viruses begun. Once people realized that these invisible agents could cause disease, efforts were made to prevent their spread from sick to healthy people. The great successes that have taken place in the area of human health in the past 100 years have resulted largely from advances in the prevention and treatment of infectious disease. We can consider the eradication of smallpox, a viral disease, as a prime example. The agent that causes this disease is one of the greatest killers the world has ever known—and was probably the greatest single incentive towards the formalization of the specialized study of immunology. Research into the mechanism of Edward Jenner's "vaccination" discovery—he found that of a patient injected with cow-pox produces immunity to smallpox—laid the foundations for the understanding of the immune system and the possibility of dealing with other diseases in a similar way. Because of an active worldwide vaccination program, no cases of smallpox have been reported since 1977. (This does not mean, however, that the disease cannot reappear, whether by natural processes or bioterror.)

Another disease that had a huge social impact was bubonic plague, a bacterial disease. Its effects were devastating in the Middle Ages. Between 1346 and 1350, one third of the entire population of Europe died of bubonic plague. Now generally less than 100 people die each year from this disease. The discovery of antibiotics in the early twentieth century provided an increasingly important weapon against bacterial diseases, and they have been instrumental in preventing similar plague epidemics.

Although progress in the application of immunological research has been impressive, a great deal still remains to be done, especially in the treatment of viral diseases (which do not respond to antibiotics) and of the diseases prevalent in developing countries. Also, seemingly "new" diseases continue to arise. Indeed, there has been much media coverage in the past twenty years in the U.S. of several "new" diseases, including Legionnaires' disease, toxic shock syndrome, Lyme disease, and acquired immunodeficiency syndrome (AIDS). Three other diseases emerged in 1993. In the summer of that year a mysterious flu-like disease struck the Southwest, resulting in 33 deaths. The causative agent was identified as a virus, hantavirus, carried by deer mice and spread in their droppings. In the same year, more than 500 residents of the state of Washington became ill with a strain of *Escherichia coli* present in undercooked beef prepared at a fast-food restaurant. The organism synthesized a potent toxin and caused haemolytic-uremic syndrome. Three children died. In 1993, 400,000 people in Milwaukee became ill with a diarrheal disease, cryptosporidiosis, that resulted from the improper chlorination of the water supply.

It is a great credit to the biomedical research community that the causative agents for all these diseases were identified very soon after the outbreaks. The bacteria causing Legionnaires' disease and Lyme disease have only been isolated in the past few decades, as have the viruses that cause AIDS. A number of factors account for the fact that seemingly "new" diseases arise almost spontaneously, even in industrially advanced countries. As people live longer, their ability to ward off infectious agents is impaired and, as a result, the organisms that usually are unable to cause disease become potentially deadly agents. Also, lifestyles change and new opportunities arise for deadly agents. For example, the use of vaginal tampons by women has resulted in an environment in which the Staphylococcus bacterium can grow and produce a toxin causing toxic shock syndrome. New diseases can also emerge because some agents have the ability to change abruptly and thereby gain the opportunity to infect new hosts. It is possible that one of the agents that causes AIDS arose from a virus that at one time could only infect other animals.

Not only are new diseases appearing but many infectious diseases that were on the wane in the U.S. have started to increase again. One reason for this resurgence is that thousands of U.S. citizens and foreign visitors enter the country daily. About one in five visitors now come from a country where diseases such as malaria, cholera, plague, and yellow fever still exist. In developed countries these diseases have been largely eliminated through sanitation, vaccination, and quarantine. Ironically, another reason why certain diseases are on the rise is the very success of past vaccination programs: because many childhood diseases (including measles, mumps, whooping cough, and diphtheria) have been effectively controlled in both developed and developing countries, some parents now opt not to vaccinate their children. Thus if the disease suddenly appears, many more children are susceptible.

A third reason for the rise of infectious diseases is that the increasing use of medications that prolong the life of the elderly, and of treatments that lower the disease resistance of patients, generally weaken the ability of the immune system to fight diseases. People infected with human immunodeficiency virus (HIV), the virus responsible for AIDS, are a high-risk group for infections that their immune systems would normally resist. For this reason, tuberculosis (TB) has increased in the U.S. and worldwide. Nearly half the world's population is infected with the bacterium causing TB, though for most people the infection is inactive. However, many thousands of new cases of TB are reported in the U.S. alone, primarily among the elderly, minority groups, and people infected with HIV. Furthermore, the organism causing these new cases of TB is resistant to the antibiotics that were once effective in treating the disease. This phenomenon is the result of the uncontrolled overuse of antibiotics over the last 70 years.

Until a few years ago, it seemed possible that the terrible loss of life associated with the plagues of the Middle Ages or with the pandemic influenza outbreak of 1918 and 1919 would never recur. However, the emergence of AIDS dramatizes the fact that microorganisms can still cause serious, incurable, life-threatening diseases. With respect to disease control, there is still much microbiological research to be done, especially in relation to the fields of immunology and chemotherapy.

Recent advances in laboratory equipment and techniques have allowed rapid progress in the articulation and understanding of the human immune system and of the elegance of the immune response. In addition, rapidly developing knowledge of the human genome offers hope for treatments designed to effectively fight disease and debilitation both by directly attacking the causative pathogens, and by strengthening the body's own immune response.

Because information in immunology often moves rapidly from the laboratory to the clinical setting, it is increasingly important that scientifically literate citizens—those able to participate in making critical decisions regarding their own health care—hold a fundamental understanding of the essential concepts in both microbiology and immunology.

Alas, as if the challenges of nature were not sufficient, the evolution of political realities in the last half of the twentieth century clearly points toward the probability that, within the first half of the twenty-first century, biological weapons will surpass nuclear and chemical weapons as a threat to civilization. Accordingly, informed public policy debates on issues of biological warfare and bioterrorism can only take place when there is a fundamental understanding of the science underpinning competing arguments.

The editors hope that *World of Microbiology and Immunology* inspires a new generation of scientists who will join in the exciting worlds of microbiological and immunological research. It is also our modest wish that this book provide valuable information to students and readers regarding topics that play an increasingly prominent role in our civic debates, and an increasingly urgent part of our everyday lives.

K. Lee Lerner & Brenda Wilmoth Lerner, editors
St. Remy, France
June 2002

Editor's note: *World of Microbiology and Immunology* is not intended to be a guide to personal medical treatment or emergency procedures. Readers desiring information related to personal issues should always consult with their physician. The editors respectfully suggest and recommend that readers desiring current information related to emergency protocols—especially with regard to issues and incidents related to bioterrorism—consult the United States Centers for Disease Control and Prevention (CDC) website at http://www.cdc.gov/.

How to Use the Book

The articles in the book are meant to be understandable by anyone with a curiosity about topics in microbiology or immunology. Cross-references to related articles, definitions, and biographies in this collection are indicated by **bold-faced type**, and these cross-references will help explain and expand the individual entries. Although far from containing a comprehensive collection of topics related to genetics, *World of Microbiology and Immunology* carries specifically selected topical entries that directly impact topics in microbiology and immunology. For those readers interested in genetics, the editors recommend Gale's *World of Genetics* as an accompanying reference. For those readers interested in additional information regarding the human immune system, the editors recommend Gale's *World of Anatomy and Physiology*.

This first edition of *World of Microbiology and Immunology* has been designed with ready reference in mind:

- **Entries are arranged alphabetically** rather than chronologically or by scientific field. In addition to classical topics, *World of Microbiology and Immunology* contains many articles addressing the impact of advances in microbiology and immunology on history, ethics, and society.

- **Bold-faced terms** direct the reader to related entries.
- **"See also" references** at the end of entries alert the reader to related entries not specifically mentioned in the body of the text.
- A **Sources Consulted** section lists the most worthwhile print material and web sites we encountered in the compilation of this volume. It is there for the inspired reader who wants more information on the people and discoveries covered in this volume.
- The **Historical Chronology** includes many of the significant events in the advancement of microbiology and immunology. The most current entries date from just days before *World of Microbiology and Immunology* went to press.
- A **comprehensive General Index** guides the reader to topics and persons mentioned in the book. Bolded page references refer the reader to the term's full entry.

Although there is an important and fundamental link between the composition and shape of biological molecules and their functions in biological systems, a detailed understanding of biochemistry is neither assumed or required for *World of Microbiology and Immunology*. Accordingly, students and other readers should not be intimidated or deterred by the complex names of biochemical molecules (especially the names for particular proteins, enzymes, etc.). Where necessary, sufficient information regarding chemical structure is provided. If desired, more information can easily be obtained from any basic chemistry or biochemistry reference.

Advisory Board

In compiling this edition we have been fortunate in being able to rely upon the expertise and contributions of the following scholars who served as academic and contributing advisors for *World of Microbiology and Immunology*, and to them we would like to express our sincere appreciation for their efforts to ensure that *World of Microbiology and Immunology* contains the most accurate and timely information possible:

Robert G. Best, Ph.D.
Director, Division of Genetics, Department of Obstetrics and Gynecology
University of South Carolina School of Medicine
Columbia, South Carolina

Antonio Farina, M.D., Ph.D.
Visiting Professor, Department of Pathology and Laboratory Medicine
Brown University School of Medicine
Providence, Rhode Island
Professor, Department of Embryology, Obstetrics, and Gynecology
University of Bologna
Bologna, Italy

Brian D. Hoyle, Ph.D.
Microbiologist

Member, American Society for Microbiology and the Canadian Society of Microbiologists
Nova Scotia, Canada

Eric v.d. Luft, Ph.D., M.L.S.
Curator of Historical Collections
SUNY Upstate Medical University
Syracuse, New York

Danila Morano, M.D.
University of Bologna
Bologna, Italy

Judyth Sassoon, Ph.D., ARCS
Department of Biology & Biochemistry
University of Bath
Bath, England

Constance K. Stein, Ph.D.
Director of Cytogenetics, Assistant Director of Molecular Diagnostics
SUNY Upstate Medical University
Syracuse, New York

Acknowledgments

In addition to our academic and contributing advisors, it has been our privilege and honor to work with the following contributing writers, and scientists: Sherri Chasin Calvo; Sandra Galeotti, M.S.; Adrienne Wilmoth Lerner; Jill Liske, M.Ed.; and Susan Thorpe-Vargas, Ph.D.

Many of the advisors for *World of Microbiology and Immunology* authored specially commissioned articles within their field of expertise. The editors would like to specifically acknowledge the following contributing advisors for their special contributions:

Robert G. Best, Ph.D.
Immunodeficiency disease syndromes
Immunodeficiency diseases, genetic

Antonio Farina, M.D., Ph.D.
Reproductive immunology

Brian D. Hoyle, Ph.D.
Anthrax, terrorist use of as a biological weapon

Eric v.d. Luft, Ph.D., M.L.S.
The biography of Dr. Harry Alfred Feldman

Danila Morano, M.D.
Rh and Rh incompatibility

Judyth Sassoon, Ph.D.
BSE and CJD disease, ethical issues and socio-economic impact

Constance K. Stein, Ph.D.
Genetic identification of microorganisms

Susan Thorpe-Vargas, Ph.D
Immunology, nutritional aspects

The editors would like to extend special thanks Dr. Judyth Sassoon for her contributions to the introduction to *World of Microbiology and Immunology*. The editors also wish to acknowledge Dr. Eric v.d. Luft for his diligent and extensive research related to the preparation of many difficult biographies. The editors owe a great debt of thanks to Dr. Brian Hoyle for his fortitude and expertise in the preparation and review of a substantial number of articles appearing in *World of Microbiology and Immunology*.

The editors gratefully acknowledge the assistance of many at Gale for their help in preparing *World of Microbiology and Immunology*. The editors thank Ms. Christine Jeryan and Ms. Meggin Condino for their faith in this project. Special thanks are offered to Ms. Robyn Young and the Gale Imaging Team for their guidance through the complexities and difficulties related to graphics. Most directly, the editors wish to acknowledge and thank the Project Editor, Mr. Brigham Narins for his good nature, goods eyes, and intelligent sculptings of *World of Microbiology and Immunology*.

The editors dedicate this book to Leslie Moore, M.D., James T. Boyd, M.D., E.M. Toler, M.D., and to the memory of Robert Moore, M.D. Their professional skills and care provided a safe start in life for generations of children, including our own.

The editors and authors also dedicate this book to the countless scientists, physicians, and nurses who labor under the most dangerous and difficult of field conditions to bring both humanitarian assistance to those in need, and to advance the frontiers of microbiology and immunology.

ACKNOWLEDGMENTS

A group of seven exiled lepers, photograph. © Michael Maslan Historic Photographs/Corbis. Reproduced by permission.—A hand holds an oyster on the half-shell, photograph. © Philip Gould/Corbis. Reproduced by permission.—A magnified virus called alpha-plaque, photograph. © Lester V. Bergman/Corbis. Reproduced by permission.—A paramecium protozoan, photograph. © Lester V. Bergman/Corbis. Reproduced by permission.—A paramecium undergoing a sexual reproductive fission, photograph. © Lester V. Bergman/Corbis. Reproduced by permission.—A tubular hydrothermal, photograph. © Ralph White/Corbis. Reproduced by permission.—About 600 sheep from France and Great Britain, burning as precaution against spread of foot-and-mouth disease, photograph by Michel Spinger. AP/Wide World Photos. Reproduced by permission.—Aerial view shows the oil slick left behind by the Japanese fishing training vessel Ehime Maru, photograph. © AFP/Corbis. Reproduced by permission.—An employee of the American Media building carries literature and antibiotics after being tested for anthrax, photograph. © AFP/Corbis. Reproduced by permission.—An under-equipped system at the Detroit Municipal Sewage Water Treatment Plant, photograph. © Ted Spiegel/Corbis. Reproduced by permission.—Anthrax, photograph by Kent Wood. Photo Researcher, Inc. Reproduced by permission.—Arneson, Charlie, photograph. © Roger Ressmeyer/Corbis. Reproduced by permission.—Beer vats in brewery, Czechoslovakia, photograph by Liba Taylor. Corbis-Bettmann. Reproduced by permission.—Bellevue-Stratford Hotel, photograph. © Bettmann/Corbis. Reproduced by permission.—Bison grazing near Hot Springs, photograph. © Michael S. Lewis/Corbis. Reproduced by permission.—Boat collecting dead fish, photograph. AP/Wide World Photos. Reproduced by permission.—Bottles of the antibiotic Cipro, photograph. © FRI/Corbis Sygma. Reproduced by permission.—Bousset, Luc, photograph. © Vo Trung Dung/Corbis. Reproduced by permission.—Budding yeast cells, photograph. © Lester V. Bergman/Corbis. Reproduced by permission.—Chlorophyll, false-colour transmission electron micrograph of stacks of grana in a chloroplast, photograph by Dr. Kenneth R. Miller. Reproduced by permission.—Close-up of Ebola virus in the blood stream, photograph. © Institut Pasteur/Corbis Sygma. Reproduced by permission.—Close-up of Ebola virus, photograph. © Corbis Sygma/Corbis. Reproduced by permission.—Close-up of prion structure examined in 3-D, photograph. © CNRS/Corbis Sygma. Reproduced by permission.—Colonies of Penicillium Notatus, photograph. © Bettmann/Corbis. Reproduced by permission.—Colored fluids in chemical beakers, photograph. © Julie Houck/Corbis. Reproduced by permission.—Colored high resolution scanning electron micrograph of the nuclear membrane surface of a pancreatic acinar cell, photograph by P. Motta & T. Naguro/Science Photo Library/Photo Researchers, Inc. Reproduced by permission.—Composite image of three genetic researchers, photograph. Dr. Gopal Murti/Science Photo Library. Reproduced by permission.—Compost pile overflowing in community garden, photograph. © Joel W. Rogers/Corbis. Reproduced by permission.—Cosimi, Benedict, photograph. © Ted Spiegel/Corbis. Reproduced by permission.—Court In Open Air During 1918 Influenza Epidemic, photograph. © Bettmann/Corbis. Reproduced by permission.—Cringing girl getting vaccination injection against Hepatitis B, photograph. © Astier Frederik/Corbis Sygma. Reproduced by permission.—Crustose Lichen, photograph. © Richard P. Jacobs/JLM Visuals. Reproduced by permission.—Crying girl getting vaccination injection against Hepatitis B, photograph. © Astier Frederik/Corbis Sygma. Reproduced by permission.—Cultures of Photobacterium NZ-11 glowing in petri dishes, photograph. © Roger Ressmeyer/Corbis. Reproduced by permission.—Darwin, Charles, photograph. Popperfoto/Archive Photos. © Archive Photos, Inc. Reproduced by permission.—Detail view of an employee's hands using a pipette in a laboratory, photograph. © Bob Rowan; Progressive Image/Corbis. Reproduced by permission.—Diagram depicting DNA and RNA with an inset on the DNA side showing specific Base Pairing, diagram by Argosy Publishing. The Gale Group.—Diagram of DNA Replication I, inset showing Semiconservative Replication (DNA Replication II), diagram by Argosy Publishing. The Gale Group.—Diagram of the Central Dogma of Molecular Biology, DNA to RNA to Protein, diagram by Argosy Publishing. The Gale Group.—Diatom Plankton, circular, transparent organisms, photograph. Corbis/Douglas P. Wilson; Frank Lane Picture Agency. Reproduced by permission.—Dinoflagellate Peridinium sp., scanning electron micrograph. © Dr. Dennis Kunkel/Phototake. Reproduced by permission.—E. coli infection, photograph by Howard Sochurek. The Stock Market. Reproduced by permission.—Electron micrographs, hanta virus, and ebola virus, photograph. Delmar Publishers, Inc. Reproduced by permission.—Electron Microscope views Martian meteorite, photograph. © Reuters NewMedia Inc./Corbis. Reproduced by permission.—Elementary school student receiving a Vaccine, photograph. © Bob Krist/Corbis. Reproduced by permission.—Enzyme-lines immunoabsorbent assay (ELISA), photograph. © Lester V. Bergman/Corbis. Reproduced by permission.—False-color transmission electron micrograph of the aerobic soil bacterium, photograph by Dr. Tony Brain. Photo Researchers, Inc. Reproduced by permission.—Farmers feeding chickens, photograph. USDA—Firefighters preparing a decontamination chamber for FBI investigators, photograph. © Randall Mark/Corbis Sygma. Reproduced by permission.—First photographed view of the influenza virus, photograph. © Bettmann/Corbis. Reproduced by permission.—First sightings of actual antibody antigen docking seen on x-ray crystallography, photograph. © Ted Spiegel/Corbis. Reproduced by permission.—Fleming, Alexander, photograph. The Bettmann Archive/Corbis-Bettmann. Reproduced by permission.—Fleming, Sir Alexander, photograph. Corbis-Bettmann. Reproduced by permission.—Friend, Charlotte, photograph. The Library of Congress. Reproduced by permission.—Fungal skin infection causing Tinea, photograph. © Lester V. Bergman/Corbis. Reproduced by permission.—Fungus colony grown in a petri dish, photograph.© Lester V. Bergman/Corbis. Reproduced by permission.—Gambierdiscus toxicus, scanning electron micrograph by Dr. Dennis Kunkel. © Dr. Dennis Kunkel/Phototake. Reproduced by permission.—Genetic code related to models of amino acids inserting into a protein chart, diagram by Argosy Publishing. The Gale Group.—German firefighters remove suspicious looking packets from a post office distribution center, photograph. © Reuters NewMedia Inc./Corbis. Reproduced by permission.—Giardia, cells shown through a microscope, photograph by J. Paulin. Reproduced by permission.—Golden lichen, photograph. © Don Blegen/JLM Visuals. Reproduced by permission.—Hay fever allergy attack triggered by oilseed rape plants, photograph. © Niall Benvie/Corbis. Reproduced by permission.—Hemolytic Staphyloccoccus Streak Plate, photograph. © Lester V. Bergman/Corbis. Reproduced by permission.—Human Immunodeficiency Virus in color imaging, photograph. © Michael Freeman/Corbis. Reproduced by permission.—Industrial Breweries, man filling kegs, photograph. Getty Images. Reproduced by permission.—Investigators

wearing hazardous materials suits, U.S. Post Office in West Trenton, New Jersey, photograph. © AFP/Corbis. Reproduced by permission.—Iron lungs, photograph. UPI/Corbis-Bettmann. Reproduced by permission.—Jacob, Francois, photograph. The Library of Congress.—Jenner, Edward, photograph. Corbis-Bettmann. Reproduced by permission.—Kiefer, Sue, Dr., photograph. © James L. Amos/Corbis. Reproduced by permission.—Koch, Robert, studying Rinderpest in laboratory, photograph. © Bettmann/Corbis. Reproduced by permission.—Koch, Robert, photograph. The Library of Congress.—Laboratory technician doing medical research, photograph. © Bill Varie/Corbis. Reproduced by permission.—Laboratory technician performing a density test from urine samples, photograph. AP/Wide World Photos. Reproduced by permission.—Laboratory technician working with restriction enzymes, photograph. © Ted Spiegel/Corbis. Reproduced by permission.—Landsteiner, Karl, photograph. The Library of Congress.—Lederberg, Joshua and Esther, photograph, 1958. UPI-Corbis-Bettmann. Reproduced by permission.—Leeuwenhoek, Anton Van, photograph. Getty Images. Reproduced by permission.—Lightning strikes on Tucson horizon, photograph. Photo Researchers, Inc. Reproduced by permission.—Lister, Joseph, photograph. © Bettmann/Corbis. Reproduced by permission.—Magnification of a gram stain of pseudomonas aeruginosa, photograph. © Lester V. Bergman/Corbis. Reproduced by permission.—Magnification of bacillus, or rodlike bacteria, photograph. © Lester V. Bergman/Corbis. Reproduced by permission.—Magnification of human immunodeficiency virus (HIV), photograph. © Lester V. Bergman/Corbis. Reproduced by permission.—Magnification of klebsiella bacteria, photograph. © Lester V. Bergman/Corbis. Reproduced by permission.—Magnified fungi cells called Candida albicans sac, photograph. © Lester V. Bergman/Corbis. Reproduced by permission.—Making of a genetic marker, with an individual DNA sequence to indicate specific genes, photograph. © Richard T. Nowitz/Corbis. Reproduced by permission.—Mallon, Mary (Typhoid Mary), 1914, photograph. Corbis Corporation. Reproduced by permission.—Man carries stretcher with patient, dysentery epidemic amongst Hutu refugees, photograph. © Baci/Corbis. Reproduced by permission.—Man washing his hands, photograph. © Dick Clintsman/Corbis. Reproduced by permission.—Marine Plankton, green organisms with orange spots, photograph by Douglas P. Wilson. Corbis/Douglas P. Wilson; Frank Lane Picture Agency. Reproduced by permission.—Measles spots on child's back, photograph. © John Heselltine/Corbis. Reproduced by permission.—Medical Researcher, fills a sample with a pipette at the National Institute of Health Laboratory, photograph. © Paul A. Souders/Corbis. Reproduced by permission.—Medical researcher dills sample trays with a pipette in a laboratory, photograph. © Paul A. Souders/Corbis. Reproduced by permission.—Milstein, Cesar, photograph. Photo Researchers, Inc. Reproduced by permission.—Mitosis of an animal cell, immunofluorescence photomicrograph. © CNRI/Phototake. Reproduced by permission.—Mitosis telophase of an animal cell, photograph. © CNRI/Phototake. Reproduced by permission.—Montagnier, Luc, photograph by Gareth Watkins.

Reuters/Archive Photos, Inc. Reproduced by permission.—Mosquito after feeding on human, photograph by Rod Planck. National Audubon Society Collection/Photo Researchers, Inc. Reproduced by permission.—Novotny, Dr. Ergo, photograph. © Ted Spiegel/Corbis. Reproduced by permission.—Nucleus and perinuclear area-liver cell from rat, photograph by Dr. Dennis Kunkel. Phototake. Reproduced by permission.—Ocean wave curling to the left, photograph. Corbis. Reproduced by permission.—Oil slick on water, photograph. © James L. Amos/Corbis. Reproduced by permission.—Pasteur, Louis, photograph. The Library of Congress.—Patient getting vaccination injection against Hepatitis B, photograph. © Astier Frederik/Corbis Sygma. Reproduced by permission.—Patients at a Turkish Tuberculosis Hospital sit up in their beds, photograph. © Corbis. Reproduced by permission.—Petri dish culture of Klebsiella pneumoniae, photograph. © Lester V. Bergman/Corbis. Reproduced by permission.—Pharmaceutical technician, and scientist, discussing experiment results in laboratory, photograph. Martha Tabor/Working Images Photographs. Reproduced by permission.—Plague of 1665, photograph. Mary Evans Picture Library/Photo Researchers, Inc. Reproduced by permission.—Prusiner, Dr. Stanley B., photograph by Luc Novovitch. Reuters/Archive Photos, Inc. Reproduced by permission.—Raccoon in winter cottonwood, photograph by W. Perry Conway. Corbis Corporation. Reproduced by permission.—Researcher, in biochemistry laboratory using a transmission electron microscope, photograph by R. Maisonneuve. Photo Researchers, Inc. Reproduced by permission.—Resistant Staphyloccoccus Bacteria, photograph. © Lester V. Bergman/Corbis. Reproduced by permission.—Sample in a Petri Dish, photograph. © Bob Krist/Corbis. Reproduced by permission.—Scientists test water samples from a canal, photograph. © Annie Griffiths Belt, Corbis. Reproduced by permission.—Scientists wearing masks hold up beaker in a laboratory of chemicals, photograph. © Steve Chenn/Corbis. Reproduced by permission.—Sheep grazing on field, photograph. © Richard Dibon-Smith, National Audubon Society Collection/Photo Researchers, Inc. Reproduced with permission.—Shelf Fungi on Nurse Log, photograph. © Darell Gulin/Corbis. Reproduced by permission.—Silvestri, Mike, and Neil Colosi, Anthrax, Decontamination Technicians, photograph. © Mike Stocke/Corbis. Reproduced by permission.—Single mammalian tissue culture cell, color transmission electron micrograph. Dr. Gopal Murti/Science Photo Library/Photo Researchers, Inc. Reproduced by permission.—Steam rises from the surface of Yellowstone's Grand Prismatic Spring, photograph. © Roger Ressmeyer/Corbis. Reproduced by permission.—Steam rising from Therman Pool, photograph. © Pat O'Hara/Corbis. Reproduced by permission.—Streptococcus pyogenes bacteria, colored transmission electron micrograph by Alfred Pasieka. © Alfred Pasieka/Science Photo Library, Photo Researchers, Inc. Reproduced by permission.—Streptococcus viridans Bacteria in petri dish, photograph. © Lester V. Bergman/Corbis. Reproduced by permission.—Surgeons operating in surgical gowns and masks, photograph. © ER Productions/Corbis. Reproduced by permission.—Technician at American type culture collection, photograph. © Ted Spiegel/Corbis. Reproduced by permission.—Technician places culture on agar plates in laboratory, photograph. © Ian Harwood; Ecoscene/Corbis. Reproduced by permission.—The parasitic bacteria Staphylococcus magnified 1000x, photograph. © Science Pictures Limited/Corbis. Reproduced by permission.—The Plague of Florence, photograph. Corbis-Bettmann. Reproduced by permission.—Three-dimensional computer model of a protein molecule of matrix porin found in the E. Coli bacteria, photograph. © Corbis. Reproduced by permission.—Three-dimensional computer model of a protein molecule of matrix porin found in the E. Coli bacteria, photograph. © Corbis. Reproduced by permission.—Three-dimensional computer model of the enzyme acetylcholinesterase, photograph. © Corbis. Reproduced by permission.—Three-dimensional computer model of the molecule dihydrofolate reductatase enzyme, photograph. © Corbis. Reproduced by permission.—Three-dimensional computer model of the protein Alzheimer Amyloid B, photograph. © Corbis. Reproduced by permission.—Twenty most common amino acids, illustration by Robert L. Wolke. Reproduced by permission—Two brown mountain sheep, photograph. © Yoav Levy/Phototake NYC. Reproduced by permission.—United States Coast Guard hazardous material workers wearing protective suits work inside the U.S. Senate's Hart Building, photograph. © AFP/Corbis. Reproduced by permission.—Urey, Harold, photograph. The Library of Congress.—Veterinarian technicians check the blood pressure of a dog, photograph. AP/Wide World Photos. Reproduced by permission.—View of aging wine in underground cellar, photograph. Getty Images. Reproduced by permission.—Virus Plaque in an E. Coli culture, photograph. © Lester V. Bergman/Corbis. Reproduced by permission.—Visual biography of monoclonal antibody development at the Wistar Institute, photograph. © Ted Spiegel/Corbis. Reproduced by permission.—Waksman, Selman Abraham, photograph. Getty Images. Reproduced by permission.—Watson, James and Crick, Francis, photograph. Getty Images. Reproduced by permission.—Watson, James Dewey, photograph. The Library of Congress.—Wind storm on the East Coast, Cape Cod, Massachusetts, photograph. Gordon S. Smith/Photo Researchers, Inc. Reproduced by permission.—Woman clerks wearing cloth masks to protect against influenza, photograph. © Bettmann/Corbis. Reproduced by permission.—Woman scientist mixes chemicals in beaker, photograph. © Julie Houck/Corbis. Reproduced by permission.—Woman sneezing, photograph. © Michael Keller/Corbis. Reproduced by permission.—Young Children lying on beds in tuberculosis camp, photograph. © Bettmann/Corbis. Reproduced by permission.

A

ABBE, ERNST (1840-1905)
German optical engineer

Ernst Abbe was among the first optical engineers, designing and perfecting methods for manufacturing microscopes and lens systems of high quality. Though he was a great scientist in his own right, he might have remained anonymous but for the foresight of his employer, Carl Zeiss (1816–1888). In his early twenties Abbe was working as a lecturer in Jena, Germany. He was recognized as being intelligent and industrious, particularly in mathematics, but he was unable to secure a professorial position at the university. In 1855 Zeiss, the owner and operator of a local company that built optical instruments, approached him. Zeiss had realized that the dramatic rise in scientific interest and research in Europe would create a demand for precision instruments—instruments his shop could easily provide. However, neither Zeiss nor his employees possessed the scientific knowledge to design such instruments. Abbe was hired as a consultant to mathematically design lenses of unrivaled excellence.

The science of lenscrafting had stalled since the time of **Anton van Leeuwenhoek** (1632–1723), chiefly due to certain seemingly insurmountable flaws in man-made lenses. Foremost among these was the problem of chromatic aberration, which manifested itself as colored circles around the subject. Scientists were also frustrated with the poor quality of the glass used to make lenses. During the following decade, Abbe worked on new grinding procedures that might correct chromatic aberration; by combining his efforts with Zeiss's glassmaker, Otto Schott, he eventually succeeded in producing near-flawless scientific lenses of exceptionally high power. These same ten years were profitable ones for Abbe. With the increasing success of the Zeiss Works, Abbe was recognized as a scientist and was given a professorship at Jena University in 1875. Zeiss, who realized that the success of his business was in no small part due to Abbe's efforts, made the young professor a partner in 1876. Abbe's work on theoretical optics earned him international notoriety, and he was offered a position at the prestigious University of Berlin (a position he declined in order to continue his research at Zeiss).

During their collaboration Abbe and Zeiss produced thousands of scientific optical instruments. Their innovations set important standards for the development of telescopes and photographic equipment. Carl Zeiss died in 1888 leaving the entire Zeiss Works to Abbe. In addition to running the company, Abbe used his own considerable funds to set up the Carl Zeiss Foundation, an organization for the advancement of science and social improvement.

See also History of microbiology; Microscope and microscopy

ACNE, MICROBIAL BASIS OF

Acne is a condition that affects the hair follicles. A hair follicle consists of a pore the opens to the surface of the skin. The pore leads inward to a cavity that is connected to oil glands. The glands, which are called sebaceous glands, produce oil (sebum) that lubricates the skin and the hair that grows out of the cavity. As the hair grows the oil leaves the cavity and spreads out over the surface of the skin, were it forms a protective coating. However, in conditions such as acne, the oil becomes trapped in the cavities of the hair follicles. This accumulation of oil is irritating and so causes an **inflammation**. One consequence of the inflammation is an unsightly, scabby appearing crust on the surface of the skin over the inflamed follicles. This surface condition is acne.

Acne is associated with the maturation of young adults, particularly boys. Part of the maturation process involves the production or altered expression of hormones. In adolescence certain hormones called androgens are produced. Androgens stimulate the enlargement of the sebaceous glands and the resulting production of more oil, to facilitate the manufacture of more facial hair. In girls, androgen production is greater around the time of menstruation. Acne often appears in young women at the time of their monthly menstrual period.

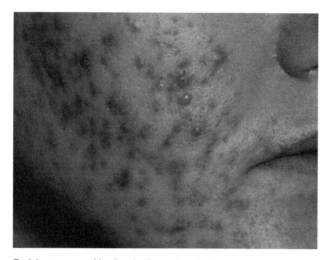

Facial acne caused by *Propionibacterium acne*.

In this altered hormonal environment, **bacteria** play a role in the development of acne. The principal bacterial species associated with acne is *Proprionibacterium acnes*. This microorganism is a normal resident on the skin and inside hair follicles. Normally, the outward flow of oil will wash the bacteria to the surface and be removed when the face is washed. However, in the androgen-altered hair follicles, the cells lining the cavity shed more frequently, stick together, mix with the excess oil that is being produced, and pile up in clumps inside the cavity. The accumulated material is a ready nutrient source for the *Proprionibacterium acnes* in the cavity. The bacteria grow and multiply rapidly.

Two other bacterial species that live and grow on the surface of the skin can be associated with acne. These are *Proprionibacterium granulosum* and *Staphylocccus epidermidis*. Their significance is less than *Proprionibacterium acnes*, however.

As the numbers of bacteria increase, the by-products of their metabolic activities cause even more inflammation. Also, the bacteria contain **enzymes** that can degrade the oil from the oil glands into what are known as free fatty acids. These free fatty acids are very irritating to the skin. Various other bacterial enzymes contribute to inflammation, including proteases and phosphatases.

The **immune system** does react to the abnormal growth of the bacteria by trying to clear the bacteria. Death of bacteria combined with the immune response generates the material known as pus. A hallmark of acne is often the pus that is exuded from the crusty sores on the skin.

The altered environment within the hair follicle that facilitates the explosive growth of *Proprionibacterium acnes* can be stimulated by factors other than the altered hormone production of puberty. The external environment, particularly a warm and moist one, is one factor.

The damage caused by bacteria in acne ranges from mild to severe. In a mild case of acne, only a so-called blackheads or whiteheads are evident on the skin. More severe cases are associated with more blackheads, whiteheads and

pimples, and also with inflammation. The most severe form, called cystic acne, may produce marked inflammation over the entire upper body, and requires a physician's attention to reduce the bacterial populations.

Reduction in the bacterial number involves slowing down the secretion of the oil from the oil glands and making the follicle pore more open, so that the normal outward flow can occur. Oil production can be slowed in the presence of 12-cis-retinoic acid (Accutane). Use of this medication is reserved for severe cases of acne, as the retinoic acid can have significant adverse side effects. Antibacterial agents can also be useful. For example, many antibacterial creams and face washes contain the compound called benzoyl peroxide, which is very active against *Proprionibacterium acnes*.

Because the bacteria active in acne are normal residents of the skin, there is no "cure" for acne. Rather, the condition is lessened until biochemical or lifestyle changes in the individual lessen or eliminate the conditions that promote bacterial overgrowth.

See also Microbial flora of the skin; Skin infections

ACRIDINE ORANGE

Acridine orange is a fluorescent dye. The compound binds to genetic material and can differentiate between **deoxyribonucleic acid (DNA)** and **ribonucleic acid (RNA)**.

A fluorescent dye such as acridine orange absorbs the energy of incoming light. The energy of the light passes into the dye molecules. This energy cannot be accommodated by the dye forever, and so is released. The released energy is at a different wavelength than was the incoming light, and so is detected as a different color.

Acridine orange absorbs the incoming radiation because of its ring structure. The excess energy effectively passes around the ring, being distributed between the various bonds that exist within the ring. However, the energy must be dissipated to preserve the stability of the dye structure.

The ring structure also confers a **hydrophobic** (water-hating) nature to the compound. When applied to a sample in solution, the acridine orange will tend to diffuse spontaneously into the membrane surrounding the **microorganisms**. Once in the interior of the cell, acridine orange can form a complex with DNA and with RNA. The chemistries of these complexes affect the wavelength of the emitted radiation. In the case of the acridine orange–DNA complex, the emitted radiation is green. In the case of the complex formed with RNA, the emitted light is orange. The different colors allow DNA to be distinguished from RNA.

Binding of acridine orange to the nucleic acid occurs in living and dead **bacteria** and other microorganisms. Thus, the dye is not a means of distinguishing living from dead microbes. Nor does acridine orange discriminate between one species of microbe versus a different species. However, acridine orange has proved very useful as a means of enumerating the total number of microbes in a sample. Knowledge of the total number of bacteria versus the number of living bacteria can be very useful in, for example, evaluating the effect of an antibacterial agent on the survival of bacteria.

Acridine orange is utilized in the specialized type of light microscopic technique called fluorescence microscopy. In addition, fluorescence of DNA or RNA can allow cells in a sample to be differentiated using the technique of flow cytometry. This sort of information allows detailed analysis of the DNA replication cycle in microorganisms such as **yeast**.

See also Laboratory techniques in microbiology

ACTINOMYCES

Actinomyces is a genus of **bacteria**. The bacteria that grouped in this genus share several characteristics. The bacteria are rod-like in shape. Under the light **microscope**, *Actinomyces* appear fungus-like. They are thin and joined together to form branching networks. Bacteria of this genus retain the primary stain in the Gram stain reaction, and so are classified as being Gram positive. *Actinomycetes* are not able to form the dormant form known as a spore. Finally, the bacteria are able to grow in the absence of oxygen.

Members of the genus *Actinomyces* are normal residents of the mouth, throat, and intestinal tract. But they are capable of causing infections both in humans and in cattle if they are able to enter other regions. This can occur as the result of an accident such as a cut or abrasion.

An infection known as *Actinomycosis* is characterized by the formation of an abscess—a process "walling off" the site of infection as the body responds to the infection—and by swelling. Pus can also be present. The pus, which is composed of dead bacteria, is granular, because of the presence of granules of sulfur that are made by the bacteria.

The diagnosis of an *Actinomyces* infection can be challenging, as the symptoms and appearance of the infection is reminiscent of a tumor or of a **tuberculosis** lesion. A well-established infection can produce a great deal of tissue damage. Additionally, the slow growth of the bacteria can make the treatment of infection with **antibiotics** very difficult, because antibiotics rely on **bacterial growth** in order to exert their lethal effect.

The culturing of *Actinomyces* in the laboratory is also challenging. The bacteria do not grow on nonselective media, but instead require the use of specialized and nutritionally complex selective media. Furthermore, incubation needs to be in the absence of oxygen. The growth of the bacteria is quite slow. Solid growth medium may need to be incubated for up to 14 days to achieve visible growth. In contrast, a bacterium like *Escherichia coli* yields visible colonies after overnight growth on a variety of nonselective media. The colonies of Actinomyces are often described as looking like bread crumbs.

Currently, identification methods such as **polymerase chain reaction** (**PCR**), chromatography to detect unique cell wall constituents, and antibody-based assays do always perform effectively with *Actinomyces*.

See also Anaerobes and anaerobic infections; Microbial flora of the oral cavity, dental caries

ACTIVE TRANSPORT • *see* CELL MEMBRANE TRANSPORT

ADENOVIRUSES

Adenoviruses are **viruses** which have twenty sides. As such they are called icosahedrons. The outer surface, the capsid, is made of particles of a protein. The protein is arranged in groups of six (hexagons) except at the twenty points where the sides meet (each is called an apex), where the particles are in a pentagon arrangement. A so-called penton fibre, which resembles a stick with a ball at the end, protrudes from each apex.

Adenoviruses contain **deoxyribonucleic acid** (DNA) as their genetic material. The **DNA** encodes 20 to 30 proteins, 15 of which are proteins that form the structure of the virus particle. Similar to other viruses, adenoviruses invade a host cell and use the host genetic machinery to manufacture new virus particles. The new viruses are released from the host cell.

Children suffer from adenovirus infections much more so than adults.

The viruses of this group infect the membranes that line the respiratory tract, the eyes, the intestines, and the urinary tract. The adenoviruses that infect humans usually cause mild maladies, including respiratory and intestinal illnesses and conjunctivitis (an **inflammation** of eye membrane, which is also commonly called "pink eye"). A more severe eye malady called keratoconjunctivitis can more widely infect the eye. The **eye infections** are very contagious and are typically a source of transmission of adenovirus from one person to another. Children can also develop a sore throat, runny nose, cough and flu-like illness. Bronchitis, an inflammation of the membranes lining the air passages in the lungs, can also result from adenovirus infection, as can an inflammation of the stomach called **gastroenteritis**. Urinary tract infections can cause pain and burning upon urination and blood in the urine. In dogs, adenovirus type 2 causes what is known as kennel cough. But curiously, the virus also protects dogs against **hepatitis**.

In the setting of the laboratory, some of the human strains of adenovirus can transform cells being grown in cell **culture**. Transformed cells are altered in their regulation of growth, such that the unrestricted growth characteristic of cancers occurs.

Adenoviruses have been known since the mid-1950s. They were first isolated from infected tonsils and adenoidal tissue in 1953. Within the next several years they had been obtained from cells involved in respiratory infections. In 1956, the multiple antigenic forms of the virus that had been discovered were classified as adenovirus. Then, in 1962, laboratory studies demonstrated that an adenovirus caused tumors in

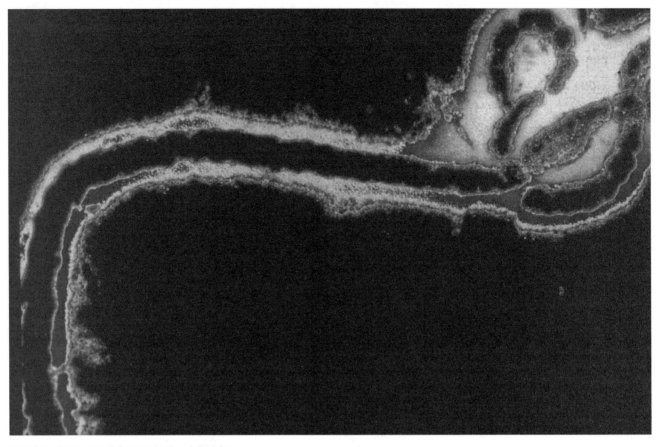

Negative stain electron micrograph of an Adenovirus.

rodents. This was the first known human virus capable of inducing tumors in animals.

More recently, the basis of the tumor-inducing activity has been unraveled. Genes that are active early in the replication cycle of adenovirus produce proteins that interfere with host proteins that are known as anti-oncogenes. Normally, the anti-oncogen proteins are responsive to cell growth, and so act as a signal to the cell to halt growth. By disrupting the anti-oncogene proteins, this stop signal is eliminated, resulting in the continued and uncontrolled growth of the cell. A tumor is produced. Thus, adenoviruses have become important as one of the central triggers of cancer development.

Such cancers may be a by-product of adenovirus infections. These infections are not by themselves serious. Most tend to appear and run their course within a few weeks. The infections are fairly common. For example, most children will have antibodies to at least four types of adenovirus. Adenovirus gains entry through a break in the skin or are inhaled. The stick-and-ball appearing penton fibers may have a role in the attachment of the virus particle to a protein on the surface of the host epithelial cell.

Adenovirus infections have contributed to the spread of bacterial **antibiotic resistance** because of the overuse of **antibiotics**. The flu-like symptoms of some adenovirus infections can lead to the prescribing of antibiotics as a treatment.

However, antibiotics are ineffective against viruses. But the circulating antibiotic can provide selective pressure on the development of resistant in bacterial populations.

See also Bacterial adaptation; Transformation

ADJUVANT

An adjuvant is any substance that enhances the response of the **immune system** to the foreign material termed an **antigen**. The particular antigen is also referred to as an immunogen. An adjuvant can also be any substance that enhances the effect of a drug on the body.

When antigen is injected into an organism being used to raise antibodies the effect is to stimulate a greater and more prolonged production of **antibody** than would otherwise occur if the antigen were injected alone. Indeed, adjuvants are very useful if a substance itself is not strongly recognized by the immune system. An example of such a weak immunogen is the capsule exopolysaccharide of a variety of **bacteria**.

Adjuvants exert their effect in several different ways. Firstly, some adjuvants retain the antigen and so "present" the antigen to the immune system over a prolonged period of time. The immune response does not occur all at once, but rather is continuous over a longer time. Secondly, an adjuvant itself can react with some of the cells of the immune system. This interaction may stimulate the immune cells to heightened activity. Thirdly, an adjuvant can also enhance the recognition and ingestion of the antigen by the immune cell known as the **phagocyte**. This enhanced **phagocytosis** presents more antigens to the other cells that form the antibody.

There are several different types of antigens. The adjuvant selected typically depends on the animal being used to generate the antibodies. Different adjuvants produce different responses in different animals. Some adjuvants are inappropriate for certain animals, due to the **inflammation**, tissue damage, and pain that are caused to the animal. Other factors that influence the choice of an adjuvant include the injection site, the manner of antigen preparation, and amount of antigen injected.

One type of adjuvant that has been of long-standing service in generating antibodies for the study of bacteria is known as Freund's Complete Adjuvant. This type of adjuvant enhances the response to the immunogen of choice via the inclusion of a type of bacteria called mycobacteria into a mixture of oil and water. Typically, there is more oil present than water. The oil and water acts to emulsify, or spread evenly throughout the suspension, the mycobacteria and the immunogen. Sometimes the mycobacteria are left out of the adjuvant. In this case, it is referred to as "incomplete" adjuvant.

See also Immunity: active, passive, and delayed

AEROBES

Aerobic **microorganisms** require the presence of oxygen for growth. Molecular oxygen functions in the respiratory pathway of the microbes to produce the energy necessary for life. **Bacteria**, yeasts, **fungi**, and algae are capable of aerobic growth.

The opposite of an aerobe is an anaerobe. An anaerobe does not require oxygen, or sometimes cannot even tolerate the presence of oxygen.

There are various degrees of oxygen tolerance among aerobic microorganisms. Those that absolutely require oxygen are known as obligate aerobes. Facultative aerobes prefer the presence of oxygen but can adjust their metabolic machinery so as to grow in the absence of oxygen. Microaerophilic organisms are capable of oxygen-dependent growth but cannot grow if the oxygen concentration is that of an air atmosphere (about 21% oxygen). The oxygen content must be lower.

Oxygen functions to accept an electron from a substance that yields an electron, typically a substance that contains carbon. Compounds called flavoproteins and cytochromes are key to this electron transport process. They act as electron carriers. By accepting an electron, oxygen enables a process known as catabolism to occur. Catabolism is the breakdown of complex structures to yield energy. The energy is used to sustain the microorganism.

A common food source for microorganisms is the sugar glucose. Compounds such as glucose store energy inside themselves, in order to bond their constituent molecules

together. When these bonds are severed, energy is released. In aerobic bacteria and other organisms, a compound called pyruvic acid retains most of the energy that is present in the glucose. The pyruvic acid in turn is broken down via a series of reactions that collectively are called the tricarboxylic acid cycle, or the Kreb's cycle (named after one the cycle's discoverers, Sir Hans Krebs). A principle product of the Kreb's cycle is a compound called nicotinamide adenine dinucleotide ($NADH_2$). The $NADH_2$ molecules feed into another chain of reactions of which oxygen is a key.

The energy-generating process in which oxygen functions is termed aerobic **respiration**. Oxygen is the final electron acceptor in the process. Anaerobic respiration exists, and involves the use of an electron acceptor other than oxygen. One of the most common of these alternate acceptors is nitrate, and the process involving it is known as denitrification.

Aerobic respiration allows a substrate to be broken down (this is also known as oxidation) to carbon dioxide and water. The complete breakdown process yields 38 molecules of adenine triphosphate (ATP) for each molecule of the sugar glucose. ATP is essentially the gasoline of the cell. Electron transport that does not involve oxygen also generates ATP, but not in the same quantity as with aerobic respiration. Thus, a facultative aerobe will preferentially use oxygen as the electron acceptor. The other so-called fermentative type of energy generation is a fall-back mechanism to permit the organism's survival in an oxygen-depleted environment.

The aerobic mode of energy production can occur in the disperse **cytoplasm** of bacteria and in the compartmentalized regions of **yeast**, fungi and algae cells. In the latter microorganisms, the structure in which the reactions take place is called the mitochondrion. The activities of the mitochondrion are coordinated with other energy-requiring processes in the cell.

See also Carbon cycle in microorganisms; Metabolism

AGAMMAGLOBULINAEMIA WITH HYPER IgM • *see* IMMUNODEFICIENCY DISEASE SYNDROMES

AGAR AND AGAROSE

Agar and agarose are two forms of solid growth media that are used for the **culture** of **microorganisms**, particularly **bacteria**. Both agar and agarose act to solidify the nutrients that would otherwise remain in solution. Both agar and agarose are able to liquefy when heated sufficiently, and both return to a gel state upon cooling.

Solid media is prepared by heating up the agar and nutrient components so that a solution results. The solution is then sterilized, typically in steam-heat apparatus known as an autoclave. The sterile medium is then poured into one half of sterile Petri plates and the lid is placed over the still hot solution. As the solution cools, the agar or agarose becomes gel-like, rendering the medium in a semi-solid. When bacteria

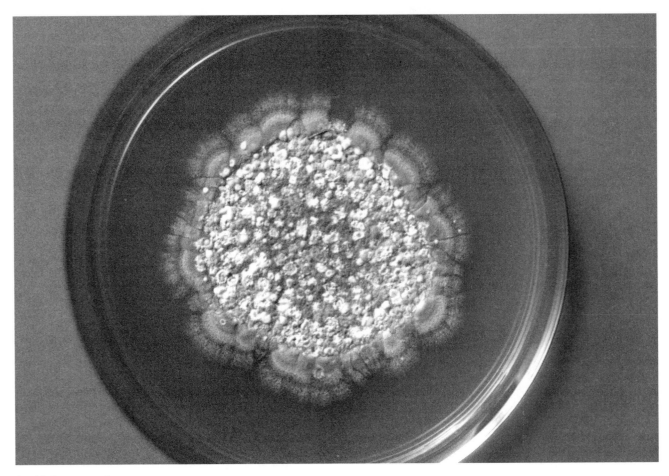

Aerobic fungus growing on agar.

contact the surface of the medium, they are able to extract the nutrients from the medium and grow as colonies.

The use of agar and agarose solid media allows for the isolation of bacteria by a streak plate technique. A similar discrimination of one bacterial species from another is not possible in liquid growth media. Furthermore, some solid growth media allows reactions to develop that cannot develop in liquid media. The best-known example is **blood agar**, where the total and partial destruction of the constituent red blood cells can be detected by their characteristic hemolytic reactions.

Agar is an uncharged network of strands of a compound called gelactose. This compound is in fact made up of two polysaccharides called agarose and agaropectin. Gelactose is extracted from a type of seaweed known as *Gelidium comeum*. The seaweed was named for the French botanist who first noted the gelatinous material that could be extracted from the **kelp**. Another seaweed called *Gracilaria verrucosa* can also be a source of agar.

Agarose is obtained by purification of the agar. The agarose component of agar is composed of repeating molecules of galactopyranose. The side groups that protrude from the galactopyranose are arranged such that two adjacent chains can associate to form a helix. The chains wrap together so tightly that water can be trapped inside the helix. As more and more helices are formed and become cross-linked, a three-dimensional network of water-containing helices is created. The entire structure has no net charge.

The history of agar and agarose extends back centuries and the utility of the compounds closely follow the emergence and development of the discipline of microbiology. The gel-like properties of agar are purported to have been first observed by a Chinese Emperor in the mid-sixteenth century. Soon thereafter, a flourishing agar manufacturing industry was established in Japan. The Japanese dominance of the trade in agar only ended with World War II. Following World War II, the manufacture of agar spread to other countries around the globe. For example, in the United States, the copious seaweed beds found along the Southern California coast has made the San Diego area a hotbed of agar manufacture. Today, the manufacture and sale of agar is lucrative and has spawned a competitive industry.

The roots of agar as an adjunct to microbiological studies dates back to the late nineteenth century. In 1882, the renowned microbiologist **Robert Koch** reported on the use of agar as a means for growing microorganisms. Since this discovery, the use of agar has become one of the bedrock techniques in microbiology. There are now hundreds of different formulations of agar-based growth media. Some are nonspecific, with a spectrum of components present. Other media are defined, with precise amounts of a few set materials included. Likewise the use of agarose has proved tremendously useful in electrophoretic techniques. By manipulation of the formulation conditions, the agarose matrix can have pores, or tunnels through the agarose strands, which can be of different size. Thus the agarose can act as a sieve, to separate molecules on the basis of the size. The uncharged nature of agarose allows a current to be passed through it, which can drive the movement of samples such as pieces of **deoxyribonucleic acid** (**DNA**) from one end of an agarose slab to the other. The speed of the molecule movement, is also related to molecular size (largest molecules moving the least).

In the non-microbiological world, agar and agarose have also found a use as stabilizers in ice cream, instant cream whips, and dessert gelatins.

See also Bacterial growth and division; Laboratory techniques in microbiology

AGAR DIFFUSION

Agar diffusion refers to the movement of molecules through the matrix that is formed by the gelling of agar. When performed under controlled conditions, the degree of the molecule's movement can be related to the concentration of the molecule. This phenomenon forms the basis of the agar diffusion assay that is used to determine the susceptibility or resistance of a bacterial strain to an antibacterial agent, (e.g., including **antibiotics**.

When the seaweed extract known as agar is allowed to harden, the resulting material is not impermeable. Rather, there are spaces present between the myriad of strands of agar that comprise the hardened polymer. Small molecules such as antibiotics are able to diffuse through the agar.

Typically, an antibiotic is applied to a well that is cut into the agar. Thus, the antibiotic will tend to move from this region of high concentration to the surrounding regions of lower antibiotic concentration. If more material is present in the well, then the zone of diffusion can be larger.

This diffusion was the basis of the agar diffusion assay devised in 1944. A bacterial suspension is spread onto the surface of the agar. Then, antibiotic is applied to a number of wells in the plate. There can be different concentrations of a single antibiotic or a number of different antibiotics present. Following a time to allow for growth of the **bacteria** then agar is examined. If **bacterial growth** is right up to the antibiotic containing well, then the bacterial strain is deemed to be resistant to the antibiotic. If there is a clearing around the antibiotic well, then the bacteria have been adversely affected by the antibiotic. The size of the inhibition zone can be measured and related to standards, in order to determine whether the bacterial strain is sensitive to the antibiotic.

This technique can also be done by placing disks of an absorbent material that have been soaked with the antibiotic of interest directly onto the agar surface. The antibiotic will subse-

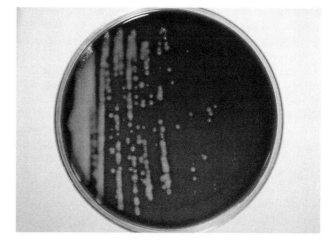

Staphylococcus colonies showing hemolytic reaction on blood agar.

quently diffuse out of the disk into the agar. This version of agar diffusion is known as the Kirby-Bauer disk-diffusion assay.

The agar diffusion assay allows bacteria to be screened in a routine, economical and easy way for the detection of resistance. More detailed analysis to ascertain the nature of the resistance can then follow.

See also Antibiotic resistance, tests for; Laboratory techniques in microbiology

AGGLUTINATION • *see* ANTIBODY-ANTIGEN, BIOCHEMICAL AND MOLECULAR REACTIONS

AIDS

The advent of AIDS (acquired **immunity** deficiency syndrome) in early 1981 surprised the scientific community, as many researchers at that time viewed the world to be on the brink of eliminating infectious disease. AIDS, an infectious disease syndrome that suppresses the **immune system**, is caused by the **Human Immune Deficiency Virus (HIV)**, part of a group of **viruses** known as **retroviruses**. The name AIDS was coined in 1982. Victims of AIDS most often die from opportunistic infections that take hold of the body because the immune system is severely impaired.

Following the discovery of AIDS, scientists attempted to identify the virus that causes the disease. In 1983 and 1984 two scientists and their teams reported isolating HIV, the virus that causes AIDS. One was French immunologist **Luc Montagnier** (1932–), working at the Pasteur Institute in Paris, and the other was American immunologist **Robert Gallo** (1937–) at the National Cancer Institute in Bethesda, Maryland. Both identified HIV as the cause of AIDS and showed the pathogen to be a retrovirus, meaning that its genetic material is **RNA** instead of **DNA**. Following the discovery, a dispute ensued over who made the initial discovery, but today Gallo and Montagnier are credited as co-discoverers.

Inside its host cell, the HIV retrovirus uses an enzyme called reverse transcriptase to make a DNA copy of its genetic material. The single strand of DNA then replicates and, in double stranded form, integrates into the chromosome of the host cell where it directs synthesis of more viral RNA. The viral RNA in turn directs the synthesis protein capsids and both are assembled into HIV viruses. A large number of viruses emerge from the host cell before it dies. HIV destroys the immune system by invading lymphocytes and macrophages, replicating within them, killing them, and spreading to others.

Scientists believe that HIV originated in the region of sub-Saharan Africa and subsequently spread to Europe and the United States by way of the Caribbean. Because viruses exist that suppress the immune system in monkeys, scientists hypothesize that these viruses mutated to HIV in the bodies of humans who ate the meat of monkeys, and subsequently caused AIDS. A fifteen-year-old male with skin lesions who died in 1969 is the first documented case of AIDS. Unable to determine the cause of death at the time, doctors froze some of his tissues, and upon recent examination, the tissue was found to be infected with HIV. During the 1960s, doctors often listed leukemia as the cause of death in many AIDS patients. After several decades however, the incidence of AIDS was sufficiently widespread to recognize it as a specific disease. Epidemiologists, scientists who study the incidence, cause, and distribution of diseases, turned their attention to AIDS. American scientist James Curran, working with the **Centers for Disease Control** and Prevention (CDC), sparked an effort to track the occurrence of HIV. First spread in the United States through the homosexual community by male-to-male contact, HIV rapidly expanded through all populations. Presently new HIV infections are increasing more rapidly among heterosexuals, with women accounting for approximately twenty percent of the AIDS cases. The worldwide AIDS epidemic is estimated to have killed more than 6.5 million people, and infected another 29 million. A new infection occurs about every fifteen seconds. HIV is not distributed equally throughout the world; most afflicted people live in developing countries. Africa has the largest number of cases, but the fastest rate of new infections is occurring in Southeast Asia and the Indian subcontinent. In the United States, though the disease was concentrated in large cities, it has spread to towns and rural areas. Once the leading cause of death among people between the ages of 25 and 44 in the Unites States, AIDS is now second to accidents.

HIV is transmitted in bodily fluids. Its main means of transmission from an infected person is through sexual contact, specifically vaginal and anal intercourse, and oral to genital contact. Intravenous drug users who share needles are at high risk of contracting AIDS. An infected mother has a 15 to 25% chance of passing HIV to her unborn child before and during birth, and an increased risk of transmitting HIV through breast-feeding. Although rare in countries such as the United States where blood is screened for HIV, the virus can be transmitted by transfusions of infected blood or blood-clotting factors. Another consideration regarding HIV transmis-

sion is that a person who has had another sexually transmitted disease is more likely to contract AIDS.

Laboratories use a test for HIV-1 that is called **Enzyme-linked immunosorbant assay (ELISA)**. (There is another type of HIV called HIV-2.) First developed in 1985 by Robert Gallo and his research team, the ELISA test is based on the fact that, even though the disease attacks the immune system, **B cells** begin to produce antibodies to fight the invasion within weeks or months of the infection. The test detects the presence of HIV-1 type antibodies and reacts with a color change. Weaknesses of the test include its inability to detect 1) patients who are infectious but have not yet produced HIV-1 antibodies, and 2) those who are infected with HIV-2. In addition, ELISA may give a false positive result to persons suffering from a disease other than AIDS. Patients that test positive with ELISA are given a second more specialized test to confirm the presence of AIDS. Developed in 1996, this test detects HIV antigens, proteins produced by the virus, and can therefore identify HIV before the patient's body produces antibodies. In addition, separate tests for HIV-1 and HIV-2 have been developed.

After HIV invades the body, the disease passes through different phases, culminating in AIDS. During the earliest phase the infected individual may experience general flu-like symptoms such as fever and headache within one to three weeks after exposure; then he or she remains relatively healthy while the virus replicates and the immune system produces antibodies. This stage continues for as long as the body's immune response keeps HIV in check. Progression of the disease is monitored by the declining number of particular antibodies called CD4-T lymphocytes. HIV attacks these immune cells by attaching to their CD4 receptor site. The virus also attacks macrophages, the cells that pass the **antigen** to helper T lymphocytes. The progress of HIV can also be determined by the amount of HIV in the patient's blood. After several months to several years, the disease progresses to the next stage in which the CD4-T cell count declines, and non-life-threatening symptoms such as weakness or swollen lymph glands may appear. The CDC has established a definition for the diagnosis of AIDS in which the CD4 T-cell count is below 200 cells per cubic mm of blood, or an opportunistic disease has set in.

Although progress has been made in the treatment of AIDS, a cure has yet to be found. In 1995 scientists developed a potent cocktail of drugs that help stop the progress of HIV. Among other substances, the cocktail combines zidovudine (AZT), didanosine (ddi), and a protease inhibitor. AZT and ddi are nucleosides that are building blocks of DNA. The enzyme, reverse transcriptase, mistakenly incorporates the drugs into the viral chain, thereby stopping DNA synthesis. Used alone, AZT works temporarily until HIV develops immunity to the nucleoside. Proteases are **enzymes** that are needed by HIV to reproduce, and when protease inhibitors are administered, HIV replicates are no longer able to infect cells. In 1995 the Federal Drug Administration approved saquinaviras, the first protease inhibitor to be used in combination with nucleoside drugs such as AZT; this was followed in 1996 by approval for the protease inhibitors ritonavir and indinavir to be used alone or in combination with nucleosides. The combination of drugs brings about a greater increase of antibodies and a greater decrease of fulminant HIV than either type of drug alone. Although patients improve on a regimen of mixed drugs, they are not cured due to the persistence of inactive virus left in the body. Researchers are looking for ways to flush out the remaining HIV. In the battle against AIDS, researchers are also attempting to develop a **vaccine**. As an adjunct to the classic method of preparing a vaccine from weakened virus, scientists are attempting to create a vaccine from a single virus protein.

In addition to treatment, the battle against AIDS includes preventing transmission of the disease. Infected individuals pass HIV-laden macrophages and T lymphocytes in their bodily fluids to others. Sexual behaviors and drug-related activities are the most common means of transmission. Commonly, the virus gains entry into the bloodstream by way of small abrasions during sexual intercourse or direct injection with an infected needle. In attempting to prevent HIV transmission among the peoples of the world, there has been an unprecedented emphasis on **public health** education and social programs; it is vitally important to increase public understanding of both the nature of AIDS and the behaviors that put individuals at risk of spreading or contracting the disease.

See also AIDS, recent advances in research and treatment; Antibody and antigen; Blood borne infections; Centers for Disease Control (CDC); Epidemics, viral; Human immunodeficiency virus (HIV); Immunodeficiency disease syndromes; Immunodeficiency diseases; Immunological analysis techniques; Infection and resistance; Infection control; Latent viruses and diseases; Sexually transmitted diseases; T cells or T lymphocytes; Viral genetics; Viral vectors in gene therapy; Virology; Virus replication; Viruses and responses to viral infection

AIDS, RECENT ADVANCES IN RESEARCH AND TREATMENT

Acquired Immune Deficiency Syndrome (**AIDS**) has only been known since the early years of the 1980s. Since that time, the number of people infected with the causative virus of the syndrome and of those who die from the various consequences of the infection, has grown considerably.

In the 1980s and 1990s, researchers were able to establish that the principle target for the maladies associated with AIDS is the **immune system**. Since then, much research has been directed towards pinpointing the changes in the human immune system due to infection, seeking ways of reversing these changes, or supplementing the compromised immune system to hold the infection in check.

The particular immune system component that has been implicated in the progression of AIDS is a type of T cell called the CDC4 T cell. This cell, which is activated following recognition of the virus by the immune system, functions in the destruction of the cells that have been infected by the virus. Over time, however, the number of CDC4 cells declines. If the decline decreases the T cell count to below 200

per microliter of blood, the number of infective virus particles goes up steeply and the immune system breaks down. This loss of the ability to fight off foreign organisms leaves the patient open to life-threatening illnesses that normally would be routinely defeated by an unimpaired immune system.

Until 2001, the prevailing view was that the decline in the number of CDC4 cells was due to a blockage of new T cell production by the infecting virus. However, the conclusions from studies published in 2001 now indicate that the production of new **T cells** is not blocked, but rather that there is acceleration in the loss of existing T cells. Even though the result is the same, namely the increased loss of the specialized AIDS-fighting T cells, the nature of the decline is crucial to determine in order to devise the most effective treatment strategy. If the reasons for the accelerated loss of the T cells can be determined, perhaps the loss can be prevented. This would better equip patients to fight the infection.

Since 1998, a multi-pronged strategy of AIDS therapy has been established. Highly Active Anti-Retroviral Therapy (HAART) consists of administering a "cocktail" of drugs targeted to the AIDS virus to a patient, even when the patient shows no symptoms of AIDS. The drug mixture typically contains a so-called nucleoside analog, which blocks genetic replication, and inhibitors of two **enzymes** that are critical enzyme in the making of new virus (protease and reverse transcriptase).

HAART has greatly reduced the loss of life due to AIDS. But, this benefit has come at the expense of side effects that can often be severe. Also, the treatment is expensive. But now, research published toward the end of 2001 indicates that the use of HAART in a "7-day-on, 7-day-off" cycle does not diminish treatment benefits, but does diminish treatment side effects. Costs of treatment has become more reasonable, as well.

Another advancement in AIDS treatment may come from the finding that the inner core of the AIDS virus, which is called the nucleocapsid, is held together by structures known as "zinc fingers." There are drugs that appear to break apart these supports. This stops the virus from functioning. Furthermore, evidence supports the view that the nucleocapsid does not change much over time. Thus, a drug that effectively targeted the nucleocapsid could be an effective drug for a long time. The drawback to this approach at the present time is that other structures in the body utilize zinc fingers. So, an anti-AIDS zinc finger strategy will have to be made very specific.

In the mid 1980s, there was great optimism that a **vaccine** for the AIDS virus would be developed within two years. However, this optimism soon disappeared. In late 2001, however, preliminary clinical trials began on a candidate vaccine. Traditional vaccines rely on the administration of a protein to stimulate the production of an **antibody** that confers protection against the disease-causing organism. The candidate vaccine works by targeting what is called cell-mediated **immunity**. This type of immunity does not prevent infection, but rather clears the virus-infected cells out of the body. Such a vaccine would be intended to prolong and enhance the quality of the lives of AIDS-infected people. Studies in monkeys have been encouraging. However, studies must still rule out the possibility that **vaccination** would create "carriers," individuals who are not sick but who are capable of spreading the disease.

There are various vaccine treatment strategies. One involves the injection of so-called "naked" **DNA**. The DNA contains genes that code for *gag*, a viral component thought to be critical to the development of AIDS. The DNA can be attached to inert particles that stimulate the response of the immune system. In another strategy, the viral **gene** is bundled into the DNA of another virus that is injected into the patient.

As of 2002, more than two dozen experimental vaccines intended to control, but not cure, AIDS infections are being studied worldwide.

Treatment strategies, vaccine-based or otherwise, will need to address the different isolates of the AIDS virus that are present in various regions of the globe. These different isolates tend to be separated into different geographical regions. Even within a geographical area, an isolate can display variation from place to place. Thus, it has become clear that a universal treatment strategy is unlikely.

See also Human immunodeficiency virus (HIV); Immune stimulation, as a vaccine; Vaccination

ALEXANDER, HATTIE ELIZABETH
(1901-1968)
American physician and microbiologist

Hattie Elizabeth Alexander was a pediatrician and microbiologist who made fundamental contributions in the early studies of the genetic basis of bacterial **antibiotic resistance**, specifically the resistance displayed by *Hemophilus influenzae*, the cause of influenzal **meningitis** (swelling of the nerves in the spinal cord and brain). Her pioneering studies paved the way for advances in treatment that have saved countless lives.

Alexander was born in Baltimore, Maryland. She received her B.A. degree from Goucher College in 1923. After working as a **public health** bacteriologist from 1923 to 1926, she entered the Johns Hopkins School of Medicine. She received her M.D. in 1930. Alexander assumed a residency at New York City Babies Hospital in 1930. She remained there for the remainder of her career, attaining the rank of Professor in 1957.

Alexander pioneered studies of the antibiotic resistance and susceptibility of *Hemophilus influenzae*. In 1939 she successfully utilized an anti-**pneumonia** serum that had been developed at Rockefeller University to cure infants of influenzal meningitis. Until then, infection with *Hemophilus influenzae* type b almost always resulted in death. Her **antiserum** reduced the death rate by almost 80%. Further research led to the use of **sulfa drugs** and other **antibiotics** in the treatment of the meningitis.

In other research, Alexander established that *Hemophilus influenzae* was the cause of a malady known as epiglottitis (also called croup). Her discovery prompted research that has led to effective treatments for croup.

In the 1950s Alexander began studies on the genetic basis of antibiotic resistance. During the next two decades she made fundamental observations concerning bacterial and **viral genetics**. She demonstrated that the ability of *Hemophilus influenzae* to cause disease rested with its genetic material. Additionally she demonstrated that the genetic material of poliovirus could infect human cells. She also proposed that the mechanisms of inheritance of traits in **microorganisms** could be similar to the mechanisms operating in humans. Time has borne out her suggestion.

In addition to her research, Alexander devoted much time to teaching and clinical duties. For her research and other professional accomplishments Alexander received many awards, honorary degrees, and other honors. Notably she became the first woman president of the American Pediatric Society in 1965.

See also Bacterial adaptation; Microbial genetics

ALGAE, ECONOMIC USES AND BENEFITS •
see ECONOMIC USES AND BENEFITS OF MICROORGANISMS

ALLERGIES

An allergy is an excessive or hypersensitive response of the **immune system** to harmless substances in the environment. Instead of fighting off a disease-causing foreign substance, the immune system launches a complex series of actions against an irritating substance, referred to as an allergen. The immune response may be accompanied by a number of stressful symptoms, ranging from mild to severe to life threatening. In rare cases, an allergic reaction leads to anaphylactic shock—a condition characterized by a sudden drop in blood pressure, difficulty in breathing, skin irritation, collapse, and possible death.

The immune system may produce several chemical agents that cause allergic reactions. Some of the main immune system substances responsible for the symptoms of allergy are the histamines that are produced after an exposure to an allergen. Along with other treatments and medicines, the use of antihistamines helps to relieve some of the symptoms of allergy by blocking out **histamine** receptor sites. The study of allergy medicine includes the identification of the different types of allergy, **immunology**, and the diagnosis and treatment of allergy.

The most common causes of allergy are pollens that are responsible for seasonal or allergic rhinitis. The popular name for rhinitis, hay fever, a term used since the 1830s, is inaccurate because the condition is not caused by fever and its symptoms do not include fever. Throughout the world during every season, pollens from grasses, trees, and weeds produce allergic reactions like sneezing, runny nose, swollen nasal tissues, headaches, blocked sinuses, and watery, irritated eyes. Of the 46 million allergy sufferers in the United States, about 25 million have rhinitis.

Dust and the house dust mite constitute another major cause of allergies. While the mite itself is too large to be inhaled, its feces are about the size of pollen grains and can lead to allergic rhinitis. Other types of allergy can be traced to the fur of animals and pets, food, drugs, insect bites, and skin contact with chemical substances or odors. In the United States, there are about 12 million people who are allergic to a variety of chemicals. In some cases an allergic reaction to an insect sting or a drug reaction can cause sudden death. Serious asthma attacks are sometimes associated with seasonal rhinitis and other allergies. About nine million people in the United States suffer from asthma.

Some people are allergic to a wide range of allergens, while others are allergic to only a few or none. The reasons for these differences can be found in the makeup of an individual's immune system. The immune system is the body's defense against substances that it recognizes as dangerous to the body. Lymphocytes, a type of white blood cell, fight **viruses**, **bacteria**, and other antigens by producing antibodies. When an allergen first enters the body, the lymphocytes produce an **antibody** called immunoglobulin E (IgE). The IgE antibodies attach to mast cells, large cells that are found in connective tissue and contain histamines along with a number of other chemical substances.

Studies show that allergy sufferers produce an excessive amount of IgE, indicating a hereditary factor for their allergic responses. How individuals adjust over time to allergens in their environments also determines their degree of susceptibility to allergic disorders.

The second time any given allergen enters the body, it becomes attached to the newly formed Y-shaped IgE antibodies. These antibodies, in turn, stimulate the mast cells to discharge its histamines and other anti-allergen substances. There are two types of histamine: H_1 and H_2. H_1 histamines travel to receptor sites located in the nasal passages, respiratory system, and skin, dilating smaller blood vessels and constricting airways. The H_2 histamines, which constrict the larger blood vessels, travel to the receptor sites found in the salivary and tear glands and in the stomach's mucosal lining. H_2 histamines play a role in stimulating the release of stomach acid, thus contributing to a seasonal stomach ulcer condition.

The simplest form of treatment is the avoidance of the allergic substance, but that is not always possible. In such cases, desensitization to the allergen is sometimes attempted by exposing the patient to slight amounts of the allergen at regular intervals.

Antihistamines, which are now prescribed and sold over the counter as a rhinitis remedy, were discovered in the 1940s. There are a number of different antihistamines, and they either inhibit the production of histamine or block them at receptor sites. After the administration of antihistamines, IgE receptor sites on the mast cells are blocked, thereby preventing the release of the histamines that cause the allergic reactions. The allergens are still there, but the body's "protective" actions are suspended for the period of time that the antihistamines are active. Antihistamines also constrict the smaller blood vessels and capillaries, thereby removing excess fluids. Recent research has identified specific receptor sites on the mast cells

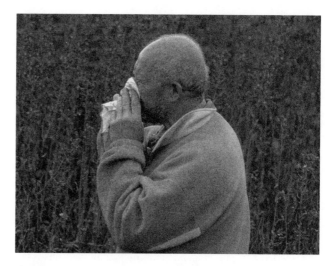

Hayfever allergy triggered by oilseed rape plants.

for the IgE. This knowledge makes it possible to develop medicines that will be more effective in reducing the symptoms of various allergies.

Corticosteroids are sometimes prescribed to allergy sufferers as anti-inflammatories. Decongestants can also bring relief, but these can be used for a short time only, since their continued use can set up a rebound effect and intensify the allergic reaction.

See also Antibody and antigen; Antibody-antigen, biochemical and molecular reactions; Antibody formation and kinetics; Antigenic mimicry; Immunology

AMEBIC DYSENTERY

Amebic (or amoebic) **dysentery**, which is also referred to as amebiasis or amoebiasis, is an **inflammation** of the intestine caused by the parasite *Entamoeba histolytica*. The severe form of the malady is characterized by the formation of localized lesions, called ulcers, in the intestine, especially in the region known as the colon, abscesses in the liver and the brain, and by vomiting, severe diarrhea with fluid loss leading to dehydration, and abdominal pain.

Amebic dysentery is one of the two most common causes of intestinal inflammation worldwide. The other is infection with **bacteria** of the *Shigella* group.

Amebiasis is contracted mainly by ingesting the parasite in contaminated food or water. Person–to–person transmission is less likely, but can occur. The disease is thus most common where sanitation is poor, in the developing world. The disease is especially prevalent in regions where untreated human waste is used as fertilizer. Run–off from fields can contaminate wells contaminating the drinking water. Amebiasis can occur anywhere in the world in almost any climate, excluding polar areas and mountainous high altitudes. Even now, approximately 500 cases are reported each year in New York State.

Those infected with the parasite may develop the severe symptoms listed above, a milder condition characterized by nausea, loose bowel movements and pain in the abdomen, or sometimes no symptoms at all. The latter is a concern to others, as the asymptomatic person can still pass the parasite in his/her feces and so potentially spread the infection to others. Indeed, such transmission can persist even years after exposure to the parasite.

Entamoeba histolytica can occur in two forms. The parasite is excreted to the environment as a so-called cyst from. This form is very hardy, and is analogous to a bacterial spore. This form is designed for longevity, to preserve the genetic material of the parasite when in inhospitable environments. Once in a more favorable environment, such as the intestinal tract of humans, the cyst resuscitates and growth resumes. The active and growing form of the parasite is known as a trophozoite. It is the trophozoite that causes the symptoms of amebiasis. Some trophozoites will re-encyst and exit via the feces, to become a potential source of further infection.

If the cyst stays in the intestinal tract after being ingested then they have little adverse effect. However, if the cysts invade the walls of the intestine, ulcers and diarrhea can be produced. Amebiasis can be fairly short in duration, lasting only a few weeks. Or, the infection may become chronic. The chronic form can be ominous, as the trophozoite can invade the blood and be carried all over the body. The abscesses formed in the liver and brain can be very destructive.

Both amebiasis and the causative parasite have been known for a long time. The parasite was described in great detail and given its name in 1903. Despite this long history, the diagnosis of the malady still relies on the visual detection of the parasite in fecal material obtained from a suspected patient. Often fecal samples need to be examined for several days to detect the presence of cysts. Amebiasis is still easily misdiagnosed, especially when no symptoms are present. Also the parasite can be visually similar to harmless normal residents of the intestinal tract, such as *Entamoeba coli*, and can co-exist with bacteria that themselves are the cause of the symptoms being experienced by the infected person.

Amebiasis is treatable, usually by a combination of drugs. An amebicide will kill the organisms in the intestinal tract, while an antibiotic will treat any bacteria that have been ingested with the feces, contaminated water, or food. Finally, if warranted, a drug can be administered to retard the spread of the infection to tissues such as the liver.

See also Parasites

AMERICAN TYPE CULTURE COLLECTION

The American Type Culture Collection, which is also known as the ATCC, is a not-for-profit bioscience organization that maintains the world's largest and most diverse collection of microbiological life. Many laboratories and institutions maintain their own stockpile of **microorganisms**, usually those that are in frequent use in the facility. Some large cul-

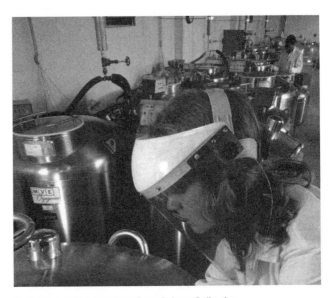

Technician at The American Type Culture Collection.

ture collections are housed and maintained, usually by universities or private enterprises. But none of these rivals the ATCC in terms of size.

The ATCC collection includes repositories of bacterial species, animal **viruses**, cell lines (which are important for the growth of certain types of viruses), **fungi**, **plant viruses**, **protists** (microscopic organisms that have a **nucleus** that is contained within a membrane), and yeasts. As well, in conjunction with researchers at George Mason University, which borders the ATCC facility, research in areas such as **bioinformatics** is carried out.

The ATCC was founded, and continues to function, to acquire, confirm the identity of, preserve and distribute biological materials to scientists worldwide. Since its inception, the mandate has expanded to now include information technology and intellectual property. Today, in addition to offering the microbiological organisms for sale, the ATCC offers technical services and educational programs to academic, government, and private organizations.

The genesis of the ATCC began in 1921. Then, the Army Medical Museum accepted a then renowned culture collection called the Winslow Culture Collection. The collection was put under the care of the Washington, D.C. members of the Society of American Bacteriologists (in time, this society grew in scope and membership to become the American Society for Microbiology). In 1925, the ATCC became an official entity with its incorporation. The burgeoning culture collection was moved to the McCormick Institute in Chicago. Twelve years later the collection returned to Washington. Space was leased to house the collection. Over the years the increasing diversification of the ATCC and the acquisition of more cultures taxed the space, so a series of moves to larger and larger sites occurred. Finally, in 1998, the organization moved to the state-of-the-art facility it continues to occupy.

The present facility is 106,000 square feet in size and has almost 35,000 square feet of laboratory space, including specialized containment facilities for more hazardous house microorganisms. Over fifty ultra-low temperature freezers are used for the long-term storage of samples. Such storage avoids changes in the organisms that could result from storage at refrigeration temperatures.

See also Cryoprotection

AMES, BRUCE N. (1928-)
American biochemist and molecular biologist

Bruce N. Ames is a professor of **biochemistry** and **molecular biology** at the University of California at Berkeley. He is best known for the development of a test used as an indicator of the carcinogenicity (cancer-causing potential) of chemicals. Known as the Ames test, it measures the rate of mutation in **bacteria** after the introduction of a test substance. Ames's research led to a greater appreciation of the role of genetic mutation in cancer and facilitated the testing of suspected cancer-causing chemicals. He also developed a database of chemicals that cause cancer in animals, listing their degree of virulence. Ames has been involved in numerous controversies involving scientific and environmental policies relevant to cancer prevention. In the 1970s he vociferously advocated strict government control of synthetic chemicals. In the 1980s, however, the discovery that many natural substances were also mutagenic (causing **gene** mutation), and thus possibly cancer causing, led him to reverse his original position.

Ames was born in New York City, the son of Dr. Maurice U. and Dorothy Andres Ames. His father taught high school science and then became assistant superintendent of schools. Ames himself graduated from the Bronx High School of Science in 1946. He received a B.A. in biochemistry from Cornell University in 1950 and a Ph.D. in the same field from the California Institute of Technology in 1953. Ames worked at the National Institutes of Health, primarily in the National Institute of Arthritis and Metabolic Diseases, from 1953 to 1967. In 1968 he moved to the Department of Biochemistry and Molecular Biology at the University of California at Berkeley as a full professor. He was Chairman of the Department from 1984 to 1989. In addition he became Director of the National Institute of Environmental Health Science at the University in 1979.

In the 1960s and early 1970s Ames developed a test that measured the degree to which synthetic chemicals cause gene mutation (a change in the **deoxyribonucleic acid**, or **DNA**, the molecule that carries genetic information). He began by deliberately mutating a *Salmonella* bacterium. The changed bacterium could not produce an amino acid called histidine that normal bacteria produce and that they need to survive. The next step was to add just enough histidine to allow the bacteria to live, and to add, as well, the synthetic chemical being tested. If the added chemical caused genetic mutation, the abnormal gene of the *Salmonella* bacteria would mutate and again be able to produce histidine. When this happened the added chemical was marked as a suspected carcinogen, because cancer is associated with somatic cell mutation (that is, mutation of any cells with the exception of germ cells).

Over eighty percent of organic chemicals known to cause cancer in humans tested positive as mutagens in the test developed by Ames and his colleagues. This result gave support to the theory that somatic mutation causes cancer and helped to validate the use of the test for initial identification of mutagens when considering synthetic chemicals for industrial and commercial use. In addition to these practical results, the research of Ames and a colleague, H. J. Whitfield, Jr., led to important advances in understanding the biochemistry of mutagenesis. Beyond his work in genetic toxicology, Ames made important discoveries in molecular biology, including ground-breaking studies on the regulation of the histidine **operon** (the gene or locus of the gene that controls histidine) and the role of transfer **ribonucleic acid** (**RNA**) in that regulation.

In the 1980s Ames set up a database of animal cancer test results with colleague Lois Swirsky Gold of Lawrence Berkeley Laboratory. The database is used to determine whether a chemical has tested positive as a carcinogen and gives the degree of its virulence. From these data Ames developed a value measuring the carcinogenic danger of a chemical to humans. HERP (daily Human Exposure dose/Rodent Potency dose) is the value determined by comparing the daily dose of a chemical that will cause cancer in half a group of test animals with the estimated daily dose to which humans are normally exposed. The result is a percentage that suggests the degree of carcinogenicity of a chemical for humans.

In the 1970s Ames was a conspicuous advocate of particular regulatory and environmental public policies that relate to the cancer-causing potential of synthetic substances. In the 1970s Ames asserted that even trace amounts of mutagenic chemicals could cause a mutation (and thus possibly cancer). He found that tris (2,3-dibromopropyl) phosphate, the chemical that was used as a flame retardant on children's pajamas, was a mutagen in the Ames test; he was instrumental in getting it banned. Similarly he found that some hair dyes contained mutagens. His advocacy led to governmental regulations that forced manufacturers to reformulate their products. In his position on the regulation of synthetic chemicals, he was a natural ally of environmentalists.

However, in the early 1980s Ames reversed his position, arguing that there is no scientific evidence that small doses of most synthetic chemicals cause human cancers; he also argued that, in the absence of such evidence, they should not be controlled. This about-face was partly a result of a growing body of knowledge concerning the mutagenic properties of numerous chemicals found in nature. Ames began arguing against the existing large public expenditures for pollution control and the regulation of synthetic chemicals, noting that cancer might just as plausibly be caused by the chemicals in plants. His arguments were based primarily on three factors: his argument that more scientific evidence should be required before controls are implemented; his attitude toward the setting of priorities, which he argued should be centered on basic research rather than regulation; and finally his belief that the large public expenditures incurred by the regulatory process hurt American economic competitiveness.

Ames and his colleague Gold have also argued that the use of bioassays (animal tests) of chemicals to predict their carcinogenic potential in humans should be abandoned. In a typical bioassay, rats are given a maximum tolerated dosage (MTD) of a particular chemical daily for a period of time (such as a year). The maximum tolerated dosage is as much as the animal can be given without immediately becoming ill or dying. At the end of the time period, the number of animals that have developed cancers is tabulated as an indicator of the cancer causing potential of the chemical being tested. Ames suggested that it is often the large dosage itself, rather than the nature of the particular chemical that induces the rat cancers. He argued that, since humans are not normally exposed to such large doses, the assays were not valid for predicting human cancers.

Ames's arguments have some support both within and outside scientific communities. However, he also has numerous critics. Those taking issue with his positions have noted that pollution control, for example, involves far more than just carcinogenicity. These critics suggest that Ames has not offered a substitute for animal assays (the Ames test has not proved to be such a substitute), and that neither he nor they have a good idea of what goes on at low dosages. Some argue that Ames has an over-simplified view of the regulatory process, which is based on a consideration of animal assays but also on other factors. It has also been argued that the discovery that many naturally occurring chemicals have a high mutagenic rate (just as synthetic chemicals) should not lead to the conclusion that synthetic chemicals pose less risk than was previously supposed. Such an assumption places too much emphasis on mutagenic rate as a sole indicator of carcinogenicity, ignoring the complex, multi-stage developmental process of the disease.

Yet the disagreements between Ames and his critics are based on several points of commonality—that cancer is a complex multi-stage process that is not fully understood; that there is no perfect test or group of tests that can fully predict the potential carcinogenicity of many substances in humans; and that public regulatory and environmental policies must be made and carried out in spite of this deficiency of knowledge. As for Ames, he has described his public-policy activism as a hobby, and he has noted that his recent scientific work includes studies in the biochemistry of aging.

Elected to the National Academy of Sciences in 1972, Ames has received many awards, including the Eli Lilly Award of the American Chemical Society (1964), the Mott Prize of the General Motors Cancer Research Foundation (1983), and the Gold Medal of the American Institute of Chemists (1991). He is the author or coauthor of more than 250 scientific articles.

See also Chemical mutagenesis; Molecular biology and molecular genetics

AMINO ACID CHEMISTRY

Amino acids are the building blocks of proteins and serve many other functions in living organisms. The prime function of **DNA** is to carry the information needed to direct the proper sequential insertion of amino acids into protein chain during **protein synthesis (translation)**.

An amino acid is a molecule that contains a terminal acidic carboxyl group (COOH) and a terminal basic amino group (NH_2). The approximately 20 amino acids (plus a few derivatives) that have been identified as protein constituents are alpha-amino acids in which the $-NH_2$ group is attached to the alpha-carbon next to the -COOH group. Thus, their basic structure is $NH_2CHRCOOH$, where R is a side chain. This side chain, which uniquely characterizes each alpha-amino acid, determines the molecules overall size, shape, chemical reactivity, and charge. There are hundreds of alpha-amino acids, both natural and synthetic.

The amino acids that receive the most attention are the alpha-amino acids that genes are codes for, and that are used to construct proteins. These amino acids include glycine NH_2CH_2COOH, alanine $CH_3CH (NH_2) COOH$, valine $(CH_3)2CHCH (NH_2)COOH$, leucine $(CH_3)_2CHCH_2CH(NH_2)COOH$, isoleucine $CH_3CH_2CH(CH_3)CH(NH_2)COOH$, methionine $CH_3SCH_2CH_2CH(NH_2)COOH$, phenylalanine $C_6H_5CH_2CH(CH_2)COOH$, proline C_4H_8NCOOH, serine $HOCH_2CH(NH_2)COOH$, threonine $CH_3CH(OH)CH(NH_2)COOH$, cysteine $HSCH_2CH(NH_2)COOH$, asparagine, glutamine $H_2NC(O)(CH_2)2CH(NH_2)COOH$, tyrosine $C_6H_4OHCH_2CHNH_2COOH$, tryptophan $C_8H_6NCH_2CHNH_2COOH$, aspartate $COOHCH_2CH(NH_2)COOH$, glutamate $COOH(CH_2)2CH(NH_2)COOH$, histidine $HOOCCH(NH_2)CH_2C_3H_3H_2$, lysine $NH_2(CH_2)_4CH(NH_2)COOH$, and arginine $(NH_2)C(NH)HNCH_2CH_2CH_2CH(NH_2)COOH$.

Proteins are one of the most common types of molecules in living matter. There are countless members of this class of molecules. They have many functions from composing cell structure to enabling cell-to-cell communication. One thing that all proteins have in common is that they are composed of amino acids.

Proteins consist of long chains of amino acids connected by peptide linkages (-CO·NH-). A protein's primary structure refers to the sequence of amino acids in the molecule. The protein's secondary structure is the fixed arrangement of amino acids that results from interactions of amide linkages that are close to each other in the protein chain. The secondary structure is strongly influenced by the nature of the side chains, which tend to force the protein molecule into specific twists and kinks. Side chains also contribute to the protein's tertiary structure, i.e., the way the protein chain is twisted and folded. The twists and folds in the protein chain result from the attractive forces between amino acid side chains that are widely separated from each other within the chain. Some proteins are composed of two of more chains of amino acids. In these cases, each chain is referred to as a subunit. The subunits can be structurally the same, but in many cases differ. The protein's quaternary structure refers to the spatial arrangement of the subunits of the protein, and

Name	The *XYZ* group is	Shorthand	Name	The *XYZ* group is	Shorthand
Glycine	—H	Gly			
Alanine	—CH₃	Ala	Glutamine	—CH₂CH₂C—NH₂	Gln
Valine	—CH—CH₃ (CH₃)	Val	Lysine	—CH₂CH₂CH₂CH₂NH₂	Lys
Leucine	—CH₂CHCH₃ (CH₃)	Leu	Arginine	—CH₂CH₂CH₂N—C—NH₂	Arg
Isoleucine	—CHCH₂CH₃ (CH₃)	Ile	Histidine	—CH₂—C—CH (HN N CH)	His
Serine	—CH₂OH	Ser			
Threonine	—CHCH₃ (OH)	Thr	Phenylalanine	—CH₂—	Phe
Cysteine	—CH₂SH	Cys	Tyrosine	—CH₂—OH	Tyr
Methionine	—CH₂CH₂SCH₃	Met			
Aspartic acid	—CH₂C—OH	Asp	Tryptophan	—CH₂—	Trp
Asparagine	—CH₂C—NH₂	Asn			
Glutamic acid	—CH₂CH₂C—OH	Glu	Proline	HO—C—CH—CH₂ (H—N CH₂ CH₂)	Pro

The twenty most common amino acids. *Illustrations reprinted by permission of Robert L. Wolke.*

describes how the subunits pack together to create the overall structure of the protein.

Even small changes in the primary structure of a protein may have a large effect on that protein's properties. Even a single misplaced amino acid can alter the protein's function. This situation occurs in certain genetic diseases such as sickle-cell anemia. In that disease, a single glutamic acid molecule has been replaced by a valine molecule in one of the chains of the hemoglobin molecule, the protein that carries oxygen in red blood cells and gives them their characteristic color. This seemingly small error causes the hemoglobin molecule to be misshapen and the red blood cells to be deformed. Such red blood cells cannot distribute oxygen properly, do not live as long as normal blood cells, and may cause blockages in small blood vessels.

Enzymes are large protein molecules that catalyze a broad spectrum of biochemical reactions. If even one amino acid in the enzyme is changed, the enzyme may lose its catalytic activity.

The amino acid sequence in a particular protein is determined by the protein's **genetic code**. The genetic code resides in specific lengths (called genes) of the polymer doxyribonucleic acid (DNA), which is made up of from 3000 to several million nucleotide units, including the nitrogeneous bases: adenine, guanine, cytosine, and thymine. Although there are only four nitrogenous bases in DNA, the order in which they appear transmits a great deal of information. Starting at one end of the **gene**, the genetic code is read three nucleotides at a time. Each triplet set of nucleotides corresponds to a specific amino acid.

Occasionally there an error, or mutation, may occur in the genetic code. This mutation may correspond to the substitution of one nucleotide for another or to the deletion of a nucleotide. In the case of a substitution, the result may be that the wrong amino acid is used to build the protein. Such a mistake, as demonstrated by sickle cell anemia, may have grave consequences. In the case of a deletion, the protein may be lose its functionality or may be completely missing.

Amino acids are also the core construction materials for neurotransmitters and hormones. Neurotransmitters are chemicals that allow nerve cells to communicate with one another and to convey information through the nervous system. Hormones also serve a communication purpose. These chemicals are produced by glands and trigger metabolic processes throughout the body. Plants also produce hormones.

Important neurotransmitters that are created from amino acids include serotonin and gamma-aminobutyric acid. Serotonin($C_{10}H_{12}N_2O$) is manufactured from tryptophan, and gamma-aminobutyric acid ($H_2N(CH_2)_3COOH$) is made from glutamic acid. Hormones that require amino acids for starting materials include thyroxine (the hormone produced by the thyroid gland), and auxin (a hormone produced by plants). Thyroxine is made from tyrosine, and auxin is constructed from tryptophan.

A class of chemicals important for both neurotransmitter and hormone construction are the catecholamines. The amino acids tyrosine and phenylalanine are the building materials for catecholamines, which are used as source material for both neurotransmitters and for hormones.

Amino acids also play a central role in the **immune system**. Allergic reactions involve the release of **histamine**, a chemical that triggers **inflammation** and swelling. Histamine is a close chemical cousin to the amino acid histidine, from which it is manufactured.

Melatonin, the chemical that helps regulate sleep cycles, and melanin, the one that determines the color of the skin, are both based on amino acids. Although the names are similar, the activities and component parts of these compounds are quite different. Melatonin uses tryptophan as its main building block, and melanin is formed from tyrosine. An individual's melanin production depends both on genetic and environmental factors.

Proteins in the diet contain amino acids that are used within the body to construct new proteins. Although the body also has the ability to manufacture certain amino acids, other amino acids cannot be manufactured in the body and must be gained through diet. Such amino acids are called the essential dietary amino acids, and include arginine, histidine, isoleucine, leucine, lysine, methionine, phenylalanine, threonine, tryptophan, and valine.

Foods such as meat, fish, and poultry contain all of the essential dietary amino acids. Foods such as fruits, vegetables, grains, and beans contain protein, but they may lack one or more of the essential dietary amino acids. However, they do not all lack the same essential dietary amino acid. For example, corn lacks lysine and tryptophan, but these amino acids can be found in soy beans. Therefore, vegetarians can meet their dietary needs for amino acids as long by eating a variety of foods.

Amino acids are not stockpiled in the body, so it is necessary to obtain a constant supply through diet. A well-balanced diet delivers more protein than most people need. In fact, amino acid and protein supplements are unnecessary for most people, including athletes and other very active individuals. If more amino acids are consumed than the body needs,

they will be converted to fat or metabolized and excreted in the urine.

However, it is vital that all essential amino acids be present in the diet if an organism is to remain healthy. Nearly all proteins in the body require all of the essential amino acids in their synthesis. If even one amino acid is missing, the protein cannot be constructed. In cases in which there is an ongoing deficiency of one or more essential amino acids, an individual may develop a condition known as kwashiorkor, which is characterized by severe weight loss, stunted growth, and swelling in the body's tissues. The situation is made even more grave because the intestines lose their ability to extract nutrients from whatever food is consumed. Children are more strongly affected by kwashiorkor than adults because they are still growing and their protein requirements are higher. Kwashiorkor often accompanies conditions of famine and starvation.

See also Bacterial growth and division; Biochemistry; Cell cycle (eukaryotic), genetic regulation of; Cell cycle (prokaryotic), genetic regulation of; Cell cycle and cell division; Chromosomes, eukaryotic; Chromosomes, prokaryotic; DNA (Deoxyribonucleic acid); Enzymes; Genetic regulation of eukaryotic cells; Genetic regulation of prokaryotic cells; Genotype and phenotype; Molecular biology and molecular genetics

AMINOGLYCOSIDE ANTIBIOTICS · *see* ANTIBIOTICS

AMYLOID PLAQUES · *see* BSE AND CJD DISEASE

ANAEROBES AND ANAEROBIC INFECTIONS

Anaerobes are **bacteria** that are either capable of growing in the absence of oxygen (referred to as facultative anaerobes) or that absolutely require the absence of oxygen (these are also called obligate anaerobes). Among the oxygen-free environments in which such bacteria can grow are deep wounds and tissues in the body. Growth in these niches can produce infections.

Examples of infections are gas gangrene (which is caused by *Streptococcus pyogenes*) and **botulism** (which is caused by *Clostridium botulinum*). Other anaerobic bacteria that are frequently the cause of clinical infections are members of the genus *Peptostreptococcus* and *Bacteroides fragilis*.

There are a number of different types of anaerobic bacteria. Two fundamental means of differentiation of these types is by their reaction to the Gram stain and by their shape. The genus *Clostridium* consists of Gram-positive rod-shaped bacteria that form spores. Gram-positive rods that do not form spores include the genera *Actinomyces*, *Bifidobacterium*, *Eubacterium*, *Propionibacterium*, and *Lactobacillus*. Gram-positive bacteria that are spherical in shape includes the genera *Peptostreptococcus*, *Streptococcus*, and *Staphylococcus*. Rod-shaped bacteria that stain Gram-negative include *Bacteroides*, *Campylobacter*, and *Fusobacterium*. Finally, Gram-negative spherical bacteria are represented by the genus *Veillonella*.

The word anaerobic means "life without air." In the human body, regions that can be devoid of oxygen include the interior of dental **plaque** that grows on the surface of teeth and gums, the gastrointestinal tract, and even on the surface of the skin. Normally the anaerobic bacteria growing in these environments are benign and can even contribute to the body's operation. Most of the bacteria in the body are anaerobes. However, if access to underlying tissues is provided due to injury or surgery, the bacteria can invade the new territory and establish an infection. Such bacteria are described as being opportunistic pathogens. That is, given the opportunity and the appropriate conditions, they are capable of causing an infection. Typically, anaerobic bacteria cause from five to ten per cent of all clinical infections.

Anaerobic infections tend to have several features in common. The infection is usually accompanied by a foul-smelling gas or pus. The infections tend to be located close to membranes, particularly mucosal membranes, as the infection typically begins by the invasion of a region that is bounded by a membrane. Anaerobic infections tend to involve the destruction of tissue, either because of bacterial digestion or because of destructive **enzymes** that are elaborated by the bacteria. This type of tissue damage is known as tissue necrosis. The tissue damage also frequently includes the production of gas or a fluid.

There are several sites in the body that are prone to infection by anaerobic bacteria. Infections in the abdomen can produce the **inflammation** of the appendix that is known as appendicitis. Lung infections can result in **pneumonia**, infection of the lining of the lung (empyema) or constriction of the small air tubes known as bronchi (bronchiectasis). In females, pelvic infections can inflame the lining of the uterus (endometritis). Mouth infections can involve the root canals or gums (gingivitis). Infections of the central nervous system can lead to brain and spinal cord infections. Infection of the skin, via bites and other routes of entry, causes open sores on the skin and tissue destruction. An example is that massive and potentially lethal tissue degradation, which is known as necrotizing fascitis, and which is caused by group A b-hemolytic *Streptococcus*. Finally, infection of the bloodstream (bacteremia) can prelude the infection of the heart (endocarditis).

The diagnosis of anaerobic infections is usually based on the symptoms, site of the infection and, if the infection is visible, on both the appearance and smell of the infected area. Most of the bacteria responsible for infection are susceptible to one or more **antibiotics**. Treatment can be prolonged, however, since the bacteria are often growing slowly and since antibiotics rely on **bacterial growth** to exert their lethal effect. In the case of infections that create tissue destruction, the removal of the affected tissue is an option to prevent the spread of the infection. Amputation of limbs is a frequent means of dealing with necrotizing fascitis, an infection that is inside of tissue (and so protected from antibiotics and the

host's immune response) and is exceptional in that it can swiftly spread.

See also Bacteria and bacterial infections

ANAPHYLACTIC SHOCK • *see* IMMUNITY: ACTIVE, PASSIVE, AND DELAYED

ANAPHYLAXIS

Anaphylaxis is a severe allergic reaction. The symptoms appear rapidly and can be life threatening.

The symptoms of anaphylaxis include the increased output of fluid from mucous membranes (e.g., passages lining the nose, mouth, and throat), skin rash (e.g., hives), itching of the eyes, gastrointestinal cramping, and stiffening of the muscles lining the throat and trachea. As a result of the latter, breathing can become difficult. These symptoms do not appear in every case. However, some sort of skin reaction is nearly always evident.

Anaphylaxis results from the exposure to an **antigen** with which the individual has had previous contact, and has developed a heightened sensitivity to the antigen. Such an antigen is also known as an allergen. The allergen binds to the specific immune cell (e.g., immunoglobulin E, also known as IgE) that was formed in response to the initial antigen exposure. IgE is also associated with other specific cells of the **immune system** that are called basophils and mast cells. The basophils and mast cells react to the binding of the allergen-IgE complex by releasing compounds that are known as mediators (e.g, **histamine**, prostaglandin D2, tryptase). Release of mediators does not occur when IgE alone binds to the basophils or mast cells.

The release of the mediators triggers the physiological reactions. For example, blood vessels dilate (become larger in diameter) and fluid can pass across the blood vessel wall more easily. Because the immune system is sensitized to the particular allergen, and because of the potent effect of mediators, the development of symptoms can be sudden and severe. A condition called anaphylactic shock can ensue, in which the body's physiology is so altered that failure of functions such as the circulatory system and breathing can occur. For example, in those who are susceptible, a bee sting, administration of a penicillin-type of antibiotic, or the ingestion of peanuts can trigger symptoms that can be fatal if not addressed immediately. Those who are allergic to bee stings often carry medication with them on hikes.

Anaphylaxis occurs with equal frequency in males and females. No racial predisposition towards anaphylaxis is known. The exact number of cases is unknown, because many cases of anaphylaxis are mistaken for other conditions (e.g., food poisoning). However, at least 100 people die annually in the United States from anaphylactic shock.

See also Allergies; Immunoglobulins and immunoglobulin deficiency syndromes

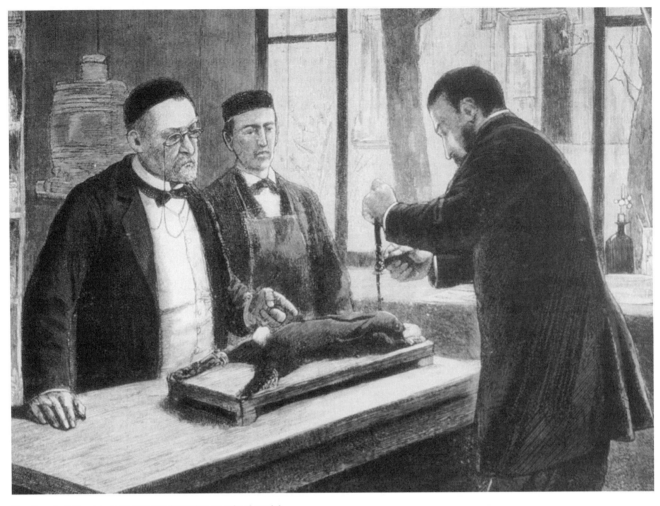

Drawing depicting Louis Pasteur (right) using an animal model.

ANIMAL MODELS OF INFECTION

The use of various animals as models for microbiological infections has been a fundamental part of infectious disease research for more than a century. Now, techniques of genetic alteration and manipulation have made possible the design of animals so as to be specifically applicable to the study of a myriad of diseases.

The intent for the use of animals as models of disease is to establish an infection that mimics that seen in the species of concern, usually humans. By duplicating the infection, the reasons for the establishment of the infection can be researched. Ultimately, the goal is to seek means by which the infection can be thwarted. Development of a **vaccine** to the particular infection is an example of the successful use of animals in infectious disease research.

The development of the idea that maladies could be caused by **bacterial infection** grow from animals studies by **Louis Pasteur** in the mid-nineteenth century. The use of animals as models of cholera and **anthrax** enabled Pasteur to develop vaccines against these diseases. Such work would not have been possible without the use of animals.

Subsequent to Pasteur, the use of animal models for a myriad of bacterial and viral diseases has led to the production of vaccines to diseases such as **diphtheria, rabies, tuberculosis, poliomyelitis, measles,** and rubella.

Animal models are also used to screen candidate drugs for their performance in eliminating the infection of concern and also to evaluate adverse effects of the drugs. While some of this work may be amenable to study using cells grown on in the laboratory, and by the use of sophisticated computer models that can make predictions about the effect of a treatment, most scientists argue that the bulk of drug evaluation still requires a living subject.

A key to developing an animal model is the selection of an animal whose physiology, reaction to an infection, and the nature of the infection itself all mirror as closely as possible the situation in humans. The study of an infection that bears no resemblance to that found in a human would be fruitless, in terms of developing treatment strategies for the human condition.

The need to mirror the human situation has led to the development of animal models that are specifically tailored for certain diseases. One example is the so-called nude mouse, which derives its name from the fact that it has no hair. Nude mice lack a thymus, and so are immunodeficient in a number of ways. Use of nude mice has been very useful in the study of **immunodeficiency** diseases in humans, such as acquired immunodeficiency syndrome. As well, this animal model lends itself to the study of opportunistic bacterial infections, which typically occur in humans whose **immune systems** are compromised.

Depending on the infection and the focus of study, other animals have proven to be useful in infectious disease research. These animals include the rabbit, rat, guinea pig, pig, dog, and monkey. The latter in particular has been utilized in the study of **AIDS**, as primates are the genetically closest relatives to humans.

The advent of molecular techniques of genetic alteration has made the development of genetically tailored animal models possible. Thus, for example, mouse models exist in which the activity of certain genes has been curtailed. These are known as transgenic animals. The involvement of the **gene** product in the infectious process is possible on a scale not possible without the use of the animal.

The data from animal models provides a means of indicating the potential of a treatment. Furthermore, if a disease in an animal does not exactly mimic the human's condition, for example cystic fibrosis in mice, the use of the animal model provides a guide towards establishing the optimal treatment in humans. In other words, the animal model can help screen and eliminate the undesirable treatments, narrowing the successful candidates for use in human studies. Further study, involving humans, is always necessary before something such as a vaccine can be introduced for general use. Such human studies are subject to rigorous control.

The use of animals in research has long been a contentious issue, mainly due to questions of ethical treatment. This climate has spawned much legislation concerning the treatment of research animals. As well, in most institutions, an evaluation committee must approve the use of animals. If the research can be accomplished in some other way than through the use of living animals, then approval for the animal study is typically denied.

See also AIDS, recent advances in research and treatment; Giardia and giardiasis; Immunodeficiency

ANIMALCULES • *see* HISTORY OF MICROBIOLOGY

ANTHRAX

Anthrax refers to a pulmonary disease that is caused by the bacterium *Bacillus anthracis*. This disease has been present since antiquity. It may be the sooty "morain" in the Book of *Exodus*, and is probably the "burning wind of plague" that

begins Homer's *Iliad*. Accounts by the Huns during their sweep across Eurasia in 80 A.D. describe mass deaths among their horse and cattle attributed to anthrax. These animals, along with sheep, are the primary targets of anthrax. Indeed, loss to European livestock in the eighteenth and nineteenth centuries stimulated the search for a cure. In 1876, **Robert Koch** identified the causative agent of anthrax.

The use of anthrax as a weapon is not a new phenomenon. In ancient times, diseased bodies were used to poison wells, and were catapulted into cities under siege. In modern times, research into the use of anthrax as a weapon was carried out during World Wars I and II. In World War II, Japanese and German prisoners were subjects of medical research, including their susceptibility to anthrax. Allied efforts in Canada, the U.S. and Britain to develop anthrax-based weapons were also active. Britain actually produced five million anthrax cakes at the Porton Down facility, to be dropped on Germany to infect the food chain.

In non-deliberate settings, humans acquire anthrax from exposure to the natural reservoirs of the microorganism; livestock such as sheep or cattle or wild animals. Anthrax has been acquired by workers engaged in shearing sheep, for example.

Human anthrax can occur in three major forms. Cutaneous anthrax refers to the entry of the organism through a cut in the skin. Gastrointestinal anthrax occurs when the organism is ingested in food or water. Finally, inhalation anthrax occurs when the organism is inhaled.

All three forms of the infection are serious, even lethal, if not treated. With prompt treatment, the cutaneous form is often cured. Gastrointestinal anthrax, however, can still be lethal in 25–75% of people who contract it. Inhalation anthrax is almost always fatal.

The inhalation form of anthrax can occur because of the changing state of the organism. *Bacillus anthracis* can live as a large "vegetative" cell, which undergoes cycles of growth and division. Or, the bacterium can wait out the nutritionally bad times by forming a spore and becoming dormant. The spore is designed to protect the genetic material of the bacterium during hibernation. When conditions are conducive for growth and reproduction the spore resuscitates and active life goes on again. The spore form can be easily inhaled. Only 8,000 spores, hardly enough to cover a snowflake, are sufficient to cause the pulmonary disease when they resuscitate in the warm and humid conditions deep within the lung.

The dangers of an airborne release of anthrax spores is well known. British open-air testing of anthrax weapons in 1941 on Gruinard Island in Scotland rendered the island uninhabitable for five decades. In 1979, an accidental release of a minute quantity of anthrax spores occurred at a bioweapons facility near the Russian city of Sverdlovsk. At least 77 people were sickened and 66 died. All the affected were some four kilometers downwind of the facility. Sheep and cattle up to 50 kilometers downwind became ill.

Three components of *Bacillus anthracis* are the cause of anthrax. First, the bacterium can form a capsule around itself. The capsule helps shield the bacterium from being recognized by the body's **immune system** as an invader, and helps fend off antibodies and immune cells that do try to deal

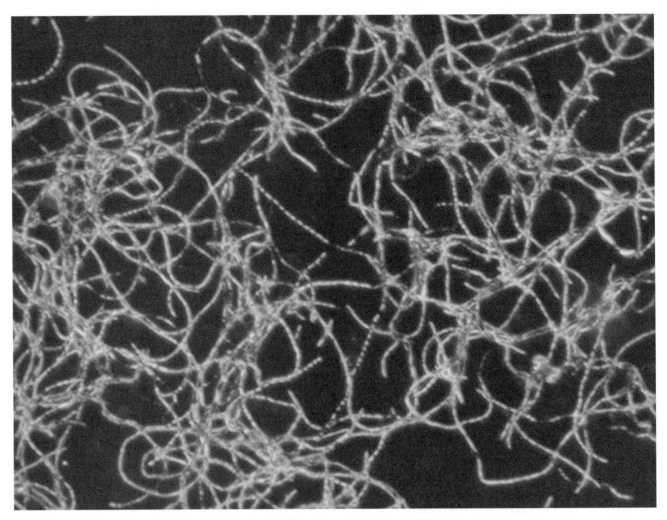

Light micrograph of *Bacillus anthracis*, showing the typical hair-like pattern of growth in a liquid.

with the bacterium. This can allow the organism to multiply to large numbers that overwhelm the immune system. The capsule also contains an **antigen** that has been designated a protective antigen. The antigen is protective, not to the host being infected, but to the bacterium. The protective antigen dissolves protein, which can allow the bacterium to "punch" through the membrane surrounding cells of the host, such as the epithelial cells that line the lung. One inside the cells, a bacterium is safe from the host's immune defenses. A second toxic component, which is called lethal factor, destroys immune cells of the host. Finally, a third toxic factor is known as edema factor (named because it results in the accumulation of fluid at the site of infection). Edema factor disables a molecule in the host called calmodulin, which is used to regulate many chemical reactions in the body. The end result of the activity of the toxic factors of *Bacillus anthracis* is to quell the immune response and so, to allow the infection to spread.

As the **bacteria** gain a foothold, toxins enter the bloodstream and circulate throughout the body causing destruction of blood cells and tissues. The damage can prove to be overwhelming to treatment efforts and death occurs.

Anthrax infections are difficult to treat because the initial symptoms are similar to other, less serious infections, such as the flu. By the time the diagnosis is made, the infection can be too advanced to treat. A **vaccine** for anthrax does exist. But to date, only those at high risk for infection (soldiers, workers in meat processing plants, anthrax research scientists) have received the vaccine, due to the possible serious side effects that can occur. Work to establish a safer vaccine is underway. The edema factor may be a potential target of a vaccine. Another promising target is the protective antigen of the capsule. If the action of this antigen could be blocked, the bacteria would not be able to hide inside host cells, and so could be more effectively dealt with by the immune response and with **antibiotics**.

See also Anthrax, terrorist use of as a biological weapon; Bioterrorism

ANTHRAX, FORENSIC IDENTIFICATION •

see GENETIC IDENTIFICATION OF MICROORGANISMS

ANTHRAX, TERRORIST USE AS A BIOLOGICAL WEAPON

During the past two decades, the potential use of biological weapons by terrorists has received a great deal of attention, particularly in the United States. The existence of an **anthrax** bioweapons development campaign by the government of Iraq was revealed during the Persian Gulf War from 1990 to 1991. Then, in the aftermath of the September 11, 2001 terrorist attacks on the World Trade Center buildings in New York City and the Pentagon in Washington, DC., letters containing a powdered form of *Bacillus anthracis*, the **bacteria** that causes anthrax, were mailed to government representatives, members of the news media, and others in the United States. The anthrax-laced powder inside the letters was aerosolized (i.e., the spores became airborne) when the letters were opened, and in a few cases were inhaled. The death of a Florida man was the first case of an inhalational anthrax death in the United States since 1978 and as of June 2002, more than 20 cases and five deaths were attributed to the terrorist attack.

Although a relatively new weapon in the hands of modern potential bioterrorists, the threat of death from the inhalation of anthrax has been part of human history since antiquity. Some scholars argue that it is the sooty "morain" in the Bible's Book of *Exodus*, and is likely the "burning wind of plague" that begins Homer's *Iliad*.

As well, the use of **microorganisms** such as the anthrax bacteria as weapons is not new. In ancient military campaigns, diseased bodies (including those who died of anthrax) were used to poison wells and were catapulted into cities under siege. Research into the military use of anthrax was carried out during World War I by combatants on all sides of the conflict, and by World War II anthrax research was actively underway. For example, Allied efforts in Canada, the United States, and Britain to develop anthrax-based weapons included the production of five million anthrax "cakes," designed to be dropped on Germany to infect wells and the food chain. The weapons were never used.

Only within the past several decades, however, have biological weapons, including anthrax, been added to the arsenal of terrorists. For example, the Japanese cult Aum Shinrikyo (which released sarin gas into the Tokyo subway system in 1995, killing 12 people and hospitalizing 5,000) was developing anthrax-based weapons. Indeed, the group had released crude anthrax preparations in Tokyo on at least eight separate occasions in 1993. These incidents were the first time that anthrax was used as a weapon against a civilian population. In addition, state-sanctioned terrorism by the government of Iraq has also, purportedly, involved the production of anthrax bioweapons, and Western intelligence sources insist that Iraq—or terrorist groups operating with Iraq's assistance—continues (despite United Nations' efforts at inspection and destruction) to develop biological weapons, including

anthrax-based weapons. Finally, during the terrorist attacks of the United States in the latter part of 2001 the use of anthrax by a terrorist or terrorists (as of June 2002, yet unidentified) pointed out how easily the lethal agent could be delivered.

This ease of delivery of anthrax is one feature that has made the bacterium an attractive weapon for terrorists. Scenarios developed by United States government agencies have shown that even a small crop dusting plane carrying only a hundred kilograms of anthrax spores flying over a city could deliver a potentially fatal dose to up to three million people in only a few hours. Although variations in weather patterns and concentration variables would substantially reduce the number of expected actual deaths, such an attack could still result in the deaths of thousands of victims and result in a devastating attack on the medical and economic infrastructure of the city attacked. In a less sophisticated effort, spores could simply be released into air intake vents or left in places like a subway tunnel, to be dispersed in the air over a much small area.

Another feature of anthrax that has led to its exploitation by terrorists is the physiology of the bacterium. *Bacillus anthracis* can live as a vegetative cell, growing and dividing in a rapid and cyclical fashion. The bacterium can also form a metabolically near-dormant form known as a spore. An individual spore is much smaller and lighter than the growing bacterium. Indeed, the spores can drift on air currents, to be inhaled into the lungs. Once in the lungs, the spores can resuscitate into an actively growing and dividing bacterium. The infections that are collectively termed anthrax can result. Although millions of spores can be released from a few grams (fractions of an ounce) of *Bacillus anthracis*, only about 5,000 to 8,000 spores are sufficient to cause the lung infection when they are inhaled. If left untreated or not promptly treated with the proper **antibiotics** (e.g., Cipro), the lung infection is almost always fatal. Non-inhalation contact with *Bacillus anthracis* can result in cutaneous anthrax—a condition more treatable with conventional antibiotic therapy.

An often-overlooked aspect of the use of anthrax as a terrorist weapon is the economic hardship that the dispersal of a small amount of the spores would exact. A report from the **Centers for Disease Control** and Prevention, entitled *The Economic Impact of a Bioterrorist Attack*, estimated the costs of dealing with an anthrax incident at a minimum of US$26 billion per 100,000 people. In just a few months in 2001 alone, a flurry of anthrax incidents, most of which turned out to be hoaxes, cost the United States government millions of dollars.

The choice of anthrax as a weapon by terrorists reflects the growing awareness of the power of biological research and **biotechnology** among the general community. The ability to grow and disperse infectious microorganisms was once restricted to specialists. However, the explosion of biotechnology in the 1980s and 1990s demonstrated that the many basic microbiological techniques are fairly simple and attainable. Experts in microbiology testifying before Congress, estimated that crude weapons could be developed with approximately $10,000 worth of equipment. A laboratory sufficient to grow and harvest the bacteria and to dry down the material to powdered form could fit into the average sized household base-

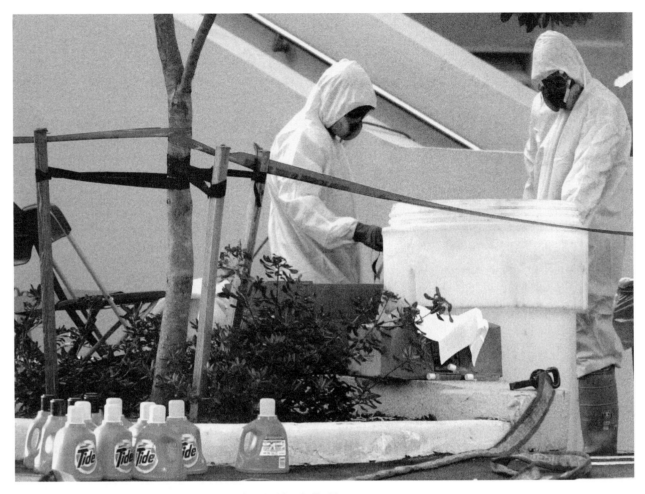

Workers in biohazard protective suits respond to an anthrax incident in Florida.

ment. The more highly trained the terrorist, the more effective weapons could be expected to be produced.

Even though *Bacillus anthracis* could be grown in such a makeshift laboratory, the preparation of the spores and the drying of the spores into a powder is not a trivial task. As an example, even after a decade of dedicated effort, United Nations inspectors who toured Iraq bioweapons facilities after the Gulf War found that Iraq had only managed to develop crude anthrax preparations. Still, the Iraq bioweapons program managed to produce 8,500 liters of concentrated anthrax.

Regardless, despite the technical challenges, the production of anthrax spores in quantities great enough to cause a huge loss of life is not beyond the capability of a small group of equipped and funded terrorists. This small size and nondescript nature of a bioweapons facility could make detection of such a lab very difficult. Accordingly, the terrorist potential of anthrax will remain a threat for the foreseeable future.

See also Bacteria and bacterial infection; Biological warfare; Bioterrorism, protective measures; Bioterrorism; Epidemics and pandemics; Vaccine

ANTI-ADHESION METHODS

The adhesion of **bacteria** and other **microorganisms** to non-living and living surfaces is a crucial part of the **contamination** and infection processes. In fact, the growth of microorganisms on surfaces is the preferred mode of existence. The ability to block adhesion would prevent surface growth.

There are numerous examples of surface growth of microorganisms. Adherence and growth of bacteria such as **Escherichia coli** on urinary catheters (synthetic tubes that are inserted into the bladder to assist hospitalized patients in removing urine from the body) is a large problem in hospitals. The chance of a urinary tract infection increases by up to10% for each day of catheterization. *Neiserria meningitidis*, the agent that causes **meningitis**, relies upon adhesion with host cells. The adhesion of this and many other bacteria, including disease causing *Escherichia coli*, is mediated by a surface tube-like protein appendage called a pilus.

Other bacterial proteins are involved in adhesion, typically by recognizing and biding to another protein on the surface of the host cell. Microorganism proteins that function in adhesion are generically known as adhesins.

Some strains of *E. coli* that infect intestinal cells do so by manufacturing and then releasing an adhesin, which is incorporated into the membrane of the host cell. Thus, the bacteria install their own receptor in the host tissue.

Adhesion need not rely on the presence of adhesins. The chemistry of the surface can also drive adhesion. For example, the surface of the spores of bacillus and the capsule surrounding *Pasteurella multocida* are described as being **hydrophobic**; that is, they tend not to associate with water. This hydrophobicity will drive the spore or bacterium to associate with a surface of similar chemistry.

In order to block adhesion that is the result of the above mechanisms, the molecular details of these mechanisms must be unraveled. This is an on-going process, but advances are being made through research.

Adhesion of *Escherichia coli* can depend on the presence of an adhesin called FimH. Antibodies to FimH can block adhesion, presumable by binding to the FimH protein, preventing that protein from binding to the receptor on the surface of the host cell. Furthermore, the three-dimensional structure of this adhesion is similar to that of adhesins from other bacteria. A **vaccine** devised against FimH might then have some protective effect against the adhesion of other bacteria.

In the case of the capsule-mediated adhesion, such as the example above, capsular antibodies may also thwart adhesion. The drawback with this approach is that capsular material is not a potent stimulator of the **immune system**.

For microorganisms that secrete their own receptor, such as *Escherichia coli*, or which have receptor molecules protruding from their own surface (an example is the **hemagglutinin** protein on the surface of *Bordetella pertussis*), adhesion could be eliminated by blocking the manufacture or the release of the receptor molecule.

In Canada, field trials began in the summer of 2001 on a vaccine to the adhesin target of *Escherichia coli O157:H7*. This pathogen, which can be permanently debilitating and even lethal to humans who ingest contaminated food or water, often lives in the intestinal tracts of cattle. By eliminating the adhesion of the bacteria, they could be "flushed" out of the cattle. Thus, a vital reservoir of infection would have been overcome. The vaccine could be ready for the market by as early as 2003.

Another anti-adhesion strategy is to out-compete the target bacteria for the available spots on the surface. This approach has been successful in preventing bacterial vaginal infections. Suppositories loaded with bacteria called **Lactobacillus** are administered. Colonization of the vaginal wall by the Lactobacillus can retard or even prevent the subsequent colonization of the wall by a harmful type of bacteria. The same bacteria are present in yogurt. Indeed, consumption of yogurt may help prevent intestinal upset due to colonization of the gut by harmful organisms.

Non-living surfaces, such as catheters and other implanted material, are colonized by, in particular, bacteria. In seeking to prevent adhesion, scientists have been experimenting with different implant materials, with the incorporation of antimicrobial compounds into the implant material, and with the "pre-coating" of the material. In the case of antimicrobial

compounds, promising results have been obtained in laboratory studies using material that can slowly release **antibiotics**. The disadvantage of this approach is that the presence of residual antibiotic could encourage the formation of resistance. Pre-coating implant material with an antimicrobial compound that is permanently bonded has also been promising in lab studies.

See also Biofilm formation and dynamic behavior; Infection and resistance; Probiotics

ANTIBIOTIC RESISTANCE, TESTS FOR

Bacteria can sometimes adapt to the **antibiotics** used to kill them. This adaptation, which can involve structural changes or the production of **enzymes** that render the antibiotic useless, can make the particular bacterial species resistant to the particular antibiotic. Furthermore, a given bacterial species will usually display a spectrum of susceptibilities to antibiotics, with some antibiotics being very effective and others totally ineffective. For another bacterial species, the pattern of antibiotic sensitivity and resistance will be different. Thus, for diagnosis of an infection and for clinical decisions regarding the best treatment, tests of an organism's response to antibiotics are essential.

A standard method of testing for antibiotic resistance involves growth of the target bacteria in the presence of various concentrations of the antibiotic of interest. Typically, this test is performed in a specially designed plastic dish that can be filled with **agar** (a Petri plate). **Contamination** of the agar, which would spoil the test results, is guaranteed by the sterility of the plate and the lid that fits over the agar-containing dish. The type of agar used is essential for the validity of the tests results. Typically, Iso-Sensitest agar is used.

The hardened agar surface receives a suspension of the test bacteria, which is then spread out evenly over the surface of the agar. The intention is to form a so-called lawn of organisms as growth occurs. Also on the agar surface are discs of an absorbent material. A plate is large enough to house six discs. Each disc has been soaked in a known and different concentration of the same or of different antibiotics.

As growth of the bacteria occurs, antibiotic diffuses out from each disc into the agar. If the concentration of the antibiotic is lethal, no growth of the bacteria will occur. Finally, the diffusing antibiotic will be below lethal concentration, so that growth of bacteria can occur. The result is a ring of no growth around a disc. From comparison with known standards, the diameter of the growth inhibition ring will indicate whether the bacteria are resistant to the antibiotic.

Automated plate readers are available that will scan the plates, measure the diameter of the growth inhibition zones and consult a standard database to indicate the antibiotic resistance or susceptibility of the sample bacteria.

In the past 15 years, the use of fluorescent indicators has become popular. A myriad of compounds are available that will fluoresce under illumination of specific wavelengths. Among the uses for the fluorescent compounds is the viability

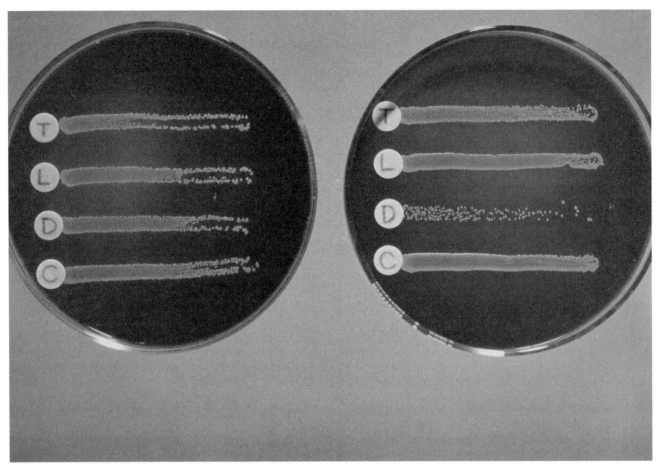

Antibiotic susceptible and resistant strains of Stapylococcus.

of a bacterium. For example, living bacteria will fluoresce in the presence of **acridine orange**, while dead bacteria will not. These probes combined with the optical technique of confocal laser microscopy, now enables populations of cells to be viewed without disrupting them to see if they fluoresce or not in the presence of an antibiotic of interest.

The ability of living bacteria to fluoresce can also be exploited by another machine called a flow cytometer. This machine operates essentially by forcing a suspension of bacteria (or other cells) through an opening so that only one bacterium at a time passes by a sensor. The sensor monitors each passing bacterium and can sort these into categories, in this case, fluorescing (living) from non-fluorescing (dead). The entire process can be completely quickly. This provides an almost "real-time" assessment of the proportion of a population that has been killed by an antibiotic. If the proportion of dead bacteria is low, resistance is indicated.

All the assessments of antibiotic effectiveness need to be done in a controlled manner. This necessitates the use of standard test types of bacteria (strains that are known to be resistant to the particular antibiotic as well as other strains that are known to be sensitive to the antibiotic). The concentration of the bacteria used is also important. Too many bacteria can "dilute" out the antibiotic, producing a false indication of

resistance. Controls need to be included to verify that the experiment was not subject to contamination, otherwise the possibility that a finding of resistance was due to a contaminating bacteria could not be discounted.

In clinical settings, a finding of resistance would prompt the search for another antibiotic. Often, identification of the bacteria will suggest, from previous documented tests of others, an antibiotic to which the organism will be susceptible. But, increasingly, formerly effective antibiotics are losing their potency as bacteria acquire resistance to them. Thus, tests of antibiotic resistance grow in importance.

ANTIBIOTICS

Antibiotics are natural or synthetic compounds that kill **bacteria**. There are a myriad of different antibiotics that act on different structural or biochemical components of bacteria. Antibiotics have no direct effect on virus.

Prior to the discovery of the first antibiotic, **penicillin**, in the 1930s, there were few effective ways of combating bacterial infections. Illnesses such as **pneumonia**, **tuberculosis**, and **typhoid fever** were virtually untreatable, and minor bacterial infections could blossom into life-threatening maladies. In the decades following the discovery of penicillin, many naturally occurring antibiotics were discovered and still more were synthesized towards specific targets on or in bacteria.

Antibiotics are manufactured by bacteria and various eukaryotic organisms, such as plants, usually to protect the organism from attack by other bacteria. The discovery of these compounds involves screening samples against bacteria for an inhibition in growth of the bacteria. In commercial settings, such screening has been automated so that thousands of samples can be processed each day. Antibiotics can also be manufactured by tailoring a compound to hone in on a selected target. The advent of molecular sequencing technology and three-dimensional image reconstruction has made the design of antibiotics easier.

Penicillin is one of the antibiotics in a class known as beta-lactam antibiotics. This class is named for the ring structure that forms part of the antibiotic molecule. Other classes of antibiotics include the tetracyclines, aminoglycosides, rifamycins, quinolones, and sulphonamides. The action of these antibiotics is varied. For example, beta-lactam antibiotics exert their effect by disrupting the manufacture of **peptidoglycan**, which is main stress-bearing network in the bacterial cell wall. The disruption can occur by blocking either the construction of the subunits of the peptidoglycan or by preventing their incorporation into the existing network. In another example, amonglycoside antibiotics can bind to a subunit of the ribosome, which blocks the manufacture of protein, or can reduce the ability of molecules to move across the cell wall to the inside of the bacterium. As a final example, the quinolone antibiotics disrupt the function of an enzyme that uncoils the double helix of **deoxyribonucleic acid**, which is vital if the **DNA** is to be replicated.

Besides being varied in their targets for antibacterial activity, different antibiotics can also vary in the range of bacteria they affect. Some antibiotics are classified as narrow-spectrum antibiotics. They are lethal against only a few types (or genera) of bacteria. Other antibiotics are active against many bacteria whose construction can be very different. Such antibiotics are described as having a broad-spectrum of activity.

In the decades following the discovery of penicillin, a myriad of different antibiotics proved to be phenomenally effective in controlling infectious bacteria. Antibiotics quickly became (and to a large extent remain) a vital tool in the physician's arsenal against many bacterial infections. Indeed, by the 1970s the success of antibiotics led to the generally held view that bacterial infectious diseases would soon be eliminated. However, the subsequent acquisition of resistance to many antibiotics by bacteria has proved to be very problematic.

Sometimes resistance to an antibiotic can be overcome by modifying the antibiotic slightly, via addition of a different chemical group. This acts to alter the tree-dimensional structure of the antibiotic. Unfortunately, such a modification tends to produce susceptibility to the new antibiotic for a relatively short time.

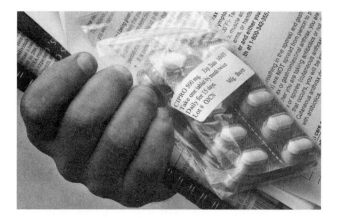

Ciprofloxacin.

Antibiotic resistance, a problem that develops when antibiotics are overused or misused. If an antibiotic is used properly to treat an infection, then all the infectious bacteria should be killed directly, or weakened such that the host's immune response will kill them. However, the use of too low a concentration of an antibiotic or stopping antibiotic therapy before the prescribed time period can leave surviving bacteria in the population. These surviving bacteria have demonstrated resistance. If the resistance is governed by a genetic alteration, the genetic change may be passed on to subsequent generations of bacterial. For example, many strains of the bacterium that causes tuberculosis are now also resistant to one or more of the antibiotics routinely used to control the lung infection. As a second example, some strains of *Staphylococcus aureus* that can cause boils, pneumonia, or bloodstream infections, are resistant to almost all antibiotics, making those conditions difficult to treat. Ominously, a strain of Staphylococcus (which so far has been rarely encountered) is resistant to all known antibiotics.

See also Bacteria and bacterial infection; Bacterial genetics; *Escherichia coli*; Rare genotype advantage

ANTIBIOTICS, HISTORY OF DEVELOPMENT • *see* HISTORY OF THE DEVELOPMENT OF ANTIBIOTICS

ANTIBODY-ANTIGEN, BIOCHEMICAL AND MOLECULAR REACTIONS

Antibodies are produced by the **immune system** in response to antigens (material perceived as foreign. The **antibody** response to a particular **antigen** is highly specific and often involves a physical association between the two molecules. This association is governed by biochemical and molecular forces.

In two dimensions, many antibody molecules present a "Y" shape. At the tips of the arms of the molecules are regions that are variable in their amino acid sequences, depending upon the antigen and the antibody formed in response. The arm-tip regions are typically those that bind to the antigen. These portions of the antibody are also known as the antigenic determinants, or the epitopes.

There are several different types of biochemical interactions between the antibody's epitopes and the target regions on the antigen. Hydrogen bonds are important in stabilizing the antibody-antigen association. In addition, other weak interactions (e.g., van der Waals forces, **hydrophobic** interactions, electrostatic forces) act to tighten the interaction between the regions on the antibody and the antigen.

The hydrogen bonds that are important in antigen-antibody bonding form between amino acids of the antibody and the antigen. Water molecules that fill in the spaces between the antibody and the antigen create other hydrogen bonds. The formation of hydrogen bonds between other regions of the **antibody and antigen**, and the water molecules stabilizes the binding of the immune molecules.

The three-dimensional shape of the molecules is also an important factor in binding between an antibody and an antigen. Frequently, the antibody molecule forms a pocket that is the right size and shape to accommodate the target region of the antigen. This phenomenon was initially described as the "lock and key" hypothesis.

The exact configuration of the antibody-antigen binding site is dependent on the particular antigen. Some antigens have a binding region that is compact. Such a region may be able to fit into a pocket or groove in the antibody molecule. In contrast, other antigen sites may be bulky. In this case, the binding site may be more open or flatter.

These various three dimensional structures for the binding site are created by the sequence of amino acids that comprise the antibody protein. Some sequences are enriched in hydrophobic (water-loving) amino acids. Such regions will tend to form flat sheets, with all the amino acids exposed to the hydrophilic environment. Other sequences of amino acids can contain both hydrophilic and hydrophobic (water-hating) amino acids. The latter will tend to bury themselves away from water via the formation of a helical shape, with the hydrophobic region on the inside. The overall shape of an antibody and antigen depends upon the number of hydrophilic and hydrophobic regions and their arrangement within the protein molecule.

The fact that the interaction between an antibody and an antigen requires a specific three-dimensional configuration is exploited in the design of some vaccines. These vaccines consist of an antibody to a region that is present on a so-called receptor protein. Antigens such as toxin molecules recognize the receptor region and bind to it. However, if the receptor region is already occupied by an antibody, then the binding of the antigen cannot occur, and the deleterious effect associated with binding of the antigen is averted.

Antibody antigen reactions tend to be irreversible under normal conditions. This is mainly due to the establishment of the various chemical bonds and interactions between the molecules. The visible clumping of the antibody-antigen complex seen in solutions and diagnostic tests such as the Ochterlony test is an example of the irreversible nature of the association.

See also Immune system; Immunoglobulins and immunoglobulin deficiency syndromes; Laboratory techniques in immunology; Protein crystallography

ANTIBODY AND ANTIGEN

Antibodies, or Y-shaped **immunoglobulins**, are proteins found in the blood that help to fight against foreign substances called antigens. Antigens, which are usually proteins or polysaccharides, stimulate the **immune system** to produce antibodies. The antibodies inactivate the antigen and help to remove it from the body. While antigens can be the source of infections from pathogenic **bacteria** and **viruses**, organic molecules detrimental to the body from internal or environmental sources also act as antigens. Genetic engineering and the use of various mutational mechanisms allow the construction of a vast array of antibodies (each with a unique genetic sequence).

Specific genes for antibodies direct the construction of antigen specific regions of the antibody molecule. Such antigen-specific regions are located at the extremes of the Y-shaped immunglobulin-molecule.

Once the immune system has created an antibody for an antigen whose attack it has survived, it continues to produce antibodies for subsequent attacks from that antigen. This long-term memory of the immune system provides the basis for the practice of **vaccination** against disease. The immune system, with its production of antibodies, has the ability to recognize, remember, and destroy well over a million different antigens.

There are several types of simple proteins known as **globulins** in the blood: alpha, beta, and gamma. Antibodies are gamma globulins produced by **B lymphocytes** when antigens enter the body. The gamma globulins are referred to as immunoglobulins. In medical literature they appear in the abbreviated form as Ig. Each antigen stimulates the production of a specific antibody (Ig).

Antibodies are all in a Y-shape with differences in the upper branch of the Y. These structural differences of amino acids in each of the antibodies enable the individual antibody to recognize an antigen. An antigen has on its surface a combining site that the antibody recognizes from the combining sites on the arms of its Y-shaped structure. In response to the antigen that has called it forth, the antibody wraps its two combining sites like a "lock" around the "key" of the antigen combining sites to destroy it.

An antibody's mode of action varies with different types of antigens. With its two-armed Y-shaped structure, the antibody can attack two antigens at the same time with each arm. If the antigen is a toxin produced by pathogenic bacteria that cause an infection like **diphtheria** or **tetanus**, the binding process of the antibody will nullify the antigen's toxin. When an antibody surrounds a virus, such as one that causes **influenza**, it prevents it from entering other body cells. Another mode of action by the antibodies is to call forth the assistance of a group of immune agents that operate in what is known as the plasma **complement** system. First, the antibodies will coat infectious bacteria and then white blood cells will complete the job by engulfing the bacteria, destroying them, and then removing them from the body.

There are five different antibody types, each one having a different Y-shaped configuration and function. They are the Ig G, A, M, D, and E antibodies.

IgG is the most common type of antibody. It is the chief Ig against microbes. It acts by coating the microbe to hasten its removal by other immune system cells. It gives lifetime or long-standing **immunity** against infectious diseases. It is highly mobile, passing out of the blood stream and between cells, going from organs to the skin where it neutralizes surface bacteria and other invading **microorganisms**. This mobility allows the antibody to pass through the placenta of the mother to her fetus, thus conferring a temporary defense to the unborn child.

After birth, IgG is passed along to the child through the mother's milk, assuming that she nurses the baby. But some of the Ig will still be retained in the baby from the placental transmission until it has time to develop its own antibodies. Placental transfer of antibodies does not occur in horses, pigs, cows, and sheep. They pass their antibodies to their offspring only through their milk.

This antibody is found in body fluids such as tears, saliva, and other bodily secretions. It is an antibody that provides a first line of defense against invading pathogens and allergens, and is the body's major defense against viruses. It is found in large quantities in the bloodstream and protects other wet surfaces of the body. While they have basic similarities, each IgA is further differentiated to deal with the specific types of invaders that are present at different openings of the body.

Since this is the largest of the antibodies, it is effective against larger microorganisms. Because of its large size (it combines five Y-shaped units), it remains in the bloodstream where it provides an early and diffuse protection against invading antigens, while the more specific and effective IgG antibodies are being produced by the plasma cells.

The ratio of IgM and IgG cells can indicate the various stages of a disease. In an early stage of a disease there are more IgM antibodies. The presence of a greater number of IgG antibodies would indicate a later stage of the disease. IgM antibodies usually form clusters that are in the shape of a star.

This antibody appears to act in conjunction with B and T-cells to help them in location of antigens. Research continues on establishing more precise functions of this antibody.

The antibody responsible for allergic reactions, IgE acts by attaching to cells in the skin called mast cells and basophil cells (mast cells that circulate in the body). In the presence of environmental antigens like pollens, foods, chemicals, and drugs, IgE releases histamines from the mast cells. The histamines cause the nasal **inflammation** (swollen tissues, running nose, sneezing) and the other discomforts of hay fever or other types of allergic responses, such as hives, asthma, and in rare cases, anaphylactic shock (a life-threatening condition brought on by an allergy to a drug or insect bite). An explanation for the role of IgE in allergy is that it was an antibody that was useful to early man to prepare the immune system to fight

parasites. This function is presently overextended in reacting to environmental antigens.

The presence of antibodies can be detected whenever antigens such as bacteria or red blood cells are found to agglutinate (clump together), or where they precipitate out of solution, or where there has been a stimulation of the plasma complement system. Antibodies are also used in laboratory tests for blood typing when transfusions are needed and in a number of different types of clinical tests, such as the Wassermann test for **syphilis** and tests for **typhoid fever** and infectious **mononucleosis**.

By definition, anything that makes the immune system respond to produce antibodies is an antigen. Antigens are living foreign bodies such as viruses, bacteria, and **fungi** that cause disease and infection. Or they can be dust, chemicals, pollen grains, or food proteins that cause allergic reactions.

Antigens that cause allergic reactions are called allergens. A large percentage of any population, in varying degrees, is allergic to animals, fabrics, drugs, foods, and products for the home and industry. Not all antigens are foreign bodies. They may be produced in the body itself. For example, cancer cells are antigens that the body produces. In an attempt to differentiate its "self" from foreign substances, the immune system will reject an organ transplant that is trying to maintain the body or a blood transfusion that is not of the same blood type as itself.

There are some substances such as nylon, plastic, or Teflon that rarely display antigenic properties. For that reason, nonantigenic substances are used for artificial blood vessels, component parts in heart pacemakers, and needles for hypodermic syringes. These substances seldom trigger an immune system response, but there are other substances that are highly antigenic and will almost certainly cause an immune system reaction. Practically everyone reacts to certain chemicals, for example, the resin from the poison ivy plant, the venoms from insect and reptile bites, solvents, formalin, and asbestos. Viral and bacterial infections also generally trigger an antibody response from the immune system. For most people **penicillin** is not antigenic, but for some there can be an immunological response that ranges from severe skin rashes to death.

Another type of antigen is found in the tissue cells of organ transplants. If, for example, a kidney is transplanted, the surface cells of the kidney contain antigens that the new host body will begin to reject. These are called **human leukocyte antigens (HLA)**, and there are four major types of HLA subdivided into further groups. In order to avoid organ rejection, tissue samples are taken to see how well the new organ tissues match for HLA compatibility with the recipient's body. Drugs will also be used to suppress and control the production of helper/suppressor T-cells and the amount of antibodies.

Red blood cells with the ABO antigens pose a problem when the need for blood transfusions arises. Before a transfusion, the blood is tested for type so that a compatible type is used. Type A blood has one kind of antigen and type B another. A person with type AB blood has both the A and B antigen. Type O blood has no antigens. A person with type A blood would require either type A or O for a successful transfusion. Type B and AB would be rejected. Type B blood would

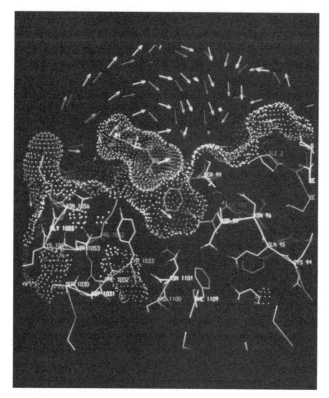

Binding of an antibody with an antigen, as detected using X-ray crystallography.

be compatible with a B donor or an O donor. Since O has no antigens, it is considered to be the universal donor. Type AB is the universal recipient because its antibodies can accept A, B, AB, or O. One way of getting around the problem of blood types in transfusion came about as a result of World War II. The great need for blood transfusions led to the development of blood plasma, blood in which the red and white cells are removed. Without the red blood cells, blood could be quickly administered to a wounded soldier without the delay of checking for the blood antigen type.

Another antigenic blood condition can affect the life of newborn babies. Rhesus disease (also called erythroblastosis fetalis) is a blood disease caused by the incompatibility of **Rh** factors between a fetus and a mother's red blood cells. When an Rh negative mother gives birth to an Rh positive baby, any transfer of the baby's blood to the mother will result in the production of antibodies against Rh positive red blood cells. At her next pregnancy the mother will then pass those antibodies against Rh positive blood to the fetus. If this fetus is Rh positive, it will suffer from Rh disease. Tests for Rh blood factors are routinely administered during pregnancy.

Western medicine's interest in the practice of vaccination began in the eighteenth century. This practice probably originated with the ancient Chinese and was adopted by Turkish doctors. A British aristocrat, Lady Mary Wortley Montagu (1689–1762), discovered a crude form of vaccination taking place in a lower-class section of the city of Constantinople while she was traveling through Turkey. She

described her experience in a letter to a friend. Children who were injected with pus from a **smallpox** victim did not die from the disease but built up immunity to it. Rejected in England by most doctors who thought the practice was barbarous, smallpox vaccination was adopted by a few English physicians of the period. They demonstrated a high rate of effectiveness in smallpox prevention.

By the end of the eighteenth century, **Edward Jenner** (1749–1823) improved the effectiveness of vaccination by injecting a subject with **cowpox**, then later injecting the same subject with smallpox. The experiment showed that immunity against a disease could be achieved by using a **vaccine** that did not contain the specific pathogen for the disease. In the nineteenth century, **Louis Pasteur** (1822–1895) proposed the **germ theory of disease**. He went on to develop a **rabies** vaccine that was made from the spinal cords of rabid rabbits. Through a series of injections starting from the weakest strain of the disease, Pasteur was able, after 13 injections, to prevent the death of a child who had been bitten by a rabid dog.

There is now greater understanding of the principles of vaccines and the immunizations they bring because of our knowledge of the role played by antibodies and antigens within the immune system. Vaccination provides active immunity because our immune systems have had the time to recognize the invading germ and then to begin production of specific antibodies for the germ. The immune system can continue producing new antibodies whenever the body is attacked again by the same organism or resistance can be bolstered by booster shots of the vaccine.

For research purposes there were repeated efforts to obtain a laboratory specimen of one single antibody in sufficient quantities to further study the mechanisms and applications of antibody production. Success came in 1975 when two British biologists, **César Milstein** (1927–) and Georges Kohler (1946–) were able to clone immunoglobulin (Ig) cells of a particular type that came from multiple myeloma cells. Multiple myeloma is a rare form of cancer in which white blood cells keep turning out a specific type of Ig antibody at the expense of others, thus making the individual more susceptible to outside infection. By combining the myeloma cell with any selected antibody-producing cell, large numbers of specific monoclonal antibodies can be produced. Researchers have used other animals, such as mice, to produce hybrid antibodies which increase the range of known antibodies.

Monoclonal antibodies are used as drug delivery vehicles in the treatment of specific diseases, and they also act as catalytic agents for protein reactions in various sites of the body. They are also used for diagnosis of different types of diseases and for complex analysis of a wide range of biological substances. There is hope that monoclonal antibodies will be as effective as **enzymes** in chemical and technological processes, and that they currently play a significant role in genetic engineering research.

See also Antibody-antigen, biochemical and molecular reactions; Antibody formation and kinetics; Antibody, monoclonal; Antigenic mimicry; Immune stimulation, as a vaccine; Immunologic therapies; Infection and resistance; Infection control; Major histocompatibility complex (MHC)

ANTIBODY FORMATION AND KINETICS

Antibody formation occurs in response to the presence of a substance perceived by the **immune system** as foreign. The foreign entity is generically called an **antigen**. There are a myriad of different antigens that are presented to the immune system. Hence, there are a myriad of antibodies that are formed.

The formation of innumerable antibodies follows the same general pattern. First, the immune system discriminates between host and non-host antigens and reacts only against those not from the host. However, malfunctions occur. An example is rheumatoid arthritis, in which a host response against self-antigens causes the deterioration of bone. Another example is heart disease caused by a host reaction to a heart muscle protein. The immune response is intended for an antigen of a bacterium called Chlamydia, which possess an antigen very similar in structure to the host heart muscle protein.

Another feature of antibody formation is that the production of an antibody can occur even when the host has not "seen" the particular antigen for a long time. In other words, the immune system has a memory for the antigenic response. Finally, the formation of an antibody is a very precise reaction. Alteration of the structure of a protein only slightly can elicit the formation of a different antibody.

The formation of antibody depends upon the processing of the incoming antigen. The processing has three phases. The first phase is the equilibration of an antigen between the inside and outside of cells. Soluble antigens that can dissolve across the cell membranes are able to equilibrate, but more bulky antigens that do not go into solution cannot. The second phase of antigen processing is known as the catabolic decay phase. Here, cells such as macrophages take up the antigen. It is during this phase that the antigen is "presented" to the immune system and the formation of antibody occurs. The final phase of antigen processing is called the immune elimination phase. The coupling between antigen and corresponding antibody occurs, and the complex is degraded. The excess antibody is free to circulate in the bloodstream.

The antibody-producing cell of the immune system is called the lymphocyte or the B cell. The presentation of a protein target stimulates the lymphocyte to divide. This is termed the inductive or lag phase of the primary antibody response. Some of the daughter cells will then produce antibody to the protein target. With time, there will be many daughter lymphocytes and much antibody circulating in the body. During this log or exponential phase, the quantity of antibody increases rapidly.

For a while, the synthesis of antibody is balanced by the breakdown of the antibody, so the concentration of antibody stays the same. This is the plateau or the steady-state phase. Within days or weeks, the production of the antibody slows. After this decline or death phase, a low, baseline concentration may be maintained.

The lymphocytes retain the memory of the target protein. If the antigen target appears, as happens in the second **vaccination** in a series, the pre-existing, "primed" lymphocytes are stimulated to divide into antibody-producing daughter cells. Thus, the second time around, a great deal more antibody is produced. This primed surge in antibody concentration is the secondary or anamnestic (memory) response. The higher concentration of antibody can be maintained for months, years, or a lifetime.

Another aspect of antibody formation is the change in the class of antibodies that are produced. In the primary response, mainly the IgM class of antibody is made. In the secondary response, IgG, IgE, or IgA types of antibodies are made.

The specificity of an antibody response, while always fairly specific, becomes highly specific in a secondary response. While in a primary response, an antibody may cross-react with antigens similar to the one it was produced in response to, such cross-reaction happens only very rarely in a secondary response. The binding between **antibody and antigen** becomes tighter in a secondary response as well.

See also Antigenic mimicry; History of immunology; Immunoglobulins and immunoglobulin deficiency syndromes; Laboratory techniques in immunology; Streptococcal antibody tests

ANTIBODY, MONOCLONAL

The **immune system** of vertebrates help keep the animal healthy by making millions of different proteins (**immunoglobulins**) called antibodies to disable antigens (harmful foreign substances such as toxins or **bacteria**). Scientists have worked to develop a method to extract large amounts of specific antibodies from clones (exact copies) of a cell created by fusing two different natural cells. Those antibodies are called monoclonal antibodies.

Antibody research began in the 1930s when the American pathologist **Karl Landsteiner** found that animal antibodies counteract specific antigens and that all antibodies have similar structures. Research by the American biochemists Rodney R. Porter (1917–1985) and **Gerald M. Edelman** (1929–) during the 1950s determined antibody structure, and particularly the active areas of individual antibodies. For their work they received the 1972 Nobel prize in physiology or medicine.

By the 1960s, scientists who studied cells needed large amounts of specific antibodies for their research, but several problems prevented them from obtaining these antibodies. Animals can be injected with antigens so they will produce the desired antibodies, but it is difficult to extract them from among the many types produced. Attempts to reproduce various antibodies in an artificial environment encountered some complications. Lymphocytes, the type of cell that produces specific antibodies, are very difficult to grow in the laboratory; conversely, tumor cells reproduce easily and endlessly, but make only their own types of antibodies. A bone marrow tumor called a myeloma interested scientists because it begins

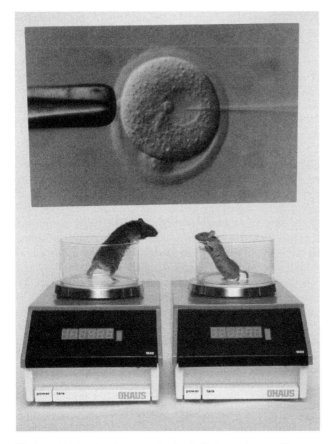

Mice used to develop the monoclonal cells that secret a specific antibody.

from a single cell that produces a single antibody, then divides many times. The cells that divided do not contain antibodies and could, therefore, be crossed with lymphocytes to produce specific antibodies. These hybrid cells are called hybridoma, and they produce monoclonal antibodies.

One molecular biologist who needed pure antibodies for a study of myeloma **mutations** was the Argentinean **César Milstein** (1927–). After receiving a doctorate in **biochemistry**, specializing in **enzymes**, from the University of Buenos Aires in 1957, he continued this study at the University of Cambridge in England. There he worked under the biochemist Frederick Sanger and earned another doctorate in 1961. Milstein had returned to Argentina, but political disturbances forced him to flee the country. He came back to Cambridge, where Sanger suggested that he work with antibodies.

In 1974, Milstein was working with **Georges Köhler** (1946–1995), a German postdoctoral student who had just received his doctorate from the University of Freiburg for work performed at the Institute for **Immunology** in Basel, Switzerland. To produce the needed antibodies, Milstein and Köhler first injected a mouse with a known **antigen**. After extracting the resulting lymphocytes from the mouse's blood, they fused one of them with a myeloma cell. The resulting hybrid produced the lymphocyte's specific antibody and reproduced endlessly. As Milstein soon realized, their tech-

nique for producing monoclonal antibodies could be used in many capacities. Milstein and Köhler shared part of the 1984 Nobel prize in physiology or medicine for their invention.

Today pure antibodies are made using the Milstein-Köhler technique and also through genetic engineering, which adds the **gene** for the desired antibody to bacteria that can produce it in large amounts. Monoclonal antibodies are instrumental in the performance of sensitive medical diagnostic tests such as: determining pregnancy with chorionic gonadotropin; determining the amino acid content of substances; classifying antigens; purifying hormones; and modifying infectious or toxic substances in the body. They are also important in cancer treatment because they can be tagged with radioisotopes to make images of tumors.

See also Antibody-antigen, biochemical and molecular reactions; Antibody and antigen; Immunity, cell mediated; Immunogenetics; Immunologic therapies; Immunological analysis techniques; *In vitro* and *in vivo* research

ANTIGEN · *see* ANTIBODY AND ANTIGEN

ANTIGENIC MIMICRY

Antigenic mimicry is the sharing of antigenic sites between **microorganisms** and mammalian tissue. An immune response can be directed both at the microorganism and at the host site that shares the antigenic determinant. This autoimmune response due to antigenic mimicry is known to be a crucial factor in the development of certain ailments in humans.

The **immune system** recognizes three-dimensional structure of protein. A protein, which is made up of a sequence of amino acids strung together, will fold up in various ways, depending on whether a section is more hydrophilic ("water loving") or **hydrophobic** ("water hating"), and depending on the function of various regions of the protein.

Proteins that adopt a similar three-dimensional configuration can stimulate a common response from the immune system. Typically, proteins that have a similar amino acid sequence will adopt the similar folded structures. For example, the **bacteria** *Chlamydia pneumoniae*, *Chlamydia psittaci*, and *Chlamydia trachomatis* possess a protein that is part of the bacterial outer membrane. This protein is similar in amino acid sequence to a portion of a protein, called alpha-myosin heavy chain, which is found specifically in the heart muscle of humans and animals such as mice. In mice, an immune reaction to Chlamydia triggers a condition known as inflammatory heart disease. A continued host autoimmune response damages the heart, leading to cardiac malfunction. Indeed, it has been shown that a significant number of patients with heart disease have antibodies to Chlamydia in their blood, indicative of a past infection with the bacteria.

Rheumatoid arthritis is another example of a malady that is the consequence of an autoimmune reaction.

The Chlamydia studies have pointed out the widespread nature of antigenic mimicry. Other bacteria, **viruses**, **fungi** and **protozoa** share the antigenic similarity with the mouse antigenic region. The bacteria include *Borrelia burgdorferi* (the agent of **Lyme disease**), *Treponema pallidum* (the causative agent of **syphilis**), and *Mycoplasma pneumoniae* (the cause of non-viral atypical **pneumonia**).

Antigenic mimicry may also be the basis of the ulcers formed upon infection of humans with *Helicobacter pylori*. The acidic environment of the stomach would exacerbate host tissue damage due to an autoimmune response.

Antigenic mimicry supports a hypothesis known as the "infection hypothesis," which proposes that common human diseases are caused by infections. If so, then treatment for heart disease and stomach ulcers would involve strategies to eliminate bacterial infections.

See also Bacteria and bacterial infection; Immunit: active, passive, and delayed

ANTISEPTICS

Antiseptics are compounds that act to counteract sepsis, which is an illness caused by a **bacterial infection** of the blood. Antiseptics are able to counteract sepsis by preventing the growth of pathogenic (disease causing) **microorganisms**. An antiseptic may kill a microorganism, but it does not necessarily have to. The treated microbes may only be weakened. The weaker, slower growing microbes may then be more susceptible to the defense mechanisms of the host.

The terms antiseptic and disinfectant are used almost interchangeably nowadays. Yet they do have different meanings. An antiseptic is a chemical or technique that is used on people. A disinfectant is a chemical that is applied to an inanimate object or surface to get rid of microorganisms. An antiseptic generally does not have the same potency as a disinfectant. Otherwise, the chemical would harm the tissues it is in contact with. For this reason, an antiseptic should not be used to treat inanimate objects. Likewise, the generally more toxic disinfectant should not be used to treat skin or areas such as the mucous membranes of the nose.

While more is known of the molecular basis of antiseptic actions, the use of antimicrobial compounds is ancient. For example, the black eye make-up known as kohl, which was used by the ancient Arabs and Egyptians, is a mixture of copper and antimony. These compounds are antiseptic. Indeed, the modern cure for trachoma (blindness caused by infection of the eyes by the bacterium *Chlamydia trachomatis*) is remarkably similar in composition to kohl.

There are a number of antiseptics and antiseptic procedures.

In a health care setting, powerful antiseptics are used to ensure that the skin is essentially sterile prior to an operation. Examples of such antiseptics include chlorhexidine and iodophors (iodine-containing compounds). Alcohol is an antiseptic, which is routinely used to swab the skin prior to an injection. Alcohol acts to coagulate the protein in **bacteria**.

The irreversible change in the protein is lethal to the bacteria. In the example of the injection, alcohol swabbing of the injection site will kill the bacteria on the skin, so that living bacteria are not carried into the body upon insertion of the needle. Dilution of alcohol, so that a solution is 30% alcohol by volume, makes this antiseptic even more potent, as it allows the alcohol to permeate into the bacteria. Pure alcohol rapidly coagulates surface proteins, producing a coagulated crust around the bacteria.

Another antiseptic is carbolic acid. This is also known as phenol. The coal tar-based product was discovered in 1834. Originally phenol was poured down sewers to kill microorganisms. Over time, its use expanded. In 1863, the British surgeon **Joseph Lister** began using a spray of phenol to disinfect open wounds during surgery. Prior to his innovation, such surgery was only performed when all other avenues of treatment had failed, since the risk of death from infection was extremely high.

Still another antiseptic compound is pine oil. It is added to household disinfectants more because of its pleasant smell than its aseptic power nowadays. In fact, it inclusion actually weakens the bacteria-killing power of the household disinfectant.

Lister's method was supplanted by the adoption of extreme cleanliness in the operating room, such as the use of sterile masks, gloves and gowns, in order to keep the surgical area free of microorganisms. This approach is known as antiseptic surgery. As strange as it may seem now, surgeons in Lister's era often did not change or clean their operating garb between operations. A surgeon would often commence an operation wearing a gown covered with the blood and germs of many previous operations. Prior to the introduction of antisepsis in the operating room, the rate of death following surgery was almost 60%. After the introduction of antisepsis, the recorded death rate in England dropped to four per cent.

Hand washing has also become standard practice in the hospital and the home.

Another antiseptic technique is **sterilization**. The use of steam at higher than atmospheric pressure is an effective means of killing many types of bacteria, including those that form spores.

In the home, antiseptics are often evident as lotions or solutions that are applied to a cut or scrape to prevent infection. For these uses, it is necessary to clean the affected area of skin first to dislodge any dirt or other material that could reduce the effectiveness of the antiseptic. Antiseptics, particularly those used in the home, are designed for a short-term use to temporarily rid the skin of microbes. The skin, being in primary contact with the environment, will quickly become recolonized with microorganisms. Long-term use of antiseptics encourages the development of populations of microorganisms that are resistant to the antiseptic. Additionally, the skin can become irritated by the long exposure to the harsh chemical. Some people can even develop **allergies** to the antiseptic.

Another hazard of antiseptics that has only become apparent since the 1990s is the **contamination** of the environment. Antiseptic solutions that are disposed of in sinks and toilets can make their way to rivers and lakes. Contamination of the aquifer (the surface or underground reserve of water from which drinking water is obtained) has become a real possibility.

See also Antibiotics; Infection control

ANTISERUM AND ANTITOXIN

Both antisera and antitoxins are means of proactively combating infections. The introduction of compounds to which the **immune system** responds is an attempt to build up protection against **microorganisms** or their toxins before the microbes actually invade the body.

The use of antiserum and antitoxin preparations is now a standard avenue of **infection control**. The beginnings of the strategies dates to the time of **Edward Jenner** in the late eighteenth century. Then, Jenner used an inoculum of **cowpox** material to elicit protection against the **smallpox** virus.

Jenner's strategy of using a live organism to elicit an **antibody** response led to a "third-party" strategy, whereby serum is obtained from an animal that has been exposed to an **antigen** or to the microorganism that contains the antigen. This so-called antiserum is injected into the human to introduce the protective antibodies directly, rather than having them manufactured by the person's own immune system.

The same strategy produces antitoxin. In this case, the material injected into the animal would consist of active toxin, but in very low quantities. The intent of the latter is to stimulate antibody production against a toxin that has not been changed by the procedures used to inactivate toxin activity.

The use of antitoxin has been largely supplanted by the injection of a crippled form of the toxin of interest (also known as a toxoid) or a particularly vital fragment of the toxin that is needed for toxic activity. The risk of the use of a toxoid or a fragment of toxin is that the antibody that is produced is sufficiently different from that produced against the real target so as to be ineffective in a person.

Since the time of Jenner, a myriad of antisera and antitoxins have been produced against bacterial, viral and protozoan diseases. The results of their use can be dramatic. For example, even in the 1930s, the form of **influenza** caused by the bacterium *Hemophilus influenzae* was almost always lethal to infants and children. Then, Elizabeth Hattie, a pediatrician and microbiologist, introduced an anti-influenzal antiserum produced in rabbits. The use of this antiserum reduced *Hemophilus influenzae* influenza-related mortality to less than twenty per cent.

Antiserum can contain just one type of antibody, which is targeted at a single antigen. This is known as monovalent antiserum. Or, the antiserum can contain multiple antibodies, which are directed at different antibody targets. This is known as polyvalent antiserum.

The indirect protective effect of antiserum and antitoxin is passive **immunity**. That is, a protective response is produced in someone who has not been immunized by direct exposure to the organism. Passive immunity provides immediate but temporary protection.

Antiserum and antitoxin are obtained from the blood of the test animal. The blood is obtained at a pre-determined time following the injection of the antigen, microorganism, or toxoid. The antiserum constitutes part of the plasma, the clear component of the blood that is obtained when the heavier blood cells are separated by spinning the blood in a machine called a centrifuge.

Examples of antisera are those against **tetanus** and **rabies**. Typically, these antisera are administered if someone has been exposed to an environment or, in the case of rabies, an animal, which makes the threat of acquiring the disease real. The antisera can boost the chances of successfully combating the infectious organism. After the threat of disease is gone, the protective effect is no longer required.

The advent of **antibiotics** has largely replaced some types of antiserum. This has been a positive development, for antiserum can cause allergic reactions that in some people are fatal. The allergic nature of antiserum, which is also known as serum shock, arises from the nature of its origin. Because it is derived from an animal, there may be components of the animal present in the antiserum. When introduced into a human, the animal proteins are themselves foreign, and so will produce an immune response. For this reason antiserum is used cautiously today, as in the above examples. The risk of the use of antiserum or antitoxin is more than compensated for by the risk of acquiring a life-threatening malady if treatment is not undertaken.

Serum sickness is a hypersensitive immune reaction to a contaminating animal protein in the antiserum. The antibodies that are produced bind to the antigen to make larger particles called immune complexes. The complexes can become deposited in various tissues, causing a variety of symptoms. The symptoms typically do not appear for a few weeks after the antiserum or antitoxin has been administered.

With the development of sophisticated techniques to examine the genetic material of microorganisms and identify genes that are responsible for the aspects of disease, the use of antiserum and antitoxin may enter a new phase of use. For example, the genetic sequences that are responsible for the protein toxins of the **anthrax** bacterium are now known. From these sequences the proteins they encode can be manufactured in pure quantities. These pure proteins can then form the basis of an antitoxin. The antibodies produced in animals can be obtained in very pure form as well, free of contaminating animal proteins. These antibodies will block the binding of the toxin to host tissue, which blocks the toxic effect. In this and other cases, such as an antitoxin being developed to *Escherichia coli O157:H7*, the use of antitoxin is superior strategy to the use of antibiotics. Antibiotics are capable of killing the anthrax bacterium. They have no effect, however, on action of the toxin that is released by the **bacteria**.

See also Anti-adhesion methods; Antiviral drugs; *E. coli O157:H7* infection; *Escharichia coli*; Immune stimulation, as a vaccine; Immunization

ANTIVIRAL DRUGS

Antiviral drugs are compounds that are used to prevent or treat viral infections, via the disruption of an infectious mechanism used by the virus, or to treat the symptoms of an infection.

Different types of antiviral drugs have different modes of operation. For example, acyclovir is a drug that is used to treat the symptoms of the infections arising from the herpes virus family. Such infection includes lesions on the genitals, oral region, or in the brain. Acyclovir is also an antiviral agent in the treatment of chickenpox in children and adults, and shingles in adults caused by the reactivation of the chickenpox virus after a period of latency. Shingles symptoms can also be treated by the administration of valacyclovir and famciclovir.

Eye infections caused by cytomegalovirus can be treated with the antiviral agent known as ganciclovir. The drug acts to lessen the further development and discomfort of the eye irritation. But, the drug may be used as a preventative agent in those people whose **immune system** will be compromised by the use of an immunosupressant.

Another category of antiviral drugs is known as the anti-retroviral drugs. These drugs target those **viruses** of clinical significance called **retroviruses** that use the mechanism of reverse **transcription** to manufacture the genetic material needed for their replication. The prime example of a retrovirus is the **Human immunodeficiency virus (HIV)**, which is the viral agent of acquired **immunodeficiency** syndrome (**AIDS**). The development of antiviral drugs has been stimulated by the efforts to combat HIV. Some anti-HIV drugs have shown promise against **hepatitis** B virus, **herpes** simplex virus, and varicella-zoster virus.

The various antiviral agents are designed to thwart the replication of whatever virus they are directed against. One means to achieve this is by blocking the virus from commandeering the host cell's nuclear replication machinery in order to have its genetic material replicated along with the host's genetic material. The virus is not killed directly. But the prevention of replication will prevent the numbers of viruses from increasing, giving the host's immune system time to deal with the stranded viruses.

The incorporation of the nucleotide building blocks into **deoxyribonucleic acid** (**DNA**) can be blocked using the drug idoxuridine or trifluridine. Both drugs replace the nucleoside thymidine, and its incorporation produces a nonfunctional DNA. However, the same thing happens to the host DNA. So, this antiviral drug is also an anti-host drug. Vidarabine is another drug that acts in a similar fashion. The drug is incorporated into DNA in place of adenine. Other drugs that mimic other DNA building blocks.

Blockage of the viral replicative pathway by mimicking nucleosides can be successful. But, because the virus utilizes the host's genetic machinery, stopping the viral replication usually affects the host cell.

Another tact for antiviral drugs is to block a viral enzyme whose activity is crucial for replication of the viral genetic material. This approach has been successfully exploited by the drug acyclovir. The drug is converted in the host cell to a compound that can out compete another compound for the binding of the viral enzyme, DNA polymerase, which is responsible for building DNA. The incorporation of the acyclovir derivative exclusively into the viral DNA stops the formation of the DNA. Acyclovir has success against herpes simplex viruses, and **Epstein-Barr virus**. Another drug that acts in a similar fashion is famciclovir.

Other antiviral drugs are directed at the **translation** process, whereby the information from the viral genome that has been made into a template is read to produce the protein product. For example, the drug ribavirin inhibits the formation of messenger **ribonucleic acid**.

Still other antiviral drugs are directed at earlier steps in the viral replication pathway. Amantadine and rimantadine block the **influenza** A virus from penetrating into the host cell and releasing the nuclear material.

Antiviral therapy also includes molecular approaches. The best example is the use of oligonucleotides. These are sequences of nucleotides that are specifically synthesized to be complimentary with a target sequence of viral ribonucleic acid. By binding to the viral **RNA**, the oligonucleotide blocks the RNA from being used as a template to manufacture protein.

The use of antiviral drugs is not without risk. Host cell damage and other adverse host reactions can occur. Thus, the use of antiviral drugs is routinely accompanied by close clinical observation.

See also Immunodeficiency diseases; Viruses and responses to viral infection

APPERT, NICOLAS FRANÇOIS (1750-1841)
French chef

Nicolas Appert gave rise to the food canning industry. Born in Châlons-sur-Marne, France, around 1750, young Appert worked at his father's inn and for a noble family as a chef and wine steward. By 1780 he had set up a confectionery shop in Paris, France.

Appert became interested in **food preservation** when the French government offered a 12,000-franc prize in 1795 to the person who could find a way to keep provisions for Napoleon's armies from spoiling in transit and storage. After years of experimentation Appert devised a method of putting food in glass bottles that were then loosely corked and immersed in boiling water for lengths of time that varied with the particular food; after boiling, the corks were sealed down tightly with wire. In an age before bacteriology, Appert did not comprehend the fact that the heat destroyed **microorganisms** in the food, but he could see that his method—which became known as appertization—preserved the food. Appert later set up his first bottling plant at Massy, south of Paris, in 1804.

The French navy successfully used Appert's products in 1807, and in 1809 Appert was awarded the 12,000-franc prize. A condition of the award was that Appert make public his discovery, which he did in his 1810 work *The Art of Preserving Animal and Vegetable Substances for Several Years,* which gave specific directions for canning over fifty different foods.

This volume spread knowledge about canning around the world and launched what would become a vast industry.

In 1812 Appert used his prize money to make his Massy plant into the world's first commercial cannery, which remained in operation until 1933. Appert, who also invented the bouillon cube, was financially ruined in 1814 when his plant was destroyed during the Napoleonic wars. He died in poverty in 1841.

See also Food preservation; Food safety

ARCHAEA

Genes that code for vital cellular functions are highly conserved through evolutionary time, and because even these genes experience random changes over time, the comparison of such genes allows the relatedness of different organisms to be assessed. American microbiologist Carl Woese and his colleagues obtained sequences of the genes coding for **RNA** in the subunit of the ribosome from different organisms to argue that life on Earth is comprised of three primary groups, or domains. These domains are the Eukarya (which include humans), **Bacteria**, and Archaea.

While Archae are **microorganisms**, they are no more related to bacteria than to **eukaryotes**. They share some traits with bacteria, such as having a single, circular molecule of **DNA**, the presence of more mobile pieces of genetic material called **plasmids**, similar **enzymes** for producing copies of DNA. However, their method of protein production and organization of their genetic material bears more similarity to eukaryotic cells.

The three domains are thought to have diverged from one another from an extinct or as yet undiscovered ancestral line. The archae and eukarya may have branched off from a common ancestral line more recently than the divergence of these two groups from bacteria. However, this view remains controversial and provisional.

The domain Archae includes a relatively small number of microooganisms. They inhabit environments which are too harsh for other microbes. Such environments include hot, molten vents at the bottom of the ocean, the highly salt water of the Great Salt Lake and the Dead Sea, and in the hot sulfurous springs of Yellowstone National Park. Very recently, it has been shown that two specific archael groups, pelagic euryarchaeota and pelagic crenarchaeota are one of the ocean's dominant cell types. Their dominance suggests that they have a fundamentally important function in that ecosystem.

See also Bacterial kingdoms; Evolution and evolutionary mechanisms; Evolutionary origin of bacteria and viruses

ARENAVIRUS

Arenavirus is a virus that belongs in a viral family known as Arenaviridae. The name arenavirus derives from the appearance of the spherical virus particles when cut into thin sections

and viewed using the transmission **electron microscope**. The interior of the particles is grainy or sandy in appearance, due to the presence of **ribosomes** that have been acquired from the host cell. The Latin designation "arena" means "sandy."

Arenaviruses contain **ribonucleic acid** (**RNA**) as their genetic material. The viral genome consists of two strands of RNA, which are designated the L and S RNA. The ribosomes of the host that are typically present inside the virus particle are used in the manufacture of the components that will be assembled to produce the new virus particles. Little is known about the actual replication of new viral components or about the assembly of these components to produce the new virus particles. It is known that the new virus exits the host by "budding" off from the surface of the host cell. When the budding occurs some of the lipid constituent from the membrane of the host forms the envelope that surrounds the virus.

Those arenaviruses that are of concern to human health are typically transmitted to humans from rats and mice. The only known exception is an arenavirus called the Tacaribe virus, which is resident in *Artibeus* bats. The association between an arenavirus type and a particular species of rodent is specific. Thus, a certain arenavirus will associate with only one species of mouse or rat. There are 15 arenaviruses that are known to infect animals. A hallmark of arenaviruses is that the infections in these rodent hosts tend not to adversely affect the rodent.

Of the fifteen **viruses** that are resident in the animals, five of these viruses are capable of being transmitted to humans. When transmitted to humans, these arenaviruses can cause illness. In contrast to the rodent hosts, the human illness can be compromising.

Most arenavirus infections produce relatively mild symptoms that are reminiscent of the flu, or produce no symptoms whatsoever. For example an arenavirus designated lymphocytic choriomeningitis virus, usually produces symptoms that are mild and are often mistaken for gastrointestinal upset. However, some infections with the same virus produce a severe illness that characterized by an **inflammation** of the sheath that surrounds nerve cells (**meningitis**). The reasons for the different outcomes of an infection with the virus is yet to be resolved.

A number of other arenaviruses are also of clinical concern to humans. These viruses include the Lassa virus (the cause of Lassa fever), Junin virus (the cause of Argentine hemorrhagic fever), Machupo virus (the cause of Bolivian hemorrhagic fever), and Guanarito virus (the cause of Venezuelan hemorrhagic fever). **Hemorrhagic fevers** are characterized by copious bleeding, particularly of internal organs. The death rate in an outbreak of these hemorrhagic fevers can be extremely high.

An arenavirus is transmitted to a human via the urine or feces of the infected rodent. The urine or feces may contaminate food or water, may accidentally contact a cut on the skin, or the virus may be inhaled from dried feces. In addition, some arenaviruses can also be transmitted from one infected person to another person. Examples of such viruses are the Lassa virus and the Machupo virus. Person-to-person transmission can involve direct contact or contact of an infected person with food implements or medical equipment, as examples.

As with other hemorrhagic fevers, treatment consists of stabilizing the patient. A **vaccine** for the Junin virus, which consists of living but weakened virus, has been developed and has been tested in a small cohort of volunteers. The results of these tests have been encouraging. Another vaccine, to the Lassa virus, consists of a protein component of the viral envelope. Tests of this vaccine in primates have also been encouraging to researchers.

Currently, the human illnesses caused by arenaviruses are best dealt with by the implementation of a rodent control program in those regions that are known to be sites of outbreaks of arenavirus illness. Because the elimination of rodents in the wild is virtually impossible, such a program is best directed at keeping the immediate vicinity of dwellings clean and rodent-free.

See also Hemorrhagic fevers and diseases; Virology, viral classification, types of viruses; Zoonoses

ARMILLARIA OSTOYAE

Armillaria ostoyae is a fungus, and is also known as the honey mushroom. The species is particularly noteworthy because of one fungus in the eastern woods of Oregon that is so far the biggest organism in the world.

Armillaria ostoyae grows from a spore by extending filaments called rhizomorphs into the surrounding soil. The rhizomorphs allow access to nutrients. The bulk of the fungus is comprised of these mycelial filaments. The filaments can also be called **hyphae**. The fungal hyphae can consist of cells each containing a **nucleus**, which are walled off from one another. Or, the cells may not be walled off, and a filament is essentially a long cell with multiple nuclei dispersed throughout its length.

For the giant fungus, using an average growth rate of the species as a gauge, scientists have estimated that the specimen in the Malheur National Forest in Oregon has been growing for some 2400 years. The growth now covers 2200 acres, an area equivalent to 1665 football fields.

Analysis of the genetic material obtained from different regions of the fungal growth has shown the **DNA** to be identical, demonstrating that the growth is indeed from the same fungus. The weight of the gigantic fungus has not been estimated.

As the giant fungus has grown the rhizomorph growth has penetrated into the interior of the tree. The fungus than draws off nutrients, suffocating the tree. As well, the mycelia can extend as deep as 10 feet into the soil, and can invade the roots of trees. When viewed from the air, the pattern of dead trees looks remarkably like a mushroom. The outline of the fungal boundary is 3.5 miles in diameter.

Scientists are studying the fungus because of the tree-killing ability it displays. Understanding more of the nature of this effect could lead to the use of the fungus to control tree growth.

The bulk of the gigantic fungus is some three feet underground. The only surface evidence of the fungus are periodic displays of golden mushrooms that are present in rainy times of the year.

Although not as well studied as the Oregon giant, another *Armillaria ostoyae* found in Washington state is even larger. Estimates put the area covered by the Washington state fungus at over 11000 acres.

See also Fungi

ASEXUAL GENERATION AND REPRODUCTION

Sexual reproduction involves the production of new cells by the fusion of sex cells (sperm and ova) to produce a genetically different cell. Asexual reproduction, on the other hand, is the production of new cells by simple division of the parent cell into two daughter cells (called binary fission). Because there is no fusion of two different cells, the daughter cells produced by asexual reproduction are genetically identical to the parent cell. The adaptive advantage of asexual reproduction is that organisms can reproduce rapidly, thus enabling the quick colonization of favorable environments.

Duplication of organisms, whether sexually or asexually, involves the partitioning of the genetic material (**chromosomes**) in the cell **nucleus**. During asexual reproduction, the chromosomes divide by mitosis, which results in the exact duplication of the genetic material into the nuclei of the two daughter cells. Sexual reproduction involves the fusion of two gamete cells (the sperm and ova), each of which has half the normal number of chromosomes, a result of reduction division known as meiosis.

Bacteria, cyanobacteria, algae, **protozoa**, **yeast**, dandelions, and flatworms all reproduce asexually. When asexual reproduction occurs, the new individuals are called clones, because they are exact duplicates of their parent cells. Mosses reproduce by forming runners that grow horizontally, produce new stalks, then decompose, leaving a new plant that is a clone of the original.

Bacteria reproducing asexually double their numbers rapidly, approximately every 20 minutes. This reproduction rate is offset by a high death rate that may be the result of the accumulation of alcohol or acids that concentrate from the bacterial colonies.

Yeasts reproduce asexually by budding; they can also reproduce sexually. In the budding process a bulge forms on the outer edge of the yeast cell as nuclear division takes place. One of these nuclei moves into the bud, which eventually breaks off completely from the parent cell. Budding also occurs in flatworms, which divide into two and then regenerate to form two new flatworms.

Bees, ants, wasps, and other insects can reproduce sexually or asexually. In asexual reproduction, eggs develop without fertilization, a process called parthenogenesis. In some

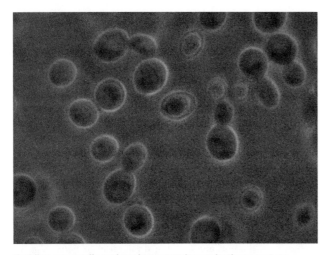

Budding yeast cells undergoing asexual reproduction; yeast are single-celled fungi.

species the eggs may or may not be fertilized; fertilized eggs produce females, while unfertilized eggs produce males.

There are a number of crop plants that are propagated asexually. The advantage of asexual propagation to farmers is that the crops will be more uniform than those produced from seed. Some plants are difficult to cultivate from seed and asexual reproduction in these plants makes it possible to produce crops that would otherwise not be available for commercial marketing. The process of producing plants asexually is called vegetative propagation and is used for such crops as potatoes, bananas, raspberries, pineapples, and some flowering plants used as ornamentals. Farmers plant the so-called "eyes" of potatoes to produce duplicates of the parent. With banana plants, the suckers that grow from the root of the plant are separated and then planted as new ones. With raspberry bushes, branches are bent and covered with soil. They then grow into a separate plant with their own root system and can eventually be detached from the parent plant.

See also Cell cycle and cell division

ASILOMAR CONFERENCE

Soon after American microbiologist Hamilton Smith's 1970 discovery of the first restriction enzyme, it became possible to combine **DNA** from different sources into one molecule, producing recombinant DNA. Concern by scientists and lay people that some of this recombinant-technology DNA might be harmful to humans prompted the research to stop until scientists could evaluate its risks.

In February 1975 over 100 internationally respected molecular biologists met at the Asilomar conference center in California. There they decided upon a set of guidelines to be followed by all scientists doing recombinant DNA research. They considered every class of experiment and assigned each a level of risk: minimal, low, moderate, or high. Each level of risk required a corresponding set of containment procedures

designed to minimize the chance of vectors (carriers) containing recombinant DNA molecules from escaping into the environment, where they could potentially harm humans or other parts of the ecosystem. Because these projected experiments had never been done, assignment to a risk category was, of course, somewhat speculative and subjective. Accordingly, the potential risks were arrived at by estimate.

At all risk levels, the guidelines called for the use of biological barriers. Bacterial host cells should be from strains unable to survive in natural environments (outside the test tube). Vectors carrying recombinant DNA, including **plasmids**, bacteriophages, and other **viruses**, were to be nontransmissible and unable to survive in natural environments.

For experiments having minimal risk, the guidelines recommended that scientists follow general microbiology safety procedures. These included not eating, drinking, or smoking in the lab; wearing laboratory coats in the work area; and promptly disinfecting contaminated materials.

Low-risk procedures required a bit more caution. For example, procedures producing aerosols, such as using a blender, were to be performed under an enclosed ventilation hood to eliminate the risk of the recombinant DNA being liberated into the air.

Moderate-risk experiments required the use of a laminar flow hood, the wearing of gloves, and the maintenance of negative air pressure in the laboratory. This would ensure that air currents did not carry recombinant DNA out of the laboratory.

Finally, in high-risk experiments, maximum precautions were specified. These included isolation of the laboratory from other areas by air locks, having researchers shower and change their clothing upon leaving the work area, and the incineration of exhaust air from the hoods.

Certain types of experiments were not to be done at all. These most potentially dangerous experiments included the **cloning** of recombinant DNA from highly pathogenic organisms or DNA containing toxin genes. Also forbidden were experiments involving the production of more than 10 liters of **culture** using recombinant DNA molecules that might render the products potentially harmful to humans, animals, or plants.

The scientists at the Asilomar conference also resolved to meet annually to re-evaluate the guidelines. As new procedures were developed and safer vectors and bacterial cells became available, it became possible to re-evaluate and relax some of the initially stringent and restrictive safety standards.

See also Recombination; Viral genetics; Viral vectors in gene therapy

ATOMIC FORCE MICROSCOPE

In 1985, the development of the atomic force **microscope** (AFM) allowed scientists to visualize the surface of cellular structures during some physiological processes. Along with the use of field ion microscopes and powerful scanning tunneling microscopes (STM), these advances in microscopy represent the most fundamental greatest advances since the development of the **electron microscope**.

Invented by Gerd Binnig and Christoph Gerber in Zurich, Switzerland, and Calvin Quate (1923–) in California, the AFM uses a tiny needle made of diamond, tungsten, or silicon, much like those used in the STM. While the STM relies upon a subject's ability to conduct electricity through its needle, the AFM scans its subjects by actually lightly touching them with the needle. Like that of a phonograph record, the AFM's needle reads the bumps on the subject's surface, rising as it hits the peaks and dipping as it traces the valleys. Of course, the topography read by the AFM varies by only a few molecules up or down, so a very sensitive device must be used to detect the needle's rising and falling. In the original model, Binnig and Gerber used an STM to sense these movements. Other AFM's later used a fine-tuned laser. The AFM has already been used to study the super-microscopic structures of living cells and other objects that could not be viewed with the STM.

American physicist Paul Hansma (1946–) and his colleagues at the University of California, Santa Barbara, conduct various studies using AFM research. In 1989, this team succeeded in observing the blood-clotting process within blood cells. Hansma's team presented their findings in a 33–minute movie, assembled from AFM pictures taken every ten seconds. Other scientists are utilizing the AFM's ability to remove samples of cells without harming the cell structure. By adding a bit more force to the scanning needle, the AFM can scrape cells, making it the world's most delicate dissecting tool.

Scientists continue to apply this method to the study of living cells, particularly fragile structures on the cell surface, whose fragility makes them nearly impossible to view without distortion.

See also Bacterial membranes and cell wall; Bacterial surface layers; Bacterial ultrastructure; Microscope and microscopy

ATTENUATION • *see* VACCINE

ATTRACTANTS AND REPELLENTS

Attractants and repellents are compounds that stimulate the directed movement of **microorganisms**, in particular **bacteria**, towards or away from the compound. The directed movement in response to the presence of the attractant or repellent compound is a feature of a bacterial behavior known as chemotaxis.

Various compounds can act as attractants. Overwhelmingly, these are nutrients for the bacterium. Attractant compounds include sugars, such as maltose, ribose, galactose, and amino acids such as L-aspartate and L-serine.

Similarly, various compounds will cause a bacterium to move away. Examples of repellents include metals that are damaging or lethal to a bacterium (e.g., cobalt, nickel), membrane-disruptive compounds such as indole, and weak acids, which can damage the integrity of the cell wall.

The presence and influence of attractants and repellents on the movement of bacteria has been known for over a century. In the 1880s experiments demonstrated that bacteria

would move into capillary tubes filled with meat extract and away from capillaries filled with acids.

Now, the molecular underpinning for this behavior is better understood. The chemotaxis process has been particularly well-studied in the related Gram-negative bacteria *Escherichia coli* and *Salmonella* typhimurium.

These bacteria are capable of self-propelled movement, by virtue of whip-like structures called flagella. Movement consists typically of a random tumbling interspersed with a brief spurt of directed movement. During the latter the bacterium senses the environment for the presence of attractants or repellents. If an attractant is sensed, the bacterium will respond by exhibiting more of the directed movement, and the movement will over time be in the direction of the attractant. If the bacterium senses a repellent, then the periods of directed movement will move the bacterium away from the compound. Both of these phenomena require mechanisms in the bacterium that can sense the presence of the compounds and can compare the concentrations of the compounds over time.

The detection of attractants and repellents is accomplished by proteins that are part of the cytoplasmic, or inner, membrane of bacteria such as *Escherichia coli* and *Salmonella typhymurium*. For example, there are four proteins that span the inner membrane, from the side that contacts the **cytoplasm** to the side that contacts the periplasmic space. These proteins are collectively called the methyl-accepting chemotaxis proteins (MCPs). The MCPs can bind different attractant and repellent compounds to different regions on their surface. For example, on of the MCPs can bind the attractants aspartate and maltose and the repellents cobalt and nickel.

The binding of an incoming attractant or repellent molecule to a MCP causes the addition or removal of a phosphate group to another molecule that is linked to the MCP on the cytoplasm side. Both events generate a signal that is transmitted to other bacterial mechanisms by what is known as a cascade. One of the results of the cascade is the control of the rotation of the flagella, so as to propel the bacterium forward or to generate the random tumbling motion.

The cascade process is exceedingly complex, with at least 50 proteins known to be involved. The proteins are also involved in other sensory events, such as to **pH**, temperature, and other environmental stresses.

The memory of a bacterium for the presence of an attractant or repellent is governed by the reversible nature of the binding of the compounds to the bacterial sensor proteins. The binding of an attractant or a repellent is only for a short time. If the particular compound is abundant in the environment, another molecule of the attractant or repellent will bind very soon after the detachment of the first attractant or repellent from the sensor. However, if the concentration of the attractant or repellent is decreasing, then the period between when the sensor-binding site becomes unoccupied until the binding of the next molecule will increase. Thus, the bacterium will have a gauge as to whether its movement is carrying the cell towards or away from the detected compound. Then, depending on whether the compound is desirable or not, corrections in the movement of the bacterium can be made.

See also Bacterial movement; Heat shock response

AUTOCLAVE • *see* STEAM PRESSURE STERILIZER

AUTOIMMUNITY AND AUTOIMMUNE DISORDERS

Autoimmune diseases are conditions in which a person's **immune system** attacks the body's own cells, causing tissue destruction. Autoimmune diseases are classified as either general, in which the autoimmune reaction takes place simultaneously in a number of tissues, or organ specific, in which the autoimmune reaction targets a single organ. Autoimmunity is accepted as the cause of a wide range of disorders, and is suspected to be responsible for many more. Among the most common diseases attributed to autoimmune disorders are rheumatoid arthritis, systemic lupus erythematosis (lupus), multiple sclerosis, myasthenia gravis, pernicious anemia, and scleroderma.

To further understand autoimmune disorders, it is helpful to understand the workings of the immune system. The purpose of the immune system is to defend the body against attack by infectious microbes (germs) and foreign objects. When the immune system attacks an invader, it is very specific—a particular immune system cell will only recognize and target one type of invader. To function properly, the immune system must not only develop this specialized knowledge of individual invaders, but it must also learn how to recognize and not destroy cells that belong to the body itself. Every cell carries protein markers on its surface that identifies it in one of two ways: what kind of cell it is (e.g., nerve cell, muscle cell, blood cell, etc.) and to whom that cell belongs. These markers are called **major histocompatibility complexes (MHCs)**. When functioning properly, cells of the immune system will not attack any other cell with markers identifying it as belonging to the body. Conversely, if the immune system cells do not recognize the cell as "self," they attach themselves to it and put out a signal that the body has been invaded, which in turn stimulates the production of substances such as antibodies that engulf and destroy the foreign particles. In case of autoimmune disorders, the immune system cannot distinguish between self cells and invader cells. As a result, the same destructive operation is carried out on the body's own cells that would normally be carried out on **bacteria**, **viruses**, and other such harmful entities.

The reason why the immune system become dysfunctional is not well understood. Most researchers agree that a combination of genetic, environmental, and hormonal factors play into autoimmunity. The fact that autoimmune diseases run in families suggests a genetic component. Recent studies have identified an antiphospholipid **antibody** (APL) that is believed to be a common thread among family members with autoimmune diseases. Among study participants, family members with elevated APL levels showed autoimmune disease, while those with other autoantibodies did not. Family members with elevated APL levels also manifested different forms of autoimmune disease, suggesting that APL may serve as a common trigger for different autoimmune diseases. Further study of the genetic patterns among unrelated family groups with APL suggests that a single genetic defect resulting in APL production may be responsible for several different autoimmune diseases. Current research focuses on finding an established APL inheritance pattern, as well as finding the autoimmune **gene** responsible for APL production.

A number of tests can help diagnose autoimmune diseases; however the principle tool used by physicians is antibody testing. Such tests involve measuring the level of antibodies found in the blood and determining if they react with specific antigens that would give rise to an autoimmune reaction. An elevated amount of antibodies indicates that a humoral immune reaction is occurring. Elevated antibody levels are also seen in common infections. These must be ruled out as the cause for the increased antibody levels. The antibodies can also be typed by class. There are five classes of antibodies and they can be separated in the laboratory. The class IgG is usually associated with autoimmune diseases. Unfortunately, IgG class antibodies are also the main class of antibody seen in normal immune responses. The most useful antibody tests involve introducing the patient's antibodies to samples of his or her own tissue—if antibodies bind to the tissue it is diagnostic for an autoimmune disorder. Antibodies from a person without an autoimmune disorder would not react to self tissue. The tissues used most frequently in this type of testing are thyroid, stomach, liver, and kidney.

Treatment of autoimmune diseases is specific to the disease, and usually concentrates on alleviating symptoms rather than correcting the underlying cause. For example, if a gland involved in an autoimmune reaction is not producing a hormone such as insulin, administration of that hormone is required. Administration of a hormone, however, will restore the function of the gland damaged by the autoimmune disease. The other aspect of treatment is controlling the inflammatory and proliferative nature of the immune response. This is generally accomplished with two types of drugs. Steroid compounds are used to control **inflammation**. There are many different steroids, each having side effects. The proliferative nature of the immune response is controlled with immunosuppressive drugs. These drugs work by inhibiting the replication of cells and, therefore, also suppress non-immune cells leading to side effects such as anemia. Prognosis depends upon the pathology of each autoimmune disease.

See also Antigens and antibodies; Antibody formation and kinetics; Antibody-antigen, biochemical and molecular reactions; Immune system; Immunity, cell mediated; Immunity, humoral regulation; Immunologic therapies; Immunosuppressant drugs; Major histocompatibility complex (MHC)

AUTOLOGOUS BANKING

Autologous banking is the recovery and storage of an individual's own blood. The blood can be from the circulating blood, and is obtained in the same way that blood is obtained during blood donation procedures. As well, blood can be recovered from the umbilical cord following the birth of an infant. In both cases, the blood is stored for future use by the individual or for the extraction of a particular form of cell known as the stem cell.

Blood and blood products (e.g., plasma) can be stored in frozen form for extended periods of time without degrading. Thus, autologous banking represents a decision by an individual to maintain his/her blood in the event of a future mishap.

One motivation for autologous blood banking can be the increased assurance that the blood that will be used in subsequent operations or blood transfusions is free of contaminating **microorganisms** (e.g., **HIV**, **hepatitis**, etc.). Regardless, even with blood screening technologies there are still several hundred thousand transfusion-associated cases of hepatitis in the United States each year. From an immunological viewpoint, another reason for autologous banking is that autologous blood will be immunologically identical to the blood present at the time of return transfusion. This eliminates the possibility of an immune reaction to blood that is antigenically different from the individual's own blood.

The autologous blood collected from the umbilical cord is a source of stem cells. Stem cells are cells that have not yet undergone differentiation into the myriad of cell types that exist in the body (e.g., red blood cells, white blood cells, tissue cells), and so retain the ability to differentiate. Thus, under appropriate conditions, stem cells can be encouraged to differentiate into whatever target cell is desired. Although this reality has not yet been fully realized, the potential of stem cell technology as a therapy for various diseases has been demonstrated.

Umbilical cord blood cells also offer the advantage of being a closer match immunologically between individuals. The differences in blood cells between individuals due to the so-called major **histocompatibility** antigen is not as pronounced in cord blood cells. Thus, umbilical cord blood cells and tissue can be used for donation and transplantation. In addition, cord blood from closely related individuals can be pooled without inducing an immune response upon the use of the blood.

See also Antibody and antigen; Histocompatibility; Immunity, cell mediated

AUTOTROPHIC BACTERIA

An autotroph is an organism able to make its own food. Autotrophic organisms take inorganic substances into their bodies and transform them into organic nourishment. Autotrophs are essential to all life because they are the primary producers at the base of all food chains. There are two categories of autotrophs, distinguished by the energy each uses to synthesize food. Photoautotrophs use light energy; chemoautotrophs use chemical energy.

Photoautotrophic organisms (e.g., green plants) have the capacity to utilize solar radiation and obtain their energy directly from sunlight.

Until recently, scientists held there existed only a few kinds of **bacteria** that used chemical energy to create their own food. Some of these bacteria were found living near vents and active volcanoes on the lightless ocean floor. The bacteria create their food using inorganic sulfur compounds gushing out of the vents from the hot interior of the planet.

In 1993, scientists found many new species of **chemoautotrophic bacteria** living in fissured rock far below the ocean floor. These bacteria take in carbon dioxide and water and convert the chemical energy in sulfur compounds to run metabolic processes that create carbohydrates and sugars. A unique characteristic of these chemoautotrophic bacteria is that they thrive at temperatures high enough to kill other organisms. Some scientists assert that these unique bacteria should be classified in their own new taxonomic kingdom.

See also Bacterial kingdoms; Biogeochemical cycles; Extremophiles

AVERY, OSWALD THEODORE (1877-1955)
Canadian-born American immunologist

Oswald Avery was one of the founding fathers of **immunochemistry** (the study of the chemical aspects of **immunology**) and a major contributor to the scientific **evolution** of microbiology. His studies of the *Pneumococcus* virus (causing acute **pneumonia**) led to further classification of the virus into many distinct types and the eventual identification of the chemical differences among various pneumococci viral strains. His work on capsular polysaccharides and their role in determining immunological specificity and virulence in pneumococci led directly to the development of diagnostic tests to demonstrate circulating **antibody**. These studies also contributed to the development of therapeutic sera used to treat the pneumonia virus. Among his most original contributions to immunology was the identification of complex carbohydrates as playing an important role in many immunological processes. Avery's greatest impact on science, however, was his discovery that **deoxyribonucleic acid** (**DNA**) is the molecular basis for passing on genetic information in biological self-replication. This discovery forced geneticists of that time to reevaluate their emphasis on the protein as the major means of transmitting hereditary information. This new focus on DNA led to **James Watson** and **Francis Crick**'s model of DNA in 1952 and an eventual revolution in understanding the mechanisms of heredity at the molecular level.

Avery was born Halifax, Nova Scotia, to Joseph Francis and Elizabeth Crowdy Avery. His father was a native of England and a clergyman in the Baptist church, with which Avery was to maintain a lifelong affiliation. In 1887 the Avery family immigrated to the United States and settled in New York City, where Avery was to spend nearly sixty-one years of his life. A private man, he guarded his personal life, even from his colleagues, and seldom spoke of his past. He stressed that research should be the primary basis of evaluation for a scientific life, extending his disregard for personal matters to the point that he once refused to include details of a colleague's personal life in an obituary. Avery's argument was that knowledge of matters outside of the laboratory have no bearing on the understanding of a scientist's accomplishments. As a result, Avery, who never married, managed to keep his own personal affairs out of the public eye.

Avery graduated with a B.A. degree from Colgate University in 1900, and he received his M.D. degree from Columbia University's College of Physicians and Surgeons in 1904. He then went into the clinical practice of general surgery for three years, soon turned to research, then became associate director of the bacteriology division at the Hoagland Laboratory in Brooklyn. Although his time at the laboratory enabled him to study species of **bacteria** and their relationship to infectious diseases, and was a precursor to his interest in immunology, much of his work was spent carrying out what he considered to be routine investigations. Eventually Rufus Cole, director of the Rockefeller Institute hospital, became acquainted with Avery's research, which included work of general bacteriological interest, such as determining the optimum and limiting hydrogen-ion concentration for *Pneumococcus* growth, developing a simple and rapid method for differentiating human and bovine *Streptococcus hemolyticus*, and studying bacterial nutrition. Impressed with Avery's analytical capabilities, Cole asked Avery to join the institute hospital in 1913, where Avery spent the remainder of his career.

At the institute Avery teamed up with A. Raymond Dochez in the study of the pneumococci (pneumonia) **viruses**, an area that was to take up a large part of his research efforts over the next several decades. Although Dochez eventually was to leave the institute, he and Avery maintained a lifelong scientific collaboration. During their early time together at the Rockefeller Institute, the two scientists further classified types of pneumococci found in patients and carriers, an effort that led to a better understanding of *Pneumococcus* lung infection and of the causes, incidence, and distribution of lobar pneumonia. During the course of these immunological classification studies, Avery and Dochez discovered specific soluble substances of *Pneumococcus* during growth in a cultured medium. Their subsequent identification of these substances in the blood and urine of lobar pneumonia patients showed that the substances were the result of a true metabolic process and not merely a result of disintegration during cell death.

Avery was convinced that the soluble specific substances present in pneumococci were somehow related to the immunological specificity of bacteria. In 1922, working with Michael Heidelberger and others at Rockefeller, Avery began to focus his studies on the chemical nature of these substances and eventually identified polysaccharides (complex carbohydrates) as the soluble specific substances of *Pneumococcus.* As a result, Avery and colleagues were the first to show that carbohydrates were involved in immune reactions. His laboratory at Rockefeller went on to demonstrate that these substances, which come from the cell wall (specifically the capsular envelopes of the bacteria), can be differentiated into several different serological types by virtue of the various chemical compositions depending on the type of *Pneumococcus.* For example, the polysaccharide in type 1 pneumococci contains nitrogen and is partly composed of

galacturonic acid. Both types 2 and 3 pneumococci contain nitrogen-free carbohydrates as their soluble substances, but the carbohydrates in type 2 are made up mainly of glucose and those of type 3 are composed of aldobionic acid units. Avery and Heidelberger went on to show that these various chemical substances account for bacterial specificity. This work opened up a new era in biochemical research, particularly in establishing the immunologic identity of the cell.

In addition to clarifying and systemizing efforts in bacteriology and immunology, Avery's work laid the foundation for modern immunological investigations in the area of antigens (parts of proteins and carbohydrates) as essential molecular markers that stimulate and, in large part, determine the success of immunological responses. Avery and his colleagues had found that specific anti-infection antibodies worked by neutralizing the bacterial capsular polysaccharide's ability to interfere with **phagocytosis** (the production of immune cells that recognize and attack foreign material). Eventually Avery's discoveries led scientists to develop immunizations that worked by preventing an antigenic response from the capsular material. Avery also oversaw studies that showed similar immunological responses in *Klebsiella* pneumonia and *Hemophilus* **influenza**. These studies resulted in highly specific diagnostic tests and preparation of immunizing antigens and therapeutic sera. The culmination of Avery's work in this area was a paper he coauthored with **Colin Munro MacLeod** and **Maclyn McCarty** in 1944 entitled "Studies on the Chemical Nature of the Substance Inducing **Transformation** of Pneumococcal Types. Induction of Transformation by a Desoxyribonucleic Fraction Isolated from *Pneumococcus* Type III." In their article, which appeared in the *Journal of Experimental Medicine,* the scientists provided conclusive data that DNA is the molecular basis for transmitting genetic information in biological self-replication.

In 1931 Avery's focus turned to transformation in bacteria, building on the studies of microbiologist Frederick Griffith showing that viruses could transfer virulence. In 1928 Griffith first showed that heat-killed virulent pneumococci could make a nonvirulent strain become virulent (produce disease). In 1932 Griffith announced that he had manipulated immunological specificity in pneumococci. At that time Avery was on leave suffering from Grave's disease. He initially denounced Griffith's claim and cited inadequate experimental controls. But in 1931, after returning to work, Avery began to study transmissible hereditary changes in immunological specificity, which were confirmed by several scientists. His subsequent investigations produced one of the great milestones in biology.

In 1933 Avery's associate, James Alloway, had isolated a crude solution of the transforming agent. Immediately the laboratory's focus turned to purifying this material. Working with type-3 capsulated *Pneumococcus,* Avery eventually succeeded in isolating a highly purified solution of the transforming agent that could pass on the capsular polysaccharides's hereditary information to noncapsulated strains. As a result the noncapsulated strains could now produce capsular polysaccharides, a trait continued in following generations. The substance responsible for the transfer of genetic information was

DNA. These studies also were the first to alter hereditary material for treatment purposes.

Avery, however, remained cautious about the implications of the discovery, suspecting that yet another chemical component of DNA could be responsible for the phenomenon. But further work by McCarty and Moses Kunitz confirmed the findings. While some scientists, such as **Peter Brian Medawar**, hailed Avery's discovery as the first step out of the "dark ages" of genetics, others refused to give up the long-held notion that the protein was the basis of physical inheritance. The subsequent modeling of the DNA molecule by James Watson and Francis Crick led to an understanding of how DNA replicates, and demonstration of DNA's presence in all animals produced clear evidence of its essential role in heredity.

See also Antibody-antigen, biochemical and molecular reactions; Antibody and antigen; Antibody formation and kinetics; History of immunology; Immunogenetics; Immunologic therapies

AZOTOBACTER

The genus *Azotobacter* is comprised of **bacteria** that require the presence of oxygen to grow and reproduce, and which are inhabitants of the soil. There are six species of *Azotobacter*. The representative species is *Azotobacter vinelandii*.

The bacteria are rod-shaped and stain negative in the **Gram staining** procedure. Some species are capable of directed movement, by means of a flagellum positioned at one end of the bacterium. Furthermore, some species produce pigments, which lend a yellow-green, red-violet, or brownish-black hue to the soil where they are located.

Relative to other bacteria, *Azotobacter* is very large. A bacterium can be almost the same size as a **yeast** cell, which is a eucaryotic single-celled microorganism.

Azotobacter has several features that allow it to survive in the sometimes harsh environment of the soil. The bacteria can round up and thicken their cell walls, to produce what is termed a cyst. A cyst is not dormant, like a spore, but does allow the bacterium to withstand conditions that would otherwise be harmful to an actively growing vegetative cell. When in a cyst form, *Azotobacter* is not capable of nitrogen fixation. The second environmentally adaptive feature of the bacterium is the large amounts of slime material that can be secreted to surround each bacterium. Slime naturally retains water. Thus, the bacterium is able to sequester water in the immediate vicinity.

A noteworthy feature of *Azotobacter* is the ability of the bacteria to "fix" atmospheric nitrogen, by the conversion of this elemental form to ammonia. Plants are able to utilize the ammonia as a nutrient. Furthermore, like the bacteria *Klebsiella pneumoniae* and *Rhizobium leguminosarum*, *Azotobacter vinelandii* is able to accomplish this chemical conversion when the bacteria are living free in the soil. In contrast to *Rhizobium leguminosarum*, however, *Azotobacter vinelandii* cannot exist in an association with plants.

Azotobacter can accomplish nitrogen fixation by using three different **enzymes**, which are termed nitrogenases. The enzyme diversity, and an extremely rapid metabolic rate (the highest of any known living organism) allow the bacterium to fix nitrogen when oxygen is present. The other nitrogen-fixing bacteria possess only a single species of nitrogenase, which needs near oxygen-free conditions in order to function. The enhanced versatility of *Azotobacter* makes the microbe attractive for agricultural purposes.

See also Aerobes; Nitrogen cycle in microorganisms; Soil formation, involvement of microorganisms

B

B CELLS OR B LYMPHOCYTES

B lymphocytes, also known as B cells, are one of the five types of white blood cells, or leukocytes, that circulate throughout the blood. They and **T-lymphocytes** are the most abundant types of white blood cells. B lymphocytes are a vital part of the body's **immune system**. They function to specifically recognize a foreign protein, designated as an **antigen**, and to aid in destroying the invader.

B lymphocytes are produced and mature in the bone marrow. The mature form of the cell is extremely diverse, with a particular B cell being tailored to recognize just a single antigen. This recognition is via a molecule on the surface of the B cell, called a B cell receptor. There are thousands of copies of the identical receptor scattered over the entire surface of a B cell. Moreover, there are many thousands of B cells, each differing in the structure of this receptor. This diversity is possible because of rearrangement of genetic material to generate genes that encode the receptors. The myriad of receptors are generated even before the body has been exposed to the protein antigen that an individual receptor will recognize. B cells thus are one means by which our immune system has "primed" itself for a rapid response to invasion.

The surface receptor is the first step in a series of reactions in the body's response to a foreign antigen. The receptor provides a "lock and key" fit for the target antigen. The antigen is soluble; that is, floating free in the fluid around the B cell. A toxin that has been released from a bacterium is an example of a soluble antigen. The binding of the antigen to the B cell receptor triggers the intake of the bound antigen into the B cell, a process called receptor-mediated endocytosis. Inside the cell the antigen is broken up and the fragments are displayed one the surface of the B cell. These are in turn recognized by a receptor on the surface of a T lymphocyte, which binds to the particular antigen fragment. There follows a series of reactions that causes the B cell to differentiate into a plasma cell, which produces and secretes large amounts of an **antibody** to the original protein antigen.

Plasma cells live in the bone marrow. They have a limited lifetime of from two to twelve weeks. Thus, they are the immune system's way of directly addressing an antigen threat. When the threat is gone, the need for plasma cells is also gone. But, B lymphocytes remain, ready to differentiate into the antibody–producing plasma cells when required.

Within the past several years, research has indicated that the deliberate depletion of B cells might aid in thwarting the progression of autoimmune disease—where the body's immune system reacts against the body's own components—and so bring relief from, for example, rheumatoid arthritis. However, as yet the data is inconclusive, and so this promising therapy remains to be proven.

See also Antibody and antigen; Antibody formation and kinetics; Immunity, active, passive and delayed; Immunity, cell mediated; Immunization

BACILLUS THURINGIENSIS, INSECTICIDE

Bacillus thuringiensis is a Gram-positive rod-shaped bacterium. This bacterium is most noteworthy because of its use to kill butterfly and moth caterpillars (Lepidoptera), the larvae of mosquitoes, and some species of black fly, that are a damage to economically important plants or a health threat.

The basis of the bacterium's insecticidal power is a protein endotoxin (an endotoxin is a toxin that remains inside the bacterium). More correctly in terms of the lethal activity, the toxin is actually a so-called protoxin. That is, the molecule must be processed to some other form before the toxic activity is present.

Inside the bacterium the protoxin molecules collect together to form a crystal. These crystals are visible as two pyramids associated with each other when the **bacteria** are examined in light microscopy. Often the bacteria contain a bright spot under light microscopic illumination. This spot is an endospore (a spore that is contained within the bacterium).

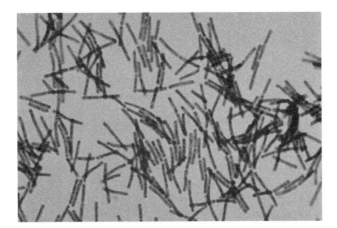

Light microscope image of Bacillus bacteria.

The presence of an endospore is very useful. Like the spores of other bacterial species, the endospore of *Bacillus thuringiensis* allows the organism to survive inhospitable conditions in a dormant state. Endospores that contain the protoxin crystal can be applied to fields via crop-dusting aircraft.

The protoxin crystal is a hardy structure, and does not readily dissolve. However, in the gut of insects, where the **pH** is very basic, the protoxin can go into solution. When this happens an insect enzyme splits the molecule. One of the toxin fragments, the delta endotoxin, confers the lethal effect to the insect.

The delta endotoxin binds to the epithelial cells lining the gut wall of the insect. By creating holes in the cells, the toxin destroys the functioning of the gut, and causes massive cell death. The larva is unable to eat. Another consequence of the destruction is a modification of the pH to a more neutral level that is hospitable for the germination of the endospores. The resuscitation and growth of *Bacillus thuringiensis* within the insect gut kills the larva.

The use of *Bacillus thuringiensis* as an insecticide has been practiced since the 1930s. In the recent three or four decades, with the advent of techniques of molecular rearrangement, the specificity of the bacterium for target insect pests has been refined. These products now represent some one percent of the worldwide use of **fungicides**, herbicides and insecticides.

See also Bacteriocidal, bacteriostatic

BACTEREMIC

Bacteremic is a term that refers to the ability of a bacterium to multiply and cause an infection in the bloodstream. The invasion of the bloodstream by the particular type of **bacteria** is also referred to as bacteremia.

If the invading bacteria also release toxins into the bloodstream, the malady can also be called blood poisoning or septicemia. *Staphylococcus* and *Streptococcus* are typically associated with septicemia.

The bloodstream is susceptible to invasion by bacteria that gain entry via a wound or abrasion in the protective skin overlay of the body, or as a result of another infection elsewhere in the body, or following the introduction of bacteria during a surgical procedure or via a needle during injection of a drug.

Depending on the identity of the infecting bacterium and on the physical state of the human host (primarily with respect to the efficiency of the **immune system**), bacteremic infections may not produce any symptoms. However, some infections do produce symptoms, ranging from an elevated temperature, as the immune system copes with the infection, to a spread of the infection to the heart (endocarditis or pericarditis) or the covering of nerve cells (**meningitis**). In more rare instances, a bacteremic infection can produce a condition known as septic shock. The latter occurs when the infection overwhelms the ability of the body's defense mechanisms to cope. Septic shock can be lethal.

Septicemic infections usually result from the spread of an established infection. Bacteremic (and septicemic) infections often arise from bacteria that are normal resident on the surface of the skin or internal surfaces, such as the intestinal tract epithelial cells. In their normal environments the bacteria are harmless and even can be beneficial. However, if they gain entry to other parts of the body, these so-called commensal bacteria can pose a health threat. The entry of these commensal bacteria into the bloodstream is a normal occurrence for most people. In the majority of people, however, the immune system is more than able to deal with the invaders. If the immune system is not functioning efficiently then the invading bacteria may be able to multiply and establish an infection. Examples of conditions that compromise the immune system are another illness (such as acquired **immunodeficiency** syndrome and certain types of cancer), certain medical treatments such as irradiation, and the abuse of drugs or alcohol.

Examples of bacteria that are most commonly associated with bacteremic infections are *Staphylococcus*, *Streptococcus*, *Pseudomonas*, *Haemophilus*, and ***Escherichia coli***.

The generalized location of bacteremia produces generalized symptoms. These symptoms can include a fever, chills, pain in the abdomen, nausea with vomiting, and a general feeling of ill health. Not all these symptoms are present at the same time. The nonspecific nature of the symptoms may not prompt a physician to suspect bacteremia until the infection is more firmly established. Septic shock produces more drastic symptoms, including elevated rates of breathing and heartbeat, loss of consciousness and failure of organs throughout the body. The onset of septic shock can be rapid, so prompt medical attention is critical.

The discovery of bacteria in the blood should be taken as grounds to suspect bacteremia, because bacteria do not typically populate blood. Antibiotic therapy is usually initiated immediately, even if other options, such as the transient entry of bacteria from a cut, have actually occurred. In addition, antibiotic therapy is prudent because many bacteremic infections arise because of an ongoing infection elsewhere in the body. Along with the prompt start of treatment, the antibiotic used must be selected with care. Use of an ineffective antibiotic can provide the bacteria with enough time to undergo explosive increases in number, whereas the use of an antibiotic to which the bacteria are susceptible can quickly quell a brewing infection.

As with many other infections, bacteremic infections can be prevented by observance of proper hygienic procedures including hand washing, cleaning of wounds, and cleaning sites of injections to temporarily free the surface of living bacteria. The rate of bacteremic infections due to surgery is much less now than in the past, due to the advent of sterile surgical procedures, but is still a serious concern.

See also Bacteria and bacterial infection; Infection and resistance

BACTERIA AND BACTERIAL INFECTION

Infectious diseases depend on the interplay between the ability of pathogens to invade and/or proliferate in the body and the degree to which the body is able to resist. If the ability of a microorganism to invade, proliferate, and cause damage in the body exceeds the body's protective capacities, a disease state occurs. Infection refers to the growth of **microorganisms** in the body of a host. Infection is not synonymous with disease because infection does not always lead to injury, even if the pathogen is potentially virulent (able to cause disease). In a disease state, the host is harmed in some way, whereas infection refers to any situation in which a microorganism is established and growing in a host, whether or not the host is harmed.

The steps of pathogenesis, the progression of a disease state, include entry, colonization, and growth. Pathogens like bacteria use several strategies to establish virulence. The bacteria must usually gain access to host tissues and multiply before damage can be done. In most cases this requires the penetration of the skin, mucous membranes, or intestinal epithelium, surfaces that normally act as microbial barriers. Passage through the skin into subcutaneous layers almost always occurs through wounds and in rare instances pathogens penetrate through unbroken skin.

Most infections begin with the adherence of bacteria to specific cells on the mucous membranes of the respiratory, alimentary, or genitourinary tract. Many bacteria possess surface macromolecules that bind to complementary acceptor molecules on the surfaces of certain animal cells, thus promoting specific and firm adherence. Certain of these macromolecules are polysaccharides and form a meshwork of fibers called the **glycocalyx**. This can be important for fixing bacteria to host cells. Other proteins are specific, e.g., M-proteins on the surface of *Streptococcus pyogenes* which facilitate binding to the respiratory mucosal receptor. Also structures known as fimbrae may be important in the attachment process. For example, the fimbrae of *Neiseria gonorrhoeae* play a key role in the attachment of this organism to the urogenital epithelium where it causes a **sexually transmitted disease**. Also, it has been shown that fimbriated strains of *Escherichia coli* are much more frequent causes of urinary tract infections than strains

lacking fimbrae, showing that these structures can indeed promote the capacity of bacteria to cause infection.

The next stage of infection is invasion that is the penetration of the epithelium to generate pathogenicity. At the point of entry, usually at small breaks or lesions in the skin or mucosal surfaces, growth is often established in the submucosa. Growth can also be established on intact mucosal surfaces, especially if the normal flora is altered or eliminated. Pathogen growth may also be established at sites distant from the original point of entry. Access to distant, usually interior, sites occurs through the blood or lymphatic system.

If a pathogen gains access to tissues by adhesion and invasion, it must then multiply, a process called colonization. Colonization requires that the pathogen bind to specific tissue surface receptors and overcome any non-specific or immune host defenses. The initial inoculum is rarely sufficient to cause damage. A pathogen must grow within host tissues in order to produce disease. If a pathogen is to grow, it must find appropriate nutrients and environmental conditions in the host. Temperature, **pH** and reduction potential are environmental factors that affect pathogen growth, but the availability of microbial nutrients in host tissues is most important. Not all nutrients may be plentiful in different regions. Soluble nutrients such as sugars, amino acids and organic acids may often be in short supply and organisms able to utilize complex nutrient sources such as glycogen may be favored. Trace elements may also be in short supply and can influence the establishment of a pathogen. For example, iron is thought to have a strong influence on microbial growth. Specific iron binding proteins called transferrin and lactoferrin exist in human cells and transfer iron through the body. Such is the affinity of these proteins for iron, that microbial iron deficiency may be common and administration of a soluble iron salt may greatly increase the virulence of some pathogens. Many bacteria produce iron-chelating compounds known as siderophores, which help them to obtain iron from the environment. Some iron chelators isolated from pathogenic bacteria are so efficient that they can actually remove iron from host iron binding proteins. For example, a siderophore called aerobactin, produced by certain strains of *E. coli* and encoded by the Col V plasmid, readily removes iron bound to transferring.

After initial entry, the organism often remains localized and multiplies, producing a small focus of infection such as a boil, carbuncle or pimple. For example, these commonly arise from Staphylococcus infections of the skin. Alternatively, the organism may pass through the lymphatic vessels and be deposited in lymph nodes. If an organism reaches the blood, it will be distributed to distal parts of the body, usually concentrating in the liver or spleen. Spread of the pathogen through the blood and lymph systems can result in generalized (systemic) infection of the body, with the organism growing in a variety of tissues. If extensive **bacterial growth** in tissues occurs, some of the organisms may be shed into the bloodstream, a condition known as bacteremia.

A number of bacteria produce extracellular proteins, which break down host tissues, encourage the spread of the organism and aid the establishment and maintenance of disease. These proteins, which are mostly **enzymes**, are called

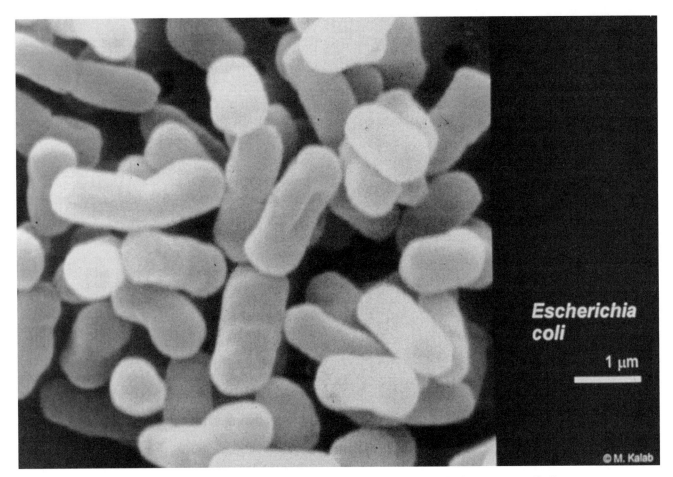

Scanning electron micrograph of *Escherichia coli*, the cause of a gastrointestinal infection that can lead to severe complications.

virulence factors. For example, **streptococci, staphylococci** and pneumococci produce hyaluronidase, an enzyme that breaks down hyaluronic acid, a host tissue cement. They also produce proteases, nucleases and lipases that depolymerize host proteins, nucleic acids and fats. Clostridia that cause gas gangrene produce collagenase, and κ-toxin, which breaks down the collagen network supporting the tissues.

The ways in which pathogens bring about damage to the host are diverse. Only rarely are symptoms of a disease due simply to the presence of a large number of microorganisms, although a large mass of bacterial cells can block vessels or heart valves or clog the air passages of the lungs. In many cases, pathogenic bacteria produce toxins that are responsible for host damage. Toxins released extracellularly are called exotoxins, and these may travel from the focus of infection to distant parts of the body and cause damage in regions far removed from the site of microbial growth. The first example of an exotoxin to be discovered was the **diphtheria** toxin produced by *Corynebacterium diphtheriae*. Some Gram negative bacteria produce lipopolysaccharides as part of their cell walls, which under some conditions can be toxic. These are called endotoxins and have been studied primarily in the genera *Escherichia, Shigella,* and *Salmonella.*

See also Anti-adhesion methods; Antibiotic resistance, tests for; Immune system; Immunofluorescence; Immunology; Infection and resistance; Infection control

BACTERIA, ECONOMIC USES AND BENE-
FITS • *see* ECONOMIC USES AND BENEFITS OF MICROORGAN-
ISMS

BACTERIAL ADAPTATION

Bacteria have been designed to be adaptable. Their surrounding layers and the genetic information for these and other structures associated with a bacterium are capable of alteration. Some alterations are reversible, disappearing when the particular pressure is lifted. Other alterations are maintained and can even be passed on to succeeding generations of bacteria.

The first antibiotic was discovered in 1929. Since then, a myriad of naturally occurring and chemically synthesized **antibiotics** have been used to control bacteria. Introduction of an antibiotic is frequently followed by the development of resistance to the agent. Resistance is an example of the adaptation of the bacteria to the antibacterial agent.

Antibiotic resistance can develop swiftly. For example, resistance to **penicillin** (the first antibiotic discovered) was recognized almost immediately after introduction of the drug. As of the mid 1990s, almost 80% of all strains of *Staphylococcus aureus* were resistant to penicillin. Meanwhile, other bacteria remain susceptible to penicillin. An example is provided by Group A *Streptococcus pyogenes*, another Grampositive bacteria.

The adaptation of bacteria to an antibacterial agent such as an antibiotic can occur in two ways. The first method is known as inherent (or natural) resistance. Gram-negative bacteria are often naturally resistant to penicillin, for example. This is because these bacteria have another outer membrane, which makes the penetration of penicillin to its target more difficult. Sometimes when bacteria acquire resistance to an antibacterial agent, the cause is a membrane alteration that has made the passage of the molecule into the cell more difficult. This is adaptation.

The second category of adaptive resistance is called acquired resistance. This resistance is almost always due to a change in the genetic make-up of the bacterial genome. Acquired resistance can occur because of mutation or as a response by the bacteria to the selective pressure imposed by the antibacterial agent. Once the genetic alteration that confers resistance is present, it can be passed on to subsequent generations. Acquired adaptation and resistance of bacteria to some clinically important antibiotics has become a great problem in the last decade of the twentieth century.

Bacteria adapt to other environmental conditions as well. These include adaptations to changes in temperature, **pH**, concentrations of ions such as sodium, and the nature of the surrounding support. An example of the latter is the response shown by *Vibrio parahaemolyticus* to growth in a watery environment versus a more viscous environment. In the more viscous setting, the bacteria adapt by forming what are called swarmer cells. These cells adopt a different means of movement, which is more efficient for moving over a more solid surface. This adaptation is under tight genetic control, involving the expression of multiple genes.

Bacteria react to a sudden change in their environment by expressing or repressing the expression of a whole lost of genes. This response changes the properties of both the interior of the organism and its surface chemistry. A well-known example of this adaptation is the so-called **heat shock response** of *Escherichia coli*. The name derives from the fact that the response was first observed in bacteria suddenly shifted to a higher growth temperature.

One of the adaptations in the surface chemistry of Gram-negative bacteria is the alteration of a molecule called lipopolysaccharide. Depending on the growth conditions or whether the bacteria are growing on an artificial growth medium or inside a human, as examples, the lipopolysaccharide chemistry can become more or less water-repellent. These changes can profoundly affect the ability of antibacterial agents or immune components to kill the bacteria.

Another adaptation exhibited by *Vibrio parahaemolyticus*, and a great many other bacteria as well, is the formation of adherent populations on solid surfaces. This mode of growth is called a biofilm. Adoption of a biofilm mode of growth induces a myriad of changes, many involving the expression of previously unexpressed genes. As well de-activation of actively expressing genes can occur. Furthermore, the pattern of **gene** expression may not be uniform throughout the biofilm. Evidence from studies where the activity of living bacteria can be measured without disturbing the biofilm is consistent with a view that the bacteria closer to the top of the biofilm, and so closer to the outside environment, are very different than the bacteria lower down in the biofilm. A critical aspect of biofilms is the ability of the adherent bacteria to sense their environment and to convert this information into signals that trigger gene expression or inhibition.

Bacteria within a biofilm and bacteria found in other niches, such as in a wound where oxygen is limited, grow and divide at a far slower speed than the bacteria found in the test tube in the laboratory. Such bacteria are able to adapt to the slower growth rate, once again by changing their chemistry and gene expression pattern. When presented with more nutrients, the bacteria can often very quickly resume the rapid growth and division rate of their test tube counterparts. Thus, even though they have adapted to a slower growth rate, the bacteria remained "primed" for the rapid another adaptation to a faster growth rate.

A further example of adaptation is the phenomenon of chemotaxis, whereby a bacterium can sense the chemical composition of the environment and either moves toward an attractive compound, or shifts direction and moves away from a compound sensed as being detrimental. Chemotaxis is controlled by more than 40 genes that code for the production of components of the flagella that propels the bacterium along, for sensory receptor proteins in the membrane, and for components that are involved in signaling a bacterium to move toward or away from a compound. The adaptation involved in the chemotactic response must have a memory component, because the concentration of a compound at one moment in time must be compared to the concentration a few moments later.

See also Antiseptics; Biofilm formation and dynamic behavior; Evolution and evolutionary mechanisms; Mutations and mutagenesis

BACTERIAL APPENDAGES

A bacterial appendage protrudes outward from the surface of the microorganism. Some are highly anchored to the surface, whereas others, like the **glycocalyx**, are loosely associated with the surface.

The entire surface of a bacterium can be covered with glycocalyx (also known as the slime layer). The layer is made of chains of sugar. Protein can also be present. The exact chemical nature of a glycocalyx varies from one species of **bacteria** to another. A glycocalyx is easily identified in light microscopy by the application of India ink. The ink does not penetrate the glycocalyx, which then appears as a halo around each bacteria.

A glycocalyx has a number of functions. It aids a bacterium in attaching to a surface. Surface contact triggers the production of a great deal of glycocalyx. The bacteria on the surface can become buried. This phenomenon has been well documented for *Pseudomonas aeruginosa*, which forms biofilms on surfaces in many environments, both within and outside of the body. The production of glycocalyx is a vital part of the biofilm formation.

By virtue of its chemical make-up, a glycocalyx will retain water near the bacteria, which protects the bacteria from drying out. Protection is also conferred against **viruses, antibiotics**, antibacterial agents such as detergents, and from the engulfing of the bacteria by immune macrophage cells (a process called **phagocytosis**). The mass of glycocalyx-enclosed bacteria becomes too large for a macrophage to engulf. For example, encapsulated strains of *Streptococcus pneumoniae* kill 90% of the animals it infects. Unencapsulated strains, however, are completely non-lethal. As another example of the protection conferred by the glycocalyx, *Pseudomonas aeruginosa* in an intact biofilm resist for hours concentrations of antibiotics up to one thousand times greater than those which kill within minutes their bacterial counterparts without glycocalyx and bacteria freed from the glycocalyx cocoon of the biofilm.

Glycocalyx material is easily removed from the bacterial surface. A glycocalyx that is more firmly anchored is known called as a capsule. Many disease causing bacteria tend to produce capsules when inside the human host, as a defense against phagocytosis.

Another type of bacterial appendage is the flagella (singular, flagellum). They appear as strings protruding outward from a bacterium. They are long, up to ten times the length of the bacterium. Each flagellum is composed of a spiral arrangement of a protein (flagellin). The flagella are closed off at the end removed from the cell. The end closest to the bacterial surface hooks into the membrane(s), where they are held by two structures termed basal bodies. The basal bodies act as bushings, allowing flagellar tube to turn clockwise and counterclockwise. By spinning around from this membrane anchor, flagella act as propellers to move a bacterium forward, or in a tumbling motion prior to a directed movement in the same or another forward path. These runs and tumbles enable a bacterium to move toward an attractant or away from a repellant. Generally termed taxis, these movements can be in response to nutrients (chemotaxis), oxygen (aerotaxis) or light (phototaxis). The tactic process is highly orchestrated, with sensory proteins detecting the signal molecule and conveying the signal into flagellar action.

Flagella are very powerful. They can propel bacteria at ten times their length per second. In contrast, an Olympic sprinter can propel himself at just over five body lengths per second. Depending upon the type of bacteria, flagella are characteristically arranged singly at only one end of the cell (monotrichous), singly at both ends of the cell (amphitrichous), in a tuft at one or a few sites (lophotrichous), or all over the bacterial surface (peritrichous).

The bacteria called **spirochetes** have a modified form of flagella, which is termed an endoflagella or an axial filament. In this case, the flagella is not an appendage, in that it is not external to the bacterium, but instead is found in the interior of the cell, running from one end of the cell to another. It is, however, similar in construction to flagella. Endoflagella attach to either end of a cell and provide the rigidity that aids a cell in turning like a corkscrew through its liquid environment.

Two other types of appendages are essentially tubes that stick out from the bacterial surface. The first of these is known as spinae (singular, spina). Spinae are cylinders that flare out at their base. They are a spiral arrangement of a single protein (spinin) that is attached only to the outer surface of the outer membrane. They have been detected in a marine pseudomonad and a freshwater bacterial species. Their formation is triggered by environmental change (**pH**, temperature, and sodium concentration). Once formed, spinae are extremely resilient, surviving treatment with harsh acids and bases. They are designed for longevity. Their function is unknown. Suggested functions include buoyancy, promoters of bacterial aggregation, and as a conduit of genetic exchange.

The appendages called pili are also tubes that protrude from the bacterial surface. They are smaller in diameter than spinae. Like spinae, pili are constructed of a protein (pilin). Unlike spinae, the functions of pili are well known. Relatively short pili are important in the recognition of receptors on the surface of a host cell and the subsequent attachment to the receptor. These are also known as fimbriae. There can be hundreds of fimbriae scattered all over the bacterial surface. Their attachment function makes fimbriae an important disease factor. An example is *Neiserria gonorrheae*, the agent of **gonorrhea**. Strains of the bacteria that produce fimbriae are more virulent than strains that do not manufacture the appendage. Not unexpectedly, such pili are a target of **vaccine** development. The second type of pili is called **conjugation** pili, sex pili, or F-pili. These are relatively long and only a few are present on a bacterium. They serve to attach bacteria together and serve as a portal for the movement of genetic material (specifically the circularly organized material called a plasmid) from one bacterium to the other. The genetic spread of **antibiotic resistance** occurs using pili.

See also Anti-adhesion methods; Bacteria and bacterial infection; Electron microscopic examination of microorganisms

BACTERIAL ARTIFICIAL CHROMOSOME (BAC)

Bacterial artificial **chromosomes** (BACs) involve a **cloning** system that is derived from a particular plasmid found in the bacterium *Escherichia coli*. The use of the BAC allows large pieces of **deoxyribonucleic acid (DNA)** from bacterial or non-bacterial sources to be expressed in *Escherichia coli*. Repeated expression of the foreign DNA produces many copies in the bacterial cells, providing enough material for analysis of the sequence of the DNA. BACs proved useful in the sequencing of the human genome.

The BAC is based on a plasmid in *Escherichia coli* that is termed the F (for fertility) plasmid. The F plasmid (or F factor) contains information that makes possible the process called **conjugation**. In conjugation, two *Escherichia coli* **bacteria** can physically connect and an exchange of DNA can occur.

A BAC contains the conjugation promoting genetic information as well as stretch of DNA that is destined for incorporation into the bacterium. The foreign DNA (e.g., portion of human genome) is flanked by sequences that mark the boundaries of the insert. The sequences are referred to as sequence tag connectors. When the BAC becomes incorporated into the genome of *Escherichia coli* the sequence tag connectors act as markers to identify the inserted foreign DNA.

Using a BAC, large stretches of DNA can be incorporated into the bacterial genome and subsequently replicated along with the bacterial DNA. In **molecular biology** terminology, pieces of DNA that contain hundreds of thousands of nucleotides (the building blocks of DNA) can be inserted into a bacterium at one time. As the process is done using different sections of the foreign DNA, the amount of DNA that can be analyzed can be very large.

BACs were developed in 1992. Since then, their usefulness has grown immensely. The primary reason for this popularity is the stability of the inserted DNA in the bacterial genome. Because the inserted DNA remains in the bacterial genome during repeated cycles of replication, the information is not lost. As well, the BAC can be sequenced using the normal tools of molecular biology.

The most dramatic recent example of the power of BACs is their use by **The Institute for Genomic Research (TIGR)** in the technique of **shotgun cloning** that was employed in the sequence determination of the human genome. Many fragments of the human genome could be incorporated into BACs. The resulting "library" could be expressed in *Escherichia coli* and the sequences determined. Subsequently, these sequences could be reconstructed to produce the orderly sequence of the actual genome. This approach proved to be less expensive and quicker than the method known as directed sequencing, where a genome was sequenced in a linear fashion starting at one end of the genome.

The total number of fragments of the DNA from the human genome that have been expressed in *Escherichia coli* by the use of BACs is now close to one million. In addition to the human genome, BACs have also been used to sequence the genome of agriculturally important plants such as corn and rice, and of animals such as the mouse.

With the realization of the sequence of the human genome, the use of BACs is becoming important in the screening of the genome for genetic abnormalities. Indeed, BAC cloning kits are now available commercially for what is termed genomic profiling.

See also Biotechnology; Plasmid and plastid

BACTERIAL EPIDEMICS • *see* EPIDEMICS, BACTERIAL

BACTERIAL FOSSILIZATION • *see* FOSSILIZATION OF BACTERIA

BACTERIAL GENETICS • *see* MICROBIAL GENETICS

BACTERIAL GROWTH AND DIVISION

The growth and division of **bacteria** is the basis of the increase of bacterial colonies in the laboratory, such as colony formation on **agar** in a liquid growth medium, in natural settings, and in infections.

A population of bacteria in a liquid medium is referred to as a **culture**. In the laboratory, where growth conditions of temperature, light intensity, and nutrients can be made ideal for the bacteria, measurements of the number of living bacteria typically reveals four stages, or phases, of growth, with respect to time. Initially, the number of bacteria in the population is low. Often the bacteria are also adapting to the environment. This represents the lag phase of growth. Depending on the health of the bacteria, the lag phase may be short or long. The latter occurs if the bacteria are damaged or have just been recovered from deep-freeze storage.

After the lag phase, the numbers of living bacteria rapidly increases. Typically, the increase is exponential. That is, the population keeps doubling in number at the same rate. This is called the log or logarithmic phase of culture growth, and is the time when the bacteria are growing and dividing at their maximum speed. For *Escherichia coli*, for example, the rate of growth and division of a single bacterium (also called the generation time) during the log phase is 15 to 20 minutes. In the log phase, most of the bacteria in a population are growing and dividing.

The explosive growth of bacteria cannot continue forever in the closed conditions of a flask of growth medium. Nutrients begin to become depleted, the amount of oxygen becomes reduced, and the **pH** changes, and toxic waste products of metabolic activity begin to accumulate. The bacteria respond to these changes in a variety of ways to do with their structure and activity of genes. With respect to bacteria numbers, the increase in the population stops and the number of living bacteria plateaus. This plateau period is called the stationary phase. Here, the number of bacteria growing and dividing is equaled by the number of bacteria that are dying.

Finally, as conditions in the culture continue to deteriorate, the proportion of the population that is dying becomes dominant. The number of living bacteria declines sharply over time in what is called the death or decline phase.

Bacteria growing as colonies on a solid growth medium also exhibit these growth phases in different regions of a **colony**. For example, the bacteria buried in the oldest part of the colony are often in the stationary or death phase, while the bacteria at the periphery of the colony are in the actively dividing log phase of growth.

Culturing of bacteria is possible such that fresh growth medium can be added at rate equal to the rate at which culture is removed. The rate at which the bacteria grow is

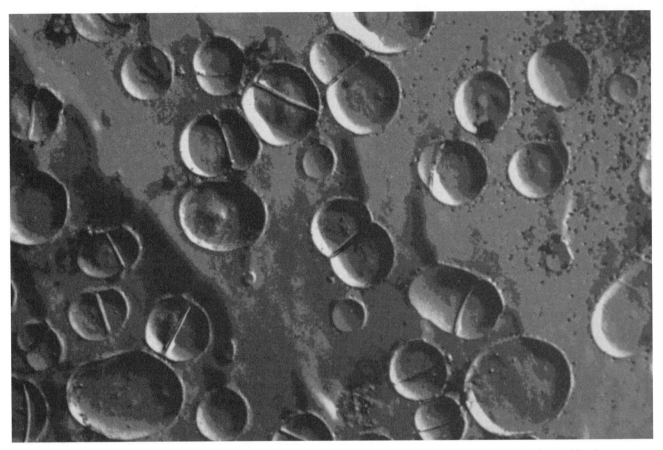

Freeze fracture electron micrograph showing dividing Streptococcus bacteria. The division plane between the daughter cells is evident in some bacteria.

dependent on the rate of addition of the fresh medium. Bacteria can be tailored to grow relatively slow or fast and, if the set-up is carefully maintained, can be maintained for a long time.

Bacterial growth requires the presence of environmental factors. For example, if a bacterium uses organic carbon for energy and structure (chemoheterotrophic bacteria) then sources of carbon are needed. Such sources include simple sugars (glucose and fructose are two examples). Nitrogen is needed to make amino acids, proteins, lipids and other components. Sulphur and phosphorus are also needed for the manufacture of bacterial components. Other elements, such as potassium, calcium, magnesium, iron, manganese, cobalt and zinc are necessary for the functioning of **enzymes** and other processes.

Growth is also often sensitive to temperature. Depending on the species, bacteria exhibit a usually limited range in temperatures in which they can growth and reproduce. For example, bacteria known as mesophiles prefer temperatures from 20°–50° C (68°–122° F). Outside this range growth and even survival is limited.

Other factors, which vary depending on species, required for growth include oxygen level, pH, osmotic pressure, light and moisture.

The obvious events of growth and division that are apparent from measurement of the numbers of living bacteria are the manifestation of a number of molecular events. At the level of the individual bacteria, the process of growth and replication is known as binary division. Binary division occurs in stages. First, the parent bacterium grows and becomes larger. Next, the genetic material inside the bacterium uncoils from the normal helical configuration and replicates. The two copies of the genetic material migrate to either end of the bacterium. Then a cross-wall known as a septum is initiated almost precisely at the middle of the bacterium. The septum grows inward as a ring from the inner surface of the membrane. When the septum is complete, an inner wall has been formed, which divides the parent bacterium into two so-called daughter bacteria. This whole process represents the generation time.

Bacterial division is initiated by as-yet unidentified sensors of either the volume or the length of the bacterium. The sensors trigger a series of events, including the formation of the septum. In septum formation are number of proteins are recruited to the site where septal formation will begin. They may be guided to the site by the concentration of a trio of proteins that either inhibit or promote the formation of a so-called Z-ring. The Z-ring is analogous to a drawstring, and is likely an integral part of the inwardly growing septum wall.

Septum formation must be coordinated with other cellular events, such as genetic replication. As well, the growth of the cell wall is a coordinated process. The **peptidoglycan** is the stress-bearing structure of a bacterium. Therefore, the insertion of new material into the existing peptidoglycan must be done in such a way that the strength of the peptidoglycan network is maintained. Otherwise, the bacterium bursts.

While proteins important in bacterial growth and division have been identified, such as the Min series of proteins active in septum formation, the nature of their actions still remains unresolved.

See also Bacterial membranes and cell wall; Colony and colony formation

BACTERIAL GROWTH CURVE · *see* BACTERIAL GROWTH AND DIVISION

BACTERIAL KINGDOMS

Bacterial kingdoms are part of the classification scheme that fits **bacteria** into appropriate groupings based on certain criteria. The kingdom is the broadest classification category.

There are two kingdoms of prokaryotes. These are the bacteria (or **eubacteria**) and the archaebacteria (or the **Archaea**). The members of these two kingdoms appear similar in shape and appearance, even under the extreme magnification of the **electron microscope**. However, they are very different from each other in a number of molecular and biochemical aspects. It is these differences that have resulted in the **microorganisms** being grouped into separate kingdoms.

For example, eubacteria contain the rigid, stress-bearing network known as the **peptidoglycan**. The only exceptions are the bacteria from the genera *Mycoplasma* and *Chlamydia*. Archaebacteria do not contain peptidoglycan. Instead, they contain a different structure that is called pseudomurein.

Another major difference in the prokaryotic kingdoms is in the sequence of a species of **ribonucleic acid** (**RNA**) known as 16S ribosomal (r) RNA. The 16 S rRNA is found in many prokaryotic and eukaryotic cells. The function it performs is vital to the life of the cell. Hence, the RNA species has not been altered very much over evolutionary time. The 16s rRNA species of eubacteria and Archaebacteria are very different. Thus, these microorganisms must have taken different evolutionary paths long ago.

Within the eubacterial kingdom are other divisions also known as kingdoms. These divisions are again determined based on the differences in the sequences of the 16S rRNA of the various bacteria. These sequence differences within the eubacterial kingdom are, however, not as pronounced as the sequences differences between the eubacteria and Archaebacteria kingdoms.

The first eubacterial kingdom is referred to as protobacteria. This designation encompasses most of the bacteria that are Gram-negative. Because a great many bacteria are Gram-negative, the protobacterial kingdom is extremely diverse in the shape and the biochemical characteristics of the bacteria. Examples of protobacteria include the photosynthetic purple bacteria, *Pseudomonas*, and bacteria that dwell in the intestinal tract of warm-blooded animals (e.g., ***Escherichia coli***, *Salmonella*, and *Shigella*.

The second eubacterial kingdom is comprised of the Gram-positive bacteria. This group is also diverse in shape and chemical character. The kingdom is further split into two major groups, based on the proportion of the nucleic acid that is composed of two particular building blocks (guanosine and cytosine). One group contains those bacteria whose **DNA** is relatively low in G and C (e.g., *Clostridium*, *Staphylococcus*, *Bacillus*, **lactic acid bacteria**, Mycoplasma). The other group is made up of bacteria whose DNA is relatively enriched in G and C (e.g., *Actinomyces*, *Streptomyces*, *Bifidobacterium*. The latter group contains most of the antibiotic-producing bacteria that are known.

The various eubacterial kingdoms, and the Archaebacterial kingdom, are markedly different in 16S rRNA sequence from the eukaryotic kingdoms (plants, **fungi**, animals). Thus, following the establishment of these life forms, the **eukaryotes** began to diverge from the evolutionary paths followed by the eubacteria and Archaebacteria.

See also Life, origin of; Microbial taxonomy

BACTERIAL MEMBRANE TRANSPORT · *see* PROKARYOTIC MEMBRANE TRANSPORT

BACTERIAL MEMBRANES AND CELL WALL

Bacteria are bounded by a cell wall. The cell wall defines the shape of the microorganism, exerts some control as to what enters and exits the bacterium, and, in the case of infectious **microorganisms**, can participate in the disease process.

Many bacteria can be classified as either Gram-positive or Gram-negative. The Gram stain is a method that differentiates bacteria based on the structure of their cell wall. Gram-positive bacteria retain the crystal violet stain that is applied to the bacteria, and appear purple. In contrast, gram-negative bacteria do not retain this stain, but are "counterstained" red by the safranin stain that is applied later. The basis of these different staining behaviors lies in the composition of the cell walls of each Gram type.

Gram-positive bacteria have a cell wall that consists of a single membrane and a thick layer of **peptidoglycan**. Gram-negative bacteria have a cell wall that is made up of two membranes that sandwich a region known as the periplasmic space or **periplasm**. The outermost membrane is designated the outer membrane and the innermost one is known as the inner membrane. In the periplasm lies a thin peptidoglycan layer, which is linked with the overlaying outer membrane.

The cell wall of Gram-positive bacteria tends to be 2 to 8 times as thick as the Gram-negative wall.

When thin sections of bacteria are viewed in the transmission **electron microscope**, the membranes appear visually similar to a railroad track. There are two parallel thickly stained lines separated by an almost transparent region. The dark regions are the charged head groups of molecules called **phospholipids**. Bacterial phospholipids consist of the charged, hydrophilic ("water-loving") head region and an uncharged, **hydrophobic** ("water-hating") tail. The tail is buried within the membrane and forms most of the electron-transparent region evident in the electron microscope.

Phospholipids make up the bulk of bacterial membranes. In Gram-positive bacteria and in the inner membrane of Gram-negative bacteria the phospholipids are arranged fairly evenly on either "leaflet" of the membrane. In contrast, the outer membrane of Gram-negative bacteria is asymmetric with respect to the arrangement of phospholipids. The majority of the phospholipids are located at the inner leaflet of the membrane. The outer leaflet contains some phospholipid, and also proteins and a lipid molecule termed lipopolysaccharide.

The asymmetrical arrangement of the Gram-negative outer membrane confers various functions to the bacterium. Proteins allow the diffusion of compounds across the outer membrane, as long as they can fit into the pore that runs through the center of the protein. In addition, other proteins function to specifically transport compounds to the inside of the bacterium in an energy-dependent manner. The lipopolysaccharide component of the outer membrane is capable of various chemical arrangements that can influence the bacterium's ability to elude host immune defenses. For example, when free of the bacterium, lipopolysaccharide is referred to as endotoxin, and can be toxic to mammals, including humans.

The presence of the outer membrane makes the existence of the periplasm possible. The periplasm was once thought to be just functionless empty space. Now, however, the periplasm is now known to have very important functions in the survival and operation of the bacterium. The region acts as a **buffer** between the very different chemistries of the external environment and the interior of the bacterium. As well, specialized transport **proteins and enzymes** are located exclusively in this region. For example, the periplasm contains proteins that function to sense the environment and help determine the response of a bacterium to environmental cues, such as occurs in the directed movement known as chemotaxis.

Not all bacteria have such a cell wall structure. For example the bacteria known as mycobacteria lack a peptidoglycan and have different components in the cell membrane. Specifically, a compound called mycolic acid is present. Other bacteria called *Mycoplasma* lack a cell wall. They need to exist inside a host cell in order to survive.

The synthesis of the cell wall and the insertion of new cell wall material into the pre-existing wall is a highly coordinated process. Incorporation of the new material must be done so as not to weaken the existing wall. Otherwise, the bacterium would lose the structural support necessary for shape and survival against the osmotic pressure difference between the interior and exterior of the bacterium. Wall synthesis and insertion involves a variety of **enzymes** that function in both the mechanics of the process and as sensors. The latter stimulate production of the cell wall as a bacterium readies for division into two daughter cells.

See also Bacterial ultrastructure; Bacterial surface layers

BACTERIAL MOVEMENT

Bacterial movement refers to the self-propelled movement of **bacteria**. This movement is also referred to motility. The jiggling movement seen in some nonmotile bacteria that are incapable of self-propelled movement is due to the bombardment of the bacteria by water molecules. This so-called Brownian motion is not considered to represent bacterial movement.

There are several types of bacteria movement. The most common occurs by the use of appendages called flagella. A bacterium can contain a single flagellum, several flagella located at one or both poles of the cell, or many flagella dispersed all over the bacterial surface. Flagella can rotate in a clockwise or counterclockwise direction. When the motion is counterclockwise, even multiple flagella can unite into a flagellar bundle that functions as a propeller. This occurs when the bacterium is moving towards a chemical attractant or away from a repellent in the behavior known as chemotaxis. If the flagella turn in the opposite direction, the coordinated motion of the flagella stops, and a bacterium will "tumble," or move in an undirected and random way.

Spirochaete bacteria have flagella that are internal. These so-called axial filaments provide the rigidity that enables the spiral bacterium to twist around the axis of the filament. As a result, the bacterium literally screws itself through the fluid. Reversal of the twist will send the bacterium in a reverse direction. Examples of bacteria that move in this manner include *Treponema pallidum* and *Rhodospirillum rubrum*.

The bacteria that are known as **gliding bacteria** exhibit another type of bacterial movement. One example of a gliding bacterium is the cyanobacterium *Oscillatoria*. Gliding movement is exactly that; a constant gliding of a bacterium over a surface. The basis of this movement is still not clear, although it is known to involve a complex of proteins.

In a human host, disease causing bacteria such as *Salmonella typhymurium* can move along the surface of the host cells. This movement is due to another bacterial appendage called a pilus. A bacterium can have numerous pili on its surface. These hair-like appendages act to bind to surface receptors and, when retracted, pull the bacteria along the surface. Movement stops when a suitable area of the host cell surface is reached.

See also Bacterial appendages

BACTERIAL SHAPES · *see* BACTERIAL ULTRASTRUCTURE

BACTERIAL SMEARS · *see* MICROSCOPE AND MICROSCOPY

BACTERIAL SURFACE LAYERS

Bacterial surface layers are regularly arranged arrays, often comprised of the same component molecule, which are located on the surface of **bacteria**. The prototype surface layer is referred to as a S layer.

S layers are found on many bacteria that are recovered their natural environment, as well as on most of the known archaebacteria. Examples of bacteria that possess S layers include *Aeromonas salmonicida*, *Caulobacter crescentus*, *Deinococcus radiodurans*, *Halobacterium volcanii*, and *Sulfolobus acidocaldarius*. In many bacteria, the production of the surface layer proteins and assembly of the surface array ceases once the bacteria are cultured in the artificial and nutrient-rich conditions of most laboratory media.

The S layer of a particular bacterium is composed entirely of one type of protein, which self-assembles into the two-dimensional array following the extrusion of the proteins to the surface of the bacterium. The array visually resembles the strings of a tennis racket, except that the spaces between adjacent proteins are very small. In some Gram-positive bacteria the surface layer proteins are also associated with the rigid **peptidoglycan** layer than lies just underneath. The combination of the two layers confers a great deal of strength and support to the bacterium.

Bacterial surface layers are the outermost surface component of bacteria. As such, they modulate the interaction of the bacterium with its external environment, and are the first line of defense against antibacterial compounds. S layers, for example, act as sieves, by virtue of the size of the holes in between adjacent protein molecules. The layer can physically restrict the passage of molecules, such as destructive **enzymes**, that are larger than the pores. The S layer around the bacterium *Bdellovibrio bacteriovorans* even precludes attack from predators of the bacterium.

Some disease-causing bacteria possess S layers. These bacteria include *Corynebacterium diphtheriae* and *Bacillus anthracis*. Microscopic examination of bacteria found in the mouth has also revealed S layers. Possession of surface layers by these bacteria aids the bacteria in avoiding the process of **phagocytosis**. This is thought to be because the protein surface layer makes the bacteria more **hydrophobic** ("water hating") than bacteria of the same species that does not have the surface layer. The increasingly hydrophobic cells are not readily phagocytosed.

BACTERIAL ULTRASTRUCTURE

Bacterial ultrastructure is concerned with the cellular and molecular construction of **bacteria**. The bulk of research in bacterial ultrastructure investigates the ultrastructure of the cell wall that surrounds bacteria.

The study of bacterial ultrastructure began with the development of the staining regimen by Danish pathologist **Christian Gram** (1853–1938) that classifies the majority of bacteria as either Gram-negative or Gram-positive. The latter

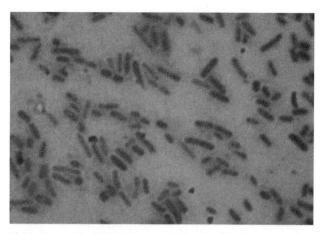

Light micrograph of *Klebsiella* bacteria showing "halo" created by the capsule.

bacteria retain the crystal violet stain, while Gram-negative bacteria do not retain this stain and are stained by the second stain that is applied, safranin. While the basis for this difference was not known at first, scientists suspected that the structure of the wall surrounding the contents of the bacteria might be involved.

Subsequent to the time of Gram, scientists have discovered that the cell wall plays only a secondary role in the Gram stain reactions. However, the cell wall of Gram-positive bacteria is indeed much different than that of Gram-negative bacteria. The study of bacterial ultrastructure relates these constituent differences to the intact cell wall. In other words, ultrastructure explores the structure of each constituent and the chemical and other associations that exist between these constituents.

The exploration of bacterial ultrastructure requires samples that are as undisturbed as possible from their natural, or so-called native, state. This has been challenging, since much of the information that has been obtained has come from the use of electron microscopy. The techniques of conventional transmission electron microscopy and scanning electron microscopy require the removal of water from the sample. Because the bulk of living things, including bacteria, are comprised of water, the removal of this fluid can have drastic consequences on the structure of the bacteria. Much effort has gone into the development of regimens that chemically "fix" bacteria, so that structure is maintained following the subsequent removal of water.

Techniques have also been developed that prepare bacteria for transmission electron microscopy without the necessity of removing water from the specimen. One technique uses an embedding resin (a substance in which the bacteria are immersed and, when the resin is hardened, allows thin slices of the bacteria to be cut) that mixes with water. This resin is harder to work with than the conventional resins that are not water-soluble. Thus, while valuable information can be obtained using water-soluble resins, a great deal of experience is necessary to produce high quality results.

A second technique of sample preparation relies on the instantaneous freezing of the bacteria. Freezing is so fast that the interior water does not extensively crystallize (which would be extremely damaging to structure). Again, an experienced analyst can produce samples that information concerning the native ultrastructure of the bacteria.

In the past several decades, other tools are increasing the ultrastructure information that can be obtained. For example, the technique of atomic force microscopy can produce information on the atomic associations between adjacent molecules on the surface of bacteria. Atomic force microscopy has been very useful in ultrastructure studies of the regularly structured surface layers on bacteria.

Modern techniques of **molecular genetics** can also yield ultrastructure information. **Mutants** can be selected or designed in which a particular **gene** or genes has been rendered incapable of producing a protein product. If the gene is involved with cell wall constituents, the analysis of the wall can reveal the alterations that have occurred in the absence of the gene product. An example are the many mutants that are defective in the construction or assembly of lipopolysaccharide, a carbohydrate and lipid constituent of the outer membrane of Gram-negative bacteria. The loss of the carbohydrate portion of lipopolysaccharide makes the outer membrane more **hydrophobic**.

One approach that has been known for decades still yields useful information concerning bacterial ultrastructure. This is the substitution of the metals present in the cell wall with other metals. Metals act like glue to hold various wall components in association with one another. Examples of such metallic species include calcium and magnesium. Out-competing these species by supplying large concentrations of another metal, the influence of the normal metallic species can be assessed. For example, replacement of metals in the Gram-negative outer membrane can cause the release of lipopolysaccharide and the formation of bubbles along the surface of the membrane, where the underlying attachment to the rigid **peptidoglycan** layer is disrupted.

The use of specific antibodies to determine the molecular arrangement of ultrastructural constituent targets greatly enhances the effectiveness of agents to be used in drug therapy.

See also Atomic force microscope; Bacterial appendages; Bacterial surface layers; Caulobacter; Electron microscope, transmission and scanning; Electron microscopic examination of microorganisms; Sheathed bacteria

BACTERIOCHLOROPHYLL • *see* PHOTOSYNTHESIS

BACTERIOCIDAL, BACTERIOSTATIC

Bacteriocidal is a term that refers to the treatment of a bacterium such that the organism is killed. Bacteriostatic refers to a treatment that restricts the ability of the bacterium to grow. A bacteriocidal treatment is always lethal and is also referred to as **sterilization**. In contrast, a bacteriocidal treatment is necessarily lethal.

Bacteriocidal methods include heat, filtration, radiation, and the exposure to chemicals. The use of heat is a very popular method of sterilization in a microbiology laboratory. The dry heat of an open flame incinerates **microorganisms** like **bacteria**, **fungi** and **yeast**. The moist heat of a device like an autoclave can cause deformation of the protein constituents of the microbe, as well as causing the microbial membranes to liquefy. The effect of heat depends on the time of exposure in addition to form of heat that is supplied. For example, in an autoclave that supplies a temperature of 121° F (49.4° C), an exposure time of 15 minutes is sufficient to kill the so-called vegetative form of bacteria. However, a bacterial spores can survive this heat treatment. More prolonged exposure to the heat is necessary to ensure that the spore will not germinate into a living bacteria after autoclaving. The relationship between the temperature and the time of exposure can be computed mathematically.

A specialized form of bacteriocidal heat treatment is called **pasteurization** after **Louis Pasteur**, the inventor of the process. Pasteurization achieves total killing of the bacterial population in fluids such as milk and fruit juices without changing the taste or visual appearance of the product.

Another bacteriocidal process, albeit an indirect one, is filtration. Filtration is the physical removal of bacteria from a fluid by the passage of the fluid through the filter. The filter contains holes of a certain diameter. If the diameter is less than the smallest dimension of a bacterium, the bacterium will be retained on the surface of the filter it contacts. The filtered fluid is sterile with respect to bacteria. Filtration is indirectly bactericidal since the bacteria that are retained on the filter will, for a time, be alive. However, because they are also removed from their source of nutrients, the bacteria will eventually die.

Exposure to electromagnetic radiation such as ultraviolet radiation is a direct means of killing bacteria. The energy of the radiation severs the strands of **deoxyribonucleic acid** in many locations throughout the bacterial genome. With only one exception, the damage is so severe that repair is impossible. The exception is the radiation resistant bacterial genus called *Deinococcus*. This genus has the ability to piece together the fragments of **DNA** in their original order and enzymatic stitch the pieces into a functional whole.

Exposure to chemicals can be bacteriocidal. For example, the gas ethylene oxide can sterilize objects. Solutions containing alcohol can also kill bacteria by dissolving the membrane(s) that surround the contents of the cell. Laboratory benches are routinely "swabbed" with an ethanol solution to kill bacteria that might be adhering to the bench top. Care must be taken to ensure that the alcohol is left in contact with the bacteria for a suitable time (e.g., minutes). Otherwise, bacteria might survive and can even develop resistance to the bactericidal agent. Other chemical means of achieving bacterial death involve the alteration of the **pH**, salt or sugar concentrations, and oxygen level.

Antibiotics are designed to be bacteriocidal. **Penicillin** and its derivatives are bactericidal because they act on the **pep-**

tidoglycan layer of Gram-positive and Gram-negative bacteria. By preventing the assembly of the peptidoglycan, penicillin antibiotics destroy the ability of the peptidoglycan to bear the stress of osmotic pressure that acts on a bacterium. The bacterium ultimately explodes. Other antibiotics are lethal because they prevent the manufacture of DNA or protein. Unlike bacteriocidal methods such as the use of heat, bacteria are able to acquire resistance to antibiotics. Indeed, such resistance by clinically important bacteria is a major problem in hospitals.

Bacteriostatic agents prevent the growth of bacteria. Refrigeration can be bacteriostatic for those bacteria that cannot reproduce at such low temperatures. Sometimes a bacteriostatic state is advantageous as it allows for the long-term storage of bacteria. Ultra-low temperature freezing and lyophilization (the controlled removal of water from a sample) are means of preserving bacteria. Another bacteriocidal technique is the storage of bacteria in a solution that lacks nutrients, but which can keep the bacteria alive. Various buffers kept at refrigeration temperatures can keep bacteria alive for weeks.

See also Bacterial growth and division; Disinfection and disinfectants; Laboratory techniques in microbiology

BACTERIOLOGY • *see* BACTERIA AND BACTERIAL INFECTION

BACTERIOPHAGE AND BACTERIOPHAGE TYPING

A bacteriophage, or phage, is a virus that infects a bacterial cell, taking over the host cell's genetic material, reproducing itself, and eventually destroying the bacterium. The word phage comes from the Greek word *phagein*, meaning "to eat." Bacteriophages have two main components, protein coat and a nucleic acid core of **DNA** or **RNA**. Most DNA phages have double-stranded DNA, whereas phage RNA may be double or single-stranded. The **electron microscope** shows that phages vary in size and shape. Filamentous or threadlike phages, discovered in 1963, are among the smallest **viruses** known. Scientists have extensively studied the phages that infect *Escherichia coli* (*E.coli*), **bacteria** that are abundant in the human intestine. Some of these phages, such as the T4 phage, consist of a capsid or head, often polyhedral in shape, that contains DNA, and an elongated tail consisting of a hollow core, a sheath around it, and six distal fibers attached to a base plate. When T4 attacks a bacterial cell, proteins at the end of the tail fibers and base plate attach to proteins located on the bacterial wall. Once the phage grabs hold, its DNA enters the bacterium while its protein coat is left outside.

Double stranded DNA phages reproduce in their host cells in two different ways: the lytic cycle and the lysogenic cycle. The lytic cycle kills the host bacterial cell. During the lytic cycle in *E.coli*, for example, the phage infects the bacte-

rial cell, and the host cell commences to transcribe and translate the viral genes. One of the first genes that it translates encodes an enzyme that chops up the *E.coli* DNA. The host now follows instructions solely from phage DNA which commands the host to synthesize phages. At the end of the lytic cycle, the phage directs the host cell to produce the enzyme, lysozyme, that digests the bacterial cell wall. As a result, water enters the cell by osmosis and the cell swells and bursts. The destroyed or lysed cell releases up to 200 phage particles ready to infect nearby cells. On the other hand, the lysogenic cycle does not kill the bacterial host cell. Instead, the phage DNA is incorporated into the host cell's chromosome where it is then called a prophage. Every time the host cell divides, it replicates the prophage DNA along with its own. As a result, the two daughter cells each contain a copy of the prophage, and the virus has reproduced without harming the host cell. Under certain conditions, however, the prophage can give rise to active phages that bring about the lytic cycle.

In 1915, the English bacteriologist Frederick Twort (1877–1950) first discovered bacteriophages. While attempting to grow *Staphylococcus aureus*, the bacteria that most often cause boils in humans, he observed that some bacteria in his laboratory plates became transparent and died. Twort isolated the substance that was killing the bacteria and hypothesized that the agent was a virus. In 1917, the French-Canadian scientist **Felix H. d'Herelle** independently discovered bacteriophages as well. The significance of this discovery was not appreciated, however, until about thirty years later when scientists conducted further bacteriophage research. One prominent scientist in the field was Salvador E. Luria (1912–1991), an Italian-American biologist especially interested in how x rays cause **mutations** in bacteriophages. Luria was also the first scientist to obtain clear images of a bacteriophage using an electron microscope. Salvador Luria emigrated to the United States from Italy and soon met Max Delbruck (1906–1981), a German-American molecular biologist. In the 1940s, Delbruck worked out the lytic mechanism by which some bacteriophages replicate. Together, Luria, Delbruck and the group of researchers that joined them studied the genetic changes that occur when viruses infect bacteria. Until 1952, scientists did not know which part of the virus, the protein or the DNA, carried the information regarding viral replication. It was then that scientists performed a series of experiments using bacteriophages. These experiments proved DNA to be the molecule that transmits the genetic information. (In 1953, the **Watson** and **Crick** model of DNA explained how DNA encodes information and replicates). For their discoveries concerning the structure and replication of viruses, Luria, Delbruck, and **Hershey** shared the Nobel Prize for physiology or medicine in 1969. In 1952, two American biologists, Norton Zinder and Joshua Lederberg at the University of Wisconsin, discovered that a phage can incorporate its genes into the bacterial chromosome. The phage genes are then transmitted from one generation to the next when the bacterium reproduces. In 1980, the English biochemist, Frederick Sanger, was awarded a Nobel Prize for determining the nucleotide sequence in DNA using bacteriophages.

In the last several decades, scientists have used phages for research. One use of bacteriophages is in genetic engineering, manipulating genetic molecules for practical uses. During genetic engineering, scientists combine genes from different sources and transfer the recombinant DNA into cells where it is expressed and replicated. Researchers often use *E. coli* as a host because they can grow it easily and the bacteria is well studied. One way to transfer the recombinant DNA to cells utilizes phages. Employing **restriction enzymes** to break into the phage's DNA, scientists splice foreign DNA into the viral DNA. The recombinant phage then infects the bacterial host. Scientists use this technique to create new medical products such as vaccines. In addition, bacteriophages provide information about genetic defects, human development, and disease. One geneticist has developed a technique using bacteriophages to manipulate genes in mice, while others are using phages to infect and kill disease-causing bacteria in mice. In addition, microbiologists found a filamentous bacteriophage that transmits the **gene** that encodes the toxin for cholera, a severe intestinal disease that kills tens of thousands worldwide each year.

See also Bacteria and bacterial infection; Biotechnology; Cell cycle (prokaryotic), genetic regulation of; Chromosomes, prokaryotic; Genetic regulation of prokaryotic cells; Laboratory techniques in microbiology; Phage genetics; Phage therapy; Viral genetics; Viral vectors in gene therapy; Virus replication; Viruses and responses to viral infection

BALTIMORE, DAVID (1938-)

American microbiologist

At the age of 37, David Baltimore was awarded the 1975 Nobel Prize in physiology or medicine for his groundbreaking work on retrovirus replication. Baltimore pioneered work on the **molecular biology** of animal **viruses**, especially poliovirus, and his investigations of how viruses interact with cells led, in 1970, to the discovery of a novel enzyme, reverse transcriptase. This enzyme transcribes **RNA** to **DNA** and permits a unique family of viruses, the **retroviruses**, to code for viral proteins. Baltimore shared the Nobel Prize with virologist Renato Dulbecco and oncologist Howard Temin, who independently discovered the same enzyme. Baltimore's achievement had profound implications for the scientific community because it challenged the central dogma of molecular biology, which stated that the flow of genetic information was unidirectional, running from DNA to RNA to proteins. His work also contributed to the understanding of certain diseases such as **AIDS**, now known to be caused by the retrovirus **HIV**.

David Baltimore was born in New York City to Richard Baltimore and Gertrude Lipschitz. Baltimore was a gifted science student while still in high school; he attended a prestigious summer program at the Jackson Laboratory in Bar Harbor, Maine, in which he studied mammalian genetics. It was during this program that he met his future colleague, Howard Temin, and decided to pursue a career in scientific research. As an undergraduate Baltimore attended Swarthmore

College in Pennsylvania and graduated in 1960 with high honors in chemistry. He started graduate work at the Massachusetts Institute of Technology (MIT), but he transferred after one year to the Rockefeller Institute, now the Rockefeller University, in New York. There he studied with Richard M. Franklin, a molecular biophysicist specializing in RNA viruses. Baltimore earned his Ph.D. in 1964 and then completed three years postdoctoral research at the Salk Institute in La Jolla, California. There he met Renato Dulbecco, who developed innovative techniques for examining animal viruses, and **Alice Shih Huang**, who later became his wife. Huang was Baltimore's postdoctoral student at Salk, collaborated in some of his viral research, and later became a full professor at the Harvard Medical School. In 1968 Baltimore joined the MIT faculty, became full professor in 1972, and in 1973 was awarded a lifetime research professorship by the American Cancer Society. After winning the Nobel Prize in 1975 Baltimore continued to be honored for his work. He was elected to the National Academy of Sciences and the American Academy of Arts and Sciences in 1974.

In the mid-1970s Baltimore turned to research in molecular **immunology**, establishing a major presence in that rapidly developing field. As a prominent figure in the scientific community, Baltimore became outspoken about the potential risks of genetic engineering. He was concerned that the rapidly developing techniques of molecular biology might be misused. In 1975 Baltimore initiated a conference in which scientists attempted to design a self-regulatory system regarding experiments with recombinant DNA. In the following year the National Institutes of Health established a committee to oversee federally funded experiments in the field of genetic engineering. Baltimore became a key link between basic molecular biology and the burgeoning **biotechnology** industry. In 1984 he was appointed founding director of the new Whitehead Institute for Biomedical Research, which is affiliated with MIT; he remained at this post until 1990. In that position Baltimore made significant advances in the field of immunology and synthetic **vaccine** research. He earned wide admiration for forging dynamically amicable relations between the two institutions, developing a high-powered young faculty and molding the Whitehead into one of the world's leading institutions of its kind. Baltimore was a major influence in shaping the Human Genome Project and is an outspoken advocate of greater national investment in AIDS research.

In July 1990 Baltimore became president of Rockefeller University, launching an energetic program of fiscal and structural reform to bring the university's finances under control and to provide greater encouragement for junior faculty members. He resigned from the presidency at the end of 1991. At the time he was caught up in a controversy that stemmed from his support of a collaborator who had been charged with scientific misconduct, but whose scientific honesty he had resolutely defended. Several years later the collaborator was found to be innocent of all the charges raised against her. Baltimore remained on the faculty of Rockefeller University until 1994, when he returned to MIT as the Ivan R. Cottrell Professor of Molecular Biology and Immunology, and then Institute Professor.

During his career, David Baltimore has served on numerous governmental advisory committees. Apart from being a member of the National Academy of Sciences, he is also affiliated with the Pontifical Academy of Sciences, the American Academy of Arts and Sciences, and the Royal Society of London. At the end of 1996 he was appointed head of the newly created AIDS Vaccine Research Committee of the National Institutes of Health, a group that supports all efforts to accelerate the discovery of a vaccine against AIDS.

See also AIDS, recent advances in research and treatment; Immunogenetics; Viral genetics; Viral vectors in gene therapy; Viruses and responses to viral infection

BASIDOMYCETES

Basidomycetes are a fungal group belonging to the Eukarya domain, which includes all life forms composed by nucleated cells. Basidomycetes are classified under the **Fungi** kingdom as belonging to the phylum –mycota (i.e., Basidomycota or Basidiomycota), class –mycetes (i.e., Basidomycetes). Fungi are frequently **parasites** that decompose organic material from their hosts, such as those growing on rotten wood, although some may cause serious plant diseases such as smuts (Ustomycetes) and rusts (Teliomycetes). Some live in a symbiotic relationship with plant roots (Mycorrhizae). A cell type termed basidium is responsible for sexual spore formation in Basidomycetes, through nuclear fusion followed by meiosis, thus forming haploid basidiospores. Fungi pertaining to the Basidomycota phylum may present dikaryotic **hyphae**, i.e., walled filamentous cylindrical structures resembling branches that are formed when the two nuclei in the apical cell of a hypha divide simultaneously. One divides in the hyphal main axis and the other into the clamp, thus giving origin to a temporary monokaryotic clamp cell that is then fused to the sub apical cell, restoring the dikaryotic status. Spores are lined next to one another on the several neighboring basidia that form the Hymenium on the mushroom gill. Each spore usually bears the haploid product of meiosis. In adverse conditions, the spores may remain dormant for long periods, from months to years. When conditions are favorable, the spores germinate into uninucleated hyphae, forming monokaryotic mycelia. A dikaryotic **mycelium** is formed as the result of the fusion of two monokaryotic mycelia. Basidomycetes' sexual spores are more often than not disseminated through the wind, either by passive or forced spore discharge.

Basidomycetes comprises over 15,000 species, belonging to 15 different orders, most of them wood-rotting species. Some examples of Basidomycetes are as follows: Coral Fungus or Ramaria, pertaining to the Hymeniales order; Stinkhorn or Phallus, from the Phallales order; Corn smut or Ustilago, from the Ustilaginales order; Puffball or Lycoperdon, from the Lycoperdales order; White Button Pizza or *Agaricus bisporus,* from the Agaricales order.

The cell walls of fungi contain distinct layers, mainly constituted by **chitin** and not by cellulose. Multicellular fungi such as mushrooms have their vegetative bodies constituted mainly by filamentous hyphae. As parasites, Basidomycota and other fungi phyla (i.e., Chytridiomycota, Zygomycota, Ascomycota), do not itlize **photosynthesis**, and therefore, lack clorophyll. They produce instead several different exoenzymes, which are released directly on their hosts through invading filaments that can reach the target substance to be enzymatically decomposed. The exoenzymes are utilized in the digestion of the available organic substance from which they absorb micronutrients to synthesize and store great amounts of glycogen, whereas plants store energy under the form of starch. They also contain in their cell membranes ergosterol, a sterol found exclusively in fungi.

See also Chitin; Eukaryotes; Fungal genetics; Mycology

BATCH AND CONTINUOUS CULTURE • *see* LABORATORY TECHNIQUES IN MICROBIOLOGY

BAYER, MANFRED E. (1928-)
German physician

While educated as a physician, Manfred Bayer is best known for the series of fundamental contributions he has made to the study of bacterial and viral ultrastructure. He was the first person to visualize the **yellow fever** virus in cultured cells, and to obtain ultrathin sections of the changes caused to the cell wall of *Escherichia coli* by the antibiotic **penicillin**. The latter achievement helped guide the development of future **antibiotics** active against the bacterial wall. In the 1960s, he identified zones of adhesion between the inner and outer membranes of *Escherichia coli*. Bayer's rigorous experiments established that these adhesion zones that were apparent in thin sections of cells examined by the technique of transmission electron microscopy had biochemical significance e.g., routing of bacterial components to the surface of the cell, route for passage of **viruses** into the bacterium, specific site of certain enzyme activity). In recognition of his efforts, the adhesion sites were dubbed "Bayer's adhesion zones."

Bayer was born in Görlitz, Prussia (now Poland). Following his high school education he enrolled in the biology program at the University of Kiel in Germany. He obtained his degree in 1949. Following this, he was accepted for medical studies at the University of Hamburg, Germany. He completed his preclinical training in 1953 and clinical training in 1955. From 1957 to 1959 he studied physics at the same university. During this same period he earned his accreditation as a physician, and undertook research studies in pathology. This research led to a Research Associate position at the University of Hamburg from 1957 to 1961. Also during this period Bayer undertook diploma studies at the university's Institute of Tropical Medicine and Parasitology. He received his diploma in 1961.

From 1960 to 1962, Bayer was an Assistant Member of the Institute of Tropical Diseases and Parasitology. Then, he immigrated to the United States to take up the position of

Research Associate with The Institute of Cancer Research in Philadelphia. He has remained at the institute ever since, as an Assistant Member (1964–1967), Associate Member (1967–1978), Member (1978–1986), Senior Member (1986 to 1997), and Senior Member Emeritus (1997 to present). As well, he was an Adjunct Professor for Microbiology at the University of Pennsylvania Medical School (1971–2000) and a Honorary Visiting Professor at Dalhousie University, Halifax (1981–present).

Another contribution that Bayer has made to the field of **bacterial ultrastructure** is in the use of water-soluble embedding resins. The resins are used to solidify samples so that thin sections can be cut for **electron microscopic examination**. Some of the early refinements to the quality of the resins and the embedding techniques were pioneered by Bayer and his colleagues.

In 1968, Bayer and his colleagues deduced the structure of the structural units that form the **hepatitis** virus. Their discovery led to the formulation of a **vaccine**.

In addition to his research activities, Bayer has been a teacher and mentor to hundreds of students over four decades.

Bayer's research and teaching accomplishments have garnered him numerous honors and awards, including the Japanese Society for the Promotion of Science (1977), fellowship in the American Academy of Microbiology, and over 15 years as an editorial member of the *Journal of Bacteriology.*

See also Bacterial ultrastructure; Electron microscopic examination of microorganisms

BEAVER FEVER · *see* GIARDIA AND GIARDIASIS

BECKWITH, JONATHAN ROGER (1935-)
American microbiologist

Jonathan Roger Beckwith is the American Cancer Society Research Professor of Microbiology and **Molecular Genetics** at Harvard Medical School in Boston, Massachusetts. He is world renowned for his studies of bacterial **gene** expression, protein secretion, the structure and function of membrane proteins, and bacterial division. He has authored over 230 scientific publications. As well, Beckwith is a commentator of the societal aspects of science, with over 70 publications to date.

Beckwith was born and educated in the Boston area. He graduated from Newton High School in 1953 and went onto Harvard College, where he graduated in 1957 with an A.B. in Chemistry. From there, he attended Harvard University, graduating with a Ph.D. in Biochemical Sciences in 1961. From 1961 until 1965, he was a National Institutes of Health postdoctoral fellow in the laboratories of Arthur Pardee (Berkeley and Princeton), William Hayes (London), Sidney Brenner (Cambridge), and Francois Jacob (Paris). In 1965, he returned to Harvard as an Associate in the Department of Bacteriology and **Immunology**, the faculty he has remained with to this day (the name of the department was changed to Microbiology and

Molecular Genetics in 1969). He became an Assistant Professor in 1966, an Associate Professor in 1968, and a Professor in 1969.

Beckwith's studies of protein expression, secretion, membrane dynamics and division in the bacterium *Escherichia coli* have been of fundamental importance in both basic bacteriology and in the development of clinical strategies to deal with *Escherichia coli* infections. As part of these studies, in 1969 Beckwith was the first person to isolate a gene.

In addition to his fundamental scientific research, Beckwith has also been an active commentator on the social impact of genetics, the need to present scientific issues and topics in language that is accessible to all, and on the political influences on scientific research.

The scope and importance of Beckwith's achievements in fundamental bacterial genetics and societal aspects of genetics have been recognized by his receipt of many awards and honors. These include a Merit Award from the National Institutes of Health (1986), the Eli Lilly Award for outstanding achievement in microbiology (1970), and the Genetics Society of America Medal (1993).

Beckwith continues to research and teach at Harvard. His laboratory remains one of the most productive and innovative **microbial genetics** labs in the world.

See also Bacterial adaptation; Microbial genetics

BEHRING, EMIL VON (1854-1917)
German bacteriologist

Emil von Behring's discovery of the **diphtheria** and **tetanus** antitoxins paved the way for the prevention of these diseases through the use of **immunization**. It also opened the door for the specific treatment of such diseases with the injection of immune serum. Behring's stature as a seminal figure in modern medicine and **immunology** was recognized in 1901, when he received the first Nobel Prize in physiology or medicine.

Emil Adolf von Behring was born in Hansdorf, West Prussia (now Germany). He was the eldest son of August Georg Behring, a schoolmaster with thirteen children, and his second wife, Augustine Zech Behring. Although his father planned for him to become a minister, young Behring had an inclination toward medicine. One of Behring's teachers, recognizing both the great promise and meager circumstances of his student, arranged for his admission to the Army Medical College in Berlin, where he was able to obtain a free medical education in exchange for future military service. Behring received his doctor of medicine degree in 1878, and two years later he passed the state examination that allowed him to practice medicine.

The army promptly sent Behring to Posen (now Poznan, Poland), then to Bonn in 1887, and finally back to Berlin in 1888. His first published papers, which date from this period, dealt with the use of iodoform as an antiseptic. After completing his military service in 1889 Behring became an assistant at the Institute of **Hygiene** in Berlin, joining a team of researchers headed by German scientist **Robert Koch** (1843–1910), a leading light in the new science of bacteriology.

It was while working in Koch's laboratory that Behring began his pioneering investigations of diphtheria and tetanus. Both of these diseases are caused by **bacteria** that do not spread widely through the body, but produce generalized symptoms by excreting toxins. Diphtheria, nicknamed the "strangling angel" because of the way it obstructs breathing, was a terrible killer of children in the late nineteenth century. Its toxin had first been detected by others in 1888. Tetanus, likewise, was fatal more often than not. In 1889 the tetanus bacillus was cultivated in its pure state for the first time by the Japanese physician **Shibasaburo Kitasato** (1852–1931), another member of Koch's team.

The next year Behring and Kitasato jointly published their classic paper, "Ueber das Zustandekommen der Diphtherie-Immunität und der Tetanus-Immunität bei Thieren" ("The Mechanism of Immunity in Animals to Diphtheria and Tetanus"). One week later Behring alone published another paper dealing with **immunity** against diphtheria and outlining five ways in which it could be achieved. These reports announced that injections of toxin from diphtheria or tetanus bacilli led animals to produce in their blood substances capable of neutralizing the disease poison.

Behring and Kitasato dubbed these substances antitoxins. Furthermore, injections of blood serum from an animal that had been given a chance to develop antitoxins to tetanus or diphtheria could confer immunity to the disease on other animals, and even cure animals that were already sick.

Several papers confirming and amplifying these results, including some by Behring himself, appeared in rapid succession. In 1893 Behring described a group of human diphtheria patients who were treated with antitoxin. That same year, he was given the title of professor. However, Behring's diphtheria antitoxin did not yield consistent results. It was the bacteriologist **Paul Ehrlich** (1854–1915), another of the talented associates in Koch's lab, who was chiefly responsible for standardizing the antitoxin, thus making it practical for widespread therapeutic use. Working together, Ehrlich and Behring also showed that high-quality antitoxin could be obtained from horses, as well as from the sheep used previously, opening the way for large-scale production of the antitoxin.

In 1894 Behring accepted a position as professor at the University of Halle. A year later he was named a professor and director of the Institute of Hygiene at the University of Marburg. Thereafter he focused much of his attention on the problem of immunization against **tuberculosis**. His assumption, unfounded as it turned out, was that different forms of the disease in humans and in cattle were closely related. He tried immunizing calves with a weakened strain of the human tuberculosis bacillus, but the results were disappointing. Although his bovine **vaccine** was widely used for a time in Germany, Russia, Sweden, and the United States, it was found that the cattle excreted dangerous **microorganisms** afterward. Nevertheless, Behring's basic idea of using a bacillus from one species to benefit another influenced the development of later vaccines.

Behring did not entirely abandon his work on diphtheria during this period. In 1913 he announced the development of a toxin-antitoxin mixture that resulted in longer-lasting immunity than did antitoxin serum alone. This approach was a forerunner of modern methods of preventing, rather than just treating, the disease. Today, children are routinely and effectively vaccinated against diphtheria and tetanus.

However, the first great drop in diphtheria mortality was due to the antitoxin therapy introduced earlier by Behring, and it is for this contribution that he is primarily remembered. The fall in the diphtheria death rate around the turn of the century was sharp. In Germany alone, an estimated 45,000 lives per year were saved. Accordingly, Behring received the 1901 Nobel Prize "for his work on serum therapy, especially its application against diphtheria, by which he... opened a new road in the domain of medical science and thereby placed in the hands of the physician a victorious weapon against illness and deaths." Behring was also elevated to the status of nobility and shared a sizable cash prize from the Paris Academy of Medicine with **Émile Roux**, the French bacteriologist who was one of the men who had discovered the diphtheria toxin in 1888. In addition, Behring was granted honorary memberships in societies in Italy, Turkey, France, Hungary, and Russia.

There were other financial rewards as well. From 1901 onward, ill health prevented Behring from giving regular lectures, so he devoted himself to research. A commercial firm in which he had a financial interest built a well-equipped laboratory for his use in Marburg, Germany. Then, in 1914, Behring established his own company to manufacture serums and vaccines. The profits from this venture allowed him to keep a large estate at Marburg, on which he grazed cattle used in experiments. This house was a gathering place of society. Behring also owned a vacation home on the island of Capri in the Mediterranean.

In 1896 Behring married the daughter of the director of a Berlin hospital. The couple had seven children. Despite outward appearances of personal and professional success, Behring was subject to frequent bouts of serious depression. He contracted **pneumonia** in 1917 and soon after died in Marburg, Germany.

See also Antibody and antigen; Antibody formation and kinetics; Bacteria and bacterial infection; History of immunology; History of microbiology; History of public health; Immune stimulation, as a vaccine; Immune system; Immunity, active, passive and delayed; Immunity, cell mediated; Immunity, humoral regulation; Immunization

BEIJERINCK, MARTINUS WILLEM (1851-1931)
Dutch botanist

Born in Amsterdam, Martinus Willem Beijerinck was the son of a tobacco dealer who went bankrupt. In response to his father's misfortune, Beijerinck would devote most of his scientific career to the **tobacco mosaic virus**, a pathogen causing an economically devastating disease that dwarfs tobacco plants and mottles their leaves.

Beijerinck, who graduated from the Delft Polytechnic School, began his research under the assumption that the tobacco mosaic disease was caused by an unidentified bacterium or a parasite. Attempting to isolate the causative agent, Beijerinck filtered the sap of an infected plant to remove all known **bacteria**; however, the resulting liquid was still infective. In addition, the filtered substance was capable of infecting another plant, which could infect another, demonstrating that the substance had the ability to multiply and grow. The Russian botanist Dmitri Ivanovsky had come up against the same type of agent, but had failed to report its existence, assuming instead that his research was flawed.

In 1898 Beijerinck published his work, which maintained that tobacco mosaic disease was caused not by bacteria, but by a living liquid virus that infected only growing plant organs where cellular division allowed it to multiply. This new agent he called a filterable virus, from Latin meaning filterable poison. **Louis Pasteur** had speculated about the existence of germs that were smaller than bacteria, but did not conduct research into this phenomenon. Beijerinck asserted that the virus was liquid, but this theory was later disproved by Wendell Stanley, who demonstrated the particulate nature of **viruses**. Beijerinck, nevertheless, set the stage for twentieth-century virologists to uncover the secrets of viral pathogens now known to cause a wide range of plant and animal (including human) diseases.

See also Virology; Virus replication; Viruses and responses to viral infection

BERG, PAUL (1926-   )
American biochemist

Paul Berg developed a technique for splicing together (DNA)—the substance that carries genetic information in living cells from generation to generation—from different types of organisms. Berg's achievement, one of the most fundamental technical contributions to the field of genetics in the twentieth century, gave scientists an invaluable tool for studying the structure of viral **chromosomes** and the biochemical basis of human genetic diseases. It also allowed researchers to turn simple organisms into chemical factories that churn out valuable medical drugs. In 1980 Berg was awarded the Nobel Prize in chemistry for pioneering this procedure, now referred to as recombinant **DNA** technology.

The commercial application of Berg's work underlies a large and growing industry dedicated to manufacturing drugs and other chemicals. Moreover, the ability to recombine pieces of DNA and transfer them into cells is the basis of an important new medical approach to treating diseases by a technique called **gene** therapy.

Berg was born in Brooklyn, New York, one of three sons of Harry Berg, a clothing manufacturer, and Sarah Brodsky, a homemaker. He attended public schools, including Abraham Lincoln High School, from which he graduated in

1943. In a 1980 interview reported in the *New York Times,* Berg credited a "Mrs. Wolf," the woman who ran a science club after school, with inspiring him to become a researcher. He graduated from high school with a keen interest in microbiology and entered Pennsylvania State University, where he received a degree in **biochemistry** in 1948.

Before entering graduate school, Berg served in the United States Navy from 1943 to 1946. On September 13, 1947, he married Mildred Levy; the couple later had one son. After completing his duty in the navy, Berg continued his study of biochemistry at Western Reserve University (now Case Western Reserve University) in Cleveland, Ohio, where he was a National Institutes of Health fellow from 1950 to 1952 and received his doctorate degree in 1952. He did postdoctoral training as an American Cancer Society research fellow, working with Herman Kalckar at the Institute of Cytophysiology in Copenhagen, Denmark, from 1952 to 1953. From 1953 to 1954 he worked with biochemist Arthur Kornberg at Washington University in St. Louis, Missouri, and held the position of scholar in cancer research from 1954 to 1957.

He became an assistant professor of microbiology at the University of Washington School of Medicine in 1956, where he taught and did research until 1959. Berg left St. Louis that year to accept the position of professor of biochemistry at Stanford University School of Medicine. Berg's background in biochemistry and microbiology shaped his research interests during graduate school and beyond, steering him first into studies of the molecular mechanisms underlying intracellular **protein synthesis**.

During the 1950s, Berg tackled the problem of how amino acids, the building blocks of proteins, are linked together according to the template carried by a form of **RNA** (**ribonucleic acid**, the "decoded" form of DNA) called messenger RNA (mRNA). A current theory, unknown to Berg at the time, held that the amino acids did not directly interact with RNA but were linked together in a chain by special molecules called joiners, or adapters. In 1956 Berg demonstrated just such a molecule, which was specific to the amino acid methionine. Each amino acid has its own such joiners, which are now called transfer RNA (tRNA).

This discovery helped to stoke Berg's interest in the structure and function of genes, and fueled his ambition to combine genetic material from different species in order to study how these individual units of heredity worked. Berg reasoned that by recombining a gene from one species with the genes of another, he would be able to isolate and study the transferred gene in the absence of confounding interactions with its natural, neighboring genes in the original organism.

In the late 1960s, while at Stanford, Berg began studying genes of the monkey tumor virus SV40 as a model for understanding how mammalian genes work. By the 1970s, he had mapped out where on the DNA the various viral genes occurred, identified the specific sequences of nucleotides in the genes, and discovered how the SV40 genes affect the DNA of host organisms they infect. It was this work with SV40 genes that led directly to the development of recombinant DNA technology. While studying how genes controlled the production of specific proteins, Berg also was trying to understand how normal cells seemed spontaneously to become cancerous. He hypothesized that cells turned cancerous because of some unknown interaction between genes and cellular biochemistry.

In order to study these issues, Berg decided to combine the DNA of SV40, which was known to cause cancer in some animals, into the common intestinal bacterium *Escherichia coli*. He thought it might be possible to smuggle the SV40 DNA into the bacterium by inserting it into the DNA of a type of virus, called a **bacteriophage**, that naturally infects *E. coli*.

A DNA molecule is composed of subunits called nucleotides, each containing a sugar, a phosphate group, and one of four nitrogenous bases. Structurally, DNA resembles a twisted ladder, or helix. Two long chains of alternating sugar and phosphate groups twist about each other, forming the sides of the ladder. A base attaches to each sugar, and hydrogen bonding between the bases—the rungs of the ladder—connects the two strands. The order or sequence of the bases determines the **genetic code**; and because bases match up in a complementary way, the sequence on one strand determines the sequence on the other.

Berg began his experiment by cutting the SV40 DNA into pieces using so-called **restriction enzymes**, which had been discovered several years before by other researchers. These **enzymes** let him choose the exact sites to cut each strand of the double helix. Then, using another type of enzyme called terminal transferase, he added one base at a time to one side of the double-stranded molecule. Thus, he formed a chain that extended out from the double-stranded portion. Berg performed the same biochemical operation on the phage DNA, except he changed the sequence of bases in the reconstructed phage DNA so it would be complementary to—and therefore readily bind to—the reconstructed SV40 section of DNA extending from the double-stranded portion. Such complementary extended portions of DNA that bind to each other to make recombinant DNA molecules are called "sticky ends."

This new and powerful technique offered the means to put genes into rapidly multiplying cells, such as **bacteria**, which would then use the genes to make the corresponding protein. In effect, scientists would be able to make enormous amounts of particular genes they wanted to study, or use simple organisms like bacteria to grow large amounts of valuable substances like human growth hormone, **antibiotics**, and insulin. Researchers also recognized that genetic engineering, as the technique was quickly dubbed, could be used to alter soil bacteria to give them the ability to "fix" nitrogen from the air, thus reducing the need for artificial fertilizers.

Berg had planned to inject the monkey virus SV40-bacteriophage DNA hybrid molecule into *E. coli*. But he realized the potential danger of inserting a mammalian tumor gene into a bacterium that exists universally in the environment. Should the bacterium acquire and spread to other *E. coli* dangerous, pathogenic characteristics that threatened humans or other species, the results might be catastrophic. In his own case, he feared that adding the tumor-causing SV40 DNA into such a common bacterium would be equivalent to planting a ticking cancer time bomb in humans who might subsequently become infected by altered bacteria that escaped from the lab. Rather

than continue his ground-breaking experiment, Berg voluntarily halted his work at this point, concerned that the tools of genetic engineering might be leading researchers to perform extremely dangerous experiments.

In addition to this unusual voluntary deferral of his own research, Berg led a group of ten of his colleagues from around the country in composing and signing a letter explaining their collective concerns. Published in the July 26, 1974, issue of the journal *Science,* the letter became known as the "Berg letter." It listed a series of recommendations supported by the Committee on Recombinant DNA Molecules Assembly of Life Sciences (of which Berg was chairman) of the National Academy of Sciences.

The Berg letter warned, "There is serious concern that some of these artificial recombinant DNA molecules could prove biologically hazardous." It cited as an example the fact that *E. coli* can exchange genetic material with other types of bacteria, some of which cause disease in humans. "Thus, new DNA elements introduced into *E. coli* might possibly become widely disseminated among human, bacterial, plant, or animal populations with unpredictable effects." The letter also noted certain recombinant DNA experiments that should not be conducted, such as recombining genes for **antibiotic resistance** or bacterial toxins into bacterial strains that did not at present carry them; linking all or segments of DNA from cancer-causing or other animal **viruses** into **plasmids** or other viral DNAs that could spread the DNA to other bacteria, animals or humans, "and thus possibly increase the incidence of cancer or other disease."

The letter also called for an international meeting of scientists from around the world "to further discuss appropriate ways to deal with the potential biohazards of recombinant DNA molecules." That meeting was held in Pacific Grove, California, on February 27, 1975, at **Asilomar** and brought together a hundred scientists from sixteen countries. For four days, Berg and his fellow scientists struggled to find a way to safely balance the potential hazards and inestimable benefits of the emerging field of genetic engineering. They agreed to collaborate on developing safeguards to prevent genetically engineered organisms designed only for laboratory study from being able to survive in humans. And they drew up professional standards to govern research in the new technology, which, though backed only by the force of moral persuasion, represented the convictions of many of the leading scientists in the field. These standards served as a blueprint for subsequent federal regulations, which were first published by the National Institutes of Health in June 1976. Today, many of the original regulations have been relaxed or eliminated, except in the cases of recombinant organisms that include extensive DNA regions from very pathogenic organisms. Berg continues to study genetic recombinants in mammalian cells and gene therapy. He is also doing research in **molecular biology** of HIV–1.

The Nobel Award announcement by the Royal Swedish Academy of Sciences cited Berg "for his fundamental studies of the biochemistry of nucleic acids with particular regard to recombinant DNA." Berg's legacy also includes his principled actions in the name of responsible scientific inquiry.

Berg was named the Sam, Lula, and Jack Willson Professor of Biochemistry at Stanford in 1970, and was chairman of the Department of Biochemistry there from 1969 to 1974. He was also director of the Beckman Center for Molecular and Genetic Medicine (1985), senior postdoctoral fellow of the National Science Foundation (1961–68), and nonresident fellow of the Salk Institute (1973–83). He was elected to the advisory board of the Jane Coffin Childs Foundation of Medical Research, serving from 1970 to 1980. Other appointments include the chair of the scientific advisory committee of the Whitehead Institute (1984–90) and of the national advisory committee of the Human Genome Project (1990). He was editor of *Biochemistry and Biophysical Research Communications* (1959–68), and a trustee of Rockefeller University (1990–92). He is a member of the international advisory board, Basel Institute of **Immunology**.

Berg received many awards in addition to the Nobel Prize, among them the American Chemical Society's Eli Lilly Prize in biochemistry (1959); the V. D. Mattia Award of the Roche Institute of Molecular Biology (1972); the Albert Lasker Basic Medical Research Award (1980); and the National Medal of Science (1983). He is a fellow of the American Academy of Arts and Sciences, and a foreign member of the Japanese Biochemistry Society and the Académie des Sciences, France.

See also Asilomar conferences; Bacteriophage and bacteriophage typing; Immunodeficiency disease syndromes; Immunogenetics

BERGEY, DAVID HENDRICKS (1860-1937)
American bacteriologist

David Hendricks Bergey was an American bacteriologist. He was the primary author of *Bergey's Manual of Determinative Bacteriology*, which has been a fundamentally important reference book for the identification and classification of **bacteria** since its publication in 1923.

Bergey was born in the state of Pennsylvania where he remained his entire life. In his early years, Bergey was a schoolteacher he taught in schools of Montgomery Country.

He left this occupation to attend the University of Pennsylvania. In 1884 he receive both a B.S. and M.D. degrees. From then until 1893 he was a practicing physician. In 1893 he became a faculty member at his alma mater. The following year he was appointed the Thomas A. Scott fellow in the Laboratory of **Hygiene**.

In 1916, he received a doctor of **public health** degree. His career at the university flourished. He was professor of hygiene and bacteriology in the undergraduate and graduate schools, and became director of the Laboratory of Hygiene in 1929. He served as director and had other university appointments from 1929 until his retirement in 1932.

From 1932 until his death in 1937 he was director of biological research at the National Drug Company in Philadelphia.

During his years at the University of Pennsylvania, Bergey was a prolific and varied researcher. His research included **tuberculosis**, food preservatives, the engulfment of particles and foreign organisms by immune cells (a phenomenon termed **phagocytosis**), and the enhanced immune reaction of an organism to an antigenic target (called **anaphylaxis**). He was also responsible for determining the interrelations and differences that helped identify the organisms in a class called Schizomycetes.

This latter research activity also formed the basis for his most well known accomplishment. In the early years of the twentieth century Bergey became chair of an organizational committee whose mandate was to devise a classification scheme for all known bacteria, a scheme that could be used to identify unknown bacteria based on various criteria (such as Gram stain reaction, shape, appearance of colonies, and on a variety of biochemical reactions). In 1923, he and four other bacteriologists published the first edition of *Bergey's Manual of Determinative Bacteriology*.

The first three editions of the *Manual* were published by the Society of American Bacteriologists (now called the American Society for Microbiology). During the preparation of the fourth edition in 1934 it became apparent that the financial constraints of the Society were making publication of the *Manual* difficult. Subsequently, it was agreed by the Society and Bergey that he would assume all rights, title and interest in the *Manual*. In turn, an educational trust was created to oversee and fund the publication of future editions of the *Manual*. The Bergey's Trust continues to the present day.

From the first edition to the present day, the Bergey's manual has continued to be updated and new revisions published every few years. In addition to the *Manual*, Bergey published the *Handbook of Practical Hygiene* in 1899 and *The Principles of Hygiene* in 1901.

See also History of public health

BERKELEY, REVEREND M. J. (1803-1889)
British cleric and fungal researcher and classifier

M.J. Berkeley lived in Britain during the nineteenth century. An ordained minister, he is best known for his contributions to the study and classification of **fungi**. He compiled a number of volumes of literature on fungi. One of the best-known examples is the massive and well-illustrated *Outlines of British Fungology*, which was published in 1860. In this volume, Berkeley detailed a thousand species of fungi then known to be native to the British Isles. He was involved active in chronicling the discoveries of others. As examples, he co-authored a paper that described the findings of a United States–Japan expedition that found many species of fungi in the North Pacific in 1852–1853, and wrote several treatises on botanic expeditions to New Zealand and Antarctica.

Another of Berkeley's important contributions were connected to the Irish potato famine. From 1846 to 1851, the loss of the potato crops in Ireland resulted in the death due to starvation of at least one million people, and the mass emigration of people to countries including the United States and Canada. The famine was attributed to many sources, many of which had no basis in scientific reason. Dr. C. Montane, a physician in the army of Napoleon, first described the presence of fungus on potatoes after a prolonged period of rain. He shared this information with Berkeley, who surmised that the fungus was the cause of the disease. Berkeley was alone in this view. Indeed, Dr. John Lindley, a botany professor at University College in London, and a professional rival of Berkeley's, hotly and publicly disputed the idea. Lindley blamed the famine on the damp weather of Ireland. Their differing opinions were published in *The Gardener's Chronicles*.

With time, Berkeley's view was proven to be correct. A committee formed to arbitrate the debate sided with Berkeley. On the basis of the decision, farmers were advised to store their crop in well-ventilated pits, which aided against fungal growth.

The discovery that the fungus *Phytophthora infestans* was the basis of the potato blight represented the first disease known to be caused by a microorganism, and marked the beginning of the scientific discipline of plant pathology.

Berkeley also contributed to the battle against poultry mildew, a fungal disease that produced rotting of vines. The disease could e devastating. For example, the appearance of poultry mildew in Madeira in the 1850s destroyed the local wine-based economy, which led to widespread starvation and emigration. Berkeley was one of those who helped established the cause of the infestation.

BEVERIDGE, TERRANCE J. (1945-)

Canadian microbiologist

Terrance (Terry) J. Beveridge has fundamentally contributed to the understanding of the structure and function of **bacteria**.

Beveridge was born in Toronto, Ontario, Canada. His early schooling was also in that city. He graduated with a B.Sc. from the University of Toronto in 1968, a Dip. Bact. in 1969, and an M.Sc. in oral microbiology in 1970. Intending to become a dentist, he was drawn to biological research instead. This interest led him to the University of Western Ontario laboratory of Dr. **Robert Murray**, where he completed his Ph.D. dissertation in 1974.

His Ph.D. research focused on the use of various techniques to probe the structure of bacteria. In particular, he developed an expertise in electron microscopy. His research interest in the molecular structure of bacteria was carried on in his appointment as an Assistant Professor at the University of Guelph in 1975. He became an Associate Professor in 1983 and a tenured Professor in 1986. He has remained at the University of Guelph to the present day.

Beveridge's interest in **bacterial ultrastructure** had led to many achievements. He and his numerous students and research colleagues pioneered the study of the binding of metals by bacteria, and showed how these metals function to

cement components of the cell wall of Gram-negative and Gram-positive bacteria together. Bacteria were shown to be capable of precipitating metals from solution, producing what he termed microfossils. Indeed, Beveridge and others have discovered similar appearing microfossils in rock that is millions of years old. Such bacteria are now thought to have played a major role in the development of conditions suitable for the explosive diversity of life on Earth.

In 1981, Beveridge became Director of a Guelph-based electron microscopy research facility. Using techniques including scanning tunneling microscopy, atomic force microscopy and confocal microscopy, the molecular nature of regularly-structured protein layers on a number of bacterial species have been detailed. Knowledge of the structure is allowing strategies to overcome the layer's role as a barrier to antibacterial compounds. In another accomplishment, the design and use of metallic probes allowed Beveridge to deduce the actual mechanism of operation of the Gram stain. The mechanism of the stain technique, of bedrock importance to microbiology, had not been known since the development of the stain in the nineteenth century.

In the 1980s, in collaboration with Richard Blakemore's laboratory, used electron microscopy to reveal the structure, arrangement and growth of the magnetically-responsive particles in *Aquaspirillum magnetotacticum*. In the past decade, Beveridge has discovered how bacterial life manages to survive in a habitat devoid of oxygen, located in the Earth's crust miles beneath the surface. These discoveries have broadened human knowledge of the diversity of life on the planet.

Another accomplishment of note has been the finding that portions of the bacterial cell wall that are spontaneously released can be used to package **antibiotics** and deliver them to the bacteria. This novel means of killing bacteria shows great potential in the treatment of bacterial infections.

These and other accomplishment have earned Beveridge numerous awards. In particular, he received the Steacie Award in 1984, an award given in recognition of outstanding fundamental research by a researcher in Canada, and the Culling Medal from the National Society of Histotechnology in 2001.

See also Bacterial ultrastructure; Electron microscope examination of microorganisms; Magnetotactic bacteria

BIOCHEMICAL ANALYSIS TECHNIQUES

Biochemical analysis techniques refer to a set of methods, assays, and procedures that enable scientists to analyze the substances found in living organisms and the chemical reactions underlying life processes. The most sophisticated of these techniques are reserved for specialty research and diagnostic laboratories, although simplified sets of these techniques are used in such common events as testing for illegal drug abuse in competitive athletic events and monitoring of blood sugar by diabetic patients.

To perform a comprehensive biochemical analysis of a biomolecule in a biological process or system, the biochemist

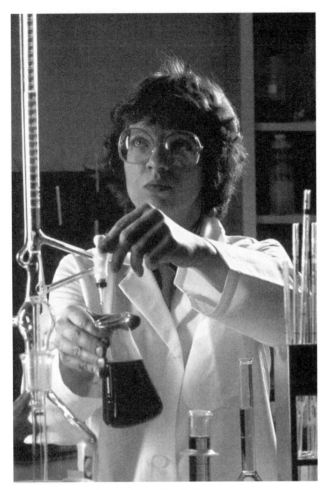

Technician performing biochemical analysis.

typically needs to design a strategy to detect that biomolecule, isolate it in pure form from among thousands of molecules that can be found in an extracts from a biological sample, characterize it, and analyze its function. An assay, the biochemical test that characterizes a molecule, whether quantitative or semi-quantitative, is important to determine the presence and quantity of a biomolecule at each step of the study. Detection assays may range from the simple type of assays provided by spectrophotometric measurements and gel staining to determine the concentration and purity of proteins and nucleic acids, to long and tedious bioassays that may take days to perform.

The description and characterization of the molecular components of the cell succeeded in successive stages, each one related to the introduction of new technical tools adapted to the particular properties of the studied molecules. The first studied biomolecules were the small building blocks of larger and more complex macromolecules, the amino acids of proteins, the bases of nucleic acids and sugar monomers of complex carbohydrates. The molecular characterization of these elementary components was carried out thanks to techniques used in organic chemistry and developed as early as the nineteenth century. Analysis and characterization of com-

plex macromolecules proved more difficult, and the fundamental techniques in protein and nucleic acid and protein purification and sequencing were only established in the last four decades.

Most biomolecules occur in minute amounts in the cell, and their detection and analysis require the biochemist to first assume the major task of purifying them from any **contamination**. Purification procedures published in the specialist literature are almost as diverse as the diversity of biomolecules and are usually written in sufficient details that they can be reproduced in different laboratory with similar results. These procedures and protocols, which are reminiscent of recipes in cookbooks have had major influence on the progress of biomedical sciences and were very highly rated in scientific literature.

The methods available for purification of biomolecules range from simple precipitation, centrifugation, and gel **electrophoresis** to sophisticated chromatographic and affinity techniques that are constantly undergoing development and improvement. These diverse but interrelated methods are based on such properties as size and shape, net charge and bioproperties of the biomolecules studied.

Centrifugation procedures impose, through rapid spinning, high centrifugal forces on biomolecules in solution, and cause their separations based on differences in weight. Electrophoresis techniques take advantage of both the size and charge of biomolecules and refer to the process where biomolecules are separated because they adopt different rates of migration toward positively (anode) or negatively (cathode) charged poles of an electric field. Gel electrophoresis methods are important steps in many separation and analysis techniques in the studies of **DNA**, proteins and lipids. Both western blotting techniques for the assay of proteins and southern and northern analysis of DNA rely on gel electrophoresis. The completion of DNA sequencing at the different human genome centers is also dependent on gel electrophoresis. A powerful modification of gel electrophoresis called two-dimensional gel electrophoresis is predicted to play a very important role in the accomplishment of the proteome projects that have started in many laboratories.

Chromatography techniques are sensitive and effective in separating and concentrating minute components of a mixture and are widely used for quantitative and qualitative analysis in medicine, industrial processes, and other fields. The method consists of allowing a liquid or gaseous solution of the test mixture to flow through a tube or column packed with a finely divided solid material that may be coated with an active chemical group or an adsorbent liquid. The different components of the mixture separate because they travel through the tube at different rates, depending on the interactions with the porous stationary material. Various chromatographic separation strategies could be designed by modifying the chemical components and shape of the solid adsorbent material. Some chromatographic columns used in gel chromatography are packed with porous stationary material, such that the small molecules flowing through the column diffuse into the matrix and will be delayed, whereas larger molecules flow through the column more quickly. Along with ultracentrifugation and gel electrophoresis, this is one of the methods used to determine the molecular weight of biomolecules. If the stationary material is charged, the chromatography column will allow separation of biomolecules according to their charge, a process known as ion exchange chromatography. This process provides the highest resolution in the purification of native biomolecules and is valuable when both the purity and the activity of a molecule are of importance, as is the case in the preparation of all **enzymes** used in **molecular biology**. The biological activity of biomolecules has itself been exploited to design a powerful separation method known as affinity chromatography. Most biomolecules of interest bind specifically and tightly to natural biological partners called ligands: enzymes bind substrates and cofactors, hormones bind receptors, and specific **immunoglobulins** called antibodies can be made by the **immune system** that would in principle interact with any possible chemical component large enough to have a specific conformation. The solid material in an affinity chromatography column is coated with the ligand and only the biomolecule that specifically interact with this ligand will be retained while the rest of a mixture is washed away by excess solvent running through the column.

Once a pure biomolecule is obtained, it may be employed for a specific purpose such as an enzymatic reaction, used as a therapeutic agent, or in an industrial process. However, it is normal in a research laboratory that the biomolecule isolated is novel, isolated for the first time and, therefore, warrants full characterization in terms of structure and function. This is the most difficult part in a biochemical analysis of a novel biomolecule or a biochemical process, usually takes years to accomplish, and involves the collaboration of many research laboratories from different parts of the world.

Recent progress in biochemical analysis techniques has been dependant upon contributions from both chemistry and biology, especially **molecular genetics** and molecular biology, as well as engineering and information technology. Tagging of proteins and nucleic acids with chemicals, especially **fluorescent dyes**, has been crucial in helping to accomplish the sequencing of the human genome and other organisms, as well as the analysis of proteins by chromatography and mass spectrometry. Biochemical research is undergoing a change in paradigm from analysis of the role of one or a few molecules at a time, to an approach aiming at the characterization and functional studies of many or even all biomolecules constituting a cell and eventually organs. One of the major challenges of the post-genome era is to assign functions to all of the **gene** products discovered through the genome and cDNA sequencing efforts. The need for functional analysis of proteins has become especially eminent, and this has led to the renovated interest and major technical improvements in some protein separation and analysis techniques. Two-dimensional gel electrophoresis, high performance liquid and capillary chromatography as well as mass spectrometry are proving very effective in separation and analysis of abundant change in highly expressed proteins. The newly developed hardware and software, and the use of automated systems that allow analysis of a huge number of samples simultaneously, is making it possible to analyze a large number of proteins in a shorter time and

with higher accuracy. These approaches are making it possible to study global protein expression in cells and tissues, and will allow comparison of protein products from cells under varying conditions like differentiation and activation by various stimuli such as stress, hormones, or drugs. A more specific assay to analyze protein function *in vivo* is to use expression systems designed to detect protein-protein and DNA-protein interactions such as the **yeast** and bacterial hybrid systems. Ligand-receptor interactions are also being studied by novel techniques using biosensors that are much faster than the conventional immunochemical and colorimetric analyzes.

The combination of large scale and automated analysis techniques, bioinformatic tools, and the power of genetic manipulations will enable scientists to eventually analyze processes of cell function to all depths.

See also Bioinformatics and computational biology; Biotechnology; Fluorescence *in situ* hybridization; Immunological analysis techniques; Luminescent bacteria

BIOCHEMISTRY

Biochemistry seeks to describe the structure, organization, and functions of living matter in molecular terms. Essentially two factors have contributed to the excitement in the field today and have enhanced the impact of research and advances in biochemistry on other life sciences. First, it is now generally accepted that the physical elements of living matter obey the same fundamental laws that govern all matter, both living and non-living. Therefore the full potential of modern chemical and physical theory can be brought in to solve certain biological problems. Secondly, incredibly powerful new research techniques, notably those developing from the fields of biophysics and **molecular biology**, are permitting scientists to ask questions about the basic process of life that could not have been imagined even a few years ago.

Biochemistry now lies at the heart of a revolution in the biological sciences and it is nowhere better illustrated than in the remarkable number of Nobel Prizes in Chemistry or Medicine and Physiology that have been won by biochemists in recent years. A typical example is the award of the 1988 Nobel Prize for Medicine and Physiology, to **Gertrude Elion** and George Hitchings of the United States and Sir James Black of Great Britain for their leadership in inventing new drugs. Elion and Hitchings developed chemical analogs of nucleic acids and vitamins which are now being used to treat leukemia, bacterial infections, **malaria**, gout, herpes virus infections and **AIDS**. Black developed beta-blockers that are now used to reduce the risk of heart attack and to treat diseases such as asthma. These drugs were designed and not discovered through random organic synthesis. Developments in knowledge within certain key areas of biochemistry, such as protein structure and function, nucleic acid synthesis, enzyme mechanisms, receptors and metabolic control, vitamins, and coenzymes all contributed to enable such progress to be made.

Two more recent Nobel Prizes give further evidence for the breadth of the impact of biochemistry. In 1997, the

Chemistry Prize was shared by three scientists: the American Paul Boyer and the British J. Walker for their discovery of the "rotary engine" that generates the energy-carrying compound ATP, and the Danish J. Skou, for his studies of the "pump" that drives sodium and potassium across membranes. In the same year, the Prize in Medicine and Physiology went to **Stanley Prusiner**, for his studies on the prion, the agent thought to be responsible for "mad cow disease" and several similar human conditions.

Biochemistry draws on its major themes from many disciplines. For example from organic chemistry, which describes the properties of biomolecules; from biophysics, which applies the techniques of physics to study the structures of biomolecules; from medical research, which increasingly seeks to understand disease states in molecular terms and also from nutrition, microbiology, physiology, cell biology and genetics. Biochemistry draws strength from all of these disciplines but is also a distinct discipline, with its own identity. It is distinctive in its emphasis on the structures and relations of biomolecules, particularly **enzymes** and biological catalysis, also on the elucidation of metabolic pathways and their control and on the principle that life processes can, at least on the physical level, be understood through the laws of chemistry. It has its origins as a distinct field of study in the early nineteenth century, with the pioneering work of Freidrich Wöhler. Prior to Wöhler's time it was believed that the substance of living matter was somehow quantitatively different from that of nonliving matter and did not behave according to the known laws of physics and chemistry. In 1828 Wöhler showed that urea, a substance of biological origin excreted by humans and many animals as a product of nitrogen **metabolism**, could be synthesized in the laboratory from the inorganic compound ammonium cyanate. As Wöhler phrased it in a letter to a colleague, "I must tell you that I can prepare urea without requiring a kidney or an animal, either man or dog." This was a shocking statement at the time, for it breached the presumed barrier between the living and the nonliving. Later, in 1897, two German brothers, Eduard and Hans Buchner, found that extracts from broken and thoroughly dead cells from **yeast**, could nevertheless carry out the entire process of **fermentation** of sugar into ethanol. This discovery opened the door to analysis of biochemical reactions and processes in vitro (Latin "in glass"), meaning in the test tube rather than in vivo, in living matter. In succeeding decades many other metabolic reactions and reaction pathways were reproduced in vitro, allowing identification of reactants and products and of enzymes, or biological catalysts, that promoted each biochemical reaction.

Until 1926, the structures of enzymes (or "ferments") were thought to be far too complex to be described in chemical terms. But in 1926, J.B. Sumner showed that the protein urease, an enzyme from jack beans, could be crystallized like other organic compounds. Although proteins have large and complex structures, they are also organic compounds and their physical structures can be determined by chemical methods.

Today, the study of biochemistry can be broadly divided into three principal areas: (1) the structural chemistry of the components of living matter and the relationships of biological function to chemical structure; (2) metabolism, the totality of chemical reactions that occur in living matter; and (3) the chemistry of processes and substances that store and transmit biological information. The third area is also the province of **molecular genetics**, a field that seeks to understand heredity and the expression of genetic information in molecular terms.

Biochemistry is having a profound influence in the field of medicine. The molecular mechanisms of many diseases, such as sickle cell anemia and numerous errors of metabolism, have been elucidated. Assays of enzyme activity are today indispensable in clinical diagnosis. To cite just one example, liver disease is now routinely diagnosed and monitored by measurements of blood levels of enzymes called transaminases and of a hemoglobin breakdown product called bilirubin. **DNA** probes are coming into play in diagnosis of genetic disorders, infectious diseases and cancers. Genetically engineered strains of **bacteria** containing recombinant DNA are producing valuable proteins such as insulin and growth hormone. Furthermore, biochemistry is a basis for the rational design of new drugs. Also the rapid development of powerful biochemical concepts and techniques in recent years has enabled investigators to tackle some of the most challenging and fundamental problems in medicine and physiology. For example in embryology, the mechanisms by which the fertilized embryo gives rise to cells as different as muscle, brain and liver are being intensively investigated. Also, in anatomy, the question of how cells find each other in order to form a complex organ, such as the liver or brain, are being tackled in biochemical terms. The impact of biochemistry is being felt in many areas of human life through this kind of research, and the discoveries are fuelling the growth of the life sciences as a whole.

See also Antibody-antigen, biochemical and molecular reactions; Biochemical analysis techniques; Biogeochemical cycles; Bioremediation; Biotechnology; Immunochemistry; Immunological analysis techniques; Miller-Urey experiment; Nitrogen cycle in microorganisms; Photosynthesis

BIODEGRADABLE SUBSTANCES

The increase in public environmental awareness and the recognition of the urgent need to control and reduce pollution are leading factors in the recent augment of scientific research for new biodegradable compounds. Biodegradable compounds could replace others that harm the environment and pose hazards to **public health**, and animal and plant survival. Biodegradation, i.e., the metabolization of substances by **bacteria, yeast, fungi**, from which these organisms obtain nutrients and energy, is an important natural resource for the development of new environmental-friendly technologies with immediate impact in the chemical industry and other economic activities. Research efforts in this field are two-fold: to identify and/or develop transgenic biological agents that digest specific existing compounds in polluted soils and water, and to develop new biodegradable compounds to replace hazardous chemicals in industrial activity. Research is, therefore, aimed at **bioremediation**, which could identify biological agents that rapidly degrade existing pollutants in the environment, such as heavy metals and toxic chemicals in soil and water, explosive residues, or spilled petroleum. Crude oil however, is naturally biodegradable, and species of hydrocarbon-degrading bacteria are responsible for an important reduction of petroleum levels in reservoirs, especially at temperatures below 176° F (80° C). The **selection**, **culture**, and even genetic manipulation of some of these species may lead to a bioremediation technology that could rapidly degrade oil accidentally spilled in water.

The search for a biodegradable substitute for plastic polymers, for instance, is of high environmental relevance, since plastic waste (bags, toys, plastic films, packing material, etc.) is a major problem in garbage disposal and its recycling process is not pollution-free. In the 1980s, research of polyhydroxybutyrate, a biodegradable thermoplastic derived from bacterial **metabolism** was started and then stalled due to the high costs involved in **fermentation** and extraction. Starch is another trend of research in the endeavor to solve this problem, and starch-foamed packing material is currently in use in many countries, as well as molded starch golf tees. However, physical and chemical properties of starch polymers have so far prevented its use for other industrial purposes in replacement of plastic. Some scientists suggest that polyhydroxybutyrate research should now be increased to benefit from new biotechnologies, such as the development of transgenic corn, with has the ability to synthesize great amounts of the compound. This corn may one day provide a cost-effective biodegradable raw material to a new biodegradable plastics industry.

Another field for biodegradable substances usage is the pharmaceutical industry, where biomedical research focuses on non-toxic polymers with physicochemical thermo-sensitivity as a matrix for drug delivering. One research group at the University of Utah at Salt Lake City in 1997, for instance, synthesized an injectable polymer that forms a non-toxic biodegradable hydro gel that acts as a sustained-release matrix for drugs.

Transgenic plants expressing microbial genes whose products are degradative **enzymes** may constitute a potential solution in the removal of explosive residues from water and soils. A group of University of Cambridge and University of Edinburgh scientists in the United Kingdom developed transgenic tobacco plants that express an enzyme (pentaerythritol tetranitrate reductase) that degrades nitrate ester and nitro aromatic explosive residues in contaminated soils.

Another environmental problem is the huge amounts of highly stable and non-biodegradable hydrocarbon compounds that are discarded in landfills, and are known as polyacrylates. Polyacrylates are utilized as absorbent gels in disposable diapers, and feminine **hygiene** absorbents, as well as added to detergents as dispersants, and are discharged through sewage into underwater sheets, rivers, and lakes. A biodegradable substitute, however, known as polyaspartate, already exists, and is presently utilized in farming and oil drilling. Polyaspartate polymers are degradable by bacteria because the molecular backbone is constituted by chains of amino acids; whereas polyacrylates have backbones made of hydrocarbon compounds.

The main challenge in the adoption of biodegradable substances as a replacement for existing hazardous chemicals and technologies is cost effectiveness. Only large-scale production of environmental friendly compounds can decrease costs. Public education and consumer awareness may be a crucial factor in the progress and consolidation of "green" technologies in the near future.

See also Amino acid chemistry; Biotechnology; Economic uses and benefits of microorganisms; Transgenics; Waste water treatment

BIOFILM FORMATION AND DYNAMIC BEHAVIOR

Biofilms are populations of **microorganisms** that form following the adhesion of **bacteria**, algae, **yeast**, or **fungi** to a surface. These surface growths can be found in natural settings, such as on rocks in streams, and in infections, such as on catheters. Both living and inert surfaces, natural and artificial, can be colonized by microorganisms.

Up until the 1980s, the biofilm mode of growth was regarded as more of a scientific curiosity than an area for serious study. Then, evidence accumulated to demonstrate that biofilm formation is the preferred mode of growth for microbes. Virtually every surface that is in contact with microorganisms has been found to be capable of sustaining biofilm formation.

The best-studied biofilms are those formed by bacteria. Much of the current knowledge of bacterial biofilm comes from laboratory studies of pure cultures of bacteria. However, biofilm can also be comprised of a variety of bacteria. Dental **plaque** is a good example. Many species of bacteria can be present in the exceedingly complex biofilm that form on the surface of the teeth and gums.

The formation of a biofilm begins with a clean, bacteria-free surface. Bacteria that are growing in solution (**planktonic bacteria**) encounter the surface. Attachment to the surface can occur specifically, via the recognition of a surface receptor by a component of the bacterial surface, or non-specifically. The attachment can be mediated by **bacterial appendages**, such as flagella, cilia, or the holdfast of *Caulobacter crescentus*.

If the attachment is not transient, the bacterium can undergo a change in its character. Genes are stimulated to become expressed by some as yet unclear aspect of the surface association. This process is referred to as auto-induction. A common manifestation of the genetic change is the production and excretion of a large amount of a sugary material. This material covers the bacterium and, as more bacteria accumulate from the fluid layer and from division of the surface-adherent bacteria, the entire mass can become buried in the sugary network. This mass represents the biofilm. The sugar constituent is known as **glycocalyx**, exopolysaccharide, or slime.

As the biofilm thickens and multiple layers of bacteria build up, the behavior of the bacteria becomes even more complex. Studies using instruments such as the confocal **microscope** combined with specific fluorescent probes of various bacterial structures and functional activities have demonstrated that the bacteria located deeper in the biofilm cease production of the slime and adopt an almost dormant state. In contrast, bacteria at the biofilm's periphery are faster-growing and still produce large quantities of the slime. These activities are coordinated. The bacteria can communicate with one another by virtue of released chemical compounds. This so-called **quorum sensing** enables a biofilm to grow and sense when bacteria should be released so as to colonize more distant surfaces.

The technique of confocal microscopy allows biofilms to be examined without disrupting them. Prior to the use of the technique, biofilms were regarded as being a homogeneous distribution of bacteria. Now it is known that this view is incorrect. In fact, bacteria are clustered together in "microcolonies" inside the biofilm, with surrounding regions of bacteria-free slime or even channels of water snaking through the entire structure. The visual effect is of clouds of bacteria rising up through the biofilm. The water channels allow nutrients and waste to pass in and out of the biofilm, while the bacteria still remain protected within the slime coat.

Bacterial biofilms have become important clinically because of the marked resistance to antimicrobial agents that the biofilm bacteria display, relative to both their planktonic counterparts and from bacteria released from the confines of the biofilm. **Antibiotics** that swiftly kill the naked bacteria do not arm the biofilm bacteria, and may even promote the development of **antibiotic resistance**. Contributors to this resistance are likely the bacteria and the cocooning slime network.

Antibiotic resistant biofilms occur on artificial heart valves, urinary catheters, gallstones, and in the lungs of those afflicted with cystic fibrosis, as only a few examples. In the example of cystic fibrosis, the biofilm also acts to shield the *Pseudomonas aeruginosa* bacteria from the antibacterial responses of the host's **immune system**. The immune response may remain in place for a long time, which irritates and damages the lung tissue. This damage and the resulting loss of function can be lethal.

See also Anti-adhesion methods; Antibiotic resistance, tests for; Bacterial adaptation

BIOGEOCHEMICAL CYCLES

The term biogeochemical cycle refers to any set of changes that occur as a particular element passes back and forth between the living and non-living worlds. For example, carbon occurs sometimes in the form of an atmospheric gas (carbon dioxide), sometimes in rocks and minerals (limestone and marble), and sometimes as the key element of which all living

organisms are made. Over time, chemical changes occur that convert one form of carbon to another form. At various points in the carbon cycle, the element occurs in living organisms and at other points it occurs in the Earth's atmosphere, lithosphere, or hydrosphere.

The universe contains about ninety different naturally occurring elements. Six elements, carbon, hydrogen, oxygen, nitrogen, sulfur, and phosphorus, make up over 95% of the mass of all living organisms on Earth. Because the total amount of each element is essentially constant, some cycling process must take place. When an organism dies, for example, the elements of which it is composed continue to move through a cycle, returning to the Earth, to the air, to the ocean, or to another organism.

All biogeochemical cycles are complex. A variety of pathways are available by which an element can move among hydrosphere, lithosphere, atmosphere, and biosphere. For instance, nitrogen can move from the lithosphere to the atmosphere by the direct decomposition of dead organisms or by the reduction of nitrates and nitrites in the soil. Most changes in the nitrogen cycle occur as the result of bacterial action on one compound or another. Other cycles do not require the intervention of **bacteria**. In the sulfur cycle, for example, sulfur dioxide in the atmosphere can react directly with compounds in the earth to make new sulfur compounds that become part of the lithosphere. Those compounds can then be transferred directly to the biosphere by plants growing in the earth.

Most cycles involve the transport of an element through all four parts of the planet—hydrosphere, atmosphere, lithosphere, and biosphere. The phosphorous cycle is an exception since phosphorus is essentially absent from the atmosphere. It does move from biosphere to the lithosphere (when organisms die and decay) to the hydrosphere (when phosphorous-containing compounds dissolve in water) and back to the biosphere (when plants incorporate phosphorus from water).

Hydrogen and oxygen tend to move together through the planet in the hydrologic cycle. Precipitation carries water from the atmosphere to the hydrosphere and lithosphere. It then becomes part of living organisms (the biosphere) before being returned to the atmosphere through **respiration**, transpiration, and evaporation.

All biogeochemical cycles are affected by human activities. As fossil fuels are burned, for example, the transfer of carbon from a very old reserve (decayed plants and animals buried in the earth) to a new one (the atmosphere, as carbon dioxide) is accelerated. The long-term impact of this form of human activity on the global environment, as well as that of other forms, is not yet known. Some scientists assert, however, that those affects can be profound, resulting in significant climate changes far into the future.

See also Biodegradable substances; Carbon cycle in microorganisms; Composting, microbiological aspects; Economic uses and benefits of microorganisms; Evolution and evolutionary mechanisms; Evolutionary origin of bacteria and viruses; Nitrogen cycle in microorganisms; Oxygen cycle in microorganisms

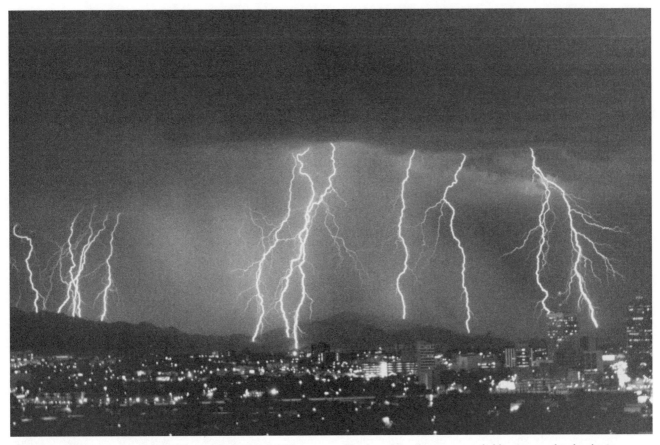

Under the proper conditions, physical phenomena such as lightning are capable of providing the energy needed for atoms and molecules to assemble into the fundamental building blocks of life.

BIOINFORMATICS AND COMPUTATIONAL BIOLOGY

Bioinformatics, or computational biology, refers to the development of new database methods to store genomic information, computational software programs, and methods to extract, process, and evaluate this information; it also refers to the refinement of existing techniques to acquire the genomic data. Finding genes and determining their function, predicting the structure of proteins and **RNA** sequences from the available **DNA** sequence, and determining the evolutionary relationship of proteins and DNA sequences are also part of bioinformatics.

The genome sequences of some **bacteria, yeast**, a nematode, the fruit fly *Drosophila* and several plants have been obtained during the past decade, with many more sequences nearing completion. During the year 2000, the sequencing of the human genome was completed. In addition to this accumulation of nucleotide sequence data, elucidation of the three-dimensional structure of proteins coded for by the genes has been accelerating. The result is a vast ever-increasing amount of databases and genetic information The efficient and productive use of this information requires the specialized computational techniques and software. Bioinformatics has developed and grown from the need to extract and analyze the reams of information pertaining to genomic information like nucleotide sequences and protein structure.

Bioinformatics utilizes statistical analysis, stepwise computational analysis and database management tools in order to search databases of DNA or protein sequences to filter out background from useful data and enable comparison of data from diverse databases. This sort of analysis is on-going. The exploding number of databases, and the various experimental methods used to acquire the data, can make comparisons tedious to achieve. However, the benefits can be enormous. The immense size and network of biological databases provides a resource to answer biological questions about mapping, **gene** expression patterns, molecular modeling, molecular **evolution**, and to assist in the structural-based design of therapeutic drugs.

Obtaining information is a multi-step process. Databases are examined, or browsed, by posing complex computational questions. Researchers who have derived a DNA or protein sequence can submit the sequence to public repositories of such information to see if there is a match or similarity with their sequence. If so, further analysis may reveal a putative structure for the protein coded for by the sequence as well as a putative function for that protein. Four primary databases, those containing one type of information (only DNA sequence data or only protein sequence data), currently available for these purposes are the European **Molecular Biology** DNA Sequence Database (EMBL), GenBank, SwissProt and the Protein Identification Resource (PIR). Secondary databases contain information derived from other databases. Specialist databases, or knowledge databases, are collections of sequence information, expert commentary and reference literature. Finally, integrated databases are collections (amalgamations) of primary and secondary databases.

The area of bioinformatics concerned with the derivation of protein sequences makes it conceivable to predict three-dimensional structures of the protein molecules, by use of computer graphics and by comparison with similar proteins, which have been obtained as a crystal. Knowledge of structure allows the site(s) critical for the function of the protein to be determined. Subsequently, drugs active against the site can be designed, or the protein can be utilized to enhanced commercial production processes, such as in pharmaceutical bioinformatics.

Bioinformatics also encompasses the field of comparative genomics. This is the comparison of functionally equivalent genes across species. A yeast gene is likely to have the same function as a worm protein with the same amino acid. Alternately, genes having similar sequence may have divergent functions. Such similarities and differences will be revealed by the sequence information. Practically, such knowledge aids in the **selection** and design of genes to instill a specific function in a product to enhance its commercial appeal.

The most widely known example of a bioinformatics driven endeavor is the Human Genome Project. It was initiated in 1990 under the direction of the National Center for Human Genome Research with the goal of sequencing the entire human genome. While this has now been accomplished, the larger aim of determining the function of each of the approximately 50,000 genes in the human genome will require much further time and effort. Work related to the Human Genome Project has allowed dramatic improvements in molecular biological techniques and improved computational tools for studying genomic function.

See also Hazard Analysis and Critical Point Program (HAACP); Immunological analysis techniques; The Institute for Genomic Research (TIGR); Medical training and careers in microbiology; Transplantation genetics and immunology

BIOLOGICAL WARFARE

Biological warfare, as defined by The United Nations, is the use of any living organism (e.g. bacterium, virus) or an infective component (e.g., toxin), to cause disease or death in humans, animals, or plants. In contrast to **bioterrorism**, biological warfare is defined as the "state-sanctioned" use of biological weapons on an opposing military force or civilian population.

Biological weapons include **viruses**, **bacteria**, **rickettsia**, and biological toxins. Of particular concern are genetically altered **microorganisms**, whose effect can be made to be group-specific. In other words, persons with particular traits are susceptible to these microorganisms.

The use of biological weapons by armies has been a reality for centuries. For example, in ancient records of battles exist the documented use of diseased bodies and cattle that had died of microbial diseases to poison wells. There are even records that infected bodies or carcasses were catapulted into cities under siege.

In the earliest years of the twentieth century, however, weapons of biological warfare were specifically developed by modern methods, refined, and stockpiled by various governments.

During World War I, Germany developed a biological warfare program based on the **anthrax** bacillus (*Bacillus anthracis*) and a strain of *Pseudomonas* known as *Burkholderia mallei*. The latter is also the cause of Glanders disease in cattle.

Allied efforts in Canada, the United States, and Britain to develop anthrax-based weapons were also active in World War II During World War II, Britain actually produced five million anthrax cakes at the U.K. Chemical and Biological Defense Establishment at Porton Down facility that were intended to be dropped on Germany to infect the food chain. The weapons were never used. Against their will, prisoners in German Nazi concentration camps were maliciously infected with pathogens, such as **hepatitis** A, *Plasmodia* spp., and two types of *Rickettsia* bacteria, during studies allegedly designed to develop vaccines and antibacterial drugs. Japan also conducted extensive biological weapon research during World War II in occupied Manchuria, China. Unwilling prisoners were infected with a variety of pathogens, including *Neisseria meningitis*, *Bacillus anthracis*, *Shigella spp*, and *Yersinia pestis*. It has been estimated that over 10,000 prisoners died as a result of either infection or execution following infection. In addition, biological agents contaminated the water supply and some food items, and an estimated 15 million potentially plague-infected fleas were released from aircraft, affecting many Chinese cities. However, as the Japanese military found out, biological weapons have fundamental disadvantages: they are unpredictable and difficult to control. After infectious agents were let loose in China by the Japanese, approximately 10,000 illnesses and 1,700 deaths were estimated to have occurred among Japanese troops.

A particularly relevant example of a microorganism used in biological warfare is *Bacillus anthracis*. This bacterium causes anthrax. *Bacillus anthracis* can live as a vegetative cell, growing and dividing as bacteria normally do. The organism has also evolved the ability to withstand potentially lethal environmental conditions by forming a near-dormant, highly resistant form known as a spore. The spore is designed to hibernate until conditions are conducive for growth and reproduction. Then, the spore resuscitates and active metabolic life resumes. The spore form can be easily inhaled to produce a highly lethal inhalation anthrax. The spores quickly and easily resuscitate in the warm and humid conditions of the lung. Contact with spores can also produce a less lethal but dangerous cutaneous anthrax infection.

One of the "attractive" aspects of anthrax as a weapon of biological warfare is its ability to be dispersed over the enemy by air. Other biological weapons also have this capacity. The dangers of an airborne release of bioweapons are well documented. British open-air testing of anthrax weapons in 1941 on Gruinard Island in Scotland rendered the island inhabitable for five decades. The US Army conducted a study in 1951-52 called "Operation Sea Spray" to study wind currents that might carry biological weapons. As part of the project design, balloons were filled with *Serratia marcescens* (then thought to be harmless) and exploded over San Francisco. Shortly thereafter, there was a corresponding dramatic increase in reported **pneumonia** and urinary tract infections. And, in 1979, an accidental release of anthrax spores, a gram at most and only for several minutes, occurred at a bioweapons facility near the Russian city of Sverdlovsk. At least 77 people were sickened and 66 died. All the affected were some 4 kilometers downwind of the facility. Sheep and cattle up to 50 kilometers downwind became ill.

The first diplomatic effort to limit biological warfare was the Geneva Protocol for the Prohibition of the Use in War of Asphyxiating, Poisonous or Other Gases, and of Bacteriological Methods of Warfare. This treaty, ratified in 1925, prohibited the use of biological weapons. The treaty has not been effective. For example, during the "Cold War" between the United States and the then Soviet Union in the 1950s and 1960s, the United States constructed research facilities to develop antisera, vaccines, and equipment for protection against a possible biological attack. As well, the use of microorganisms as offensive weapons was actively investigated.

Since then, other initiatives to ban the use of biological warfare and to destroy the stockpiles of biological weapons have been attempted. For example, in 1972 more than 100 countries, including the United States, signed the Convention on the Prohibition of the Development Production, and the Stockpiling of Bacteriological (Biological) and Toxin Weapons and on Their Destruction. Although the United States formally stopped biological weapons research in 1969 (by executive order of then President Richard M. Nixon), the Soviet Union carried on biological weapons research until its demise. Despite the international prohibitions, the existence of biological weapons remains dangerous reality.

See also Anthrax, terrorist use of as a biological weapon; Bacteria and bacterial infection; Bioterrorism, protective measures; Bioterrorism; Infection and resistance; Viruses and response to viral infection

BIOLOGICAL WEAPONS CONVENTION (BWC)

The Biological Weapons Convention (more properly but less widely known as The Biological and Toxin Weapons Convention) is an international agreement that prohibits the development and stockpiling of biological weapons. The language of the Biological Weapons Convention (BWC) describes biological weapons as "repugnant to the conscience of mankind." Formulated in 1972, the treaty has been signed (as of June 2002) by more than 159 countries; 141 countries have formally ratified the BWC.

The BWC broadly prohibits the development of pathogens—disease-causing **microorganisms** such as **viruses** and bacteria—and biological toxins that do not have established prophylactic merit (i.e., no ability to serve a protective immunological role), beneficial industrial use, or use in medical treatment.

The United States renounced the first-use of biological weapons and restricted future weapons research programs to issues concerning defensive responses (e.g., **immunization**, detection, etc.), by executive order in 1969.

Although the BWC disarmament provisions stipulated that biological weapons stockpiles were to have been destroyed by 1975, most Western intelligence agencies openly question whether all stockpiles have been destroyed. Despite the fact that it was a signatory party to the 1972 Biological and Toxin Weapons Convention, the former Soviet Union maintained a well-funded and high-intensity biological weapons program throughout the 1970s and 1980s, producing and stockpiling biological weapons including **anthrax** and **smallpox** agents. US intelligence agencies openly raise doubt as to whether successor Russian biological weapons programs have been completely dismantled. In June 2002, traces of biological and chemical weapon agents were found in Uzbekistan on a military base used by U.S. troops fighting in Afghanistan. Early analysis dates and attributes the source of the **contamination** to former Soviet Union or successor Russian biological and chemical weapons programs that utilized the base.

As of 2002, intelligence estimates compiled from various agencies provide indications that more than two dozen countries are actively involved in the development of biological weapons. The US Office of Technology Assessment and the United States Department of State have identified a list of potential enemy states developing biological weapons. Such potentially hostile nations include Iran, Iraq, Libya, Syria, North Korea, and China.

The BWC prohibits the offensive weaponization of biological agents (e.g., anthrax spores). The BWC also prohibits the **transformation** of biological agents with established legitimate and sanctioned purposes into agents of a nature and quality that could be used to effectively induce illness or death. In addition to offensive weaponization of microorganisms or toxins, prohibited research procedures include concentrating a strain of bacterium or virus, altering the size of aggregations of potentially harmful biologic agents (e.g., refining anthrax spore sizes to spore sizes small enough to be effectively and widely carried in air currents), producing strains capable of withstanding normally adverse environmental conditions (e.g., disbursement weapons blast), and the manipulation of a number of other factors that make biologic agents effective weapons.

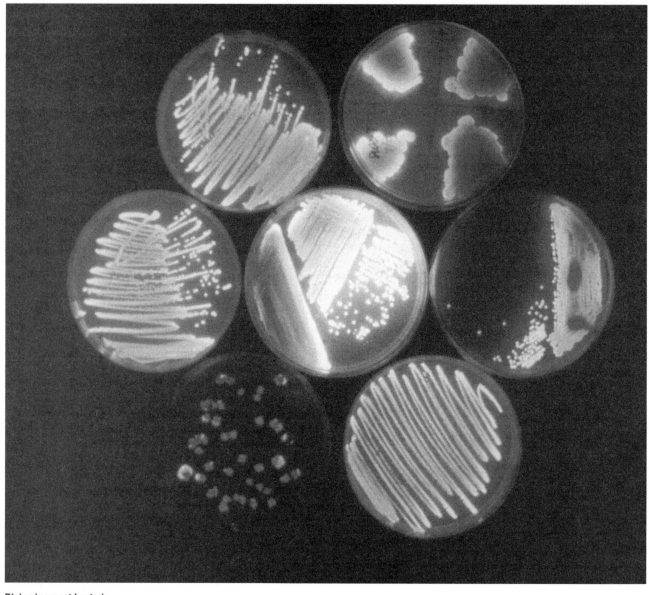

Bioluminescent bacteria.

Although there have been several international meetings designed to strengthen the implementation and monitoring of BWC provisions, BWC verification procedures are currently the responsibility of an ad hoc commission of scientists. Broad international efforts to coordinate and strengthen enforcement of BWC provisions remains elusive.

See also Anthrax, terrorist use of as a biological weapon; Bacteria and bacterial infection; Biological warfare; Epidemics and pandemics; Vaccine

BIOLOGY, CENTRAL DOGMA OF · *see*

MOLECULAR BIOLOGY AND MOLECULAR GENETICS

BIOLUMINESCENCE

Bioluminescence is the production of light by living organisms. Some single-celled organisms (**bacteria** and protista) as well as many multicellular animals and **fungi** demonstrate bioluminescence.

Light is produced by most bioluminescent organisms when a chemical called luciferin reacts with oxygen to produce light and oxyluciferin. The reaction between luciferin and oxygen is catalyzed by the enzyme luciferase. Luciferases, like luciferins, usually have different chemical structures in different organisms. In addition to luciferin, oxygen, and luciferase, other molecules (called cofactors) must be present for the bioluminescent reaction to proceed. Cofactors are molecules required by an enzyme (in this case luciferase) to perform its catalytic function. Common cofactors required for bioluminescent reactions are calcium and ATP, a molecule used to store and release energy that is found in all organisms.

The terms luciferin and luciferase were first introduced in 1885. The German scientist Emil du Bois-Reymond obtained two different extracts from bioluminescent clams and beetles. When Dubois mixed these extracts they produced light. He also found that if one of these extracts was first heated, no light would be produced upon mixing. Heating the other extract had no effect on the reaction, so Dubois concluded that there were at least two components to the reaction. Dubois hypothesized that the heat-resistant chemical undergoes a chemical change during the reaction, and called this compound luciferin. The heat sensitive chemical, Dubois concluded, was an enzyme which he called luciferase.

The two basic components needed to produce a bioluminescent reaction, luciferin and luciferase, can be isolated from the organisms that produce them. When they are mixed in the presence of oxygen and the appropriate cofactors, these components will produce light with an intensity dependent on the quantity of luciferin and luciferase added, as well as the oxygen and cofactor concentrations. Luciferases isolated from fireflies and other beetles are commonly used in research.

Scientists have used isolated luciferin and luciferase to determine the concentrations of important biological molecules such as ATP and calcium. After adding a known amount of luciferin and luciferase to a blood or tissue sample, the cofactor concentrations may be determined from the intensity of the light emitted. Scientists have also found numerous other uses for the bioluminescent reaction such as using it to quantify specific molecules that do not directly participate in the bioluminescence reaction. To do this, scientists attach luciferase to antibodies—molecules produced by the **immune system** that bind to specific molecules called antigens. The antibody-luciferase complex is added to a sample where it binds to the molecule to be quantified. Following washing to remove unbound antibodies, the molecule of interest can be quantified indirectly by adding luciferin and measuring the light emitted. Methods used to quantify particular compounds in biological samples such as the ones described here are called assays.

In recent studies, luciferase has been used to study viral and bacterial infections in living animals and to detect bacterial contaminants in food. The luciferase reaction also is used to determine **DNA** sequences, the order of the four types of molecules that comprise DNA and code for proteins.

Luciferase is often used as a "reporter gene" to study how individual genes are activated to produce protein or repressed to stop producing protein. Most genes are turned on and off by DNA located in front of the part of the **gene** that codes for protein. This region is called the gene promoter. A specific gene promoter can be attached to the DNA that codes for firefly luciferase and introduced into an organism. The activity of the gene promoter can then be studied by measuring the bioluminescence produced in the luciferase reaction. Thus, the luciferase gene can be used to "report" the activity of a promoter for another gene.

Bioluminescent organisms in the terrestrial environment include species of fungi and insects. The most familiar of these is the firefly, which can often be seen glowing during the warm summer months. In some instances organisms use bioluminescence to communicate, such as in fireflies, which use light to attract members of the opposite sex. Marine environments support a number of bioluminescent organisms including species of bacteria, **dinoflagellates**, jellyfish, coral, shrimp, and fish. On any given night one can see the luminescent sparkle produced by the single-celled dinoflagellates when water is disturbed by a ship's bow or a swimmer's motions.

See also Antibiotic resistance, tests for; Biotechnology; Food safety; Immunoflorescence; Microbial genetics

BIOREMEDIATION

Bioremediation is the use of living organisms or ecological processes to deal with a given environmental problem. The most common use of bioremediation is the metabolic breakdown or removal of toxic chemicals before or after they have been discharged into the environment. This process takes advantage of the fact that certain **microorganisms** can utilize toxic chemicals as metabolic substrates and render them into less toxic compounds. Bioremediation is a relatively new and actively developing technology. Increasingly, microorganisms and plants are being genetically engineered to aide in their ability to remove deleterious substances.

In general, bioremediation methodologies focus on one of two approaches. The first approach, bioaugmentation, aims to increase the abundance of certain species or groups of microorganisms that can metabolize toxic chemicals. Bioaugmentation involves the deliberate addition of strains or species of microorganisms that are effective at treating particular toxic chemicals, but are not indigenous to or abundant in the treatment area. Alternatively, environmental conditions may be altered in order to enhance the actions of such organisms that are already present in the environment. This process is known as biostimulation and usually involves fertilization, aeration, or irrigation. Biostimulation focuses on rapidly increasing the abundance of naturally occurring microorganisms capable of dealing with certain types of environmental problems.

Accidental spills of petroleum or other hydrocarbons on land and water are regrettable but frequent occurrences. Once spilled, petroleum and its various refined products can be persistent environmental contaminants. However, these organic chemicals can also be metabolized by certain microorganisms, whose processes transform the toxins into more simple compounds, such as carbon dioxide, water, and other inorganic chemicals. In the past, concentrates of **bacteria** that are highly efficient at metabolizing hydrocarbons have been "seeded" into spill areas in an attempt to increase the rate of degradation of the spill residues. Although this technique has occasionally been effective, it commonly fails because the large concentrations of hydrocarbons stimulates rapid growth of indigenous microorganisms also capable of utilizing hydrocarbons as metabolic substrates. Consequently, seeding of microorgan-

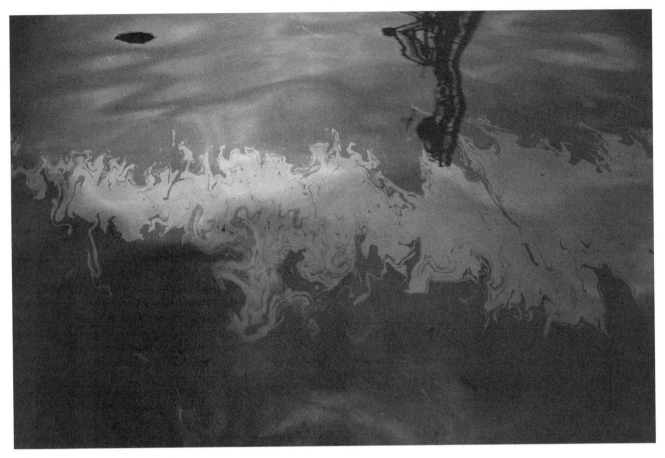

An oil spill. The oil does not mix with the water.

isms that are metabolically specific to hydrocarbons often does not affect the overall rate of degradation.

Environmental conditions under which spill residues occur are often sub-optimal for toxin degradation by microorganisms. Most commonly the rate is limited by the availability of oxygen or of certain nutrients such as nitrate and phosphate. Therefore the microbial breakdown of spilled hydrocarbons on land can be greatly enhanced by aeration and fertilization of the soil.

Metals are common pollutants of water and land because they are emitted by many industrial, agricultural, and domestic sources. In some situations organisms can be utilized to concentrate metals that are dispersed in the environment. For example, metal-polluted waste waters can be treated by encouraging the vigorous growth of certain types of vascular plants. This bioremediation system, also known as phytoremediation, works because the growing plants accumulate high levels of metals in their shoots, thereby reducing the concentration in the water to a more tolerable range. The plants can then be harvested to remove the metals from the system.

Many advanced sewage-treatment technologies utilize microbial processes to oxidize organic matter associated with fecal wastes and to decrease concentrations of soluble compounds or ions of metals, pesticides, and other toxic chemicals. Decreasing the aqueous concentrations of toxic chemicals is accomplished by a combination of chemical adsorption as well as microbial biodegradation of complex chemicals into their inorganic constituents.

If successful, bioremediation of contaminated sites can offer a cheaper, less environmentally damaging alternative to traditional clean-up technologies.

See also Economic uses and benefits of microorganisms; Microbial genetics; Waste water treatment; Water purification; Water quality

BIOTECHNOLOGY

The word biotechnology was coined in 1919 by Karl Ereky to apply to the interaction of biology with human technology. Today, it comes to mean a broad range of technologies from genetic engineering (recombinant **DNA** techniques), to animal breeding and industrial **fermentation**. Accurately, biotechnology is defined as the integrated use of **biochemistry**, microbiology, and engineering sciences in order to achieve technological (industrial) application of the capabilities of **microorganisms**, cultured tissue cells, and parts thereof.

The nature of biotechnology has undergone a dramatic change in the last half century. Modern biotechnology is greatly based on recent developments in **molecular biology**, especially those in genetic engineering. Organisms from **bacteria** to cows are being genetically modified to produce pharmaceuticals and foods. Also, new methods of disease **gene** isolation, analysis, and detection, as well as gene therapy, promise to revolutionize medicine.

In theory, the steps involved in genetic engineering are relatively simple. First, scientists decide the changes to be made in a specific DNA molecule. It is desirable in some cases to alter a human DNA molecule to correct errors that result in a disease such as diabetes. In other cases, researchers might add instructions to a DNA molecule that it does not normally carry: instructions for the manufacture of a chemical such as insulin, for example, in the DNA of bacteria that normally lack the ability to make insulin. Scientists also modify existing DNA to correct errors or add new information. Such methods are now well developed. Finally, scientists look for a way to put the recombinant DNA molecule into the organisms in which it is to function. Once inside the organism, the new DNA molecule give correct instructions to cells in humans to correct genetic disorders, in bacteria (resulting in the production of new chemicals), or in other types of cells for other purposes.

Genetic engineering has resulted in a number of impressive accomplishments. Dozens of products that were once available only from natural sources and in limited amounts are now manufactured in abundance by genetically engineered microorganisms at relatively low cost. Insulin, human growth hormone, tissue plasminogen activator, and alpha interferon are examples. In addition, the first trials with the alteration of human DNA to cure a genetic disorder began in 1991.

Molecular geneticists use molecular **cloning** techniques on a daily basis to replicate various genetic materials such as gene segments and cells. The process of molecular cloning involves isolating a DNA sequence of interest and obtaining multiple copies of it in an organism that is capable of growth over extended periods. Large quantities of the DNA molecule can then be isolated in pure form for detailed molecular analysis. The ability to generate virtually endless copies (clones) of a particular sequence is the basis of recombinant DNA technology and its application to human and medical genetics.

A technique called positional cloning is used to map the location of a human disease gene. Positional cloning is a relatively new approach to finding genes. A particular DNA marker is linked to the disease if, in general, family members with certain nucleotides at the marker always have the disease, and family members with other nucleotides at the marker do not have the disease. Once a suspected linkage result is confirmed, researchers can then test other markers known to map close to the one found, in an attempt to move closer and closer to the disease gene of interest. The gene can then be cloned if the DNA sequence has the characteristics of a gene and it can be shown that particular **mutations** in the gene confer disease.

Embryo cloning is another example of genetic engineering. Agricultural scientists are experimenting with embryo cloning processes with animal embryos to improve upon and increase the production of livestock. The first successful attempt at producing live animals by embryo cloning was reported by a research group in Scotland on March 6, 1997.

Although genetic engineering is a very important component of biotechnology, it is not alone. Biotechnology has been used by humans for thousands of years. Some of the oldest manufacturing processes known to humankind make use of biotechnology. Beer, wine, and bread making, for example, all occur because of the process of fermentation. As early as the seventeenth century, bacteria were used to remove copper from its ores. Around 1910, scientists found that bacteria could be used to decompose organic matter in sewage. A method that uses microorganisms to produce glycerol synthetically proved very important in the World War I since glycerol is essential to the manufacture of explosives.

See also Fermentation; Immune complex test; Immunoelectrophoresis; Immunofluorescence; Immunogenetics; Immunologic therapies; Immunological analysis techniques; Immunosuppressant drugs; *In vitro* and *in vivo* research

BIOTERRORISM

Bioterrorism is the use of a biological weapon against a civilian population. As with any form of terrorism, its purposes include the undermining of morale, creating chaos, or achieving political goals. Biological weapons use **microorganisms** and toxins to produce disease and death in humans, livestock, and crops.

Biological, chemical, and nuclear weapons can all be used to achieve similar destructive goals, but unlike chemical and nuclear technologies that are expensive to create, biological weapons are relatively inexpensive. They are easy to transport and resist detection by standard security systems. In general, chemical weapons act acutely, causing illness in minutes to hours at the scene of release. For example, the release of sarin gas by the religious sect Aum Shinrikyo in the Tokyo subway in 1995 killed 12 and hospitalized 5,000 people. In contrast, the damage from biological weapons may not become evident until weeks after an attack. If the pathogenic (disease-causing) agent is transmissible, a bioterrorist attack could eventually kill thousands over a much larger area than the initial area of attack.

Bioterrorism can also be enigmatic, destructive, and costly even when targeted at a relatively few number of individuals. Starting in September 2001, bioterrorist attacks with anthrax-causing **bacteria** distributed through the mail targeted only a few U.S. government leaders, media representatives, and seemingly random private citizens. As of June 2002, these attacks remain unsolved. Regardless, in addition to the tragic deaths of five people, the terrorist attacks cost the United States millions of dollars and caused widespread concern. These attacks also exemplified the fact that bioterrorism can strike at the political and economic infrastructure of a targeted country.

Although the deliberate production and stockpiling of biological weapons is prohibited by the 1972 **Biological Weapons Convention** (BWC)—the United States stopped for-

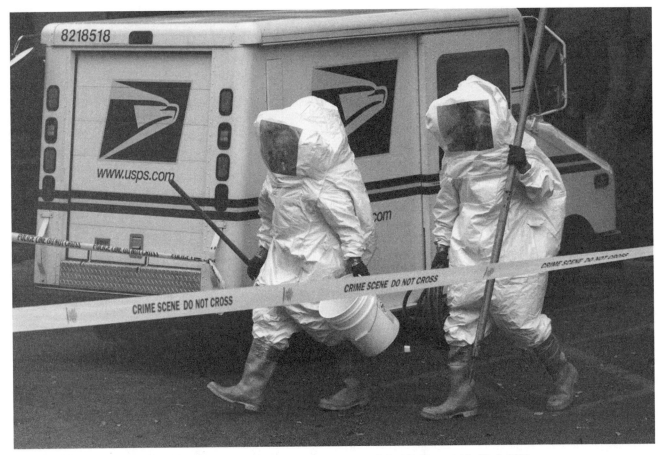

A decontamination crew responds to a possible release of anthrax by terrorists at a United States postal facility in 2001.

mal bioweapons programs in 1969—unintended byproducts or deliberate misuse of emerging technologies offer potential bioterrorists opportunities to prepare or refine biogenic weapons. Genetic engineering technologies can be used to produce a wide variety of bioweapons, including organisms that produce toxins or that are more weaponizable because they are easier to aerosolize (suspend as droplets in the air). More conventional laboratory technologies can also produce organisms resistant to **antibiotics**, routine vaccines, and therapeutics. Both technologies can produce organisms that cannot be detected by antibody-based sensor systems.

Among the most serious of potential bioterrorist weapons are those that use **smallpox** (caused by the **Variola virus**), **anthrax** (caused by *Bacillus anthracis*), and plague (caused by *Yersinia pestis*). During naturally occurring **epidemics** throughout the ages, these organisms have killed significant portions of afflicted populations. With the advent of vaccines and antibiotics, few U.S. physicians now have the experience to readily recognize these diseases, any of which could cause catastrophic numbers of deaths.

Although the last case of smallpox was reported in Somalia in 1977, experts suspect that smallpox **viruses** may be in the biowarfare laboratories of many nations around the world. At present, only two facilities—one in the United States and one in Russia—are authorized to store the virus. As

recently as 1992, United States intelligence agencies learned that Russia had the ability to launch missiles containing weapons-grade smallpox at major cities in the U.S. A number of terrorist organizations—including the radical Islamist Al Qaeda terrorist organization—actively seek the acquisition of state-sponsored research into weapons technology and pathogens.

There are many reasons behind the spread of biowarfare technology. Prominent among them are economic incentives; some governments may resort to selling bits of scientific information that can be pieced together by the buyer to create biological weapons. In addition, scientists in politically repressive or unstable countries may be forced to participate in research that eventually ends up in the hands of terrorists.

A biological weapon may ultimately prove more powerful than a conventional weapon because its effects can be far-reaching and uncontrollable. In 1979, after an accident involving *B. anthracis* in the Soviet Union, doctors reported civilians dying of anthrax **pneumonia** (i.e., inhalation anthrax). Death from anthrax pneumonia is usually swift. The bacilli multiply rapidly and produce a toxin that causes breathing to stop. While antibiotics can combat this bacillus, supplies adequate to meet the treatment needs following an attack on a large urban population would need to be delivered and distributed within 24 to 48 hours of exposure. The National Pharmaceutical Stockpile Program (NPS) is designed to enable such a response to a bioterrorist attack.

Preparing a strategy to defend against these types of organisms, whether in a natural or genetically modified state, is difficult. Some of the strategies include the use of bacterial **RNA** based on structural templates to identify pathogens; increased abilities for rapid **genetic identification of microorganisms**; developing a database of virtual pathogenic molecules; and development of antibacterial molecules that attach to pathogens but do not harm humans or animals. Each of these is an attempt to increase—and make more flexible—identification capabilities.

Researchers are also working to counter potential attacks using several innovative technological strategies. For example, promising research is being done with biorobots or microchip-mechanized insects, which have computerized artificial systems that mimic biological processes such as neural networks, can test responses to substances of biological or chemical origin. These insects can, in a single operation, process **DNA**, screen blood samples, scan for disease genes, and monitor genetic cell activity. The robotics program of the Defense Advanced Research Project (DARPA) works to rapidly identify bio-responses to pathogens, and to design effective and rapid treatment methods.

Biosensor technology is the driving force in the development of biochips for detection of biological and chemical contaminants. Bees, beetles, and other insects outfitted with sensors are used to collect real-time information about the presence of toxins or similar threats. Using fiber optics or electrochemical devices, biosensors have detected microorganisms in chemicals and foods, and they offer the promise of rapid identification of biogenic agents following a bioterrorist attack. The early accurate identification of biogenic agents is critical to implementing effective response and treatment protocols.

To combat biological agents, bioindustries are developing a wide range of antibiotics and vaccines. In addition, advances in **bioinformatics** (i.e., the computerization of information acquired during, for example, genetic screening) also increases flexibility in the development of effective counters to biogenic weapons.

In addition to detecting and neutralizing attempts to weaponize biogenic agents (i.e., attempts to develop bombs or other instruments that could effectively disburse a bacterium or virus), the major problem in developing effective counter strategies to bioterrorist attacks involves the breadth of organisms used in **biological warfare**. For example, researchers are analyzing many pathogens in an effort to identify common genetic and cellular components. One strategy is to look for common areas or vulnerabilities in specific sites of DNA, RNA, or proteins. Regardless of whether the pathogens evolve naturally or are engineered, the identification of common traits will assist in developing counter measures (i.e., specific vaccines or antibiotics).

See also Anthrax, terrorist use of as a biological weapon; Biological warfare; Contamination, bacterial and viral; Genetic identification of microorganisms; Public health, current issues

BIOTERRORISM, IDENTIFICATION OF MICROORGANISMS • *see* GENETIC IDENTIFICATION OF MICROORGANISMS

BIOTERRORISM, PROTECTIVE MEASURES

In the aftermath of the September 11, 2001 terrorist attacks on the United States and the subsequent anthrax attacks on U.S. government officials, media representatives, and citizens, the development of measures to protect against biological terrorism became an urgent and contentious issue of public debate. Although the desire to increase readiness and response capabilities to possible nuclear, chemical, and biological attacks is widespread, consensus on which preventative measures to undertake remains elusive.

The evolution of political realities in the last half of the twentieth century and events of 2001 suggest that, within the first half of the twenty-first century, biological weapons will surpass nuclear and chemical weapons as a threat to the citizens of the United States.

Although a range of protective options exists—from the stockpiling of **antibiotics** to the full-scale resumption of biological weapons programs—no single solution provides comprehensive protection to the complex array of potential biological agents that might be used as terrorist weapons. Many scientists argue, therefore, that focusing on one specific set of protective measures (e.g., broadly inoculating the public against the virus causing **smallpox**) might actually lower overall preparedness and that a key protective measure entails upgrading fundamental research capabilities.

The array of protective measures against **bioterrorism** are divided into strategic, tactical, and personal measures.

Late in 2001, the United States and its NATO (North Atlantic Treaty Organization) allies reaffirmed treaty commitments that stipulate the use of any weapon of mass destruction (i.e., biological, chemical, or nuclear weapons) against any member state would be interpreted as an attack against all treaty partners. As of June 2002, this increased strategic deterrence was directed at Iraq and other states that might seek to develop or use biological weapons—or to harbor or aid terrorists seeking to develop weapons of mass destruction. At the tactical level, the United States possesses a vast arsenal of weapons designed to detect and eliminate potential biological weapons. Among the tactical non-nuclear options is the use of precision-guided conventional thermal fuel-air bombs capable of destroying both biological research facilities and biologic agents.

Because terrorist operations are elusive, these large-scale military responses offer protection against only the largest, identifiable, and targetable enemies. They are largely ineffective against small, isolated, and dispersed "cells" of hostile forces, which operate domestically or within the borders of other nations. When laboratories capable of producing low-grade weaponizable anthrax-causing spores can be established in the basement of a typical house for less than $10,000,

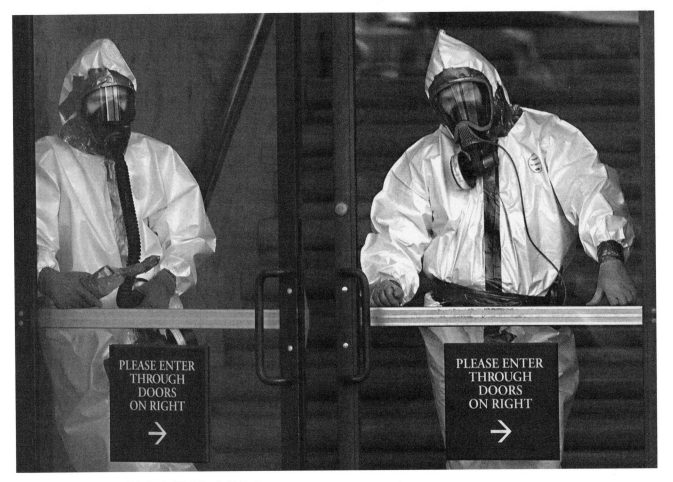

Bioterrorist attack on the U.S. Capitol Building in 2001.

the limitations of full-scale military operations become apparent.

Many scientists and physicians argue that the most extreme of potential military responses, the formal resumption of biological weapons programs—even with a limited goal of enhancing understanding of potential biological agents and weapons delivery mechanisms—is unneeded and possibly detrimental to the development of effective protective measures. Not only would such a resumption be a violation of the **Biological Weapons Convention** to which the United States is a signatory and which prohibits such research, opponents of such a resumption argue any such renewal of research on biological weapons will divert critical resources, obscure needed research, and spark a new global biological arms race.

Most scientific bodies, including the National Institutes of Health, **Centers for Disease Control** and Prevention, advocate a balanced scientific and medical response to the need to develop protective measures against biological attack. Such plans allow for the maximum flexibility in terms of effective response to a number of disease causing pathogens.

In addition to increased research, preparedness programs are designed to allow a rapid response to the terrorist use of biological weapons. One such program, the National

Pharmaceutical Stockpile Program (NPS) provides for a ready supply of antibiotics, vaccines, and other medical treatment countermeasures. The NPS stockpile is designed to be rapidly deployable to target areas. For example, in response to potential exposures to the *Bacillus anthracis* (the bacteria that causes anthrax) during the 2001 terrorist attacks, the United States government and some state agencies supplied Cipro, the antibiotic treatment of choice, to those potentially exposed to the bacterium. In addition to increasing funding for the NPS, additional funds have already been authorized to increase funding to train medical personnel in the early identification and treatment of disease caused by the most likely pathogens.

Despite this increased commitment to preparedness, medical exerts express near unanimity in doubting whether any series of programs or protocols can adequately provide comprehensive and effective protection to biological terrorism. Nonetheless, advocates of increased research capabilities argue that laboratory and hospital facilities must be expanded and improved to provide maximum scientific flexibility in the identification and response to biogenic threats. For example, the Centers for Disease Control and Prevention (CDC), based in Atlanta, Georgia, has established a bioterrorism response program that includes increased testing and treatment capacity. The CDC plan also calls for an increased emphasis on epidemiological detection and surveillance, along with the development of a public heath infrastructure capable of providing accurate information and treatment guidance to both medical professionals and the general public.

Because an informed and watchful public is key element in early detection of biological pathogens, the CDC openly identifies potential biological threats and publishes a list of those biological agents most likely to be used on its web pages. As of July 2002, the CDC identified approximately 36 microbes including **Ebola virus** variants and plague bacterium, that might be potentially used in a bioterrorist attack

Other protective and emergency response measures include the development of the CDC Rapid Response and Advanced Technology Laboratory, a Health Alert Network (HAN), National Electronic Data Surveillance System (NEDSS), and Epidemic Information Exchange (Epi-X) designed to coordinate information exchange in efforts to enhance early detection and identification of biological weapons.

Following the September 11, 2001 terrorist attacks on the United States, additional funds were quickly allocated to enhance the United States Department of Health and Human Services 1999 Bioterrorism Initiative. One of the key elements of the Bioterrorism Preparedness and Response Program (BPRP) increases the number and capacity of laboratory test facilities designed to identify pathogens and find effective countermeasures. In response to a call from the Bush administration, in December 2001, Congress more than doubled the previous funding for bioterrorism research.

Advances in effective therapeutic treatments are fundamentally dependent upon advances in the basic biology and pathological mechanisms of **microorganisms**. In response to terrorist attacks, in February 2002, the US National Institute of Allergy and Infectious Diseases (NIAID) established a group of experts to evaluate changes in research in order to effectively anticipate and counter potential terrorist threats. As a result, research into smallpox, anthrax, **botulism**, plague, **tularemia**, and viral **hemorrhagic fevers** is now given greater emphasis.

In addition to medical protective measures, a terrorist biological weapon attack could overburden medical infrastructure (e.g., cause an acute shortage of medical personnel and supplies) and cause economic havoc. It is also possible that an effective biological weapon could have no immediate effect upon humans, but could induce famine in livestock or ruin agricultural production. A number of former agreements between federal and state governments involving response planning will be subsumed by those of the Department of Homeland Security.

On a local level, cities and communities are encouraged to develop specific response procedures in the event of bioterrorism. Most hospitals are now required to have response plans in place as part of their accreditation requirements.

In addition to airborne and surface exposure, biologic agents may be disseminated in water supplies. Many communities have placed extra security on water supply and treatment facilities. The U.S. Environmental Protection Agency (EPA) has increased monitoring and working with local water suppliers to develop emergency response plans.

Although it is beyond the scope of this article to discuss specific personal protective measures—nor given the complexities and ever-changing threat would it be prudent to offer such specific medical advice—there are a number of general issues and measures that can be discussed. For example, the public has been specifically discouraged from buying often antiquated military surplus gas masks, because they can provide a false sense of protection. In addition to issues of potency decay, the hoarding of antibiotics has is also discouraged because inappropriate use can lead to the development of bacterial resistance and a consequential lowering of antibiotic effectiveness.

Generally, the public is urged to make provisions for a few days of food and water and to establish a safe room in homes and offices that can be temporarily sealed with duct tape to reduce outside air infiltration.

More specific response plans and protective measures are often based upon existing assessments of the danger posed by specific diseases and the organisms that produce the disease. For example, anthrax (*Bacillus anthracis*), botulism (*Clostridium botulinum* toxin), plague (*Yersinia pestis*), smallpox (*Variola major*), tularemia (*Francisella tularensis)*, and viral hemorrhagic fevers (e.g., Ebola, Marburg), and arenaviruses (e.g., Lassa) are considered high-risk and high-priority. Although these biogenic agents share the common attributes of being easily disseminated or transmitted and all can result in high mortality rates, the disease and their underlying microorganisms are fundamentally different and require different response procedures.

Two specific protective measures, smallpox and anthrax vaccines, remain highly controversial. CDC has adopted a position that, in the absence of a confirmed case of smallpox, the risks of resuming general smallpox **vaccination** far outweigh the potential benefits. In addition, **vaccine** is still maintained and could be used in the event of a bioterrorist emergency. CDC has also accelerated production of a smallpox vaccine. Moreover, vaccines delivered and injected during the incubation period for smallpox (approximately 12 days) convey at least some protection from the ravages of the disease.

Also controversial remains the safety and effectiveness of an anthrax vaccine used primarily by military personnel.

See also Anthrax, terrorist use of as a biological weapon; Bacteria and bacterial infection; Biological warfare; Epidemics and pandemics; Vaccine

BLACK DEATH • *see* BUBONIC PLAGUE

BLACK LIPID BILAYER MEMBRANE • *see* LABORATORY TECHNIQUES IN MICROBIOLOGY

BLACK SMOKER BACTERIA · *see*

EXTREMOPHILES

BLOOD AGAR, HEMOLYSIS, AND HEMOLYTIC REACTIONS

Blood **agar** is a solid growth medium that contains red blood cells. The medium is used to detect **bacteria** that produce **enzymes** to break apart the blood cells. This process is also termed hemolysis. The degree to which the blood cells are hemolyzed is used to distinguish bacteria from one another.

The blood agar medium is prepared in a two-step process. First, a number of ingredients are added to water, including heart infusion, peptone, and sodium chloride. This solution is sterilized. Following **sterilization**, a known amount of sterile blood is added. The blood can be from rabbit or sheep. Rabbit blood is preferred if the target bacterium is from the group known as group A *Streptococcus*. Sheep blood is preferred if the target bacterium is *Haemophilus parahaemolyticus*.

Blood agar is a rich food source for bacteria. So, it can be used for primary culturing, that is, as a means of obtaining as wide a range of **bacterial growth** from a sample as possible. It is typically not used for this purpose, however, due to the expense of the medium. Other, less expensive agars will do the same thing. What blood agar is uniquely suited for is the determination of hemolysis.

Hemolysis is the break down of the membrane of red blood cells by a bacterial protein known as hemolysin, which causes the release of hemoglobin from the red blood cell. Many types of bacterial posses hemolytic proteins. These proteins are thought to act by integrating into the membrane of the red blood cell and either punching a hole through the membrane or disrupting the structure of the membrane in some other way. The exact molecular details of hemolysin action is still unresolved.

The blood used in the agar is also treated beforehand to remove a molecule called fibrin, which participates in the clotting of blood. The absence of fibrin ensures that clotting of the blood does not occur in the agar, which could interfere with the visual detection of the hemolytic reactions.

There are three types of hemolysis, designated alpha, beta and gamma. Alpha hemolysis is a greenish discoloration that surrounds a bacterial **colony** growing on the agar. This type of hemolysis represents a partial decomposition of the hemoglobin of the red blood cells. Alpha hemolysis is characteristic of *Streptococcus pneumonia* and so can be used as a diagnostic feature in the identification of the bacterial strain.

Beta hemolysis represents a complete breakdown of the hemoglobin of the red blood cells in the vicinity of a bacterial colony. There is a clearing of the agar around a colony. Beta hemolysis is characteristic of *Streptococcus pyogenes* and some strains of*Staphylococcus aureus.*

The third type of hemolysis is actually no hemolysis at all. Gamma hemolysis is a lack of hemolysis in the area around a bacterial colony. A blood agar plate displaying

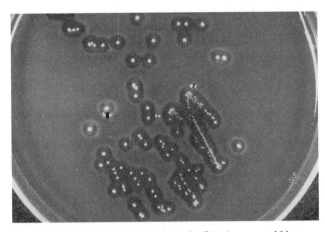

Beta hemolysis produced on blood agar by *Streptococcus viridans*.

gamma hemolysis actually appears brownish. This is a normal reaction of the blood to the growth conditions used (37° C in the presence of carbon dioxide). Gamma hemolysis is a characteristic of *Enterococcus faecalis*.

Hemolytic reactions can also display some synergy. That is, the combination of reactions produces a reaction that is stronger than either reaction alone. Certain species of bacteria, such as group B Strep (n example is *Streptococcus agalactiae*) are weakly beta-hemolytic. However, if the bacteria are in close proximity with a strain of Staphylococcus the beta-hemolysins of the two organisms can combine to produce an intense beta hemolytic reaction. This forms the basis of a test called the CAMP test (after the initials of its inventors).

The determination of hemolysis and of the hemolytic reactions is useful in distinguishing different types of bacteria. Subsequent biochemical testing can narrow down the identification even further. For example, a beta hemolytic reaction is indicative of a Streptococcus. Testing of the Streptococcus organisms with bacitracin is often the next step. Bacitracin is an antimicrobial that is produced by the bacterium *Bacillus subtilis*. *Streptococcus pyogenes* strains are almost uniformally sensitive to bacitracin. But other antigenic groups of Streptococcus are not bacitracin sensitive.

See also Laboratory techniques in microbiology; Staphylococci and staphylococcal infections; Streptococci and streptococcal infections

BLOOD BORNE INFECTIONS

Blood borne infections are those in which the infectious agent is transmitted from one person to another in contaminated blood. Infections of the blood can occur as a result of the spread of an ongoing infection, such as with **bacteria** including bacteria such as *Yersinia pestis, Haemophilus influenzae, Staphylococcus aureus*, and *Streptococcus pyogenes*. However, the latter re considered to be separate from true bloodborne infections.

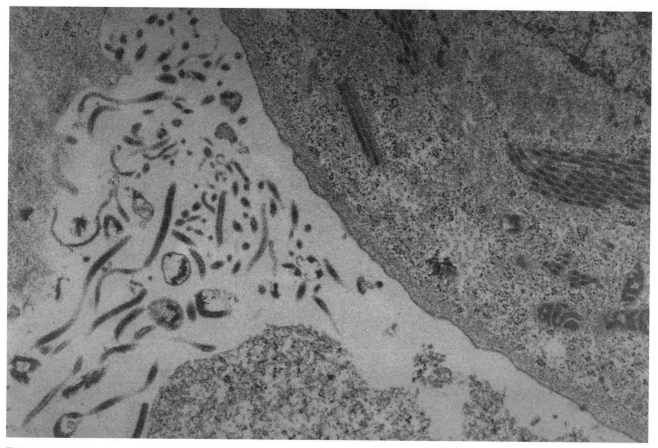

Thin section electron micrograph of Ebola virus.

Bacterial blood borne infection can occur, typically in the transfusion of blood. Such infections arise from the **contamination** of the site of transfusion. While information on the rate of such infections is scarce, the risk of transmission of bacterial infections via transfusions is thought to be at least equal to the risk of viral infection. For example, figures from the United States Food and Drug Administration indicate that bacterial infections comprise at least 10% of transfusion-related deaths in the United States each year.

Another route of entry for bacteria are catheters. For example, it has been estimated that the chances of acquiring a urinary tract infection (which can subsequently spread to the blood) rises by up to 10% for each day a hospitalized patient is catheterized.

While bacteria can be problematic in blood borne infections, the typical agents of concern in blood borne infections are **protozoa** and **viruses**. The protozoan *Trypanosoma brucei* is transmitted to humans by the bite of the tsetse fly. The subsequent infection of the blood and organs of the body produces **sleeping sickness**, al illness that still afflicts millions each year in the underdeveloped world.

With respect to viral blood borne diseases, **hepatitis** A, hepatitis C, and the **Human Immunodeficiency Virus** (**HIV**; the cause of acquired **immunodeficiency** syndrome) are the focus of scrutiny in blood donors and in the setting of a hospital. Exposure to the blood from an infected person or the sharing of needles among intravenous drug users can transmit these viruses from person to person. In Canada, the contamination of donated blood and blood products with the hepatitis viruses and HIV in the 1980s sickened thousands of people. As a result the system for blood donation and the monitoring guidelines for the blood and blood products was completely overhauled. For example, in the 1980s, monitoring for hepatitis C was in its infancy (then only a few agencies in the world tested blood for what was then termed "non-A, non-B hepatitis"). Since then, definitive tests for the hepatitis C virus at the nucleic acid level have been developed and put into routine use.

Within the past 20 years, emerging diseases such the lethal fever and tissue destruction caused by the **Ebola virus** have been important blood borne threats. These so-called **hemorrhagic fevers** may have become more prominent because of human encroachment onto formerly wild regions, particularly in Africa.

Health care workers are particularly at risk of acquiring a blood borne infection. Open wounds present an opportunity for blood to splatter on a cut or scratch of a doctor or nurse. Also, the use of needles presents a risk of accidental puncture of the skin to doctors, nurses and even to custodial workers responsible for collecting the debris of hospital care.

Another group particularly at risk of blood borne infections are hemophiliacs. The necessity of hemophiliacs to receive blood products that promote clotting leaves them vulnerable. For example, in the United States, some 20% of adult hemophiliacs are infected with HIV, about 56% are infected with the hepatitis B virus, and almost 90% are infected with the hepatitis C virus. HIV is the most common cause of death among hemophiliacs.

Other viruses pose a potential for blood borne transmission. Human herpesvirus 6 and 7, **Epstein-Barr virus** and cytomegalovirus require close contact between mucous membranes for person-to-person transfer. Abrasions in the genital area may allow for the transfer of the viruses in the blood. Parvovirus, which causes the rash known as fifth disease in children, can be transferred between adults in the blood. In adults, particularly women, the resulting infection can cause arthritis

At least in North America, the increasing urbanization is bringing people into closer contact with wildlife. This has resulted in an increase in the incidence of certain blood borne diseases that are transmitted by ticks. Mice, chipmunks, and deer are two reservoirs of *Borrelia burgdorferi*, the bacterium that causes **Lyme disease**. The increasing deer population over the past 35 years in the state of Connecticut has paralleled the increasing number of cases of Lyme disease, over 3,000 in 1996 alone.

Other blood borne disease transmitted by ticks includes Rocky Mountain Spotted Fever, human granulolytic ehrlichiosis, and babesiosis. While these diseases can ultimately affect various sites in the body, their origin is in the blood.

The institution of improved means of monitoring donated blood and blood products has lowered the number of cases of blood borne infections. However, similar success in the hospital or natural settings has not occurred, and likely will not. Avoidance of infected people and the wearing of appropriate garments (such as socks and long pants when walking in forested areas where ticks may be present) are the best strategies to avoid such blood borne infections at the present time.

See also AIDS; Hemorrhagic fevers and diseases; Transmission of pathogens

BLUE-GREEN ALGAE

Blue-green algae are actually a type of **bacteria** that is known as cyanobacteria. In their aquatic habitat, cyanobacteria are equipped to use the sun's energy to manufacture their own food through **photosynthesis**. The moniker blue-green algae came about because of the color, which was a by-product of the photosynthetic activity of the microbes, and their discovery as a algal-like scum on the surface of ponds. They were assumed to be algae until their identity as bacteria was determined.

Although the recognition of the bacterial nature of the microbe occurred recently, cyanobacteria are ancient. Fossils of cyanobacteria have been found that date back 3.5 billion years and are among the oldest fossils of any life from thus far discovered on Earth. These **microorganisms** must have developed very early following the establishment of land on Earth,

because the oldest known rocks are only slightly older at 3.8 billion years.

Modern day examples of cyanobacteria include *Nostoc*, *Oscillatoria*, *Spirulina*, *Microcystis*, and *Anabaena*

Cyanobacteria were monumentally important in shaping life on this planet. The oxygen atmosphere that supports human and other life was generated by cyanobacterial activity in the distant past. Many oil deposits that were laid down in the Proterozoic Era were due the activity of cyanobacteria. Another huge contribution of cyanobacteria is their role in the genesis of plants. The plant organelle known as a **chloroplast**, which the plant uses to manufacture food, is a remnant of a cyanobacterium that took up residence in a eukaryotic cell sometime in the Proterozoic or early Cambrian Era. The mitochondrion in eukaryotic cells also arose in this fashion.

The ability of cyanobacteria to photosynthetically utilize sunlight as an energy source is due to a pigment called phycocyanin. The microbes also contain the same **chlorophyll** a compound used by plants. Some blue-green algae possess a different photosynthetic pigment, which is known as phycoerythrin. This pigment imparts a red or pink color to the cells. An example is *Spirulina*. The pink color of African flamingos actually results, in part, from their ingestion of *Spirulina*.

Cyanobacteria tend to proliferate in very slow moving or still fresh water. Large populations can result very quickly, given the appropriate conditions of temperature and nutrient availability. This explosive growth is popularly referred to as a bloom. Accounts of blooms attributable to cyanobacteria date back to the twelfth century. The toxic capabilities of the organism have been known for over 100 years. Some species produce a toxin that can be released into the water upon the death of the microorganism. One of the cyanobacterial toxins is damaging to the liver, and so is designated a hepatotoxin. Another cyanobacterial toxin is damaging to cells of the nervous system, and so is a neurotoxin. Still other cyanobacterial toxins cause skin irritation.

A toxin of particular note is called microcystin. This toxin is produced by *Microcystis aeruginosa*. The microcystin toxin is the most common in water, likely because of its stability in this environment. One type of microcystin, which is designated microcystin-LR, is found in waters all over the world, and is a common cause of cyanobacterial poisoning of humans and animals.

At low levels, toxins such as microcystin produce more of an uncomfortable feeling than actual damage to the body. However, blue-green algae and their toxins can become concentrated in shallow, slow-moving bodies of water or in fish. Ingestion of the fish or accidental swallowing of the water while swimming can produce nausea, vomiting fever, and diarrhea. Eyes can also become irritated. These symptoms can be more exacerbated in children, because the toxin-to-body-weight ratio is higher in children than in adults. Liver damage can result in children exposed to the toxins.

In contrast to many other toxins, the cyanobacterial toxins can still remain potent after toxin-contaminated water has been boiled. Only the complete removal of the toxin from the water is an assurance of safety. Some success in the removal of toxins has been claimed by the use of charcoal and by techniques that oxidize the water.

Cyanobacteria are one of the few microorganisms that can convert inert atmospheric nitrogen into a usable form, such as nitrate or ammonia. For example, the cyanobacterium *Anabaena* co-exist with a type of fern called *Azolla*, where it supplies nitrogen to the plant. The production of rice has benefited from the fertilization capability of this bacterial-plant association. The cyanobacterium *Spirulina* is a popular, high protein food source.

See also Fossilization of bacteria; Photosynthetic microorganisms

BORDATELLA PERTUSSIS • *see* PERTUSSIS

BORDET, JULES (1870-1961)

Belgian physician

Jules Bordet's pioneering research made clear the exact manner by which serums and antiserums act to destroy **bacteria** and foreign blood cells in the body, thus explaining how human and animal bodies defend themselves against the invasion of foreign elements. Bordet was also responsible for developing **complement** fixation tests, which made possible the early detection of many disease-causing bacteria in human and animal blood. For his various discoveries in the field of **immunology**, Bordet was awarded the Nobel Prize for medicine or physiology in 1919.

Jules Jean Baptiste Vincent Bordet was born in Soignies, Belgium, a small town situated twenty-three miles southwest of Brussels. He was the second son of Charles Bordet, a schoolteacher, and Célestine Vandenabeele Bordet. The family moved to Brussels in 1874, when his father received an appointment to the École Moyenne, a primary school. Jules and his older brother Charles attended this school and then received their secondary education at the Athéné Royal of Brussels. It was at this time that Bordet became interested in chemistry and began working in a small laboratory that he constructed at home. He entered the medical program at the Free University of Brussels at the age of sixteen, receiving his doctorate of medicine in 1892. Bordet began his research career while still in medical school, and in 1892 published a paper on the adaptation of **viruses** to vaccinated organisms in the *Annales de l'Institut Pasteur* of Paris. For this work, the Belgian government awarded him a scholarship to the Pasteur Institute, and from 1894 to 1901, Bordet stayed in Paris at the laboratory of the Ukrainian-born scientist **Élie Metchnikoff**. In 1899, Bordet married Marthe Levoz; they eventually had two daughters, and a son who also became a medical scientist.

During his seven years at the Pasteur Institute, Bordet made most of the basic discoveries that led to his Nobel Prize of 1919. Soon after his arrival at the Institute, he began work on a problem in immunology. In 1894, Richard Pfeiffer, a German scientist, had discovered that when cholera bacteria was injected into the peritoneum of a guinea pig immunized against the infection, the pig would rapidly die. This bacteriolysis, Bordet discovered, did not occur when the bacteria was injected into a non-immunized guinea pig, but did so when the same animal received the **antiserum** from an immunized animal. Moreover, the bacteriolysis did not take place when the bacteria and the antiserum were mixed in a test tube unless fresh antiserum was used. However, when Bordet heated the antiserum to 55 degrees centigrade, it lost its power to kill bacteria. Finding that he could restore the bacteriolytic power of the antiserum if he added a little fresh serum from a non-immunized animal, Bordet concluded that the bacteria-killing phenomenon was due to the combined action of two distinct substances: an **antibody** in the antiserum, which specifically acted against a particular kind of bacterium; and a non-specific substance, sensitive to heat, found in all animal serums, which Bordet called "alexine" (later named "complement").

In a series of experiments conducted later, Bordet also learned that injecting red blood cells from one animal species (rabbit cells in the initial experiments) into another species (guinea pigs) caused the serum of the second species to quickly destroy the red cells of the first. And although the serum lost its power to kill the red cells when heated to 55 degrees centigrade, its potency was restored when alexine (or complement) was added. It became apparent to Bordet that hemolytic (red cell destroying) serums acted exactly as bacteriolytic serums; thus, he had uncovered the basic mechanism by which animal bodies defend or immunize themselves against the invasion of foreign elements. Eventually, Bordet and his colleagues found a way to implement their discoveries. They determined that alexine was bound or fixed to red blood cells or to bacteria during the immunizing process. When red cells were added to a normal serum mixed with a specific form of bacteria in a test tube, the bacteria remained active while the red cells were destroyed through the fixation of alexine. However, when serum containing the antibody specific to the bacteria was destroyed, the alexine and the solution separated into a layer of clear serum overlaying the intact red cells. Hence, it was possible to visually determine the presence of bacteria in a patient's blood serum. This process became known as a complement fixation test. Bordet and his associates applied these findings to various other infections, like **typhoid fever**, carbuncle, and hog cholera. **August von Wasserman** eventually used a form of the test (later known as the **Wasserman test**) to determine the presence of **syphilis** bacteria in the human blood.

Already famous by the age of thirty-one, Bordet accepted the directorship of the newly created Anti-rabies and Bacteriological Institute in Brussels in 1901; two years later, the organization was renamed the Pasteur Institute of Brussels. From 1901, Bordet was obliged to divide his time between his research and the administration of the Institute. In 1907, he also began teaching following his appointment as professor of bacteriology in the faculty of medicine at the Free University of Brussels, a position that he held until 1935. Despite his other activities, he continued his research in immunology and bacteriology. In 1906, Bordet and Octave Gengou succeeded in isolating the bacillus that causes **pertussis** (whooping cough) in children and later developed a **vaccine** against the disease. Between 1901 and 1920, Bordet conducted important studies on the coagulation of blood. When research became impossible because of the German occupation of Belgium during World War I, Bordet devoted himself to the writing of *Traité de l'immunité dans les maladies infectieuses* (1920), a classic book in the field of immunology. He was in the United States to raise money for new medical facilities for the war-damaged Free University of Brussels when he received word that he had been awarded the Nobel Prize. After 1920, he became interested in **bacteriophage**, the family of viruses that kill many types of bacteria, publishing several articles on the subject. In 1940, Bordet retired from the directorship of the Pasteur Institute of Brussels and was succeeded by his son, Paul. Bordet himself continued to take an active interest in the work of the Institute despite his failing eyesight and a second German occupation of Belgium during World War II. Many scientists, friends, and former students gathered in a celebration of his eightieth birthday at the great hall of the Free University of Brussels in 1950. He died in Brussels in 1961.

See also Antibody and antigen; B cells or B lymphocytes; Bacteria and bacterial infection; Bacteriophage and bacteriophage typing; Blood agar, hemolysis, and hemolytic reactions; Immune system; Immunity; Immunization; T cells or T lymphocytes

BOREL, JEAN-FRANÇOIS (1933-)
Belgian immunologist

Jean-François Borel is one of the discoverers of cyclosporin. The compound is naturally produced by a variety of fungus, where is acts as an antibiotic to suppress **bacterial growth**. Borel's research in the late 1970s demonstrated that in addition to the antibiotic activity, cyclosporin could act as an immunosupressant. This latter property of the compound has been exploited in limiting the rejection of transplanted organs in humans.

Borel was born in Antwerp, Belgium. After undergraduate studies in that city, he studied at the Swiss Federal Institute of Technology in Zurich. He obtained his Ph.D. in immunogenetics 1964. From there he obtained training in veterinary immunogenetics. In 1965, he moved to the Swiss Research Institute Department of Medicine where he studied **immunology**, particularly the inflammatory response. Five years later, he joined the scientific staff at Sandoz (now Novartis). He has been director of the immunology and microbiology departments at this company. Since 1983, Borel has been Vice-President of the Pharma division of Novartis. Since 1981, Borel has also been a professor of immunopharmacology in the medical faculty at the University of Bern.

In 1971, Borel isolated a compound (subsequently called cyclosporin) from a sample of the fungus *Beauvaria nivea* that was obtained during a hike by a Sandoz employee who had vacationed in the United States. Analyses by Borel showed that, unlike other immunosuppressants then known, the isolated compound selectively suppressed the **T cells** of the **immune system**. The compound was obtained in pure from in 1973. By the end of that decade, Borel had demonstrated the antirejection powers of the drug in humans.

During this period, Borel is remembered for having tested the putative immunosuppressant drug on himself. The compound was found to be insoluble. When Borel dissolved some of the compound in alcohol (subsequently, the use of olive oil as an emulsifier proved more efficient) and drank it, the compound subsequently appeared in his blood. This was a major finding, indicating that the compound might be amenable to injection so as to control the immune rejection of transplanted organs.

There has been a controversy as to whether Borel or another Sandoz scientist (Harold Stähelin) was primarily responsible for the discovery of cyclosporin. Both were actively involved at various stages in the purification and testing of the compound, and the primary contribution is difficult to assign. Nonetheless, it was Borel who first established the immunosuppressant effect of cyclosporin, during routine testing of compounds isolated from **fungi** for antibiotic activity.

Beginning in the 1980s, cyclosporin was licensed for use in transplantations. Since then, hundreds of thousands of people have successfully received organ transplants, where none would have before the discovery of cyclosporin.

The research of Borel and his colleagues inspired the search for other immunosupressant therapies. In recognition of his fundamental achievement to the advancement of organ transplantation, Borel received the prestigious Gairdner Award in 1986.

See also Antibody and antigen; Immunosuppressant drugs

BORRELIA BURGDORFERI • *see* LYME DISEASE

BOTULISM

Botulism is an illness produced by a toxin that is released by the soil bacterium *Clostridium botulinum*. One type of toxin is also produced by *Clostridium baratii*. The toxins affect nerves and can produce paralysis. The paralysis can affect the functioning of organs and tissues that are vital to life.

There are three main kinds of botulism. The first is conveyed by food containing the botulism toxin. Contaminated food can produce the illness after being ingested. Growth of the **bacteria** in the food may occur, but is not necessary for botulism. Just the presence of the toxin is sufficient. Thus, this form of botulism is a food intoxication (as compared with food poisoning, where **bacterial growth** is necessary). The second way that botulism can be produced is via infection of an open wound with *Clostridium botulinum*. Growth of the bacteria in the wound leads to the production of the toxin, which can diffuse into the bloodstream. The wound mode of toxin entry is commonly found in intravenous drug abusers. Finally, botulism can occur in young children following the consumption of the organism, typically when hands dirty from outdoor play are put into the mouth.

The latter means of acquiring botulism involves the form of the bacterium known as a spore. A spore is a biologically dormant but environmentally resilient casing around the bacterium's genetic material. The spore form allows the organism to survive through prolonged periods of inhospitable conditions. When conditions improve, such as when a spore in soil is ingested, resuscitation, growth of the bacterium, and toxin production can resume. For example, foodborne botulism is associated with canned foods where the food was not heated sufficiently prior to canning to kill the spores.

Botulism is relatively rare. In the United States, just over 100 cases are reported each year, on average. The number of cases of foodborne and infant botulism has not changed appreciably through the 1990s to the present day. Foodborne cases have tended to involve the improper preparation of home-canned foods.

There are seven known types of botulism toxin, based on their antigenic make-up. These are designated toxins A through G. Of these, only types A, B, E, and F typically cause botulism in humans, although involvement of type C toxin in infants has been reported, and may be particularly associated with the consumption of contaminated honey.

Infant botulism caused by toxin type C may be different from the other types of botulism in that the toxin is produced in the person following the ingestion of living *Clostridium botulinum.*

The toxins share similarities in their gross structure and in their mechanism of action. The toxins act by binding to the region of nerve cells that is involved in the release of a chemical known as a neurotransmitter. Neurotransmitters travel across the gap (synapse) separating neurons (nerve cells) and are essential to the continued propagation of a neural impulse. Accordingly, they are vital in maintaining the flow of a transmitted signal from nerve to nerve. Blocking nerve transmissions inhibits the means by which the body can initiate the movement of muscles. The result is paralysis. This paralysis produces a variety of symptoms including double or blurred vision, drooping eyelids, slurred speech, difficulties in swallowing, muscle weakness, paralysis of limbs and respiratory muscles.

The appearance of the symptoms of botulism vary depending on the route of toxin entry. For example, ingestion of toxin-contaminated food usually leads to symptoms within two to three days. However, symptoms can appear sooner or later depending on whether the quantity of toxin ingested is low or high.

The diagnosis of botulism and so the start of the appropriate therapy can be delayed, due to the relative infrequency of the malady and its similarity (in the early stages) with other maladies, such as Guillain-Barré syndrome and stroke. Diagnosis can involve the detection of toxin in the patient's serum, isolation of living bacteria from the feces, or by the ability of the patient's sample to produce botulism when introduced into test animals.

Clostridium botulinum requires an oxygen-free atmosphere to grow. Growth of the bacteria is associated with the production of gas. Thus, canned foods can display a bulging lid, due to the build-up of internal pressure. Recognition of this phenomenon and discarding of the unopened can is always a safe preventative measure.

Studies conducted by United States health authorities have shown that the different forms of the botulism toxin display some differences in their symptomatology and geographic distribution. Type A associated botulism is most prevalent in the western regions of the US, particularly in the Rocky Mountains. This toxin produces the most severe and long-lasting paralysis. Type B toxin is more common in the eastern regions of the country, especially in the Allegheny mountain range. The paralysis produced by type B toxin is less severe than with type A toxin. Type E botulism toxin is found more in the sediments of fresh water bodies, such as the Great Lakes. Finally, type F is distinctive as it is produced by *Clostridium baratii.*

Treatment for botulism often involves the administration of an antitoxin, which acts to block the binding of the toxin to the nerve cells. With time, paralysis fades. However, recovery can take a long time. If botulism is suspected soon after exposure to the bacteria, the stomach contents can be pumped out to remove the toxic bacteria, or the wound can be cleaned and disinfected. In cases of respiratory involvement, the patient may need mechanical assistance with breathing until lung function is restored. These measures have reduced the death rate from botulism to 8% from 50% over the past half century.

As dangerous as botulinum toxin is when ingested or when present in the bloodstream, the use of the toxin has been a boon to those seeking non-surgical removal of wrinkles. Intramuscular injection of the so-called "Botox" relaxes muscles and so relieves wrinkles. Thus far, no ill effects of the cosmetic enhancement have appeared. As well, Botox may offer relief to those suffering from the spastic muscle contractions that are a hallmark of cerebral palsy.

See also Bacteria and bacterial diseases; Bioterrorism; Food safety

BOVINE SPONGIFORM ENCEPHALOPATHY (BSE) • *see* BSE AND CJD DISEASE

BOYER, HERBERT WAYNE (1936-)

American molecular geneticist

In 1973 Herbert Boyer was part of the scientific team that first described the complete process of **gene** splicing, which is a basic technique of genetic engineering (recombinant **DNA**). Gene splicing involves isolating DNA, cutting out a piece of it at known locations with an enzyme, then inserting the fragment into another individual's genetic material, where it functions normally.

Boyer was born in Pittsburgh and received a bachelor's degree in 1958 from St. Vincent College. At the University of

Pittsburgh he earned an M.S. in 1960 and a Ph.D. in bacteriology in 1963. In 1966 Boyer joined the **biochemistry** and biophysics faculty at the University of California, San Francisco, where he continues his research.

Boyer performed his work with Stanley Cohen from the Stanford School of Medicine and other colleagues from both Stanford and the University of California, San Francisco. The scientists began by isolating a plasmid (circular DNA) from the **bacteria** *E. coli* that contains genes for an **antibiotic resistance** factor. They next constructed a new plasmid in the laboratory by cutting that plasmid with restriction endonucleases (**enzymes**) and joining it with fragments of other **plasmids**.

After inserting the engineered plasmid into *E. coli* bacteria, the scientists demonstrated that it possessed the DNA nucleotide sequences and genetic functions of both original plasmid fragments. They recognized that the method allowed bacterial **plasmids** to replicate even though sequences from completely different types of cells had been spliced into them.

Boyer and his colleagues demonstrated this by **cloning** DNA from one bacteria species to another and also cloning animal genes in *E. coli*.

Boyer is a co-founder of the genetic engineering firm Genentech, Inc. and a member National Academy of Sciences. His many honors include the Albert and Mary Lasker Basic Medical Research Award in 1980, the National Medal of Technology in 1989, and the National Medal of Science in 1990.

See also Molecular biology and molecular genetics

BRENNER, SYDNEY (1927-　)
South African–English molecular biologist

Sydney Brenner is a geneticist and molecular biologist who has worked in the laboratories of Cambridge University since 1957. Brenner played an integral part in the discovery and understanding of the triplet **genetic code** of **DNA**. He was also a member of the first scientific team to introduce messenger **RNA**, helping to explain the mechanism by which genetic information is transferred from DNA to the production of **proteins and enzymes**. In later years, Brenner conducted a massive, award-winning research project, diagramming the nervous system of a particular species of worm and attempting to map its entire genome.

Brenner was born in Germiston, South Africa. His parents were neither British nor South African—Morris Brenner was a Lithuanian exile who worked as a cobbler, and Lena Blacher Brenner was a Russian immigrant. Sydney Brenner grew up in his native town, attending Germiston High School. At the age of fifteen, he won an academic scholarship to the University of the Witwatersrand in Johannesburg, where he earned a master's degree in medical biology in 1947. In 1951, Brenner received his bachelor's degree in medicine, the qualifying degree for practicing physicians in Britain and many of its colonies. The South African university system could offer him no further education, so he embarked on independent research. Brenner studied **chromosomes**, cell structure, and

staining techniques, built his own centrifuge, and laid the foundation for his interest in **molecular biology**.

Frustrated by lack of resources and eager to pursue his interest in molecular biology, Brenner decided to seek education elsewhere, and was encouraged by colleagues to contact Cyril Hinshelwood, professor of physical chemistry at Oxford University. In 1952, Hinshelwood accepted Brenner as a doctoral candidate and put him to work studying a **bacteriophage**, a virus that had become the organism of choice for studying molecular biology in living systems. Brenner's change of location was an important boost to his career; while at Oxford he met Seymour Benzer, with whom Brenner collaborated on important research into **gene** mapping, sequencing, **mutations** and colinearity. He also met and exchanged ideas with **James Watson** and **Francis Crick**, the Cambridge duo who published the first paper elucidating the structure of DNA, or **deoxyribonucleic acid**, the basic genetic molecule. Brenner and Crick were to become the two most important figures in determining the general nature of the genetic code.

Brenner earned his Ph.D. from Oxford in 1954, while still involved in breakthrough research in molecular biology. His colleagues tried to find a job for him in England, but he accepted a position as lecturer in physiology at the University of the Witwatersrand and returned to South Africa in 1955. Brenner immediately set up a laboratory in Johannesburg to continue his phage research, but missed the resources he had enjoyed while in England. Enduring almost three years of isolation, Brenner maintained contact with his colleagues by mail.

In January 1957, Brenner was appointed to the staff of the Medical Research Council's Laboratory of Molecular Biology at Cambridge, and he and his family were able to settle in England permanently. Brenner immediately attended to theoretical research on the characteristics of the genetic code that he had begun in Johannesburg, despite the chaotic atmosphere. At the time, the world's foremost geneticists and molecular biologists were debating about the manner in which the sequences of DNA's four nucleotide bases were interpreted by an organism. The structure of a DNA molecule is a long, two-stranded chain that resembles a twisted ladder. The sides of the ladder are formed by alternating phosphate and sugar groups. The nucleotide bases adenine, guanine, thymine, and cytosine—or A, G, T, and C—form the rungs, a single base anchored to a sugar on one side of the ladder and linked by hydrogen bonds to a base similarly anchored on the other side. Adenine bonds only with thymine and guanine only with cytosine, and this complementarity is what makes it possible to replicate DNA. Most believed that the bases down the rungs of the ladder were read three at a time, in triplets such as ACG, CAA, and so forth. These triplets were also called codons, a term coined by Brenner. Each codon represented an amino acid, and the amino acids were strung together to construct a protein. The problem was in understanding how the body knew where to start reading; for example, the sequence AAC-CGGTT could be read in several sets of three-letter sequences. If the code were overlapping, it could be read AAC, ACC, CCG, and so forth.

Brenner's contribution was his simple theoretical proof that the base triplets must be read one after another and could not overlap. He demonstrated that an overlapping code would put serious restrictions on the possible sequences of amino acids. For example, in an overlapping code the triplet AAA, coding for a particular amino acid, could only be followed by an amino acid coded by a triplet beginning with AA—AAT, AAA, AAG, or AAC. After exploring the amino acid sequences present in naturally occurring proteins, Brenner concluded that the sequences were not subject to these restrictions, eliminating the possibility of an overlapping code. In 1961, Brenner, in collaboration with Francis Crick and others, confirmed his theory with bacteriophage research, demonstrating that the construction of a bacteriophage's protein coat could be halted by a single "nonsense" mutation in the organism's genetic code, and the length of the coat when the **transcription** stopped corresponded to the location of the mutation. Interestingly, Brenner's original proof was written before scientists had even determined the universal genetic code, although it opened the door for sequencing research.

Also in 1961, working with Crick, **François Jacob**, and **Matthew Meselson,** Brenner made his best-known contribution to molecular biology, the discovery of the messenger RNA (mRNA). Biologists knew that DNA, which is located in the **nucleus** of the cell, contains a code that controlled the production of protein. They also knew that protein is produced in structures called **ribosomes** in the cell **cytoplasm**, but did not know how the DNA's message is transmitted to, or received by, the ribosomes. RNA had been found within the ribosomes, but did not seem to relate to the DNA in an interesting way. Brenner's team, through original research and also by clever interpretation of the work of others, discovered a different type of RNA, mRNA, which was constructed in the nucleus as a template for a specific gene, and was then transported to the ribosomes for transcription. The RNA found within the ribosomes, rRNA, was only involved in the construction of proteins, not the coding of them. The ribosomes were like protein factories, following the instructions delivered to them by the messenger RNA. This was a landmark discovery in genetics and cell biology for which Brenner earned several honors, including the Albert Lasker Medical Research Award in 1971, one of America's most prestigious scientific awards.

In 1963 Brenner set out to expand the scope of his research. For most of his career, he had concentrated on the most fundamental chemical processes of life, and now he wanted to explore how those processes governed development and regulation within a living organism. He chose the nematode *Caenorhabditis elegans,* a worm no more than a millimeter long. As reported in *Science,* Brenner had initially told colleagues, "I would like to tame a small metazoan," expecting that the simple worm would be understood after a small bit of research. As it turned out, the nematode project was to span three decades, involve almost one hundred laboratories and countless researchers, make *C. elegans* one of the world's most studied and best understood organisms, and become one of the most important research projects in the history of genetics.

Brenner's nematode was an ideal subject because it was transparent, allowing scientists to observe every cell in its body, and had a life cycle of only three days. Brenner and his assistants observed thousands of *C. elegans* through every stage of development, gathering enough data to actually trace the lineage of each of its 959 somatic cells from a single zygote. Brenner's team also mapped the worm's entire nervous system by examining electron micrographs and producing a wiring diagram that showed all the connections among all of the 309 neurons. This breakthrough research led Brenner to new discoveries concerning sex determination, brain chemistry, and programmed cell death. Brenner also investigated the genome of the nematode, a project that eventually led to another milestone, a physical map of virtually the entire genetic content of *C. elegans.* This physical map enabled researchers to find a specific gene not by initiating hundreds of painstaking experiments, but by reaching into the freezer and pulling out the part of the DNA that they desired. In fact, Brenner's team was able to distribute copies of the physical map, handing out the worm's entire genome on a postcard-size piece of filter paper.

Brenner's ultimate objective was to understand development and behavior in genetic terms. He originally sought a chemical relationship that would explain how the simple molecular mechanisms he had previously studied might control the process of development. As his research progressed, however, he discovered that development was not a logical, program-driven process—it involved a complex network of organizational principles. Brenner's worm project was his attempt to understand the next level in the hierarchy of development. What he and his assistants have learned from *C. elegans* may have broad implications about the limits and difficulties of understanding behavior through gene sequencing. The Human Genome Project, for instance, was a mammoth effort to sequence the entire human DNA. James Watson has pointed to Brenner's worm experiments as a model for the project.

Brenner's research has earned him worldwide admiration. He has received numerous international awards, including the 1970 Gregor Mendel Medal from the German Academy of Sciences, the prestigious Kyoto Prize from Japan, as well as honors from France, Switzerland, Israel, and the United States. He has been awarded honorary degrees from several institutions, including Oxford and the University of Chicago, and has taught at Princeton, Harvard, and Glasgow Universities. Brenner is known for his aggressiveness, intelligence, flamboyance, and wit. His tendency to engage in remarkably ambitious projects such as the nematode project, as well as his ability to derive landmark discoveries from them, led *Nature* to claim that Brenner is "alternatively molecular biology's favorite son and *enfant terrible."*

While still in Johannesburg in 1952, Brenner married May Woolf Balkind. He has two daughters, one son, and one stepson. In 1986, the Medical Research Council at Cambridge set up a new **molecular genetics** unit, and appointed Brenner to a lifelong term as its head. Research at the new unit is centered on Brenner's previous work on *C. elegans* and the mapping and **evolution** of genes.

See also Bacteriophage and bacteriophage typing; Genetic code; Genetic identification of microorganisms; Genetic mapping; Microbial genetics

BROCK, THOMAS D. (1926-   )

American bacteriologist

Thomas D. Brock was born in Cleveland, Ohio, and has lived in the midwestern states of the United States all his life. Brock's 1967 summary article in *Science,* entitled "Life at High Temperatures" generated a great deal of interest, and spawned the branch of microbiology concerned with **bacteria** that live in extreme environments.

After graduating from high school in Chillicothe, Ohio, Brock enlisted in the Navy. As a veteran, he enrolled at Ohio State University in 1946. He graduated with a degree in botany in 1949, a MS degree and a Ph.D. in 1952. After graduation he joined the **antibiotics** research department at the Upjohn Company. His relative lack of microbiology training to that point necessitated that he learn on the job. This embracing of new aspects of research continued throughout his microbiology career. Leaving Upjohn after five years, he accepted a position at Western Reserve University (now Case Western University). In 1960 he moved to Indiana University as an Assistant Professor of Bacteriology. He remained there until 1971.

In 1963, Brock had the opportunity to pursue **marine microbiology** research at the Friday Harbor Laboratories of the University of Washington. There he studied *Leucothrix mucor.* His diagrams of the twisted configurations called "knots" formed by the growing organisms became a cover story in *Science* and were featured in the *New York Times*. This work also stimulated his interest in the microbial ecology of sulfur springs, which led him to conduct research at Yellowstone National Park over the next decade.

Beginning in the mid 1960s, Brock began field research in Yellowstone National Park, Montana. At the time of these studies, bacterial life was not thought to be possible at growth temperatures above about 80° C. Brock found **microorganisms** that were capable of growth and division at temperatures of nearly 100° C, the temperature at which water boils.

In particular, Brock isolated and named the bacterium *Thermus aquaticus*. This microbe was the first so-called archaebacteria to be discovered. Archaebacteria are now known to be a very ancient form of life, and may even constitute a separate kingdom of life. The discovery of *Thermus aquaticus* is thus, one of the fundamental milestones of microbiology.

Brock's discovery has also had a significant impact in the field of **biotechnology**. The **enzymes** of the bacterium are designed to work at high temperatures. In particular, a polymerase is the basis of the **polymerase chain reaction** that is used to artificially amplify the amount of **deoxyribonucleic acid**. The use of **PCR** has spawned a multi-billion dollar biotechnology industry.

In 1971, Brock moved to the Department of Bacteriology at the University of Wisconsin-Madison. He is currently E.B. Fred Professor of Natural Sciences-Emeritus at Wisconsin.

Brock has also been a prolific writer and scientific historian. His numerous books include volumes on the biology of microorganisms, the principles of microbial ecology, the mile-

stones in microbiology, and a profile of **Robert Koch**. In the 1980s, he formed his own scientific publishing company, which continues to the present day.

For his groundbreaking research and publishing efforts, Brock has received many scientific achievement and education awards in the United States and worldwide.

See also Extremophiles; Tag enzyme

BROTH • *see* GROWTH AND GROWTH MEDIA

BROWNIAN MOTION • *see* BACTERIAL MOVEMENT

BRUCELLOSIS

Brucellosis is a disease caused by **bacteria** in the genus Brucella. The disease infects animals such as swine, cattle, and sheep; humans can become infected indirectly through contact with infected animals or by drinking Brucella-contaminated milk. In the United States, most domestic animals are vaccinated against the bacteria, but brucellosis remains a risk with imported animal products.

Brucella are rod-shaped bacteria that lack a capsule around their cell membranes. Unlike most bacteria, Brucella cause infection by actually entering host cells. As the bacteria cross the host cell membrane, they are engulfed by host cell vacuoles called phagosomes. The presence of Brucella within host cell phagosomes initiates a characteristic immune response, in which infected cells begin to stick together and form aggregations called granulomas.

Three species of Brucella cause brucellosis in humans: *Brucella melitensis,* which infects goats; *B. abortis,* which infects cattle and, if the animal is pregnant, causes the spontaneous abortion of the fetus; and *B. suis,* which infects pigs. In animals, brucellosis is a self-limiting disease, and usually no treatment is necessary for the resolution of the disease. However, for a period of time from a few days to several weeks, infected animals may continue to excrete brucella into their urine and milk. Under warm, moist conditions, the bacteria may survive for months in soil, milk, and even seawater.

Because the bacteria are so hardy, humans may become infected with Brucella by direct contact with the bacteria. Handling or cleaning up after infected animals may put a person in contact with the bacteria. Brucella are extremely efficient in crossing the human skin barrier through cuts or breaks in the skin.

The incubation period of Brucella, the time from exposure to the bacteria to the start of symptoms, is typically about three weeks. The primary complaints are weakness and fatigue. An infected person may also experience muscle aches, fever, and chills.

The course of the disease reflects the location of the Brucella bacteria within the human host. Soon after the Brucella are introduced into the bloodstream, the bacteria seek out the nearest lymph nodes and invade the lymph node cells.

From the initial lymph node, the Brucella spread out to other organ targets, including the spleen, bone marrow, and liver. Inside these organs, the infected cells form granulomas.

Diagnosing brucellosis involves culturing the blood, liver, or bone marrow for Brucella organisms. A positive **culture** alone does not signify brucellosis, since persons who have been treated for the disease may continue to harbor Brucella bacteria for several months. Confirmation of brucellosis, therefore, includes a culture positive for Brucella bacteria as well as evidence of the characteristic symptoms and a history of possible contact with infected milk or other animal products.

In humans, brucellosis caused by *B. abortus* is a mild disease that resolves itself without treatment. Brucellosis caused by *B. melitensis* and *B. suis,* however, can be chronic and severe. Brucellosis is treated with administration of an antibiotic that penetrates host cells to destroy the invasive bacteria.

Since the invention of an animal **vaccine** for brucellosis in the 1970s, the disease has become somewhat rare in the United States. Yet the vaccine cannot prevent all incidence of brucellosis. The **Centers for Disease Control** usually reports fewer than 100 total cases per year in the United States. Most of these were reported in persons who worked in the meat processing industry. Brucellosis remains a risk for those who work in close contact with animals, including veterinarians, farmers, and dairy workers.

Brucellosis also remains a risk when animal products from foreign countries are imported into the United States. Outbreaks of brucellosis have been linked to unpasteurized feta and goat cheeses from the Mediterranean region and Europe. In the 1960s, brucellosis was linked to bongo drums imported from Africa; drums made with infected animal skins can harbor Brucella bacteria, which can be transmitted to humans through cuts and scrapes in the human skin surface.

In the United States, preventive measures include a rigorous **vaccination** program that involves all animals in the meat processing industry. On an individual level, people can avoid the disease by not eating animal products imported from countries where brucellosis is frequent, and by avoiding foods made with unpasteurized milk.

See also Bacteria and bacterial infection; Food safety; Infection and resistance; Pasteurization

BSE AND CJD DISEASE

Bovine spongiform encephalopathy (BSE) and Creutzfeldt-Jakob Disease (CJD) are ailments in which the functioning of the brain is progressively impaired. Both diseases are associated with visually abnormal pinpoints (or plaques) in the brain, and in a changed texture of the brain tissue. The brain tissue, particularly in the cortex and cerebellum, becomes filled with large open spaces (vacuoles) and becomes spongy in texture. The "spongiform" part of BSE comes from this texture characteristic.

BSE is a disease of animals such as cattle and sheep, while CJD is associated with humans. However, the two diseases may have a common cause. The cause of BSE and CJD, and of other diseases such as scrapie, transmissible mink encephalopathy, fatal familial insomnia, and kuru, are **prions**. Prions are particles that are made solely of protein. Even though they lack genetic material, they are infectious.

Both BSE and CJD are characterised by a loss of coordination and the control over functions such as grasping and holding, dementia, paralysis, eventually leading to death. There is no cure for either disease, and no are vaccines available.

CJD derives its name from its discoverers. Progressive and ultimately fatal dementia that was accompanied by other neurological abnormalities was described in six patients in the 1920s by two German neuroscientists, Hans Gerhard Creutzfeldt and Alphons Maria Jakob. In the 1960s, the neurological changes associated with the development of CJD had become accepted by the medical community.

The average incidence rate for CJD over time is about one person per million. Clusters of CJD do occur. The most recent example is the 48 confirmed cases that were diagnosed in Britain between 1996 and 2001. There is no evident predilection for a gender, any ethnic group, or for geographical location. However, the incidence in those over 55 years of age is far higher (over 30 times) than for those under 55 years.

Three means of acquiring CJD have been identified. First, the disease can be genetically inherited. This is also described as familial CJD. Secondly, the disease can appear with no exact origin being known. About 85% of CJD cases are of this unknown variety. Lastly, the disease can be acquired during surgery. This so-called iatrogenic form is typically a result of CJD-contaminated equipment or tissue (brain and corneal grafts are two examples).

There is no cure for CJD. Treatment consists of managing the patient so that his/her increasingly impaired mental faculties do not result in injury, and in personal care as these functions become impossible for the person to perform themselves.

BSE causes a progressive neurological deterioration in cattle that is similar to the course of CJD in humans. Cattle with BSE are more temperamental, have problems with their posture and coordination, have progressively greater difficulty in rising off the ground and walking, produce less milk, have severe twitching of muscles, and loss weight even though their appetite is undiminished. The so-called incubation period, the time from when the animal is first infected until symptoms appear, ranges from two to eight years. After appearance of symptoms, deterioration is rapid and the animal dies or is destroyed within six months. The disease is one of several so-called transmissible spongiform encephalopathies (TSEs) in animals.

BSE was confirmed as a disease of cattle in November of 1996. Since then, almost all reported cases have been in cattle born in the United Kingdom. Other countries in Europe and Asia have reported BSE, but in far fewer numbers than in Britain. No cases have been detected in the United States (the U.S. has not imported U.K. beef since 1985 and maintains a rigorous surveillance program). As of November 2001, the total number of confirmed cases of BSE in U.K. cattle was just over 181,000. In 1993, a BSE epidemic in the U.K. peaked at almost 1,000 new cases per week. While the cause of this near-exclusivity has yet to be conclusively determined, the

2001 outbreak of hoof and mouth disease in the United Kingdom revealed that a common practice has been to feed cattle "offal," the ground up waste from the slaughter process. Experience with kuru has shown that consumption of prion-infected tissue is a means of spreading the disease.

This method of transmission is suspected of being important, if not principle, for BSE. The exact origin of the prions is not known. Sheep are considered a likely source.

Until the 1900s, scientists believed that the transmission of the BSE agent to humans did not occur. However, several studies conducted in the latter years of the 1990s has cast doubt on this assumption. Studies using mice showed that the brain injuries caused in BSE and CJD are identical. Moreover, these brain alterations occurred in mice injected with either brain tissue from BSE-diseased cattle, which was expected, or with brain tissue from CJD-diseased animals, which was unexpected. Thus, development of CJD could be due to human consumption of BSE-diseased meat.

The currently held view is that prions from cattle infected with BSE are capable of infecting humans and causing what is termed a variant CJD (vCJD) disease in humans. There is evidence that the suspect vCJD has a different infectious behavior than CJD. For instance, younger people can be infected, and the neurological symptoms differ.

The existence of a vCJD is based mainly on epidemiological evidence. If the existence of vCJD is proven, then the species barrier for the transmission of BSE and CJD does not exist. However, the possibility still remains that the contaminating agent in the meat is really a prion that causes normally CJD, and that this prion is naturally present in cattle but has escaped detection until now. If so, then BSE and CJD infections could indeed be confined to non-human and human mammals, respectively.

See also BSE and CJD disease, advances in research; BSE and CJD disease, ethical issues and socio-economic impact; Latent viruses and diseases

BSE AND CJD: ETHICAL ISSUES AND SOCIO-ECONOMIC IMPACT

The outbreak of bovine spongiform encephalopathy (BSE) or "mad cow disease" in the United Kingdom and continental Europe continues to concern beef and dairy producers and the general public in the United States. This concern has increased recently because of the continued spread of the disease on the European continent and the development of a similar disease that has appeared in people, mostly in the U.K. The new disease known as variant Creutzfeldt-Jakob disease (vCJD) appears to be more closely related to BSE in its pathology than to traditional CJD. It is therefore assumed that vCJD has crossed the species barrier from cattle to Man.

BSE and CJD are prion diseases, a group of rapidly progressive, fatal, untreatable neurodegenerative syndromes characterized by the accumulation in the brain of a protease-resistant protein that is the main (or only) macromol-

ecule of the transmissible agent. The prototypical prion disease of animals is scrapie, which has been long recognized in sheep and goats as a common and economically important disorder. Following 1988, BSE has given rise to considerable economic and political turmoil in the United Kingdom as it developed in more than 150 000 cattle. At the peak of the epidemic in 1993, approximately 700 cattle were newly affected each week. The epidemic has been linked to changes in the rendering of sheep or cattle carcasses for use as protein supplements to feed-meal, suggesting that inadequately inactivated scrapie agent from sheep, cattle or both was the initial cause. Following a legislation banning the feeding of ruminant offal to livestock, the rate of diagnosed BSE has decreased. It is still uncertain whether the origins of BSE lie in a mutant form of scrapie or if it developed naturally in cattle.

A number of human prion diseases exist including CJD, kuru, Gerstmann-Sträussler-Scheinker (GSS) syndrome and fatal familial insomnia (FFI). These diseases are rare and, until recently, were not considered of any great socio-economic significance. However, in the wake of the BSE crisis in the U.K. and the suspicion that contaminated beef may lie at the root of it, many people now fear that an epidemic may be imminent. The infectivity of prion diseases appears to reside in the prion protein designated PrPSc. PrPSc is the abnormal, protease-resistant isoform of a normal cellular membrane protein designated PrPC. **Stanley B. Prusiner** of the University of California at San Francisco has long contended that changes in conformation underlie the dramatic differences in the properties of the two isoforms; by abnormal molecular folding, PrPSc acquires protease resistance and a "catalytic" ability to recruit more conformational copies of itself from PrPC. PrPSc is remarkably resistant to many procedures that inactivate conventional infectious agents and, therefore, problems have been encountered in decontamination procedures of, for example, surgical instruments. Although 90% of prion disease cases arise sporadically and a further 10% arise where the family has some history of the disease, it is an unfortunate fact that about eighty cases of CJD have arisen iatrogenically, that is, as a result of exposure to medical treatment, facilities, or personnel. Cases of transmission by corneal transplant, transplant of dura mater, exposure to infected neurosurgical instruments and electroencephalogram probes, and transplantation of human growth hormone have been confirmed.

The indestructibility of **prions** creates real problems in sterilizing surgical instruments; it is basically impossible, and equipment has retained infectivity and caused infection in patients even after repeated "sterilizations." Currently in the U.K., scientists are considering making all surgical instruments disposable. Neurosurgical equipment is already disposed of after each patient. Since vCJD is carried heavily by the lymphoreticular (blood/lymph) systems, the tonsils, appendix, and most recently, the lymph nodes of vCJD patients have been found to be full of prions, unlike in patients with classical CJD. This has brought about the worrisome debate in the U.K. that all surgical equipment, not just neurosurgical, could be contaminated and has brought on calls to destroy all surgical equipment after use or to use disposable instruments only. The U.K. has also banned the reuse of contact "fitting" lenses by

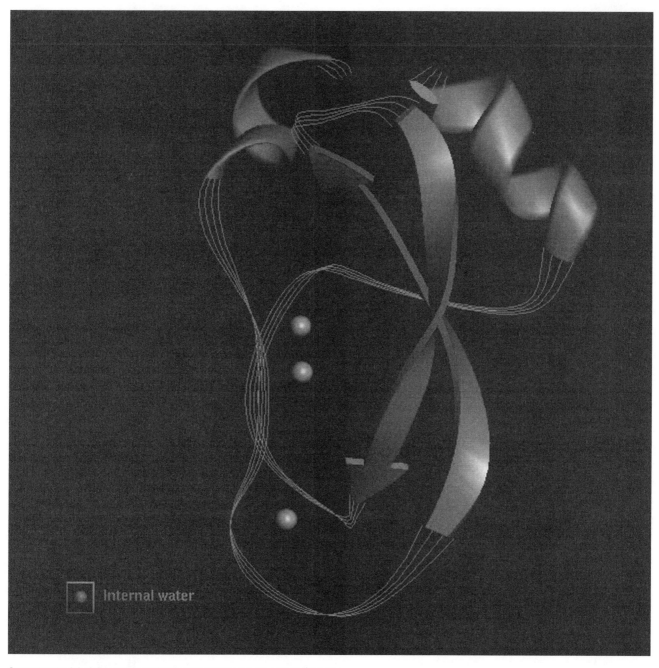

Internal water

Computer model of the protein molecule responsible for plaques in the brain.

optometrists and opthamologists—hard lenses that are "sterilized" between patient use in clinics that fit contact lenses. The eye has a direct neural link with the brain and is one of the most highly infectious organs of the body in CJD and vCJD, after the brain and spinal cord. There is concern that these lenses could spread iatrogenic vCJD. Additionally "touch" tonometry has been banned in the UK, only the "air puff" method is allowed now. And, of course, ophthalmological surgery could be a prime candidate for this as well. However, nothing is being

done in this regard in the U.S. to screen U.K. patients, or U.S. patients who have lived abroad.

A new fear is that blood supplies may be contaminated with prions and that Creutzfeldt-Jakob disease (CJD) will join **hepatitis** and **AIDS** in the public and medical consciousness as the next infectious disease epidemic which may be contracted through donated blood and tissue. In view of the theoretical risk of blood-borne transmission of CJD, some experts recommend that the following groups of people not donate blood: all people with CJD; first-degree relatives of CJD patients with familial disease (determined by genetic testing, by identifying two or more first-degree relatives with CJD or, if there is no information, by a precautionary assumption of familial disease); recipients of products derived from human pituitary glands; and recipients of corneal or dura-mater grafts.

The risk of transmission of CJD through blood, blood products, and organ or tissue transplants, is being addressed by, for example, the Laboratory Centre for Disease Control (LCDC) in Canada. They are planning to initiate an enhanced surveillance system for CJD throughout Canada. Cases will be reported to the surveillance system by specialists in neurology, neuropathology and geriatrics. Through record review, interview, genetic sequencing and neuropathological examination, extensive information about every person suspected of having CJD will be collected and compared with data from a control population to ascertain the relative risk of CJD associated with exposure to blood and blood products. In addition, Canada has been invited to participate in European Concerted Action on CJD, an international surveillance program for variant CJD coordinated by investigators in Edinburgh. This obviously has ethical implications for patient privacy and it is questionable if such extreme measures are really necessary. The prion agent is not new unlike **HIV** and other emerging agents and there is an absence of any recorded cases of CJD among people with hemophilia and recipients of multiple transfusions or people who abuse injection drugs. Also, a small case-controlled study in Britain revealed no risk for the subsequent development of CJD associated with receiving blood.

See also BSE and CJD: recent advances in research; Public health, current issues

BSE, SCRAPIE, AND CJD: RECENT ADVANCES IN RESEARCH

Bovine spongiform encephalopathy (BSE) in cows, scrapie in sheep, and Creutzfeldt-Jakob disease (CJD) in humans are examples of prion diseases. The central event in the pathogenesis of these fatal disorders is hypothesized to be the post-translational conversion of a normal host protein of unknown function, termed PrPC into an abnormal isoform called PrPSc. The idea that protein alone can carry information sufficient to ensure its own propagation was an unprecedented challenge to the "central dogma" of **molecular biology** which essentially states that nucleic acids, not proteins, are the biological information carriers. The work that led to current understanding of prion diseases originated more than four decades ago. In the 1960s, Tikvah Alper and her co-workers reported that the scrapie agent was extremely resistant to treatments that normally destroy nucleic acids, but sensitive to procedures that damage proteins. Furthermore, the minimum molecular size needed in maintaining infectivity was too small to be a virus or other known infectious agent. These results led J. Griffith to propose that the material responsible for transmitting scrapie could be a protein that has the unusual ability to replicate itself in the body. Extensive work by **Stanley Prusiner** finally led to

the purification of the PrP protein. For the next two decades, most research on prion diseases has focussed on the abnormal PrPSc and consequently, the functional role of PrPC has remained an enigma. Recent advances in the field of prion research, however, suggest that PrPC is a copper binding protein and has a modulating role in brain oxidative homeostasis. On the basis of *in vitro* studies by D. R. Brown at the University of Cambridge, it would appear that PrPC may act as an antioxidant enzyme in a similar manner to superoxide dismutase. The presence of the copper ion is essential for such a function.

Much recent evidence suggests that alterations in metallochemical processes could be a contributing factor for the pathological process in neurodegenerative disorders, including Alzheimer's disease and now possibly prion diseases. The PrPC protein has recently been found to have a region at its N-terminus, which is able to bind copper tightly and other metals, such as nickel, zinc and manganese, less tightly. One of the biochemical differences between the PrPC and PrPSc that was recognized very early is the surprising resistance of PrPSc to proteases (**enzymes** able to degrade proteins). *In vitro* studies have shown that if manganese ions replace the copper ions in the PrPC protein, it undergoes a structural change and becomes protease resistant. Furthermore, the binding of manganese to PrP dramatically reduces its superoxide-dismutase activity, suggesting that its cellular function may be affected under these conditions. Whether these *in vitro* changes brought about by different metal ions resemble the changes in PrP during prion disease is still to be confirmed, but the results are certainly suggestive. Research in this direction is progressing in several institutions in the UK at the moment.

High concentrations of metals are found in the brain and to prevent neuronal damage triggered by these elevated concentrations, the brain has evolved efficient mechanisms to regulate the availability of these metals. Metals are required for the normal functioning of the brain, such as the proper transmission of synaptic signals, which involve the release of zinc, copper and iron by neurons. At the same time, metals are an integral part of the cellular defense system, as they are often bound to antioxidant proteins and protect the brain from damage by free radicals. Although metals are essential to the normal functioning of the brain, perturbation in metal levels can upset cellular protein behaviour and possibly lead to neurological disorders. In Alzheimer's disease, for example, the levels of copper, zinc, and iron were found to alter in severely degenerated brain regions. In the hippocampus and amygdala regions, the levels of both zinc and iron were increased while the levels of copper were decreased.

In the 1970s, Pattison and Jebbett showed that when mice were fed with cuprizone, a copper chelator, it induced histopathological changes reminiscent of scrapie in sheep and further analysis indicated similar biochemical changes. Also a recent report by Mark Purdey showed that in the ecosystem supporting isolated clusters of sporadic prion diseases in Colorado, Iceland, and Slovakia, a consistent elevation of manganese concentration in relation to normal levels recorded in adjoining prion disease-free localities were detected. Evidence has also emerged concerning the metal content of the brains of animals and humans with prion diseases. The most alarming finding is preliminary evidence from two independent groups that CJD patients have a ten-fold increase in the levels of manganese in their brains. This increase is unprecedented in any other diseases—except cases of manganese poisoning—implying that high brain manganese might be a specific hallmark of prion diseases. This has prompted intensive work on the relationship between prion diseases and environmental pollution. It is proposed that in regions where manganese levels are abnormally high, the manganese may bind to the normal brain PrPC protein and alter its structure into the abnormal PrPSc form. Under these circumstances, the PrPC would lose its protective antioxidant function and predispose the brain to increased oxidative damage.

Many questions concerning the connection between metals and prion diseases remain to be answered. What is clear is that metals can be both beneficial and malicious to the structure and function of PrP. It is important to elucidate the mechanisms involved in these brain metal perturbations and their role in modulating the structure of PrP. Furthermore, it is also essential to determine the structural and functional changes induced by different metals on PrP at the molecular level and the resultant phenotypic features. Conclusive evidence that the loss of PrPC function contributes to prion diseases requires further experiments, possibly with animal models. What is certain is that the next few years will be crucial and exciting in deducing whether brain metal abnormalities constitute a mechanism in the development of prion disease.

See also BSE and CJD: Socio-economic impact and ethical issues; BSE and CJD; Slow virus and viral diseases

BUBONIC PLAGUE

Bubonic plague is a disease that is typically passed from rodents to other animals and humans via the bite of a flea. The flea acquires the bacterium that causes the disease as it lives on the skin of the rodent. Humans can also acquire the disease by direct contact with infected tissue. The bacterium is called *Yersinia pestis*, after one of its co-discoverers, Alexandre Yersin.

The disease is named because of the symptoms. The **bacterial infection** produces a painful swelling of the lymph nodes. These are called buboes. Often the first swelling is evident in the groin. During the Middle Ages, an huge epidemic of bubonic plague was referred to as the Black Death, because of the blackening of the skin due to the dried blood that accumulated under the skin's surface.

The bubonic plague has been a significant cause of misery and death throughout recorded history. The Black Death was only one of many **epidemics** of plague that extend back to the beginning of recorded history. Biblical descriptions of some disease outbreaks likely involved bubonic plague. The first recorded outbreak of bubonic plague was in 542–543. This plague destroyed the attempts of the Roman emperor of the day to re-establish a Roman empire in Europe.

This is only one example of how bubonic plague has changed the course of history.

The plague of London in 1665 killed over 17,000 people (almost twenty percent of the city's population). This outbreak was quelled by a huge fire that destroyed most of the city.

The disease remains present to this day. In North America, the last large epidemic occurred in Los Angeles in 1925. With the advent of the antibiotic, era bubonic plague has been controlled in the developed world. However, sporadic cases (e.g., 10 to 15 cases each year) still occur in the western United States. In less developed countries (e.g., in Africa, Bolivia, Peru, Ecuador, Brazil) thousands of cases are reported each year.

The infrequent outbreaks of bubonic plague does not mean the disease disappears altogether. Rather, the disease normally exists in what is called an enzootic state. That is, a few individuals of a certain community (e.g., rodents) harbor the disease. Sometimes, however, environmental conditions cause the disease to spread through the carrier population, causing loss of life. As the rodent populations dies, the fleas that live on them need to find other food sources. This is when the interaction with humans and non-rodent animals can occur. Between outbreaks, *Yersinia pestis* infects rodents without causing much illness. Thus, the rodents become a reservoir of the infection.

Symptoms of infection in humans begin within days after **contamination** with the plague bacterium. The **bacteria** enter the bloodstream and travels to various organs (e.g., kidney, liver, spleen, lungs) as well as to the brain. Symptoms include shivering, nausea with vomiting, headache, intolerance to light, and a whitish-appearing tongue. Buboes then appear, followed by rupture of blood vessels. The released blood can coagulate and turn black.

If the infection is untreated, the death rate in humans approaches 75%. Prompt treatment most often leads to full recovery and a life-long **immunity** from further infection. Prevention is possible, since a **vaccine** is available. Unfortunately, the vaccine is protective for only a few months. Use of the vaccine is usually reserved for those who will be at high risk for acquiring the bacterial infection (e.g., soldiers, travelers to an outbreak region). **Antibiotics** such as tetracycline or sulfonamide are used more commonly as a precaution for those who might be exposed to the bacterium. Such use of antibiotics should be stopped once the risk of infection is gone, to avoid the development of resistance in other bacteria resident in the body.

These modern day treatment and preventative measures are a marked improvement from earlier times. In the fourteenth century, treatments included bathing in human urine, wearing feces, having a dead animal present in the home, and drinking concoctions of molten gold and crushed emeralds. As time progressed, even though the cause of the disease was still unknown, the preventative measures became more constructive. By the fifteenth century, for example, incoming ships were required to anchor offshore for 40 days before cargo or people could disembark. Quarantine is still practiced today as a protective measure for some diseases.

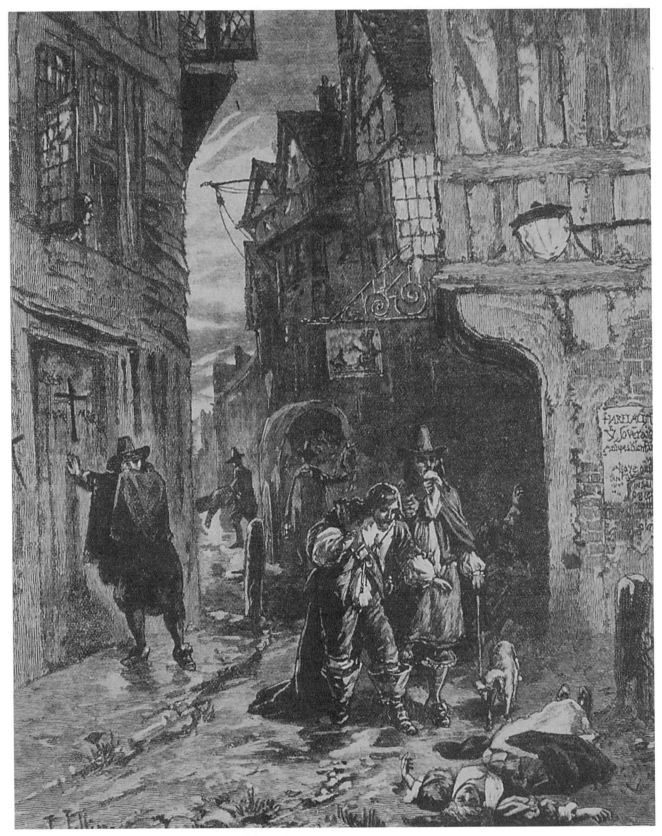

Drawing depicting the effect of Bubonic plague in eighteenth-century London.

The most effective way to prevent bubonic plague is the maintenance of adequate sanitary conditions. This acts to control the rodent population, especially in urban centers.

See also Bacteria and bacterial infection; Epidemics and pandemics; Zoonoses

BUCHANAN, ROBERT EARLE (1883-1972)
American microbial taxonomist

Robert Earle Buchanan's contributions to the wider world of microbiology involve the classification of **microorganisms** and his activity in the expansion of the Society of American Bacteriologists. This expansion was one of the important events that led the Society to become the American Society for Microbiology, the paramount microbiology society in the world.

Buchanan was educated at Iowa State University and subsequently became a faculty member there. He received a B.S. degree in 1904, and a M.S. degree in 1906. After joining the faculty, he became the first head of the Bacteriology Department in 1910. He remained head until his retirement in 1948. He was also the first dean of Industrial Science, first dean of the Graduate College (1919–1948), and was Director of the Agriculture Experiment Station from 1933 until 1948.

In his research life, Buchanan was a microbial taxonomist, concerned with the classification of microorganisms. This interest led him to serve on the Board of Trustees of the *Bergey's Manual of Determinative Bacteriology,* and to assume the responsibilities of co-editor of the eighth edition of the manual in 1974. The Manual is the definitive reference volume on bacterial classification. Buchanan was also one of the founders of the *International Bulletin of Bacterial Nomenclature and Taxonomy* in 1951. He served on the first editorial board of the journal. The journal is still published, now as the *International Journal of Systematic and Evolutionary Bacteriology.*

In 1934, the Society of American Bacteriologists began the process of expansion by adding a branch that represented bacteriologists in Iowa, Minnesota, North Dakota, South Dakota, and Wisconsin. Buchanan became the first President of the Northwest Branch of the Society in 1935.

Buchanan also founded the Iowa State *Journal of Science* in 1926. The journal was intended as a forum for the rapid publication of research papers that were too lengthy for publication in other scientific journals. The journal published works from the biological and agricultural sciences and, in 1972, research from the humanities. The journal ceased publication in 1988.

Another landmark publication of Buchanan was in 1960. Then, he published an essay listing the correct Latin forms of chemical elements and compounds that are used in the naming of **bacteria**, yeasts, many filamentous **fungi** and some **protozoa**. This article has proven vital to several generations of bacterial taxonomists.

Buchanan was also active in other international agencies, including the National Research Council, Inter-American Institute of Agricultural Sciences, the President's Committee on Foreign Aid. His service on missions to Greece, the Middle East, and India spread agricultural technology and knowledge of microbiological diseases of agricultural crops around the developing world.

BUDDING · *see* YEAST

BUFFER

A buffer is a solution that resists changes in **pH** upon the addition of acid or base. Buffers typically contain several species that react with added acid and base.

Buffers are important in maintaining the proper environment within **microorganisms** and within other cells, including those in man. In the microbiology laboratory, many solutions and growth media are buffered to prevent sudden and adverse changes in the acidity or alkalinity of the environment surrounding the microorganisms.

Blood is an example of a natural buffer. In water, small volumes of an acid or base solution can greatly change the pH (measure of the hydrogen ion concentration). If the same amount of the acid or base solution is added to blood, the normal pH of the blood (7.4) changes only marginally. Blood and many other bodily fluids are naturally buffered to resist changes in pH.

In order to explain the properties of a buffer, it is useful to consider a specific example, the acetic acid/acetate buffer system. When acid (e.g., HCl, hydrochloric acid) is added to this buffer, the added hydronium ion (H^+) reacts with the strongest base in the medium, namely the acetate ion, to form more acetic acid. This reaction uses up the added hydronium ion, preventing the pH from rising drastically, and is responsible for the buffering effect. As a result of adding acid to the buffer, the concentration of acetate decreases and the concentration of acetic acid increases. The solution acts as a buffer because nearly all of the added hydronium ion is consumed by reaction with acetate. As the hydrogen ion concentration increases, the acetate concentration and acetic acid concentration must adjust. The pH changes slightly to reflect the shift in the concentrations, but the change is much smaller than in the absence of the buffer because most of the added acid is consumed by its reaction with the acetate ion. This example of an acetic acid/acetate ion buffer is typical of other buffer systems.

Buffers are vitally important in living prokaryotic and eukaryotic systems. The rates of various biochemical reactions are very sensitive to the availability of hydronium ions. Many biochemical reactions (e.g., **metabolism**, **respiration**, the transmission of nerve impulses, and muscle contraction and relaxation) take place only within a narrow range of pH.

An important buffer in the blood is the bicarbonate ion and dissolved carbon dioxide in the form of carbonic acid. The acidity or alkalinity of the blood can be altered by the ingestion of acidic or basic substances. The carbonate/bicarbonate buffer system compensates for such additions and maintains the pH within the required range.

This buffering system is intimately tied to respiration, and an exceptional feature of pH control by this system is the role of ordinary breathing in maintaining the pH. Carbon dioxide is a normal product of metabolism. It is transported to the lungs, where it is eliminated from the body with every exhalation. However, carbon dioxide in blood is converted to carbonic acid, which dissociates to produce the hydrogen carbonate ion and the hydronium ion. If a chemical reaction or the ingestion of an acidic material increases the hydronium ion concentration in the blood, bicarbonate ion reacts with the added hydronium ion and is transformed into carbonic acid. As a result the concentration of dissolved carbon dioxide in the blood increases. Respiration increases, and more carbon dioxide is expelled from the lungs. Conversely, if a base is ingested, the hydronium ion reacts with it, causing a decrease in the concentration of hydronium ion. More carbonic acid dissociates to restore the hydronium ion consumed by the base. This requires more carbon dioxide to be dissolved in the blood, so respiration is decreased and more gas is retained.

To act as a buffer, a solution must maintain a nearly constant pH when either acid or base is added. Two considerations must be made when a buffer is prepared: (1) Which pH is desired to maintain? The desired pH defines the range of the buffer. (2) How much acid or base does the solution need to consume without a significant change in pH? This defines the capacity of the buffer. The desired pH also determines the compounds used in making up the buffer. The quantity of acid or base the buffer must be able to consume determines the concentrations of the components that must be used, and which allows biological reactions to take place consistently.

See also Biochemical analysis techniques; Laboratory techniques in microbiology

BURNET, FRANK MACFARLANE
(1899-1985)
Australian immunologist and virologist

While working at the University of Melbourne's Walter and Eliza Hall Institute for Medical Research in the 1920s, Frank Macfarlane Burnet became interested in the study of **viruses** and **bacteriophage** (viruses that attack **bacteria**). That interest eventually led to two major and related accomplishments. The first of these was the development of a method for cultivating viruses in chicken embryos, an important technological step forward in the science of **virology**. The second accomplishment was the development of a theory that explains how an organism's body is able to distinguish between its own cells and those of another organism. For this research, Burnet was awarded a share of the 1960 Nobel Prize for physiology or medicine (with **Peter Brian Medawar**).

Burnet was born in Traralgon, Victoria, Australia. His father was Frank Burnet, manager of the local bank in Traralgon, and his mother was the former Hadassah Pollock MacKay. As a child, Burnet developed an interest in nature, particularly in birds, butterflies, and beetles. He carried over that interest when he entered Geelong College in Geelong, Victoria, where he majored in biology and medicine.

In 1917, Burnet continued his education at Ormond College of the University of Melbourne, from which he received his bachelor of science degree in 1922 and then, a year later, his M.D. degree. Burnet then took concurrent positions as resident pathologist at the Royal Melbourne Hospital and as researcher at the University of Melbourne's Hall Institute for Medical Research. In 1926, Burnet received a Beit fellowship that permitted him to spend a year in residence at the Lister Institute of Preventive Medicine in London. The work on viruses and bacteriophage that he carried out at Lister also earned him a Ph.D. from the University of London in 1927. At the conclusion of his studies in England in 1928, Burnet returned to Australia, where he became assistant director of the Hall Institute. He maintained his association with the institute for the next thirty-seven years, becoming director there in 1944. In the same year, he was appointed professor of experimental medicine at the University of Melbourne.

Burnet's early research covered a somewhat diverse variety of topics in virology. For example, he worked on the classification of viruses and bacteriophage, on the occurrence of psittacosis in Australian parrots, and on the **epidemiology** of **herpes** and **poliomyelitis**. His first major contribution to virology came, however, during his year as a Rockefeller fellow at London's National Institute for Medical Research from 1932 to 1933. There he developed a method for cultivating viruses in chicken embryos. The Burnet technique was an important breakthrough for virologists since viruses had been notoriously difficult to **culture** and maintain in the laboratory.

Over time, Burnet's work on viruses and bacteriophage led him to a different, but related, field of research, the vertebrate **immune system**. The fundamental question he attacked is one that had troubled biologists for years: how an organism's body can tell the difference between "self" and "not-self." An organism's immune system is a crucial part of its internal hardware. It provides a mechanism for fighting off invasions by potentially harmful—and sometimes fatal—foreign organisms (antigens) such as bacteria, viruses, and **fungi**. The immune system is so efficient that it even recognizes and fights back against harmless invaders such as pollen and dust, resulting in allergic reactions.

Burnet was attracted to two aspects of the phenomenon of **immunity**. First, he wondered how an organism's body distinguishes between foreign invaders and components of its own body, the "self" versus "not-self" problem. That distinction is obviously critical, since if the body fails to recognize that difference, it may begin to attack its own cells and actually destroy itself. This phenomenon does, in fact, occur in some cases of **autoimmune disorders**.

The second question on which Burnet worked was how the immune system develops. The question is complicated by the fact that a healthy immune system is normally able to recognize and respond to an apparently endless variety of antigens, producing a specific chemical (**antibody**) to combat each **antigen** it encounters. According to one theory, these antibodies are present in an organism's body from birth, prior to birth, or an early age. A second theory suggested that antibodies are produced "on the spot" as they are needed and in response to an attack by an antigen.

For more than two decades, Burnet worked on resolving these questions about the immune system. He eventually developed a complete and coherent explanation of the way the system develops in the embryo and beyond, how it develops the ability to recognize its own cells as distinct from foreign cells, and how it carries with it from the very earliest stages the templates from which antibodies are produced. For this work, Burnet was awarded a share of the 1960 Nobel Prize in physiology or medicine. Among the other honors he received were the Royal Medal and the Copley Medal of the Royal Society (1947 and 1959, respectively) and the Order of Merit in 1958. He was elected a fellow of the Royal Society in 1947 and knighted by King George V in 1951.

Burnet retired from the Hall Institute in 1965, but continued his research activities. His late work was in the area of autoimmune disorders, cancer, and aging. He died of cancer in Melbourne in 1985. Burnet was a prolific writer, primarily of books on science and medicine, during his lifetime.

See also Antigens and antibodies; Autoimmune disorders; Bacteriophage and bacteriophage typing; Immunity, cell mediated; Immunity, humoral regulation; Virology; Virus replication; Viruses and responses to viral infection

C

CAMPYLOBACTERIOSIS

Campylobacteriosis is a **bacterial infection** of the intestinal tract of humans. The infection, which typically results in diarrhea, is caused by members of the genus *Campylobacter*. In particular, *Campylobacter jejuni* is the most commonly cause of bacterial diarrhea in the United States (and likely other countries as well), with more occurrences than **salmonella** (another prominent disease causing **bacteria** associated with food poisoning). Worldwide, approximately five to fourteen per cent of all diarrhea is thought to be the result of campylobacteriosis.

Humans contract campylobacteriosis by eating or drinking contaminated food or water. Less often, direct contact with infected people or animals can spread the infection. The infection begins from two to five days after the contaminated food or water has been ingested.

The illness caused by *Campylobacter* bacteria has been known for decades, and was recognized as a cause of disease in animals since 1909. However, it is only in the last two decades of the twentieth century that the bacteria were identified as the cause of the human disease campylobacteriosis. Over 10,000 cases are now reported to the Unites States **Centers for Disease Control** (CDC) each year. As the illness is often not identified, the actual number of cases is much higher. Indeed, CDC estimates that 2 million people contract campylobacteriosis each year in the United States.

In under-developed countries, campylobacteriosis is a significant health threat. Organization such as the **World Health Organization** have devoted much effort to improving the **water quality** of villages in an effort to decrease the incidence of water-borne campylobacteriosis.

The *Campylobacter* organism is distinctive on several counts. The bacteria have a spiral shape. Also, they are fragile, not tolerating drying or the presence of pure oxygen.

As with other bacterial intestinal upsets, campylobacteriosis is more of a transient inconvenience than a dire health threat in the developed world. The symptoms of the disease (malaise, fever, abdominal cramps, diarrhea, nausea, vomiting) are often mistaken for stomach flu. Still, severe forms of the infection can produce bloody diarrhea. In some people, especially in infants, the elderly, and those whose immune systems are not operating efficiently, the resulting diarrhea and fluid loss can produce dehydration if fluid intake is not maintained during the period of illness. Very rarely, seizures can occur due to high fever or because of the exacerbation of a neurological disorder such as Guillain-Barre syndrome. Guillan-Barre syndrome occurs when a person's own **immune system** begins to attack the body's own nerves. Paralysis can result. It has been estimated that one in every 1000 cases of campylobacteriosis leads to Guillain-Barre syndrome.

Most people afflicted with campylobacteriosis recover on their own. Occasionally, **antibiotics** need to be given to rid the body of the infection. While the main bout of the malady passes in about a week, abdominal cramps can recur for up to three months after an infection.

Campylobacteriosis is an example of a zoonosis (an ailment passed to humans via animals or animal products). *Campylobacter* bacteria naturally inhabit the intestinal tract of many animals, including swine, cattle, ostriches, dogs, shellfish and poultry. These creatures can carry the bacteria without displaying any symptoms of illness. Soil is another habitat. A principle reason for the wide distribution of *Campylobacter* is the ability of the bacteria to survive anywhere there is moisture, food source, less than an atmospheric level of oxygen and room temperature conditions. In particular, poultry are a reservoir of the microorganism. These sources can contaminate meat products, water and milk. Studies monitoring poultry carcasses in processing plants have demonstrated that over 50% of raw chicken is contaminated with *Campylobacter*.

The prevalence of *Campylobacter jejuni* in poultry carcasses results from the **contamination** of the meat by the intestinal contents of the bird (including the bacteria) when an infected bird is slaughtered. Because chickens can carry the organism without showing any symptoms of infection, they can escape inspection.

Despite the high contamination rate of foodstuffs such as poultry, *Campylobacter jejuni* does not grow readily on or in foods. Furthermore, the organism is sensitive to temperatures much above room temperature. Proper cooking of food will readily destroy the bacteria. Other sensible hygienic practices, such as washing the cutting board after dealing with a chicken, also reduce the chances of illness. Unfortunately, undercooking of foods such as poultry, poor **hygiene**, and inadequate **disinfection** of drinking water accounts for most of the cases of campylobacteriosis.

See also Food safety; Water quality

CANDIDIASIS

Candidiasis is an infection that is caused by members of the fungal genus *Candida*.

The two most common species associated with Candidiasis are *Candida albicans* and *Candida glabrata*. Less commonly, but still able to cause the infection, are *Candida tropicalis*, *Candida parapsilosis*, *Candida guilliermondi*, and *Candida krusei*.

The fungus is a normal resident of the body, typically in the mouth and the gastrointestinal tract. In these habitats, the microorganism normally colonizes the cell surface. In healthy people in the United States, *Candida* species colonize more than half of these individuals. The presence of the fungus is beneficial. Invading **bacteria** are recognized by the *Candida* cells and are destroyed. Thus, the **fungi complement** the **immune system** and other defenses of the body against infection.

When the body is in proper balance with respect to the microbial flora, the fungi exist as a so-called **yeast** form. These are not capable of invasion. However, *Candida* can infect areas of the body that are warm and moist. These include the eye (conjunctivitis), fingernails, rectum, folds in the skin, and, in infants, the skin irritation in infants known commonly as diaper rash. Typically, such infections are more of an inconvenience than a dangerous health concern.

However, in people whose immune systems are compromised in some way, or when the normal balance of the microbial flora has been disrupted by, for example, antibiotic therapy, *Candida* can establish an infection. For example, an infection of the mouth region, which is referred to as oropharyngeal infection, was a very common infection in those whose immune system was deficient due to infection with the **Human immunodeficiency virus**. More aggressive antiviral therapy has reduced the incidence of the infection.

Such infections are associated with the change from the *Candida* cells from the yeast form to a so-called mycelial fungal form. The mycelia produce long, root-like structures that are called rhizoids. The rhizoids can penetrate through the mucous cells that line the inside of the mouth and vagina, and through the epithelial cells that line the intestinal tract. This invasion can spread the infection to the bloodstream. As well, the microscopic holes that are left behind in the cell walls can be portals for the entry of toxins, undigested food, bacteria, and yeast.

In countries around the world where fungal infections are widespread in the populations, *Candida* species have overtaken *Cryptococcus* species as the most common cause of infections that affect the central nervous system of immunocompromised people.

Besides the oropharyngeal infection, *Candida* can also commonly cause a vaginal infection. Both infections are evident by the development of a fever and chills that, because of the fungal genesis of the infections, are unaffected by antibacterial therapy. Visually, white patches appear on the surface of the cells lining the mouth and oral cavity and the vagina. More rarely, the infections may spread to the bloodstream. Examples of the infections that can result include the kidney, spleen, nerve cells (**meningitis**), heart (endocarditis). Arthritis may even develop. Immunocompromised individuals are especially susceptible to these infections.

The **contamination** of the bloodstream by *Candida* occurs most commonly in the hospital setting, where a patient is being treated for Candidiasis or other malady. Indeed, this type of bloodstream infection is the fourth most common cause of hospital-acquired bloodstream infections in the United States. The death rate from the infection can approach 40 per cent.

Treatment for *Candida* infections consist of the administration of antifungal drugs. Examples of the drugs of choice include amphotericin B, fluconazole, ketoconazole, and nystatin. The real possibility of the development of irritative side effects makes monitoring during therapy a prudent precaution.

See also Fungi; Immunodeficiency

CAPSID AND CAPSULE · *see* GLYCOCALYX

CARBON CYCLE IN MICROORGANISMS

The carbon cycle in **microorganisms** is part of a larger cycling of carbon that occurs on the global scale. The actions of microorganisms help extract carbon from non-living sources and make the carbon available to living organisms (including themselves).

The cycling of carbon by microorganisms, including a variety of **bacteria** and **fungi**, occurs in aquatic habitats. Even relatively oxygen-free zones such as in the deep mud of lakes, ponds and other water bodies can be regions where the anaerobic conversion of carbon takes place.

Much of the carbon that enters the carbon cycle of microorganisms is carbon dioxide. This form of carbon exists as a gas in the atmosphere and can be dissolved in water. The atmospheric carbon dioxide can be converted to organic material in the process of **photosynthesis**. Photosynthetic algae are important microorganisms in this regard. As well, chemoautotrophs, primarily bacteria and archae are capable of carbon dioxide conversion. In both systems the carbon dioxide is converted to chains that are comprised of sugars that have the structure CH_2O.

Both types of conversion take place in the presence and the absence of oxygen. Algal involvement is an aerobic process. The conversion of carbon dioxide to sugar is an energy-requiring process that generates oxygen as a by-product. This **evolution** of oxygen also occurs in plants and is one of the recognized vital benefits of trees to life on Earth.

The carbon available in the carbohydrate sugar molecules is cycled further by microorganisms in a series of reactions that form the so-called tricarboxylic acid (or TCA) cycle. The breakdown of the carbohydrate serves to supply energy to the microorganism. This process is also known as **respiration**. In anaerobic environments, microorganisms can cycle the carbon compounds to yield energy in a process known as **fermentation**.

Carbon dioxide can be converted to another gas called methane (CH_4). This occurs in anaerobic environments, such as deep compacted mud, and is accomplished by bacteria known as methanogenic bacteria. The conversion, which requires hydrogen, yields water and energy for the methanogens. To complete the recycling pattern another group of methane bacteria called methane-oxidizing bacteria or methanotrophs (literally "methane eaters") can convert methane to carbon dioxide. This conversion, which is an aerobic (oxygen-requiring) process, also yields water and energy. Methanotrophs tend to live at the boundary between aerobic and anaerobic zones. There they have access to the methane produced by the anaerobic methanogenic bacteria, but also access to the oxygen needed for their conversion of the methane.

Other microorganisms are able to participate in the cycling of carbon. For example the green and purple sulfur bacteria are able to use the energy they gain from the degradation of a compound called hydrogen sulfide to degrade carbon compounds. Other bacteria such as *Thiobacillus ferrooxidans* uses the energy gained from the removal of an electron from iron-containing compounds to convert carbon.

The anerobic degradation of carbon is done only by microorganisms. This degradation is a collaborative effort involving numerous bacteria. Examples of the bacteria include *Bacteroides succinogenes*, *Clostridium butyricum*, and *Syntrophomonas sp.* This bacterial collaboration, which is termed interspecies hydrogen transfer, is responsible for the bulk of the carbon dioxide and methane that is released to the atmosphere.

See also Bacterial growth and division; Chemoautotrophic and chemolithotrophic bacteria; Metabolism; Methane oxidizing and producing bacteria; Nitrogen cycle in microorganisms

CAULOBACTER

Caulobacter crescentus is a Gram-negative rod-like bacterium that inhabits fresh water. It is noteworthy principally because of the unusual nature of its division. Instead of dividing two form two identical daughter cells as other **bacteria** do (a process termed binary division), *Caulobacter crescentus* undergoes what is termed symmetric division. The parent bacterium divides to yield two daughter cells that differ from one another structurally and functionally.

When a bacterium divides, one cell is motile by virtue of a single flagellum at one end. This daughter cell is called a swarmer cell. The other cell does not have a flagellum. Instead, at one end of the cell there is a stalk that terminates in an attachment structure called a holdfast. This daughter cell is called the stalk cell. The stalk is an outgrowth of the cell wall, and serves to attach the bacterium to plants or to other microbes in its natural environment (lakes, streams, and sea water).

Caulobacter crescentus exhibits a distinctive behavior. The swarmer cell remains motile for 30 to 45 minutes. The cell swims around and settles onto a new surface where the food supply is suitable. After settling, the flagellum is shed and the bacterium differentiates into a stalk cell. With each division cycle the stalk becomes longer and can grow to be several times as long as the body of the bacterium.

The regulation of **gene** expression is different in the swarmer and stalk cells. Replication of the genetic material occurs immediately in the stalk cell but for reasons yet to be determined is repressed in the swarmer cell. However, when a swarmer cell differentiates into a stalk cell, replication of the genetic material immediately commences. Thus, the transition to a stalk cell is necessary before division into the daughter swarmer and stalk cells can occur.

The genetics of the swarmer to stalk **cell cycle** are complex, with at least 500 genes known to play a role in the structural transition. The regulation of these activities with respect to time are of great interest to geneticists.

Caulobacter crescentus can be grown in the laboratory so that all the bacteria in the population undergoes division at the same time. This type of growth is termed **synchronous growth**. This has made the bacterium an ideal system to study the various events in gene regulation necessary for growth and division.

See also Bacterial appendages; Bacterial surface layers; Cell cycle (prokaryotic), genetic regulation of; Phenotypic variation

CDC · *see* CENTERS FOR DISEASE CONTROL (CDC)

CECH, THOMAS R. (1947-   )
American biochemist

The work of Thomas R. Cech has revolutionized the way in which scientists look at **RNA** and at proteins. Up to the time of Cech's discoveries in 1981 and 1982, it had been thought that genetic coding, stored in the **DNA** of the **nucleus**, was imprinted or transcribed onto RNA molecules. These RNA molecules, it was believed, helped transfer the coding onto proteins produced in the **ribosomes**. The DNA/RNA nexus was thus the information center of the cell, while protein molecules in the form of **enzymes** were the workhorses, catalyzing the thousands of vital chemical reactions that occur in the cell. Conventional wisdom held that the two functions were separate—that there was a delicate division of labor. Cech and his colleagues at the University of Colorado established, however, that this picture of how RNA functions was incorrect; they proved that in the absence of other enzymes RNA acts as its own catalyst. It was a discovery that reverberated throughout the scientific community, leading not only to new technologies in RNA engineering but also to a revised view of the **evolution** of life. Cech shared the 1989 Nobel Prize for Chemistry with Sidney Altman at Yale University for their work regarding the role of RNA in cell reactions.

Cech was born in Chicago, Illinois, to Robert Franklin Cech, a physician, and Annette Marie Cerveny Cech. Cech recalled in an autobiographical sketch for *Les Prix Nobel,* he grew up in "the safe streets and good schools" of Iowa City, Iowa. His father had a deep and abiding interest in physics as well as medicine, and from an early age Cech took an avid interest in science, collecting rocks and minerals and speculating about how they had been formed. In junior high school he was already conferring with geology professors from the nearby university. Cech went to Grinnell College in 1966; at first attracted to physical chemistry, he soon concentrated on biological chemistry, graduating with a chemistry degree in 1970.

It was at Grinnell that he met Carol Lynn Martinson, who was a fellow chemistry student. They married in 1970 and went together to the University of California at Berkeley for graduate studies. His thesis advisor there was John Hearst who, Cech recalled in *Les Prix Nobel,* "had an enthusiasm for chromosome structure and function that proved infectious." Both Cech and his wife were awarded their Ph.D. degrees in 1975, and they moved to the east coast for postdoctoral positions—Cech at the Massachusetts Institute of Technology (MIT) under Mary Lou Pardue, and his wife at Harvard. At MIT Cech focused on the DNA structures of the mouse genome, strengthening his knowledge of biology at the same time.

In 1978, both Cech and his wife were offered positions at the University of Colorado in Boulder; he was appointed assistant professor in chemistry. By this time, Cech had decided that he would like to investigate more specific genetic material. He was particularly interested in what enables the DNA molecule to instruct the body to produce the various parts of itself—a process known as **gene** expression. Cech set out to discover the proteins that govern the DNA **transcription** process onto RNA, and in order to do this he decided to use nucleic acids from a single-cell **protozoa,** *Tetrahymena thermophila.* Cech chose *Tetrahymena* because it rapidly reproduced genetic material and because it had a structure which allowed for the easy extraction of DNA.

By the late 1970s, much research had already been done on DNA and its transcription partner, RNA. It had been determined that there were three types of RNA: messenger RNA, which relays the transcription of the DNA structure by attaching itself to the ribosome where **protein synthesis** occurs; ribosomal RNA, which imparts the messenger's structure within the ribosome; and transfer RNA, which helps to establish amino acids in the proper order in the protein chain as it is being built. Just prior to the time Cech began his work, it was discovered that DNA and final-product RNA (after copying or transcription) actually differed. In 1977, Phillip A. Sharp and

others discovered that portions of seemingly noncoded DNA were snipped out of the RNA and the chain was spliced back together where these intervening segments had been removed. These noncoded sections of DNA were called introns.

Cech and his coworkers were not initially interested in such introns, but they soon became fascinated with their function and the splicing mechanism itself. In an effort to understand how these so-called nonsense sequences, or introns, were removed from the transcribed RNA, Cech and his colleague Arthur Zaug decided to investigate the pre-ribosomal RNA of the *Tetrahymena,* just as it underwent transcription. In order to do this, they first isolated unspliced RNA and then added some *Tetrahymena* nuclei extract. Their assumption was that the catalytic agent or enzyme would be present in such an extract. The two scientists also added small molecules of salts and nucleotides for energy, varying the amounts of each in subsequent experiments, even excluding one or more of the additives. But the experiment took a different turn than was expected.

Cech and Zaug discovered instead that RNA splicing occurred even without the nucleic material being present. This was a development they did not understand at first; it was a long-held scientific belief that proteins in the form of enzymes had to be present for catalysis to occur. Presenting itself was a situation in which RNA appeared to be its own catalytic motivator. At first they suspected that their experiment had been contaminated. Cech did further experiments involving recombinant DNA in which there could be no possibility of the presence of splicing enzymes, and these had the same result: the RNA spliced out its own intron. Further discoveries in Cech's laboratory into the nature of the intron led to his belief that the intron itself was the catalytic agent of RNA splicing, and he decided that this was a sort of RNA enzyme which they called the ribozyme.

Cech's findings of 1982 met with heated debate in the scientific community, for it upset many beliefs about the nature of enzymes. Cech's ribozyme was in fact not a true enzyme, for thus far he had shown it only to work upon itself and to be changed in the reaction; true enzymes catalyze repeatedly and come out of the reaction unchanged. Other critics argued that this was a freak bit of RNA on a strange microorganism and that it would not be found in other organisms. The critics were soon proved wrong, however, when scientists around the world began discovering other RNA enzymes. In 1984, Sidney Altman proved that RNA carries out enzyme-like activities on substances other than itself.

The discovery of catalytic RNA has had profound results. In the medical field alone RNA enzymology may lead to cures of viral infections. By using these rybozymes as gene scissors, the RNA molecule can be cut at certain points, destroying the RNA molecules that cause infections or genetic disorders. In life sciences, the discovery of catalytic RNA has also changed conventional wisdom. The old debate about whether proteins or nucleic acids were the first bit of life form seems to have been solved. If RNA can act as a catalyst and a genetic template to create proteins as well as itself, then it is rather certain that RNA was first in the chain of life.

Cech and Altman won the Nobel Prize for chemistry in 1989 for their independent discoveries of catalytic RNA. Cech has also been awarded the Passano Foundation Young Scientist Award and the Harrison Howe Award in 1984; the Pfizer Award in Enzyme Chemistry in 1985; the U. S. Steel Award in **Molecular Biology**; and the V. D. Mattia Award in 1987. In 1988, he won the Newcombe-Cleveland Award, the Heineken Prize, the Gairdner Foundation International Award, the Louisa Gross Horwitz Prize, and the Albert Lasker Basic Medical Research Award; he was presented with the Bonfils-Stanton Award for Science in 1990.

Cech was made full professor in the department of chemistry at the University of Colorado in 1983. Cech and his wife have two daughters. In the midst of his busy research career, Cech finds time to enjoy skiing and backpacking.

See also Viral genetics

CELL-MEDIATED IMMUNE RESPONSE • *see* IMMUNITY, CELL MEDIATED

CELL CYCLE AND CELL DIVISION

The series of stages that a cell undergoes while progressing to division is known as cell cycle. In order for an organism to grow and develop, the organism's cells must be able to duplicate themselves. Three basic events must take place to achieve this duplication: the **deoxyribonucleic acid DNA**, which makes up the individual **chromosomes** within the cell's **nucleus** must be duplicated; the two sets of DNA must be packaged up into two separate nuclei; and the cell's **cytoplasm** must divide itself to create two separate cells, each complete with its own nucleus. The two new cells, products of the single original cell, are known as daughter cells.

Although prokaryotes (e.g. **bacteria**, non-nucleated unicellular organisms) divide through binary fission, **eukaryotes** (including, of course, human cells) undergo a more complex process of cell division because DNA is packed in several chromosomes located inside a cell nucleus. In eukaryotes, cell division may take two different paths, in accordance with the cell type involved. Mitosis is a cellular division resulting in two identical nuclei that takes place in somatic cells. Sex cells or gametes (ovum and spermatozoids) divide by meiosis. The process of meiosis results in four nuclei, each containing half of the original number of chromosomes. Both prokaryotes and eukaryotes undergo a final process, known as cytoplasmatic division, which divides the parental cell in new daughter cells.

Mitosis is the process during which two complete, identical sets of chromosomes are produced from one original set. This allows a cell to divide during another process called cytokinesis, thus creating two completely identical daughter cells.

During much of a cell's life, the DNA within the nucleus is not actually organized into the discrete units known as chromosomes. Instead, the DNA exists loosely within the nucleus, in a form called chromatin. Prior to the major events of mitosis, the DNA must replicate itself, so that each cell has twice as much DNA as previously.

Cells undergoing division are also termed competent cells. When a cell is not progressing to mitosis, it remains in phase G0 ("G" zero). Therefore, the cell cycle is divided into two major phases: interphase and mitosis. Interphase includes the phases (or stages) G1, S and G2 whereas mitosis is subdivided into prophase, metaphase, anaphase and telophase.

Interphase is a phase of cell growth and metabolic activity, without cell nuclear division, comprised of several stages or phases. During Gap 1 or G1 the cell resumes protein and **RNA** synthesis, which was interrupted during previous mitosis, thus allowing the growth and maturation of young cells to accomplish their physiologic function. Immediately following is a variable length pause for DNA checking and repair before cell cycle transition to phase S during which there is synthesis or semi-conservative replication or synthesis of DNA. During Gap 2 or G2, there is increased RNA and **protein synthesis**, followed by a second pause for proofreading and eventual repairs in the newly synthesized DNA sequences before transition to mitosis.

The cell cycle starts in G1, with the active synthesis of RNA and proteins, which are necessary for young cells to grow and mature. The time G1 lasts, varies greatly among eukaryotic cells of different species and from one tissue to another in the same organism. Tissues that require fast cellular renovation, such as mucosa and endometrial epithelia, have shorter G1 periods than those tissues that do not require frequent renovation or repair, such as muscles or connective tissues.

The first stage of mitosis is called prophase. During prophase, the DNA organizes or condenses itself into the specific units known as chromosomes. Chromosomes appear as double-stranded structures. Each strand is a replica of the other and is called a chromatid. The two chromatids of a chromosome are joined at a special region, the centromere. Structures called centrioles position themselves across from each other, at either end of the cell. The nuclear membrane then disappears.

During the stage of mitosis called metaphase, the chromosomes line themselves up along the midline of the cell. Fibers called spindles attach themselves to the centromere of each chromosome.

During the third stage of mitosis, called anaphase, spindle fibers will pull the chromosomes apart at their centromere (chromosomes have two complementary halves, similar to the two nonidentical but complementary halves of a zipper). One arm of each chromosome will migrate toward each centriole, pulled by the spindle fibers.

During the final stage of mitosis, telophase, the chromosomes decondense, becoming unorganized chromatin again. A nuclear membrane forms around each daughter set of chromosomes, and the spindle fibers disappear. Sometime during telophase, the cytoplasm and cytoplasmic membrane of the cell split into two (cytokinesis), each containing one set of chromosomes residing within its nucleus.

Cells are mainly induced into proliferation by growth factors or hormones that occupy specific receptors on the surface of the cell membrane, being also known as extra-cellular

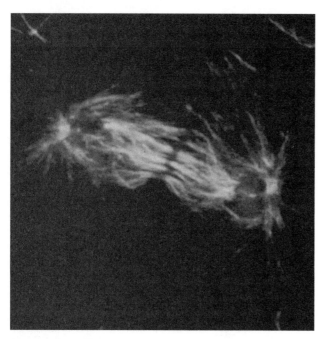

Segregation of eukaryotic genetic material during mitosis.

ligands. Examples of growth factors are as such: epidermal growth factor (EGF), fibroblastic growth factor (FGF), platelet-derived growth factor (PDGF), insulin-like growth factor (IGF), or by hormones. PDGF and FGF act by regulating the phase G2 of the cell cycle and during mitosis. After mitosis, they act again stimulating the daughter cells to grow, thus leading them from G0 to G1. Therefore, FGF and PDGF are also termed competence factors, whereas EGF and IGF are termed progression factors, because they keep the process of cellular progression to mitosis going on. Growth factors are also classified (along with other molecules that promote the cell cycle) as pro-mitotic signals. Hormones are also pro-mitotic signals. For example, thyrotrophic hormone, one of the hormones produced by the pituitary gland, induces the proliferation of thyroid gland's cells. Another pituitary hormone, known as growth hormone or somatotrophic hormone (STH), is responsible by body growth during childhood and early adolescence, inducing the lengthening of the long bones and protein synthesis. Estrogens are hormones that do not occupy a membrane receptor, but instead, penetrate the cell and the nucleus, binding directly to specific sites in the DNA, thus inducing the cell cycle.

Anti-mitotic signals may have several different origins, such as cell-to-cell adhesion, factors of adhesion to the extracellular matrix, or soluble factor such as TGF beta (tumor growth factor beta), which inhibits abnormal cell proliferation, proteins p53, p16, p21, APC, pRb, etc. These molecules are the products of a class of genes called tumor suppressor genes. Oncogenes, until recently also known as proto-oncogenes, synthesize proteins that enhance the stimuli started by growth factors, amplifying the mitotic signal to the nucleus, and/or promoting the accomplishment of a necessary step of the cell cycle. When each phase of the cell cycle is completed, the pro-

teins involved in that phase are degraded, so that once the next phase starts, the cell is unable to go back to the previous one. Next to the end of phase G1, the cycle is paused by tumor suppressor **gene** products, to allow verification and repair of DNA damage. When DNA damage is not repairable, these genes stimulate other intra-cellular pathways that induce the cell into suicide or apoptosis (also known as programmed cell death). To the end of phase G2, before the transition to mitosis, the cycle is paused again for a new verification and "decision": either mitosis or apoptosis.

Along each pro-mitotic and anti-mitotic intra-cellular signaling pathway, as well as along the apoptotic pathways, several gene products (**proteins and enzymes**) are involved in an orderly sequence of activation and inactivation, forming complex webs of signal transmission and signal amplification to the nucleus. The general goal of such cascades of signals is to achieve the orderly progression of each phase of the cell cycle.

Mitosis always creates two completely identical cells from the original cell. In mitosis, the total amount of DNA doubles briefly, so that the subsequent daughter cells will ultimately have the exact amount of DNA initially present in the original cell. Mitosis is the process by which all of the cells of the body divide and therefore reproduce. The only cells of the body that do not duplicate through mitosis are the sex cells (egg and sperm cells). These cells undergo a slightly different type of cell division called meiosis, which allows each sex cell produced to contain half of its original amount of DNA, in anticipation of doubling it again when an egg and a sperm unite during the course of conception.

Meiosis, also known as reduction division, consists of two successive cell divisions in diploid cells. The two cell divisions are similar to mitosis, but differ in that the chromosomes are duplicated only once, not twice. The result of meiosis is four haploid daughter cells. Because meiosis only occurs in the sex organs (gonads), the daughter cells are the gametes (spermatozoa or ova), which contain hereditary material. By halving the number of chromosomes in the sex cells, meiosis assures that the fusion of maternal and paternal gametes at fertilization will result in offspring with the same chromosome number as the parents. In other words, meiosis compensates for chromosomes doubling at fertilization. The two successive nuclear divisions are termed as meiosis I and meiosis II. Each is further divided into four phases (prophase, metaphase, anaphase, and telophase) with an intermediate phase (interphase) preceding each nuclear division.

The events that take place during meiosis are similar in many ways to the process of mitosis, in which one cell divides to form two clones (exact copies) of itself. It is important to note that the purpose and final products of mitosis and meiosis are very different.

Meiosis I is preceded by an interphase period in which the DNA replicates (makes an exact duplicate of itself), resulting in two exact copies of each chromosome that are firmly attached at one point, the centromere. Each copy is a sister chromatid, and the pair are still considered as only one chromosome. The first phase of meiosis I, prophase I, begins as the chromosomes come together in homologous pairs in a process known as synapsis. Homologous chromosomes, or homologues, consist of two chromosomes that carry genetic information for the same traits, although that information may hold different messages (e.g., when two chromosomes carry a message for eye color, but one codes for blue eyes while the other codes for brown). The fertilized eggs (zygotes) of all sexually reproducing organisms receive their chromosomes in pairs, one from the mother and one from the father. During synapsis, adjacent chromatids from homologous chromosomes "cross over" one another at random points and join at spots called chiasmata. These connections hold the pair together as a tetrad (a set of four chromatids, two from each homologue). At the chiasmata, the connected chromatids randomly exchange bits of genetic information so that each contains a mixture of maternal and paternal genes. This "shuffling" of the DNA produces a tetrad, in which each of the chromatids is different from the others, and a gamete that is different from others produced by the same parent. Crossing over does explain why each person is a unique individual, different even from those in the immediate family. Prophase I is also marked by the appearance of spindle fibers (strands of microtubules) extending from the poles or ends of the cell as the nuclear membrane disappears. These spindle fibers attach to the chromosomes during metaphase I as the tetrads line up along the middle or equator of the cell. A spindle fiber from one pole attaches to one chromosome while a fiber from the opposite pole attaches to its homologue. Anaphase I is characterized by the separation of the homologues, as chromosomes are drawn to the opposite poles. The sister chromatids are still intact, but the homologous chromosomes are pulled apart at the chiasmata. Telophase I begins as the chromosomes reach the poles and a nuclear membrane forms around each set. Cytokinesis occurs as the cytoplasm and organelles are divided in half and the one parent cell is split into two new daughter cells. Each daughter cell is now haploid (n), meaning it has half the number of chromosomes of the original parent cell (which is diploid-2n). These chromosomes in the daughter cells still exist as sister chromatids, but there is only one chromosome from each original homologous pair.

The phases of meiosis II are similar to those of meiosis I, but there are some important differences. The time between the two nuclear divisions (interphase II) lacks replication of DNA (as in interphase I). As the two daughter cells produced in meiosis I enter meiosis II, their chromosomes are in the form of sister chromatids. No crossing over occurs in prophase II because there are no homologues to synapse. During metaphase II, the spindle fibers from the opposite poles attach to the sister chromatids (instead of the homologues as before). The chromatids are then pulled apart during anaphase II. As the centromeres separate, the two single chromosomes are drawn to the opposite poles. The end result of meiosis II is that by the end of telophase II, there are four haploid daughter cells (in the sperm or ova) with each chromosome now represented by a single copy. The distribution of chromatids during meiosis is a matter of chance, which results in the concept of the law of independent assortment in genetics.

The events of meiosis are controlled by a protein enzyme complex known collectively as maturation promoting factor (MPF). These **enzymes** interact with one another and with cell organelles to cause the breakdown and reconstruction of the nuclear membrane, the formation of the spindle fibers, and the final division of the cell itself. MPF appears to work in a cycle, with the proteins slowly accumulating during interphase, and then rapidly degrading during the later stages of meiosis. In effect, the rate of synthesis of these proteins controls the frequency and rate of meiosis in all sexually reproducing organisms from the simplest to the most complex.

Meiosis occurs in humans, giving rise to the haploid gametes, the sperm and egg cells. In males, the process of gamete production is known as spermatogenesis, where each dividing cell in the testes produces four functional sperm cells, all approximately the same size. Each is propelled by a primitive but highly efficient flagellum (tail). In contrast, in females, oogenesis produces only one surviving egg cell from each original parent cell. During cytokinesis, the cytoplasm and organelles are concentrated into only one of the four daughter cells—the one that will eventually become the female ovum or egg. The other three smaller cells, called polar bodies, die and are reabsorbed shortly after formation. The concentration of cytoplasm and organelles into the oocyte greatly enhances the ability of the zygote (produced at fertilization from the unification of the mature ovum with a spermatozoa) to undergo rapid cell division.

The control of cell division is a complex process and is a topic of much scientific research. Cell division is stimulated by certain kinds of chemical compounds. Molecules called **cytokines** are secreted by some cells to stimulate others to begin cell division. Contact with adjacent cells can also control cell division. The phenomenon of contact inhibition is a process where the physical contact between neighboring cells prevents cell division from occurring. When contact is interrupted, however, cell division is stimulated to close the gap between cells. Cell division is a major mechanism by which organisms grow, tissues and organs maintain themselves, and wound healing occurs.

Cancer is a form of uncontrolled cell division. The cell cycle is highly regulated by several enzymes, proteins, and cytokines in each of its phases, in order to ensure that the resulting daughter cells receive the appropriate amount of genetic information originally present in the parental cell. In the case of somatic cells, each of the two daughter cells must contain an exact copy of the original genome present in the parental cell. Cell cycle controls also regulate when and to what extent the cells of a given tissue must proliferate, in order to avoid abnormal cell proliferation that could lead to dysplasia or tumor development. Therefore, when one or more of such controls are lost or inhibited, abnormal overgrowth will occur and may lead to impairment of function and disease.

See also Amino acid chemistry; Bacterial growth and division; Cell cycle (eukaryotic), genetic regulation of; Cell cycle (prokaryotic), genetic regulation of; Chromosomes, eukaryotic; Chromosomes, prokaryotic; DNA (Deoxyribonucleic acid); Enzymes; Genetic regulation of eukaryotic cells; Genetic regulation of prokaryotic cells; Molecular biology and molecular genetics

CELL CYCLE (EUKARYOTIC), GENETIC REGULATION OF

Although prokaryotes (i.e., non-nucleated unicellular organisms) divide through binary fission, **eukaryotes** undergo a more complex process of cell division because **DNA** is packed in several **chromosomes** located inside a cell **nucleus**. In eukaryotes, cell division may take two different paths, in accordance with the cell type involved. Mitosis is a cellular division resulting in two identical nuclei is performed by somatic cells. The process of meiosis results in four nuclei, each containing half of the original number of chromosomes. Sex cells or gametes (ovum and spermatozoids) divide by meiosis. Both prokaryotes and eukaryotes undergo a final process, known as cytoplasmatic division, which divides the parental cell into new daughter cells.

The series of stages that a cell undergoes while progressing to division is known as **cell cycle**. Cells undergoing division are also termed competent cells. When a cell is not progressing to mitosis, it remains in phase G0 ("G" zero). Therefore, the cell cycle is divided into two major phases: interphase and mitosis. Interphase includes the phases (or stages) G1, S and G2 whereas mitosis is subdivided into prophase, metaphase, anaphase and telophase.

The cell cycle starts in G1, with the active synthesis of **RNA** and proteins, which are necessary for young cells to grow and mature. The time G1 lasts, varies greatly among eukaryotic cells of different species and from one tissue to another in the same organism. Tissues that require fast cellular renovation, such as mucosa and endometrial epithelia, have shorter G1 periods than those tissues that do not require frequent renovation or repair, such as muscles or connective tissues.

The cell cycle is highly regulated by several **enzymes**, proteins, and **cytokines** in each of its phases, in order to ensure that the resulting daughter cells receive the appropriate amount of genetic information originally present in the parental cell. In the case of somatic cells, each of the two daughter cells must contain an exact copy of the original genome present in the parental cell. Cell cycle controls also regulate when and to what extent the cells of a given tissue must proliferate, in order to avoid abnormal cell proliferation that could lead to dysplasia or tumor development. Therefore, when one or more of such controls are lost or inhibited, abnormal overgrowth will occur and may lead to impairment of function and disease.

Cells are mainly induced into proliferation by growth factors or hormones that occupy specific receptors on the surface of the cell membrane, and are also known as extra-cellular ligands. Examples of growth factors are as such: epidermal growth factor (EGF), fibroblastic growth factor (FGF), platelet-derived growth factor (PDGF), insulin-like growth factor (IGF), or by hormones. PDGF and FGF act by regulating the phase G2 of the cell cycle and during mitosis. After mitosis, they act again stimulating the daughter cells to grow, thus leading them from G0 to G1. Therefore, FGF and PDGF are also termed competence factors, whereas EGF and IGF are termed progression factors, because they keep the process of cellular progression to mitosis going on. Growth factors are also classified (along with other

molecules that promote the cell cycle) as pro-mitotic signals. Hormones are also pro-mitotic signals. For example, thyrotrophic hormone, one of the hormones produced by the pituitary gland, induces the proliferation of thyroid gland's cells. Another pituitary hormone, known as growth hormone or somatotrophic hormone (STH), is responsible by body growth during childhood and early adolescence, inducing the lengthening of the long bones and **protein synthesis**. Estrogens are hormones that do not occupy a membrane receptor, but instead, penetrate the cell and the nucleus, binding directly to specific sites in the DNA, thus inducing the cell cycle.

Anti-mitotic signals may have several different origins, such as cell-to-cell adhesion, factors of adhesion to the extracellular matrix, or soluble factor such as TGF beta (tumor growth factor beta), which inhibits abnormal cell proliferation, proteins p53, p16, p21, APC, pRb, etc. These molecules are the products of a class of genes called tumor suppressor genes. Oncogenes, until recently also known as proto-oncogenes, synthesize proteins that enhance the stimuli started by growth factors, amplifying the mitotic signal to the nucleus, and/or promoting the accomplishment of a necessary step of the cell cycle. When each phase of the cell cycle is completed, the proteins involved in that phase are degraded, so that once the next phase starts, the cell is unable to go back to the previous one. Next to the end of phase G1, the cycle is paused by tumor suppressor **gene** products, to allow verification and repair of DNA damage. When DNA damage is not repairable, these genes stimulate other intra-cellular pathways that induce the cell into suicide or apoptosis (also known as programmed cell death). To the end of phase G2, before the transition to mitosis, the cycle is paused again for a new verification and "decision": either mitosis or apoptosis.

Along each pro-mitotic and anti-mitotic intra-cellular signaling pathway, as well as along the apoptotic pathways, several gene products (**proteins and enzymes**) are involved in an orderly sequence of activation and inactivation, forming complex webs of signal transmission and signal amplification to the nucleus. The general goal of such cascades of signals is to achieve the orderly progression of each phase of the cell cycle.

Interphase is a phase of cell growth and metabolic activity, without cell nuclear division, comprised of several stages or phases. During Gap 1 or G1 the cell resumes protein and RNA synthesis, which was interrupted during mitosis, thus allowing the growth and maturation of young cells to accomplish their physiologic function. Immediately following is a variable length pause for DNA checking and repair before cell cycle transition to phase S during which there is synthesis or semiconservative replication or synthesis of DNA. During Gap 2 or G2, there is increased RNA and protein synthesis, followed by a second pause for proofreading and eventual repairs in the newly synthesized DNA sequences before transition to Mitosis.

At the start of mitosis the chromosomes are already duplicated, with the sister-chromatids (identical chromosomes) clearly visible under a light **microscope**. Mitosis is subdivided into prophase, metaphase, anaphase and telophase.

During prophase there is a high condensation of chromatids, with the beginning of nucleolus disorganization and nuclear membrane disintegration, followed by the start of cen-

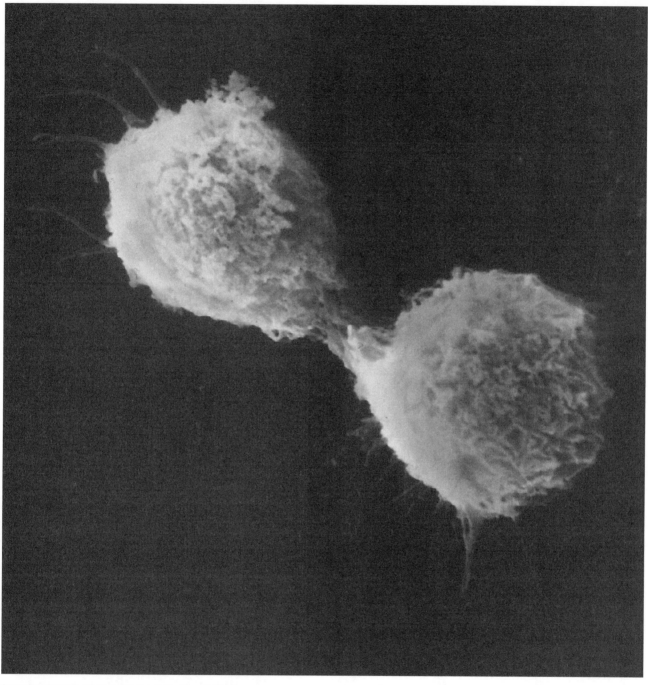

Scanning electron micrograph of eukaryotic cell division.

trioles' migration to opposite cell poles. During metaphase the chromosomes organize at the equator of a spindle apparatus (microtubules), forming a structure termed metaphase plate. The sister-chromatids are separated and joined to different centromeres, while the microtubules forming the spindle are attached to a region of the centromere termed kinetochore. During anaphase there are spindles, running from each opposite kinetochore, that pull each set of chromosomes to their respective cell poles, thus ensuring that in the following phase each new cell will ultimately receive an equal division of chromosomes. During telophase, kinetochores and spindles disintegrate, the reorganization of nucleus begins, chromatin becomes less condensed, and the nucleus membrane start forming again around each set of chromosomes. The cytoskeleton is reorganized and the somatic cell has now doubled its volume and presents two organized nucleus.

Cytokinesis usually begins during telophase, and is the process of cytoplasmatic division. This process of division varies among species but in somatic cells, it occurs through the equal division of the cytoplasmatic content, with the plasma membrane forming inwardly a deep cleft that ultimately divides the parental cell in two new daughter cells.

The identification and detailed understanding of the many molecules involved in the cell cycle controls and intracellular signal **transduction** is presently under investigation by several research groups around the world. This knowledge is crucial to the development of new anti-cancer drugs as well as to new treatments for other genetic diseases, in which a gene over expression or deregulation may be causing either a chronic or an acute disease, or the impairment of a vital organ function. Scientists predict that the next two decades will be dedicated to the identification of gene products and their respective function in the cellular microenvironment. This new field of research is termed **proteomics**.

See also Cell cycle (Prokaryotic) genetic regulation of; Genetic regulation of eukaryotic cells; Genetic regulation of prokaryotic cells

CELL CYCLE (PROKARYOTIC), GENETIC REGULATION OF

Although prokaryotes do not have an organized **nucleus** and other complex organelles found in eukaryotic cells, prokaryotic organisms share some common features with **eukaryotes** as far as cell division is concerned. For example, they both replicate **DNA** in a semi conservative manner, and the segregation of the newly formed DNA molecules occurs before the cell division takes place through cytokinesis. Despite such similarities, the prokaryotic genome is stored in a single DNA molecule, whereas eukaryotes may contain a varied number of DNA molecules, specific to each species, seen in the interphasic nucleus as **chromosomes**. Prokaryotic cells also differ in other ways from eukaryotic cells. Prokaryotes do not have cytoskeleton and the DNA is not condensed during mitosis. The prokaryote chromosomes do not present histones, the complexes of histonic proteins that help to pack eukaryotic DNA into a condensate state. Prokaryotic DNA has one single promoter site that initiates replication, whereas eukaryotic DNA has multiple promoter sites. Prokaryotes have a lack of spindle apparatus (or microtubules), which are essential structures for chromosome segregation in eukaryotic cells. In prokaryotes, there are no membranes and organelles dividing the cytosol in different compartments. Although two or more DNA molecules may be present in a given prokaryotic cell, they are genetically identical. They may contain one extra circular strand of genes known as plasmid, much smaller than the genomic DNA, and **plasmids** may be transferred to another prokaryote through bacterial **conjugation**, a process known as horizontal **gene** transfer.

The prokaryotic method of reproduction is asexual and is termed binary fission because one cell is divided in two new identical cells. Some prokaryotes also have a plasmid. Genes in **plasmids** are extra-chromosomal genes and can either be separately duplicated by a class of gene known as **transposons** Type II, or simply passed on to another individual. Transposons Type I may transfer and insert one or more genes from the plasmid to the cell DNA or vice-versa causing mutation through genetic **recombination**. The chromosome is attached to a region of the internal side of the membrane, forming a nucleoide. Some bacterial cells do present two or more nucleoides, but the genes they contain are identical.

The prokaryotic **cell cycle** is usually a fast process and may occur every 20 minutes in favorable conditions. However, some **bacteria**, such as *Mycobacterium leprae* (the cause of **leprosy**), take 12 days to accomplish replication in the host's leprous lesion. Replication of prokaryotic DNA, as well as of eukaryotic DNA, is a semi- conservative process, which means that each newly synthesized strand is paired with its complementary parental strand. Each daughter cell, therefore, receives a double-stranded circular DNA molecule that is formed by a new strand is paired with an old strand.

The cell cycle is regulated by genes encoding products (i.e., **enzymes** and proteins) that play crucial roles in the maintenance of an orderly sequence of events that ensures that each resultant daughter cell will inherit the same amount of genetic information. Cell induction into proliferation and DNA replication are controlled by specific gene products, such as enzyme DNA polymerase III, that binds to a promoter region in the circular DNA, initiating its replication. However, DNA polymerase requires the presence of a pre-existing strand of DNA, which serves as a template, as well as **RNA** primers, to initiate the polymerization of a new strand. Before replication starts, timidine-H³, (a DNA precursor) is added to a Y-shaped site where the double helices were separated, known as the replicating fork. The DNA strands are separated by enzyme helicases and kept apart during replication by single strand proteins (or ss DNA-binding proteins) that binds to DNA, while the enzyme topoisomerase further unwinds and elongates the two strands to undo the circular ring.

DNA polymerase always makes the new strand by starting from the extremity 5' and terminating at the extremity 3'. Moreover, the two DNA strands have opposite directions (i.e., they keep an anti-parallel arrangement to each other). Therefore, the new strand 5' to 3' that is complementary to the old strand 3' to 5' is synthesized in a continuous process (leading strand synthesis), whereas the other new strand (3' to 5') is synthesized in several isolated fragments (lagging strand synthesis) that will be later bound together to form the whole strand. The new 3' to 5' strand is complementary to the old 5' to 3'. However, the lagging fragments, known as Okazaki's fragments, are individually synthesized in the direction 5' to 3' by DNA polymerase III. RNA polymerases produce the RNA primers that help DNA polymerases to synthesize the leading strand. Nevertheless, the small fragments of the lagging strand have as primers a special RNA that is synthesized by another enzyme, the primase. Enzyme topoisomerase III does the proofreading of the newly transcribed sequences and eliminates those wrongly transcribed, before DNA synthesis may continue. RNA primers are removed from the newly synthesized sequences by ribonuclease H. Polymerase I fills the gaps and DNA ligase joins the lagging strands.

After DNA replication, each DNA molecule is segregated, i.e., separated from the other, and attached to a different region of the internal face of the membrane. The formation of a septum, or dividing internal wall, separates the cell into halves, each containing a nucleotide. The process of splitting the cell in two identical daughter cells is known as cytokinesis.

See also Bacterial growth and division; Biochemistry; Cell cycle (eukaryotic), genetic regulation of; Cell cycle and cell division; Chromosomes, eukaryotic; Chromosomes, prokaryotic; DNA (Deoxyribonucleic acid); Enzymes; Genetic regulation of eukaryotic cells; Genetic regulation of prokaryotic cells; Genotype and phenotype; Molecular biology and molecular genetics

CELL MEMBRANE TRANSPORT

The cell is bound by an outer membrane that, in accord with the fluid mosaic model, is comprised of a phospholipid lipid bilayer with proteins—molecules that also act as receptor sites—interspersed within the phospholipid bilayer. Varieties of channels exist within the membrane. There are a number of internal cellular membranes that partially partition the intercellular matrix, and that ultimately become continuous with the nuclear membrane.

There are three principal mechanisms of outer cellular membrane transport (i.e., means by which molecules can pass through the boundary cellular membrane). The transport mechanisms are passive, or gradient diffusion, facilitated diffusion, and active transport.

Diffusion is a process in which the random motions of molecules or other particles result in a net movement from a region of high concentration to a region of lower concentration. A familiar example of diffusion is the dissemination of floral perfumes from a bouquet to all parts of the motionless air of a room. The rate of flow of the diffusing substance is proportional to the concentration gradient for a given direction of diffusion. Thus, if the concentration of the diffusing substance is very high at the source, and is diffusing in a direction where little or none is found, the diffusion rate will be maximized. Several substances may diffuse more or less independently and simultaneously within a space or volume of liquid. Because lightweight molecules have higher average speeds than heavy molecules at the same temperature, they also tend to diffuse more rapidly. Molecules of the same weight move more rapidly at higher temperatures, increasing the rate of diffusion as the temperature rises.

Driven by concentration gradients, diffusion in the cell usually takes place through channels or pores lined by proteins. Size and electrical charge may inhibit or prohibit the passage of certain molecules or electrolytes (e.g., sodium, potassium, etc.).

Osmosis describes diffusion of water across cell membranes. Although water is a polar molecule (i.e., has overall partially positive and negative charges separated by its molecular structure), transmembrane proteins form hydrophilic (water loving) channels to through which water molecules may move.

Facilitated diffusion is the diffusion of a substance not moving against a concentration gradient (i.e., from a region of low concentration to high concentration) but which require the assistance of other molecules. These are not considered to be energetic reactions (i.e., energy in the form of use of adenosine triphosphate molecules (ATP) is not required. The facilitation or assistance—usually in physically turning or orienting a molecule so that it may more easily pass through a membrane—may be by other molecules undergoing their own random motion.

Transmembrane proteins establish pores through which ions and some small hydrophilic molecules are able to pass by diffusion. The channels open and close according to the physiological needs and state of the cell. Because they open and close transmembrane proteins are termed "gated" proteins. Control of the opening and closing mechanism may be via mechanical, electrical, or other types of membrane changes that may occur as various molecules bind to cell receptor sites.

Active transport is movement of molecules across a cell membrane or membrane of a cell organelle, from a region of low concentration to a region of high concentration. Since these molecules are being moved against a concentration gradient, cellular energy is required for active transport. Active transport allows a cell to maintain conditions different from the surrounding environment.

There are two main types of active transport; movement directly across the cell membrane with assistance from transport proteins, and endocytosis, the engulfing of materials into a cell using the processes of pinocytosis, **phagocytosis**, or receptor-mediated endocytosis.

Transport proteins found within the phospholipid bilayer of the cell membrane can move substances directly across the cell membrane, molecule by molecule. The sodium-potassium pump, which is found in many cells and helps nerve cells to pass their signals in the form of electrical impulses, is a well-studied example of active transport using transport proteins. The transport proteins that are an essential part of the sodium-potassium pump maintain a higher concentration of potassium ions inside the cells compared to outside, and a higher concentration of sodium ions outside of cells compared to inside. In order to carry the ions across the cell membrane and against the concentration gradient, the transport proteins have very specific shapes that only fit or bond well with sodium and potassium ions. Because the transport of these ions is against the concentration gradient, it requires a significant amount of energy.

Endocytosis is an infolding and then pinching in of the cell membrane so that materials are engulfed into a vacuole or vesicle within the cell. Pinocytosis is the process in which cells engulf liquids. The liquids may or may not contain dissolved materials. Phagocytosis is the process in which the materials that are taken into the cell are solid particles. With receptor-mediated endocytosis the substances that are to be transported into the cell first bind to specific sites or receptor proteins on the outside of the cell. The substances can then be engulfed into the cell. As the materials are being carried into the cell, the cell membrane pinches in forming a vacuole or other vesicle. The materials can then be used inside the cell.

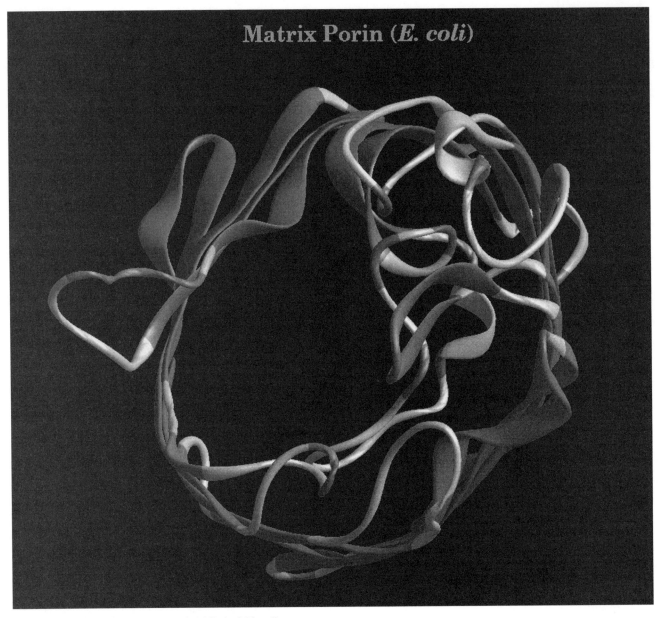

Matrix Porin (*E. coli*)

View down the channel of the matrix porin of *Escherichia coli*.

Because all types of endocytosis use energy, they are considered active transport.

See also Bacterial growth and division; Biochemistry; Cell cycle and cell division; Enzymes; Molecular biology and molecular genetics

CENTERS FOR DISEASE CONTROL

The Centers for Disease Control and Prevention (CDC) is one of the primary **public health** institutions in the world. CDC is headquartered in Atlanta, Georgia, with facilities at 9 other sites in the United States. The centers are the focus of the United States government efforts to develop and implement prevention and control strategies for diseases, including those of microbiological origin.

The CDC is home to 11 national centers that address various aspects of health care and disease prevention. Examples of the centers include the National Center for Chronic Disease Prevention and Health promotion, National Center for Infectious Diseases, National **Immunization** Program, and the National Center for **HIV**, STD, and TB Prevention.

CDC was originally the acronym for The Communicable Disease Center. This center was a redesignation of an existing facility known as the Malaria Control in War Areas. The malaria control effort had been mandated to eradicate

malaria from the southern United States during World War II. The Communicable Disease Center began operations in Atlanta on July 1, 1946, under the direction of Dr. Joseph M. Mountin.

Initially, the center was very small and was staffed mainly by engineers and entomologists (scientists who study insects). But under Mountin's direction, an expansion program was begun with the intent of making the center the predominant United States center of **epidemiology**. By 1950 the center had opened a disease surveillance unit that remains a cornerstone of CDC's operations today. Indeed, during the Korean War, the Epidemiological Intelligence Service was created, to protect the United States from the immigration of disease causing **microorganisms**.

Two events in the 1950s brought the CDC to national prominence and assured the ongoing funding of the center. The first event was the outbreak of **poliomyelitis** in children who had received an inoculation with the recently approved Salk polio **vaccine**. A Polio Surveillance Unit that was established at CDC confirmed the cause of the cases to be due to a contaminated batch of the vaccine. With CDC's help, the problem was solved and the national polio **vaccination** program recommenced. The other event was a massive outbreak of influenzae. Data collected by CDC helped pave the way for the development of **influenza** vaccines and inoculation programs.

In the 1950s and 1960s, CDC became the center for venereal disease, **tuberculosis**, and immunization programs. The centers also played a pivotal role in the eradication of **smallpox**, through the development of a vaccine and an inoculation instrument. Other accomplishments include the identification of **Legionnaire's disease** and **toxic shock syndrome** in the 1970s and 1980s, hantavirus pulmonary syndrome in 1993, and, beginning in 1981, a lead role in the research and treatment of Acquired **Immunodeficiency** Syndrome.

In 1961, CDC took over the task of publishing *Morbidity and Mortality Weekly Report*. Then as now, the MMWR is a definitive weekly synopsis of data on deaths and selected diseases from every state in the United States. A noteworthy publication in MMWR was the first report in a 1981 issue of the disease that would come to be known as Acquired Immunodeficiency Syndrome.

Another advance took place in 1978, with the opening of a containment facility that could be used to study the most lethal **viruses** known to exist (e.g., Ebola). Only a few such facilities exist in the world. Without such high containment facilities, hemorrhagic viruses could not be studied, and development of vaccines would be impossible.

Ultimately, CDC moved far beyond its original mandate as a communicable disease center. To reflect this change, the name of the organization was changed in 1970 to the Center for Disease Control. In 1981, the name was again changed to the Centers for Disease Control. The subsequent initiation of programs designed to target chronic diseases, breast and cervical cancers and lifestyle issues (e.g., smoking) extended CDC's mandate beyond disease control. Thus, in 1992, the organization became the Centers for Disease Control and Prevention (the acronym CDC was retained).

Today, CDC is a world renowned center of excellence for public health research, disease detection, and dissemination of information on a variety of diseases and health issues.

See also AIDS, recent advances in research and treatment; Bacteria and bacterial infection; History of public health; Public health, current issues

CEPHALOSPORINS • *see* ANTIBIOTICS

CHAGAS DISEASE

Chagas disease is a human infection that is caused by a microorganism that establishes a parasitic relationship with a human host as part of its life cycle. The disease is named for the Brazilian physician Carlos Chagas, who described in 1909 the involvement of the flagellated protozoan known as *Trypanosoma cruzi* in a prevalent disease in South America.

The disease is confined to North, South, and Central America. Reflecting this, and the similarity of the disease to trypanosomiasis, a disease that occurs on the African continent, Chagas disease has also been dubbed American trypanosomiasis. The disease affects some 16 to 18 million each year, mainly in Central and South American. Indeed, in these regions the prevalence of Chagas disease in the population is higher than that of the **Human Immunodeficiency Virus** and the **Hepatitis** B and C **viruses**. Of those who acquire Chagas disease, approximately 50,000 people die each year.

The agent of Chagas disease, *Trypanosoma cruzi*, is a member of a division, or phylum, called Sarcomastigophora. The protozoan is spread to human via a bug known as Reduviid bugs (or "kissing bugs"). These bugs are also known as triatomines. Examples of species include *Triatoma infestans*, *Triatoma brasiliensis*, *Triatoma dimidiata*, and *Triatoma sordida*.

The disease is spread because of the close proximity of the triatomine bugs and humans. The bugs inhabit houses, particularly more substandard houses where cracks and deteriorating framework allows access to interior timbers. Biting an already infected person or animal infects the bugs themselves. The protozoan lives in the digestive tract of the bug. The infected bug subsequently infects another person by defecating on them, often while the person is asleep and unaware of the bug's presence. The trypanosomes in the feces gain entry to the bloodstream when feces are accidentally rubbed into the bite, or other orifices such as the mouth or eyes.

Chagas disease can also be transmitted in the blood. Acquisition of the disease via a blood transfusion occurs in thousands of people each year.

The association between the Reduviid bug and poor quality housing tends to make Chagas disease prevalent in underdeveloped regions of Central and South America. To add to the burden of these people, some 30% of those who are infected in childhood develop a chronic form of the disease 10

•

to 20 years later. This long-lasting form of Chagas disease reduces the life span by almost a decade.

Chagas disease may be asymptomatic (without symptoms)—or can produce a variety of symptoms. The form of the disease that strikes soon after infection with *Trypanosoma cruzi* tends to persist only for a few months before disappearing. Usually, no treatment is necessary for relief from the infection. Symptoms of this type of so-called acute infection include swelling at the site of the bug bite, tiredness, fever, enlarged spleen or liver, diarrhea, and vomiting. Infants can experience a swelling of the brain that can be fatal.

The chronic form of Chagas disease can produce more severe symptoms, including an enlarged heart, irregularities in heart function, and the enlargement and malfunction of the digestive tract. These symptoms are of particular concern in those people whose **immune system** is not functioning properly.

Currently, there is no **vaccine** or other preventative treatment for Chagas disease. Avoidance of habitats where the Reduviid bug lives is the most prudent precaution. Unfortunately, given the economic circumstances of those most at risk, this option is not easily attainable. *Trypanosoma cruzi* can also be transmitted in the blood. Therefore, screening of blood and blood products for the presence of the protozoan is wise. Once again, however, the poverty that often plays a role in the spread of Chagas disease may also be reflected in less than adequate medical practices, including blood screening.

See also Parasites; Zoonoses

CHAIN, ERNST BORIS (1906-1979)

German–born English biochemist

Ernst Chain was instrumental in the creation of **penicillin**, the first antibiotic drug. Although the Scottish bacteriologist **Alexander Fleming** discovered the *penicillium notatum* **mold** in 1928, it was Chain who, together with **Howard Florey**, isolated the breakthrough substance that has saved countless victims of infections. For their work, Chain, Florey, and Fleming were awarded the Nobel Prize in physiology or medicine in 1945.

Chain was born in Berlin to Michael Chain and Margarete Eisner Chain. His father was a Russian immigrant who became a chemical engineer and built a successful chemical plant. The death of Michael Chain in 1919, coupled with the collapse of the post–World War I German economy, depleted the family's income so much that Margarete Chain had to open up her home as a guesthouse.

One of Chain's primary interests during his youth was music, and for a while it seemed that he would embark on a career as a concert pianist. He gave a number of recitals and for a while served as music critic for a Berlin newspaper. A cousin, whose brother–in–law had been a failed conductor, gradually convinced Chain that a career in science would be more rewarding than one in music. Although he took lessons in conducting, Chain graduated from Friedrich–Wilhelm University in 1930 with a degree in chemistry and physiology.

Chain began work at the Charite Hospital in Berlin while also conducting research at the Kaiser Wilhelm Institute for Physical Chemistry and Electrochemistry. But the increasing pressures of life in Germany, including the growing strength of the Nazi party, convinced Chain that, as a Jew, he could not expect a notable professional future in Germany. Therefore, when Hitler came to power in January 1933, Chain decided to leave. Like many others, he mistakenly believed the Nazis would soon be ousted. His mother and sister chose not to leave, and both died in concentration camps.

Chain arrived in England in April 1933, and soon acquired a position at University College Hospital Medical School. He stayed there briefly and then went to Cambridge to work under the biochemist Frederick Gowland Hopkins. Chain spent much of his time at Cambridge conducting research on **enzymes**. In 1935, Howard Florey became head of the Sir William Dunn School of Pathology at Oxford. Florey, an Australian–born pathologist, wanted a top–notch biochemist to help him with his research, and asked Hopkins for advice. Without hesitation, Hopkins suggested Chain.

Florey was actively engaged in research on the bacteriolytic substance lysozyme, which had been identified by Fleming in his quest to eradicate infection. Chain came across Fleming's reports on the penicillin mold and was immediately intrigued. He and Florey both saw great potential in the further investigation of penicillin. With the help of a Rockefeller Foundation grant, the two scientists assembled a research team and set to work on isolating the active ingredient in *Penicillium notatum*.

Fleming, who had been unable to identify the antibacterial agent in the mold, had used the mold broth itself in his experiments to kill infections. Assisted in their research by fellow scientist Norman Heatley, Chain and Florey began their work by growing large quantities of the mold in the Oxford laboratory. Once there were adequate supplies of the mold, Chain began the tedious process of isolating the "miracle" substance. Succeeding after several months in isolating small amounts of a powder that he obtained by freeze–drying the mold broth, Chain was ready for the first practical test. His experiments with laboratory mice were successful, and it was decided that more of the substance should be produced to try on humans. To do this, the scientists needed to ferment massive quantities of mold broth; it took 125 gallons of the broth to make enough penicillin powder for one tablet. By 1941, Chain and his colleagues had finally gathered enough penicillin to conduct experiments with patients. The first two of eight patients died from complications unrelated to their infections, but the remaining six, who had been on the verge of death, were completely cured.

One potential use for penicillin was the treatment of wounded soldiers, an increasingly significant issue during the Second World War. For penicillin to be widely effective, however, the researchers needed to devise a way to mass–produce the substance. Florey and Heatley went to the United States in 1941 to enlist the aid of the government and of pharmaceutical houses. New ways were found to yield more and stronger penicillin from mold broth, and by 1943, the drug went into regular medical use for Allied troops. After the war, penicillin was made available for civilian use. The ethics of whether to make penicillin research universally available posed a particularly difficult problem for the scientific community during the war years. While some believed that the research should not be shared with the enemy, others felt that no one should be denied the benefits of penicillin. This added layers of political intrigue to the scientific pursuits of Chain and his colleagues. Even after the war, Chain experienced firsthand the results of this dilemma. As chairman of the **World Health Organization** in the late 1940s, Chain had gone to Czechoslovakia to supervise the operation of penicillin plants established there by the United Nations. He remained there until his work was done, even though the Communist coup occurred shortly after his arrival. When Chain applied for a visa to visit the United States in 1951, his request was denied by the State Department. Though no reason was given, many believed his stay in Czechoslovakia, however apolitical, was a major factor.

After the war, Chain tried to convince his colleagues that penicillin and other antibiotic research should be expanded, and he pushed for more state-of-the-art facilities at Oxford. Little came of his efforts, however, and when the Italian State Institute of Public Health in Rome offered him the opportunity to organize a biochemical and microbiological department along with a pilot plant, Chain decided to leave Oxford.

Under Chain's direction, the facilities at the State Institute became known internationally as a center for advanced research. While in Rome, Chain worked to develop new strains of penicillin and to find more efficient ways to produce the drug. Work done by a number of scientists, with Chain's guidance, yielded isolation of the basic penicillin molecule in 1958, and hundreds of new penicillin strains were soon synthesized.

In 1963, Chain was persuaded to return to England. The University of London had just established the Wolfson Laboratories at the Imperial College of Science and Technology, and Chain was asked to direct them. Through his hard work the Wolfson Laboratories earned a reputation as a first–rate research center.

In 1948, Chain had married Anne Beloff, a fellow biochemist, and in the following years she assisted him with his research. She had received her Ph.D. from Oxford and had worked at Harvard in the 1940s. The couple had three children.

Chain retired from Imperial College in 1973, but continued to lecture. He cautioned against allowing the then-new field of **molecular biology** to downplay the importance of **biochemistry** to medical research. He still played the piano, for which he had always found time even during his busiest research years. Over the years, Chain also became increasingly active in Jewish affairs. He served on the Board of Governors of the Weizmann Institute in Israel, and was an outspoken supporter of the importance of providing Jewish education for young Jewish children in England and abroad—all three of his children received part of their education in Israel.

In addition to the Nobel Prize, Chain received the Berzelius Medal in 1946, and was made a commander of the Legion d'Honneur in 1947. In 1954, he was awarded the **Paul Ehrlich** Centenary Prize. Chain was knighted by Queen Elizabeth II in 1969. Chain died of heart failure at age 73.

See also Antibiotic resistance, tests for; Bacteria and responses to bacterial infection; Chronic bacterial disease; Staphylococci and staphylococcal infections

CHAPERONES

The last two decades of the twentieth century saw the discovery of the heat-shock or cell-stress response, changes in the expression of certain proteins, and the unraveling of the function of proteins that mediate this essential cell-survival strategy. The proteins made in response to the stresses are called heat-shock proteins, stress proteins, or molecular chaperones. A large number of chaperones have been identified in **bacteria** (including archaebacteria), **yeast**, and eukaryotic cells. Fifteen different groups of proteins are now classified as chaperones. Their expression is often increased by cellular stress. Indeed, many were identified as heat-shock proteins, produced when cells were subjected to elevated temperatures. Chaperones likely function to stabilize proteins under less than ideal conditions.

The term chaperone was coined only in 1978, but the existence of chaperones is ancient, as evidenced by the conservation of the peptide sequences in the chaperones from prokaryotic and eukaryotic organisms, including humans.

Chaperones function 1) to stabilize folded proteins, 2) unfold them for translocation across membranes or for degradation, or 3) to assist in the proper folding of the proteins during assembly. These functions are vital. Accumulation of unfolded proteins due to improper functioning of chaperones can be lethal for cells. **Prions** serve as an example. Prions are an infectious agent composed solely of protein. They are present in both healthy and diseased cells. The difference is that in diseased cells the folding of the protein is different. Accumulation of the misfolded proteins in brain tissue kills nerve cells. The result for the affected individual can be dementia and death, as in the conditions of kuru, Creutzfeld-Jakob disease and "mad cow" disease (bovine spongiform encephalopthy).

Chaperones share several common features. They interact with unfolded or partially folded protein subunits, nascent chains emerging from the ribosome, or extended chains being translocated across subcellular membranes. They do not, however, form part of the final folded protein molecule. Chaperones often facilitate the coupling of cellular energy sources (adenosine triphosphate; ATP) to the folding process. Finally, chaperones are essential for viability.

Chaperones differ in that some are non-specific, interacting with a wide variety of polypeptide chains, while others are restricted to specific targets. Another difference concerns their shape; some are donut-like, with the central zone as the direct interaction region, while others are block-like, tunnel-like, or consist of paired subunits.

The reason for chaperone's importance lies with the environment within cells. Cells have a watery environment, yet many of the amino acids in a protein are **hydrophobic** (water hating). These are hidden in the interior of a correctly folded protein, exposing the hydrophilic (water loving) amino acids to the watery interior solution of the cell. If folded in such a correct manner, tensions are minimized and the three-dimensional structure of the protein is stable. Chaperons function to aid the folding process, ensuring protein stability and proper function.

Protein folding occurs by trial and error. If the protein folds the wrong way, it is captured by a chaperone, and another attempt at folding can occur. Even correctly folded proteins are subject to external stress that can disrupt structure. The chaperones, which are produced in greater amounts when a cell is exposed to higher temperatures, function to stabilize the unraveling proteins until the environmental crisis passes.

Non-biological molecules can also participate as chaperones. In this category, protein folding can be increased by the addition of agents such as glycerol, guanidium chloride, urea, and sodium chloride. Folding is likely due to an electrostatic interaction between exposed charged groups on the unfolded protein and the anions.

Increasing attention is being paid to the potential roles of chaperones in human diseases, including infection and idiopathic conditions such as arthritis and atherosclerosis. One subgroup of chaperones, the chaperonins, has received the most attention in this regard, because, in addition to facilitating protein folding, they also act as cell-to-cell signaling molecules.

See also Proteins and enzymes

CHASE, MARTHA COWLES (1927-)
American geneticist

Martha Cowles Chase is remembered for a landmark experiment in genetics carried out with American geneticist **Alfred Day Hershey** (1908–1997). Their experiment indicated that, contrary to prevailing opinion in 1952, **DNA** was genetic material. A year later, **James D. Watson** and British biophysicist **Francis Crick** proposed their double helical model for the three-dimensional structure of structure of DNA. Hershey was honored as one of the founders of **molecular biology**, and shared the 1969 Nobel Prize in medicine or physiology with Salvador Luria and Max Delbrück.

Martha Chase was born in Cleveland, Ohio. She earned a bachelor's degree from the College of Wooster in 1950 and her doctoral degree from the University of Southern California in 1964. Having married and changed her name to Martha C. Epstein (Martha Cowles Chase Epstein), she later returned to Cleveland Heights, Ohio, where she lived with her father, Samuel W. Chase. After graduating from college, Chase worked as an assistant to Alfred Hershey at the Carnegie Institution of Washington in Cold Spring Harbor, New York. This was a critical period in the history of modern genetics and the beginning of an entirely new phase of research that established the science of molecular biology. Including the name of an assistant or technician on a publication, especially one that was certain to become a landmark in the history of molecular biology, was unusual during the 1960s. Thus, it is remarkable that Martha

Chase's name is inextricably linked to all accounts of the path to the demonstration that DNA is the genetic material.

During the 1940s, most chemists, physicists, and geneticists thought that the genetic material must be a protein, but research on the **bacteria** that cause **pneumonia** suggested the nucleic acids played a fundamental role in inheritance. The first well-known series of experiments to challenge the assumption that genes must be proteins or nucleoproteins was carried out by **Oswald T. Avery** (1877–1955) and his co-workers **Colin Macleod**, and **Maclyn McCarty** in 1944. Avery's work was a refinement of observations previously reported in 1928 by Fred Griffith (1877–1941), a British bacteriologist. Avery identified the transforming principle of bacterial types as DNA and noted that further studies of the chemistry of DNA were required in order to explain its biological activity.

Most geneticists were skeptical about the possibility that DNA could serve as the genetic material until the results of the Hershey-Chase experiments of 1952 were reported. Their experiments indicated that bacteriophages (**viruses** that attack bacteria) might act like tiny syringes containing the genetic material and the empty virus containers might remain outside the bacterial cell after the genetic material of the virus had been injected. To test this possibility, Hershey and Chase used radioactive sulfur to label **bacteriophage** proteins and radioactive phosphate to label their DNA. After allowing viruses to attack the bacterial cells, the bacterial cultures were spun in a blender and centrifuged in order to separate intact bacteria from smaller particles.

Hershey and Chase found that most of the bacteriophage DNA remained with the bacterial cells while their protein coats were released into the medium. They concluded that the protein played a role in adsorption to the bacteria and helped inject the viral DNA into the bacterial cell. Thus, it was the DNA that was involved in the growth and multiplication of bacteriophage within the infected bacterial cell. Friends of Alfred Hershey recalled that when he was asked for his concept of the greatest scientific happiness, he said it would be to have an experiment that works. The Hershey-Chase experiments became a proverbial example of what his friends and colleagues called "Hershey Heaven."

See also Bacteriophage and bacteriophage typing; DNA (Deoxyribonucleic acid); Molecular biology and molecular genetics; Molecular biology, central dogma of; Viral genetics

CHEMICAL MUTAGENESIS

The interaction of certain environmental chemical compounds and cell **metabolism** may result in genetic changes in **DNA** structure, affecting one or more genes. These chemical-induced **mutations** are known as chemical mutagenesis. Many cancers and other degenerative diseases result from acquired genetic mutations due to environmental exposure, and not as an outcome of inherited traits. Chemicals capable of inducing genetic mutation (i.e., chemical mutagens or genotoxic compounds) are present in both natural and man-made environments and products.

Many plants, including edible ones, produce discreet amounts of some toxic compound that plays a role in plant protection against some natural predator. Some of these natural compounds may also be genotoxic for humans and animals, when that plant is consumed frequently and in great amounts. For instance, most edible mushrooms contain a family of chemical mutagenes known as hydrazines; but once mushrooms are cooked, most hydrazines evaporate or are degraded into less toxic compounds.

Among the most aggressive man-made chemical mutagenes are:

- asbestos
- DDT
- insecticides and herbicides containing arsenic
- industrial products containing benzene
- formaldehyde
- diesel and gasoline exhaust
- polychlorinated biphenyl (PCB)

Exposure to some of these compounds may occur in the work place, others can be present in the polluted air of great cities and industrial districts. For instance, insecticide and herbicide sprayers on farms, tanners, and oil refinery workers are frequently exposed to arsenic and may suffer mutations that lead to lung or skin cancers. Insulation and demolition workers are prone to **contamination** with asbestos and may eventually develop lung cancer. Painters, dye users, furniture finishers, and rubber workers are often exposed to benzene, which can induce mutations in stem cells that generate white blood cells, thus causing myelogenous leukemia. People working in the manufacture of wood products, paper, textiles and metallurgy, as well as hospital and laboratory workers, are frequently in contact with formaldehyde and can thus suffer mutations leading to nose and nasopharynx tumors. Cigarette and cigar smoke contains a class of chemical mutagenes, known as PAH (polycyclic aromatic hydrocarbons), that leads to mutation in lung cells. PAH is also present in gas and diesel combustion fumes.

Except for the cases of accidental high exposure and contamination, most chemical mutagenes or their metabolites (i.e., cell-transformed by-products) have a progressive and gradual accumulation in DNA, throughout years of exposition. Some individuals are more susceptible to the effects of cumulative contamination than others. Such individual degrees of susceptibility are due to discreet genetic variations, known as polymorphism, meaning several forms or versions of a given group of genes. Depending on the polymorphic version of Cytochrome P450 genes, an individual may metabolize some mutagenes faster than others. Polymorphism in another group of genes, NAT (N-acetyltransferase), is also implied in different individual susceptibilities to chemical exposure and mutagenesis.

See also Immunogenetics; Mutants, enhanced tolerance or sensitivity to temperature and pH ranges; Mutations and mutagenesis

CHEMOAUTOTROPHIC AND CHEMOLITHOTROPHIC BACTERIA

Autotrophic bacteria obtain the carbon that they need to sustain survival and growth from carbon dioxide (CO_2). To process this carbon source, the **bacteria** require energy. Chemoautotrophic bacteria and chemolithotrophic bacteria obtain their energy from the oxidation of inorganic (non-carbon) compounds. That is, they derive their energy from the energy already stored in chemical compounds. By oxidizing the compounds, the energy stored in chemical bonds can be utilized in cellular processes. Examples of inorganic compounds that are used by these types of bacteria are sulfur, ammonium ion (NH_4^+), and ferrous iron (Fe^{2+}).

The designation autotroph means "self nourishing." Indeed, both chemoautotrophs and chemolithotrophs are able to grow on medium that is free of carbon. The designation lithotrophic means "rock eating," further attesting to the ability of these bacteria to grow in seemingly inhospitable environments.

Most bacteria are chemotrophic. If the energy source consists of large chemicals that are complex in structure, as is the case when the chemicals are derived from once-living organisms, then it is the chemoautotrophic bacteria that utilize the source. If the molecules are small, as with the elements listed above, they can be utilized by chemolithotrophs.

Only bacteria are chemolithotrophs. Chemoautotrophs include bacteria, **fungi**, animals, and **protozoa**.

There are several common groups of chemoautotrophic bacteria. The first group is the colorless sulfur bacteria. These bacteria are distinct from the sulfur bacteria that utilize sunlight. The latter contain the compound **chlorophyll**, and so appear colored. Colorless sulfur bacteria oxidize hydrogen sulfide (H_2S) by accepting an electron from the compound. The acceptance of an electron by an oxygen atom creates water and sulfur. The energy from this reaction is then used to reduce carbon dioxide to create carbohydrates. An example of a colorless sulfur bacteria is the genus *Thiothrix*.

Another type of chemoautotroph is the "iron" bacteria. These bacteria are most commonly encountered as the rusty coloured and slimy layer that builds up on the inside of toilet tanks. In a series of chemical reactions that is similar to those of the sulfur bacteria, iron bacteria oxidize iron compounds and use the energy gained from this reaction to drive the formation of carbohydrates. Examples of iron bacteria are *Thiobacillus ferrooxidans* and *Thiobacillus thiooxidans*. These bacteria are common in the runoff from coal mines. The water is very acidic and contains ferrous iron. Chemoautotrophs thrive in such an environment.

A third type of chemoautotrophic bacteria includes the nitrifying bacteria. These chemoautotrophs oxidize ammonia (NH_3) to nitrate (NO_3^-). Plants can use the nitrate as a nutrient source. These nitrifying bacteria are important in the operation of the global nitrogen cycle. Examples of chemoautotrophic nitrifying bacteria include Nitrosomonas and Nitrobacter.

The **evolution** of bacteria to exist as chemoautotrophs or chemolithotrophs has allowed them to occupy niches that would otherwise be devoid of bacterial life. For example, in recent years scientists have studied a cave near Lovell, Wyoming. The groundwater running through the cave contains a strong sulfuric acid. Moreover, there is no sunlight. The only source of life for the thriving bacterial populations that adhere to the rocks are the rocks and the chemistry of the groundwater.

The energy yield from the use of inorganic compounds is not nearly as great as the energy that can be obtained by other types of bacteria. But, chemoautotrophs and chemolithotrophs do not usually face competition from other **microorganisms**, so the energy they are able to obtain is sufficient to sustain their existence. Indeed, the inorganic processes associated with chemoautotrophs and chemolithotrophs may make these bacteria one of the most important sources of weathering and erosion of rocks on Earth.

The ability of chemoautotrophic and chemolithotrophic bacteria to thrive through the energy gained by inorganic processes is the basis for the metabolic activities of the so-called **extremophiles**. These are bacteria that live in extremes of **pH**, temperature of pressure, as three examples. Moreover, it has been suggested that the metabolic capabilities of extremophiles could be duplicated on extraterrestrial planetary bodies.

See also Metabolism

CHEMOSTAT AND TURBIDOSTAT · *see* LABORATORY TECHNIQUES IN MICROBIOLOGY

CHEMOTAXIS · *see* BACTERIAL MOVEMENT

CHEMOTHERAPY

Chemotherapy is the treatment of a disease or condition with chemicals that have a specific effect on its cause, such as a microorganism or cancer cell. The first modern therapeutic chemical was derived from a synthetic dye. The sulfonamide drugs developed in the 1930s, **penicillin** and other **antibiotics** of the 1940s, hormones in the 1950s, and more recent drugs that interfere with cancer cell **metabolism** and reproduction have all been part of the chemotherapeutic arsenal.

The first drug to treat widespread **bacteria** was developed in the mid-1930s by the German physician-chemist Gerhard Domagk. In 1932, he discovered that a dye named prontosil killed streptococcus bacteria, and it was quickly used medically on both streptococcus and staphylococcus. One of the first patients cured with it was Domagk's own daughter. In 1936, the Swiss biochemist Daniele Bovet, working at the Pasteur Institute in Paris, showed that only a part of prontosil was active, a sulfonamide radical long known to chemists. Because it was much less expensive to produce, sulfonamide soon became the basis for several widely used "sulfa drugs" that revolutionized the treatment of formerly fatal diseases. These included **pneumonia**, **meningitis**, and puerperal

("childbed") fever. For his work, Domagk received the 1939 Nobel Prize in physiology or medicine. Though largely replaced by antibiotics, **sulfa drugs** are still commonly used against urinary tract infections, Hanson disease (**leprosy**), **malaria**, and for burn treatment.

At the same time, the next breakthrough in chemotherapy, penicillin, was in the wings. In 1928, the British bacteriologist **Alexander Fleming** noticed that a **mold** on an uncovered laboratory dish of staphylococcus destroyed the bacteria. He identified the mold as *Penicillium notatum*, which was related to ordinary bread mold. Fleming named the mold's active substance penicillin, but was unable to isolate it.

In 1939, the American microbiologist **René Jules Dubos** (1901–1982) isolated from a soil microorganism an antibacterial substance that he named tyrothricin. This led to wide interest in penicillin, which was isolated in 1941 by two biochemists at Oxford University, **Howard Florey** and **Ernst Chain**.

The term antibiotic was coined by American microbiologist **Selman Abraham Waksman**, who discovered the first antibiotic that was effective on gram-negative bacteria. Isolating it from a Streptomyces fungus that he had studied for decades, Waksman named his antibiotic streptomycin. Though streptomycin occasionally resulted in unwanted side effects, it paved the way for the discovery of other antibiotics. The first of the tetracyclines was discovered in 1948 by the American botanist Benjamin Minge Duggar. Working with *Streptomyces aureofaciens* at the Lederle division of the American Cyanamid Co., Duggar discovered chlortetracycline (Aureomycin).

The first effective chemotherapeutic agent against **viruses** was acyclovir, produced in the early 1950s by the American biochemists George Hitchings and **Gertrude Belle Elion** for the treatment of **herpes**. Today's **antiviral drugs** are being used to inhibit the reproductive cycle of both **DNA** and **RNA** viruses. For example, two drugs are used against the **influenza** A virus, Amantadine and Rimantadine, and the **AIDS** treatment drug AZT inhibits the reproduction of the **human immunodeficiency virus** (**HIV**).

Cancer treatment scientists began trying various chemical compounds for use as cancer treatments as early as the mid-nineteenth century. But the first effective treatments were the sex hormones, first used in 1945, estrogens for prostate cancer and both estrogens and androgens to treat breast cancer. In 1946, the American scientist Cornelius Rhoads developed the first drug especially for cancer treatment. It was an alkylating compound, derived from the chemical warfare agent nitrogen mustard, which binds with chemical groups in the cell's DNA, keeping it from reproducing. Alkylating compounds are still important in cancer treatment.

In the next twenty years, scientists developed a series of useful antineoplastic (anti-cancer) drugs, and, in 1954, the forerunner of the National Cancer Institute was established in Bethesda, MD. Leading the research efforts were the so-called "4-H Club" of cancer chemotherapy: the Americans Charles Huggins (1901–1997), who worked with hormones; George Hitchings (1905–1998), purines and pyrimidines to interfere with cell metabolism; Charles Heidelberger, fluorinated compounds; and British scientist Alexander Haddow (1907–1976), who worked with various substances. The first widely used drug was 6-Mercaptopurine, synthesized by Elion and Hitchings in 1952.

Chemotherapy is used alone, in combination, and along with radiation and/or surgery, with varying success rates, depending on the type of cancer and whether it is localized or has spread to other parts of the body. They are also used after treatment to keep the cancer from recurring (**adjuvant** therapy). Since many of the drugs have severe side effects, their value must always be weighed against the serious short-and long-term effects, particularly in children, whose bodies are still growing and developing.

In addition to the male and female sex hormones androgen, estrogen, and progestins, scientists also use the hormone somatostatin, which inhibits production of growth hormone and growth factors. They also use substances that inhibit the action of the body's own hormones. An example is Tamoxifen, used against breast cancer. Normally the body's own estrogen causes growth of breast tissues, including the cancer. The drug binds to cell receptors instead, causing reduction of tissue and cancer cell size.

Forms of the B-vitamin folic acid were found to be useful in disrupting cancer cell metabolism by the American scientist Sidney Farber (1903–1973) in 1948. Today they are used on leukemia, breast cancer, and other cancers.

Plant alkaloids have long been used as medicines, such as colchicine from the autumn crocus. Cancer therapy drugs include vincristine and vinblastine, derived from the pink periwinkle by American Irving S. Johnson (1925–). They prevent mitosis (division) in cancer cells. VP-16 and VM-16 are derived from the roots and rhizomes of the may apple or mandrake plant, and are used to treat various cancers. Taxol, which is derived from the bark of several species of yew trees, was discovered in 1978, and is used for treatment of ovarian and breast cancer.

Another class of naturally occurring substances are anthracyclines, which scientists consider to be extremely useful against breast, lung, thyroid, stomach, and other cancers.

Certain antibiotics are also effective against cancer cells by binding to DNA and inhibiting RNA and **protein synthesis**. Actinomycin D, derived from Streptomyces, was discovered by Selman Waksman and first used in 1965 by American researcher Seymour Farber. It is now used against cancer of female reproductive organs, brain tumors, and other cancers.

A form of the metal platinum called cisplatin stops cancer cells' division and disrupts their growth pattern. Newer treatments that are biological or based on proteins or genetic material and can target specific cells are also being developed. Monoclonal antibodies are genetically engineered copies of proteins used by the **immune system** to fight disease. Rituximab was the first moncoclonal **antibody** approved for use in cancer, and more are under development. **Interferons** are proteins released by cells when invaded by a virus. Interferons serve to alert the body's immune system of an impending attack, thus causing the production of other proteins that fight off disease. Interferons are being studied for treating a number of cancers, including a form of skin cancer called multiple myeloma. A third group of drugs are called

anti-sense drugs, which affect specific genes within cells. Made of genetic material that binds with and neutralizes messenger-RNA, anti-sense drugs halt the production of proteins within the cancer cell.

Genetically engineered cancer vaccines are also being tested against several virus-related cancers, including liver, cervix, nose and throat, kidney, lung, and prostate cancers. The primary goal of genetically engineered vaccines is to trigger the body's immune system to produce more cells that will react to and kill cancer cells. One approach involves isolating white blood cells that will kill cancer and then to find certain antigens, or proteins, that can be taken from these cells and injected into the patient to spur on the immune system. A "vaccine **gene** gun" has also been developed to inject DNA directly into the tumor cell. An RNA cancer **vaccine** is also being tested. Unlike most vaccines, which have been primarily tailored for specific patients and cancers, the RNA cancer vaccine is designed to treat a broad number of cancers in many patients.

As research into cancer treatment continues, new cancer-fighting drugs will continue to become part of the medical armamentarium. Many of these drugs will come from the burgeoning **biotechnology** industry and promise to have fewer side effects than traditional chemotherapy and radiation.

See also Antibiotic resistance, tests for; Antiviral drugs; Bacteria and bacterial infection; Blood borne infections; Cell cycle and cell division; Germ theory of disease; History of microbiology; History of public health; Immunization

CHICKEN POX · *see* ANTIBIOTICS

CHITIN

Chitin is a polymer, a repeating arrangement of a chemical structure. Chitin is found in the supporting structures of many organisms. Of relevance to microbiology, chitin is present in fungal species such as mushrooms, where it can comprise from 5% to 20% of the weight of the organism.

The backbone of chitin is a six-member carbon ring that has side groups attached to some of the carbon atoms. This structure is very similar to that of cellulose. One of the side groups of chitin is known as acetamide, whereas cellulose has hydroxy (OH) side groups.

Chitin is a noteworthy biological feature because it is constructed solely from materials that are naturally available. In contrast, most polymers are man-made and are comprised of constituents that must be artificially manufactured.

The purpose of chitin is to provide support for the organism. The degree of support depends on the amount and the thickness of chitin that is present. In **fungi** such as mushrooms, chitin confers stability and rigidity, yet allows some flexibility. This allows the mushrooms to stand and still be flexible enough to sway without snapping.

The role of chitin as a support structure is analogous to the **peptidoglycan** supportive layer that is a feature of Gram-positive and Gram-negative **bacteria**. The think peptidoglycan layer in Gram-positive bacteria provides a rigid and robust support. The peptidoglycan layer in Gram-negative bacteria that is only one molecule thick does not provide the same degree of structural support. Other mechanical elements of the Gram-negative cell wall are necessary to shore up the structure.

In the ocean, where many creatures contain chitin, sea-dwelling bacteria called *Vibrio furnisii* have evolved a sensory system that detects discarded chitin. The bacteria are able to break down the polymer and use the sugar molecules as metabolic fuel.

See also Fungi

CHLAMYDIAL PNEUMONIA

Chlamydial **pneumonia** is a pneumonia cause by one of several forms of Chlamydial **bacteria**. The three major forms of *Chlamydia* responsible for pneumonia are *Chlamydia pneumoniae, Chlamydia psittaci,* and *Chlamydia trachomatis.*

In reaction to infection, infected lung tissue may become obstructed with secretions. As part of a generalized swelling or **inflammation** of the lungs, the fluid or pus secretions block the normal vascular exchanges that take place in the alveolar air sacs. Blockage of the alveoli results in a decreased oxygenation of the blood and deprivation of oxygen to tissues.

Chlamydia pneumoniae (in older literature known as "Taiwan acute respiratory agent") usually produces a condition known as "walking pneumonia," a milder form of pneumonia that may only result in a fever and persistent cough. Although the symptoms are usually mild, they can be debilitating and dangerous to at risk groups that include the elderly, young children, or to individuals already weakened by another illness. *Chlamydia pneumoniae* spreads easily and the high transmission rate means that many individuals within a population—including at risk individuals can be rapidly exposed.

Species of chlamydiae can be directly detected following cultivation in embryonated egg cultures and **immunofluorescence** staining or via **polymerase chain reaction** (**PCR**). Chlamydiae can also be detected via specific serologic tests.

Chlamydia psittaci is an avian bacteria that is transmitted by human contact with infected birds, feathers from infected birds, or droppings from infected birds. The specific pneumonia (psittacosis) may be severe and last for several weeks. The pneumonia is generally more dangerous than the form caused by *Chlamydia pneumoniae.*

Chlamydia trachomatis is the underlying bacterium responsible for one of several types of **sexually transmitted diseases** (STD). Most frequently *Chlamydia trachomatis* results in an inflammation of the urethra (nongonococcal urethritis) and pelvic inflammatory disease. Active *Chlamydia trachomatis* infections are especially dangerous during pregnancy because the newborn may come in contact with the bacteria in the vaginal canal and aspirate the bacteria into its lung tissue

from coating left on the mouth and nose. Although many newborns develop only mild pneumonia, because the lungs of a newborn are fragile, especially in pre-term babies, any infection of lung tissue is serious and can be life-threatening.

Specific **antibiotics** are used to fight chlamydial pneumonias. Erythromycin and erythromycin derivatives are used to combat *Chlamydia pneumoniae* and *Chlamydia trachomatis.* Tetracycline is usually effective against *Chlamydia psittaci.*

See also Bacteria and bacterial infection; Transmission of pathogens

CHLORAMPHENICOL · *see* ANTIBIOTICS

CHLORINATION

Chlorination refers to a chemical process that is used primarily to disinfect drinking water and spills of **microorganisms**. The active agent in chlorination is the element chlorine, or a derivative of chlorine (e.g., chlorine dioxide). Chlorination is a swift and economical means of destroying many, but not all, microorganisms that are a health-threat in fluid such as drinking water.

Chlorine is widely popular for this application because of its ability to kill **bacteria** and other disease-causing organisms at relatively low concentrations and with little risk to humans. The killing effect occurs in seconds. Much of the killing effect in bacteria is due to the binding of chlorine to reactive groups within the membrane(s) of the bacteria. This binding destabilizes the membrane, leading to the explosive death of the bacterium. As well, chlorine inhibits various biochemical reactions in the bacterium. In contrast to the rapid action of chlorine, other water **disinfection** methods, such as the use of ozone or ultraviolet light, require minutes of exposure to a microorganism to kill the organism.

In many water treatment facilities, chlorine gas is pumped directly into water until it reaches a concentration that is determined to kill microorganisms, while at the same time not imparting a foul taste or odor to the water. The exact concentration depends on the original purity of the water supply. For example, surface waters contain more organic material that acts to absorb the added chlorine. Thus, more chlorine needs to be added to this water than to water emerging from deep underground. For a particular treatment facility, the amount of chlorine that is effective is determined by monitoring the water for the amount of chlorine remaining in solution and for so-called indictor microorganisms (e.g., *Escherichia coli*).

Alternatively, chlorine can be added to water in the form of a solid compound (e.g., calcium or sodium hypochlorite). Both of these compounds react with water, releasing free chlorine. Both methods of chlorination are so inexpensive that nearly every public water purification system in the world has adopted one or the other as its primary means of destroying disease-causing organisms.

Despite this popularity, chlorination is not without drawbacks. Microorganisms such as *Cryptosporidium* and *Giardia* form dormant structures called cysts that are resistant to chlorination. The prevalence of these protozoans in worldwide drinking water supplies is increasing. Thus, the effectiveness of chlorination may be compromised in some water systems. As well, adherent bacterial populations of bacteria such as *Escherichia coli* that form in distribution pipelines are extremely resistant to chlorine, and so can contaminate the disinfected water that flows from the treatment plant to the tap. A third concern with chlorination is the reaction between chlorine and methane gas, which produces one or more chlorinated derivatives. The best known are trichloromethane (chloroform) and tetrachloromethane (carbon tetrachloride). These chlorinated hydrocarbons have been shown to have adverse health effects in humans when ingested in sufficient quantity for a long time.

Furthermore, from an engineering point of view, excess chlorine can be corrosive to pipelines. In older water treatment systems in the United States, for example, the deterioration of the water distribution pipelines is a significant problem to water delivery and **water quality**.

See also Infection control; Water quality

CHLOROPHYLL

Chlorophyll is a green pigment contained in the foliage of plants, giving them their notable coloration. This pigment is responsible for absorbing sunlight required for the production of sugar molecules, and ultimately of all biochemicals, in the plant.

Chlorophyll is found in the thylakoid sacs of the **chloroplast**. The chloroplast is a specialized part of the cell that functions as an organelle. Once the appropriate wavelengths of light are absorbed by the chlorophyll into the thylakoid sacs, the important process of **photosynthesis** is able to begin. In photosynthesis, the chloroplast absorbs light energy, and converts it into the chemical energy of simple sugars.

Vascular plants, which can absorb and conduct moisture and nutrients through specialized systems, have two different types of chlorophyll. The two types of chlorophyll, designated as chlorophyll a and b, differ slightly in chemical makeup and in color. These chlorophyll molecules are associated with specialized proteins that are able to penetrate into or span the membrane of the thylakoid sac.

When a chlorophyll molecule absorbs light energy, it becomes an excited state, which allows the initial chain reaction of photosynthesis to occur. The pigment molecules cluster together in what is called a photosynthetic unit. Several hundred chlorophyll a and chlorophyll b molecules are found in one photosynthetic unit.

A photosynthetic unit absorbs light energy. Red and blue wavelengths of light are absorbed. Green light cannot be absorbed by the chlorophyll and the light is reflected, making the plant appear green. Once the light energy penetrates these pigment molecules, the energy is passed to one chlorophyll molecule, called the reaction center chlorophyll. When this

molecule becomes excited, the light reactions of photosynthesis can proceed. With carbon dioxide, water, and the help of specialized **enzymes**, the light energy absorbed creates chemical energy in a form the cell can use to carry on its processes.

In addition to chlorophyll, there are other pigments known as accessory pigments that are able to absorb light where the chlorophyll is unable to. Carotenoids, like B-carotenoid, are also located in the thylakoid membrane. Carotenoids give carrots and some autumn leaves their color. Several different pigments are found in the chloroplasts of algae, **bacteria**, and **diatoms**, coloring them varying shades of red, orange, blue, and violet.

See also Autotrophic bacteria; Blue-green algae

CHLOROPHYTA

Chlorophyta are **microorganisms** that are grouped in the kingdom called Protista. The microbes are plant-like, in that they are able to manufacture energy from sunlight. The microbes are also commonly known as green algae

Depending on the species, Chlorophyta can be single-celled, multicelled, and can associate together in colonies. The environmental diversity of Chlorophyta is vast. Many types live in marine and fresh water. Terrestrial habitats include tree trunks, moist rocks, snowbanks, and creatures including turtles, sloths and mollusks. There are some 8,000 species of chlorophytes, ranging in size from microscopic to visibly large.

There are three classes of Chlorophyta. The first class, which contains the greatest number of organisms, is called Chlorophyceae. A notable example of an organism from this class is Chlorella, which is economically important as a dietary supplement. Another member of the class is *Volvox*, a spherical organized community containing upwards of 60,000 cells.

The second class is called Charophyceae. Members of this class have existed since prehistoric times, as evidenced by fossil finds. An example of this class is *Spirogyra*, which form slimy filaments on the surface of freshwater.

The third class is called Ulvophyceae. These are marine organisms. Some become associated with sea slugs where they provide the slug with oxygen and are in turn provided with protection and nutrients. Species of a calcium-rich green algae called *Halimeda* form the blinding white sand beaches of the Caribbean when they wash up onshore and become bleached by the sun. Another example from this class is *Ulva* that grows on rocks and wharves as green, leafy-appearing clusters.

Chlorophyta contain structures that are called chloroplasts. Within the chloroplasts two pigments (**chlorophyll** a and chlorophyll b) are responsible for the conversion of sunlight to chemical energy. The energy is typically stored as starch, and in their cell walls, which are composed of a material called cellulose. The stored material can be used for energy as needed. This process of energy generation is similar to that which occurs in plants. There is an evolutionary basis for this similarity. Available evidence indicates that members of Chlorophyta were the precursors of plants. Chlorophyte

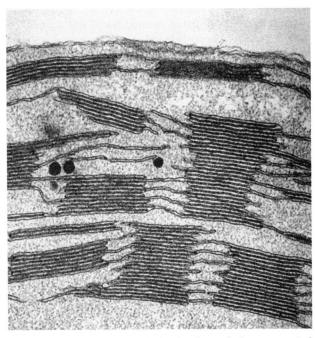

Thin section electron micrograph showing the stacked arrangement of chloroplast membranes.

fossils date from over one billion years ago, before the development of plants.

See also Photosynthesis

CHLOROPLAST

Chloroplasts are organelles—specialized parts of a cell that function in an organ-like fashion. They are found in vascular plants, mosses, liverworts, and algae. Chloroplast organelles are responsible for **photosynthesis**, the process by which sunlight is absorbed and converted into fixed chemical energy in the form of simple sugars synthesized from carbon dioxide and water.

Chloroplasts are located in the mesophyll, a green tissue area in plant leaves. Four layers or zones define the structure of a chloroplast. The chloroplast is a small lens-shaped organelle that is enclosed by two membranes with a narrow intermembrane space, known as the chloroplast envelope. Raw material and products for photosynthesis enter in and pass out through this double membrane, the first layer of the structure.

Inside the chloroplast envelope is the second layer, which is an area filled with a fluid called stroma. A series of chemical reactions involving **enzymes** and the incorporation of carbon dioxide into organic compounds occur in this region.

The third layer is a membrane-like structure of thylakoid sacs. Stacked like poker chips, the thylakoid sacs form a grana. These grana stacks are connected by membranous structures. Thylakoid sacs contain a green pigment called **chlorophyll**. In this region the thylakoid sacs, or grana, absorb

light energy using this pigment. Chlorophyll absorbs light between the red and blue spectrums and reflects green light, making leaves appear green. Once the light energy is absorbed into the final layer, the intrathylakoid sac, the important process of photosynthesis can begin.

Scientists have attempted to discover how chloroplasts convert light energy to the chemical energy stored in organic molecules for a long time. It has only been since the beginning of this century that scientists have begun to understand this process. The following equation is a simple formula for photosynthesis:

$$6CO_2 + 6H_2O \rightarrow C_6H_{12}O_6 + 6O_2.$$

Carbon dioxide plus water produce a carbohydrate plus oxygen. Simply, this means that the chloroplast is able to split water into hydrogen and oxygen.

Many questions still remain unanswered about the complete process and role of the chloroplast. Researchers continue to study the chloroplast and its **evolution**. Based on studies of the evolution of early complex cells, scientists have devised the serial endosymbiosis theory. It is suspected that primitive microbes were able to evolve into more complex microbes by incorporating other photosynthetic microbes into their cellular structures and allowing them to continue functioning as organelles. As **molecular biology** becomes more sophisticated, the origin and genetic makeup of the chloroplast will be more clearly understood.

See also Autotrophic bacteria; Blue-green algae; Evolution and evolutionary mechanisms; Evolutionary origin of bacteria and viruses

CHROMOSOMES, EUKARYOTIC

Chromosomes are microscopic units containing organized genetic information, eukaryotic chromosomes are located in the nuclei of diploid and haploid cells (e.g., human somatic and sex cells). Prokaryotic chromosomes are also present in one-cell non-nucleated (unicellular **microorganisms**) prokaryotic cells (e.g., **bacteria**). The sum-total of genetic information contained in different chromosomes of a given individual or species are generically referred to as the genome.

In humans, eukaryotic chromosomes are structurally made of roughly equal amounts of proteins and **DNA**. Each chromosome contains a double-strand DNA molecule, arranged as a double helix, and tightly coiled and neatly packed by a family of proteins called histones. DNA strands are comprised of linked nucleotides. Each nucleotide has a sugar (deoxyribose), a nitrogenous base, plus one to three phosphate groups. Each nucleotide is linked to adjacent nucleotides in the same DNA strand by phosphodiester bonds. Phosphodiester is another sugar, made of sugar-phosphate. Nucleotides of one DNA strand link to their complementary nucleotide on the opposite DNA strand by hydrogen bonds, thus forming a pair of nucleotides, known as a base pair, or nucleotide base.

Chromosomes contain the genes, or segments of DNA, that encode for proteins of an individual. Genes contain up to thousands of sequences of these base pairs. What distinguishes one **gene** from another is the sequence of nucleotides that code for the synthesis of a specific protein or portion of a protein. Some proteins are necessary for the structure of cells and tissues. Others, like **enzymes**, a class of active (catalyst) proteins, promote essential biochemical reactions, such as digestion, energy generation for cellular activity, or **metabolism** of toxic compounds. Some genes produce several slightly different versions of a given protein through a process of alternate **transcription** of bases pairs segments known as codons. When a chromosome is structurally faulty, or if a cell contains an abnormal number of chromosomes, the types and amounts of the proteins encoded by the genes are altered. Changes to proteins often result in serious mental and physical defects and disease.

Within the chromosomes, the DNA is tightly coiled around proteins (e.g., histones) allowing huge DNA molecules to occupy a small space within the **nucleus** of the cell. When a cell is not dividing, the chromosomes are invisible within the cell's nucleus. Just prior to cell division, the chromosomes uncoil and begin to replicate. As they uncoil, the individual chromosomes take on a distinctive appearance that allows physicians and scientists to classify the chromosomes by size and shape.

Numbers of autosomal chromosomes differ in cells of different species; but are usually the same in every cell of a given species. Sex determination cells (mature ovum and sperm) are an exception, where the number of chromosomes is halved. Chromosomes also differ in size. For instance, the smallest human chromosome, the sex chromosome Y, contains 50 million base pairs (bp), whereas the largest one, chromosome 1, contains 250 million base pairs. All 3 billion base pairs in the human genome are stored in 46 chromosomes. Human genetic information is therefore stored in 23 pairs of chromosomes (totaling 46), 23 inherited from the mother, and 23 from the father. Two of these chromosomes are sex chromosomes (chromosomes X and Y). The remaining 44 are autosomes (in 22 autosomal pairs), meaning that they are not sex chromosomes and are present in all somatic cells (i.e., any other body cell that is not a germinal cell for spermatozoa in males or an ovum in females). Sex chromosomes specify the offspring gender: normal females have two X chromosomes and normal males have one X and one Y chromosome. These chromosomes can be studied by constructing a karyotype, or organized depiction, of the chromosomes.

Each set of 23 chromosomes constitutes one allele, containing gene copies inherited from one of the progenitors. The other allele is complementary or homologous, meaning that they contain copies of the same genes and on the same positions, but originated from the other progenitor. As an example, every normal child inherits one set of copies of gene BRCA1, located on chromosome 13, from the mother and another set of BRCA1 from the father, located on the other allelic chromosome 13. Allele is a Greek-derived word that means "one of a pair," or any one of a series of genes having the same locus (position) on homologous chromosomes.

The first chromosome observations were made under light microscopes, revealing rod-shaped structures in varied sizes and conformations, commonly J- or V-shaped in eukaryotic cells and ring-shaped in bacteria. Staining reveals a pattern of light and dark bands. Today, those bands are known to correspond to regional variations in the amounts of the two nucleotide base pairs: Adenine-Thymine (A-T or T-A) in contrast with amounts of Guanine-Cytosine (G-C or C-G).

In humans, two types of cell division exist. In mitosis, cells divide to produce two identical daughter cells. Each daughter cell has exactly the same number of chromosomes. This preservation of chromosome number is accomplished through the replication of the entire set of chromosomes just prior to mitosis.

Two kinds of chromosome number defects can occur in humans: aneuploidy, an abnormal number of chromosomes, and polyploidy, more than two complete sets of chromosomes. Most alterations in chromosome number occur during meiosis. During normal meiosis, chromosomes are distributed evenly among the four daughter cells. Sometimes, however, an uneven number of chromosomes are distributed to the daughter cells.

Genetic abnormalities and diseases occur if chromosomes or portions of chromosomes are missing, duplicated or broken. Abnormalities and diseases may also occur if a specific gene is transferred from one chromosome to another (translocation), or there is a duplication or inversion of a segment of a chromosome. Down syndrome, for instance, is caused by trisomy in chromosome 21, the presence of a third copy of chromosome 21. Some structural chromosomal abnormalities have been implicated in certain cancers. For example, myelogenous leukemia is a cancer of the white blood cells. Researchers have found that the cancerous cells contain a translocation of chromosome 22, in which a broken segment switches places with the tip of chromosome 9.

In non-dividing cells, it is not possible to distinguish morphological details of individual chromosomes, because they remain elongated and entangled to each other. However, when a cell is dividing, i.e., undergoing mitosis, chromosomes become highly condensed and each individual chromosome occupies a well-defined spatial location.

Karyotype analysis was the first genetic screening utilized by geneticists to assess inherited abnormalities, like additional copies of a chromosome or a missing copy, as well as DNA content and gender of the individual. With the development of new molecular screening techniques and the growing number of identified individual genes, detection of other more subtle chromosomal **mutations** is now possible (e.g., determinations of gene mutations, levels of gene expression, etc.). Such data allow scientists to better understand disease causation and to develop new therapies and medicines for those diseases.

In mitosis, cells divide to produce two identical daughter cells. Each daughter cell has exactly the same number of chromosomes. This preservation of chromosome number is accomplished through the replication of the entire set of chromosomes just prior to mitosis.

Sex cells, such as eggs and sperm, undergo a different type of cell division called meiosis. Because sex cells each contribute half of a zygote's genetic material, sex cells must carry only half the full **complement** of chromosomes. This reduction in the number of chromosomes within sex cells is accomplished during two rounds of cell division, called meiosis I and meiosis II. Prior to meiosis I, the chromosomes replicate and chromosome pairs are distributed to daughter cells. During meiosis II, however, these daughter cells divide without a prior replication of chromosomes. Mistakes can occur during either meiosis I and meiosis II. Chromosome pairs can be separated during meiosis I, for instance, or fail to separate during meiosis II.

Meiosis produces four daughter cells, each with half of the normal number of chromosomes. These sex cells are called haploid cells (meaning half the number). Non-sex cells in humans are called diploid (meaning double the number) since they contain the full number of normal chromosomes.

Most alterations in chromosome number occur during meiosis. When an egg or sperm that has undergone faulty meiosis and has an abnormal number of chromosomes unites with a normal egg or sperm during conception, the zygote formed will have an abnormal number of chromosomes. If the zygote survives and develops into a fetus, the chromosomal abnormality is transmitted to all of its cells. The child that is born will have symptoms related to the presence of an extra chromosome or absence of a chromosome.

See also Cell cycle (eukaryotic), genetic regulation of; Cell cycle (prokaryotic), genetic regulation of; Chromosomes, prokaryotic; DNA (Deoxyribonucleic acid); Enzymes; Genetic regulation of eukaryotic cells; Genetic regulation of prokaryotic cells; Molecular biology and molecular genetics

CHROMOSOMES, HUMAN · *see* CHROMOSOMES, EUKARYOTIC

CHROMOSOMES, PROKARYOTIC

The genetic material of **microorganisms**, be they prokaryotic or eukaryotic, is arranged in an organized fashion. The arrangement in both cases is referred to as a chromosome.

The **chromosomes** of prokaryotic microorganisms are different from that of eukaryotic microorganisms, such as **yeast**, in terms of the organization and arrangement of the genetic material. Prokaryotic **DNA** tends to be more closely packed together, in terms of the stretches that actually code for something, than is the DNA of eukaryotic cells. Also, the shape of the chromosome differs between many prokaryotes and **eukaryotes**. For example, the **deoxyribonucleic acid** of yeast (a eukaryotic microorganism) is arranged in a number of linear arms, which are known as chromosomes. In contrast, **bacteria** (the prototypical prokaryotic microorganism) lack chromosomes. Rather, in many bacteria the DNA is arranged in a circle.

The chromosomal material of **viruses** is can adopt different structures. Viral nucleic acid, whether DNA or **ribonucleic acid (RNA)** tends to adopt the circular arrangement when

packaged inside the virus particle. Different types of virus can have different arrangements of the nucleic acid. However, viral DNA can behave differently inside the host, where it might remain autonomous or integrating into the host's nucleic acid. The changing behavior of the viral chromosome makes it more suitable to a separate discussion.

The circular arrangement of DNA was the first form discovered in bacteria. Indeed, for many years after this discovery the idea of any other arrangement of bacterial DNA was not seriously entertained. In bacteria, the circular bacterial chromosome consists of the double helix of DNA. Thus, the two strands of DNA are intertwined while at the same time being oriented in a circle. The circular arrangement of the DNA allows for the replication of the genetic material. Typically, the copying of both strands of DNA begins at a certain point, which is called the origin of replication. From this point, the replication of one strand of DNA proceeds in one direction, while the replication of the other strand proceeds in the opposite direction. Each newly made strand also helically coils around the template strand. The effect is to generate two new circles, each consisting of the intertwined double helix.

The circular arrangement of the so-called chromosomal DNA is mimicked by **plasmids**. Plasmids exist in the **cytoplasm** and are not part of the chromosome. The DNA of plasmids tends to be coiled extremely tightly, much more so than the chromosomal DNA. This feature of plasmid DNA is often described as supercoiling. Depending of the type of plasmid, replication may involve integration into the bacterial chromosome or can be independent. Those that replicate independently are considered to be minichromosomes.

Plasmids allow the genes they harbor to be transferred from bacterium to bacterium quickly. Often, such genes encode proteins that are involved in resistance to antibacterial agents or other compounds that are a threat to bacterial survival, or proteins that aid the bacteria in establishing an infection (such as a toxin).

The circular arrangement of bacterial DNA was first demonstrated by electron microscopy of ***Escherichia coli*** and *Bacillus subtilis* bacteria in which the DNA had been delicately released from the bacteria. The microscopic images clearly established the circular nature of the released DNA. In the aftermath of these experiments, the assumption was that the bacterial chromosome consisted of one large circle of DNA. However, since these experiments, some bacteria have been found to have a number of circular pieces of DNA, and even to have linear chromosomes and sometimes even linear plasmids. Examples of bacteria with more than one circular piece of DNA include *Brucella* species, *Deinococcus radiodurans*, *Leptospira interrogans*, *Paracoccus denitrificans*, *Rhodobacter sphaerodes*, and *Vibrio* species. Examples of bacteria with linear forms of chromosomal DNA are *Agrobacterium tumefaciens*, *Streptomyces* species, and *Borrelia* species.

The linear arrangement of the bacterial chromosome was not discovered until the late 1970s, and was not definitively proven until the advent of the technique of pulsed field gel **electrophoresis** a decade later. The first bacterium shown to possess a linear chromosome was *Borrelia burgdorferi*.

The linear chromosomes of bacteria are similar to those of eukaryotes such as yeast in that they have specialized regions of DNA at the end of each double strand of DNA. These regions are known as telomeres, and serve as boundaries to bracket the coding stretches of DNA. Telomeres also retard the double strands of DNA from uncoiling by essentially pinning the ends of each strand together with the complimentary strand.

There are two types of telomeres in bacteria. One type is called a hairpin telomere. As its name implies, the telomers bends around from the end of one DNA strand to the end of the complimentary strand. The other type of telomere is known as an invertron telomere. This type acts to allow an overlap between the ends of the complimentary DNA strands.

Replication of a linear bacterial chromosome proceeds from one end, much like the operation of a zipper. As replication moves down the double helix, two tails of the daughter double helices form behind the point of replication.

Research on bacterial chromosome structure and function has tended to focus on *Escherichia coli* as the model microorganism. This bacterium is an excellent system for such studies. However, as the diversity of bacterial life has become more apparent in beginning in the 1970s, the limitations of extrapolating the findings from the *Escherichia coli* chromosome to bacteria in general has also more apparent. Very little is known, for example, of the chromosome structure of the Archae, the primitive life forms that share features with prokaryotes and eukaryotes, and of those bacteria that can live in environments previously thought to be completely inhospitable for **bacterial growth**.

See also Genetic identification of microorganisms; Genetic regulation of prokaryotic cells; Microbial genetics; Viral genetics; Yeast genetics

CHRONIC BACTERIAL DISEASE

Chronic bacterial infections persist for prolonged periods of time (e.g., months, years) in the host. This lengthy persistence is due to a number of factors including masking of the **bacteria** from the **immune system**, invasion of host cells, and the establishment of an infection that is resistance to antibacterial agents.

Over the past three decades, a number of chromic bacterial infections have been shown to be associated with the development of the adherent, exopolysaccharide-encased populations that are termed biofilms. The constituents of the exopolysaccharide are poorly immunogenic. This means that the immune system does not readily recognize the exopolysaccharide as foreign material that must be cleared from the body. Within the blanket of polysaccharide the bacteria, which would otherwise be swiftly detected by the immune system, are protected from immune recognition. As a result, the infection that is established can persist for a long time.

An example of a chronic, **biofilm**-related **bacterial infection** is prostatitis. Prostatitis is an **inflammation** of the prostate gland that is common in men over 30 years of age. Symptoms of this disease can include intense pain, urinary complications, and sexual malfunction including infertility. Chronic bacterial prostatitis is generally associated with repeated urinary tract infections. The chronic infection is typically caused by biofilms of *Escherichia coli*.

A second biofilm-related chronic bacterial infection is the *Pseudomonas aeruginosa* lung infection that develops early in life in some people who are afflicted with cystic fibrosis. Cystic fibrosis is due to a genetic defect that restricts the movement of salt and water in and out of cells in the lung. The resulting build-up of mucus predisposes the lungs to bacterial infection. The resulting *Pseudomonas aeruginosa* infection becomes virtually impossible to clear, due the **antibiotic resistance** of the bacteria within the biofilm. Furthermore, the body's response to the chronic infection includes inflammation. Over time, the inflammatory response is causes breathing difficulty that can be so pronounced as to be fatal.

Another chronic bacterial infection that affects the lungs is **tuberculosis**. This disease causes more deaths than any other infectious disease. Nearly two billion people are infected with the agent of tuberculosis, the bacterium *Mycobacterium tuberculosis*. As with other chronic infections, the symptoms can be mild. But, for those with a weakened immune system the disease can become more severe. Each year some three million people die of this active form of the tuberculosis infection.

Tuberculosis has re-emerged as a health problem in the United States, particularly among the poor. The development of drug resistance by the bacteria is a factor in this re-emergence.

Beginning in the mid 1970s, there has been an increasing recognition that maladies that were previously thought to be due to genetic or environmental factors in fact have their basis in chronic bacterial infections. A key discovery that prompted this shift in thinking concerning the origin of certain diseases was the demonstration by **Barry Marshall** that a bacterium called *Helicobacter pylori* is the major cause of stomach ulcers. Furthermore, there is now firm evidence of an association with chronic *Helicobacter pylori* stomach and intestinal infections and the development of certain types of intestinal cancers.

At about the same time the bacterium called *Borrelia burgdorferi* was established to be the cause of a debilitating disease known as **Lyme disease**. The spirochaete is able to establish a chronic infection in a host. The infection and the host's response to the infection, causes arthritis and long-lasting lethargy.

As a final recent example, **Joseph Penninger** has shown that the bacterium *Chlamydia trachomatis* is the agent that causes a common form of heart disease. The bacterium chronically infects a host and produces a protein that is very similar in three-dimensional structure to a protein that composed a heart valve. The host's immune response to the bacterial protein results in the deterioration of the heart protein, leading to heart damage.

Evidence is accumulating that implicates chronic bacterial infection with other human ailments including schizophrenia and Alzheimer's disease. While not yet conclusive, the involvement of chronic bacterial infections in maladies that have hitherto not been suspected of having a bacterial origin will not be surprising.

Research efforts to prevent chronic bacterial infections are focusing on the prevention of the surface adhesion that is a hallmark of many such infections. Molecules that can competitively block the sites to which the disease-causing bacteria bind have shown promising results in preventing infections in the laboratory setting.

See also Bacteria and bacterial infection; Biofilm formation and dynamic behavior; Immunity, active, passive and delayed

CJD DISEASE • *see* BSE AND CJD DISEASE

CLINICAL MICROBIOLOGY • *see* MICROBIOLOGY, CLINICAL

CLINICAL TRIALS, TYPES • *see* MICROBIOLOGY, CLINICAL

CLONING: APPLICATIONS TO BIOLOGICAL PROBLEMS

Human proteins are often used in the medical treatment of various human diseases. The most common way to produce proteins is through human cell **culture**, an expensive approach that rarely results in adequate quantities of the desired protein. Larger amounts of protein can be produced using **bacteria** or **yeast**. However, proteins produced in this way lack important post-translational modification steps necessary for protein maturation and proper functioning. Additionally, there are difficulties associated with the purification processes of proteins derived from bacteria and yeast. Scientists can obtain proteins purified from blood but there is always risk of **contamination**. For these reasons, new ways of obtaining low-cost, high-yield, purified proteins are in demand.

One solution is to use transgenic animals that are genetically engineered to express human proteins. **Gene** targeting using nuclear transfer is a process that involves removing nuclei from cultured adult cells engineered to have human genes and inserting the nuclei into egg cells void of its original **nucleus**.

Transgenic cows, sheep, and goats can produce human proteins in their milk and these proteins undergo the appropriate post-translational modification steps necessary for therapeutic efficacy. The desired protein can be produced up to 40 grams per liter of milk at a relatively low expense. Cattle and other animals are being used experimentally to express specific genes, a process known as "pharming." Using cloned transgenic animals facilitates the large-scale introduction of foreign genes into animals. Transgenic animals are cloned using nuclear gene transfer, which reduces the amount of

experimental animals used as well as allows for specification of the sex of the progeny resulting in faster generation of breeding stocks.

Medical benefits from cloned transgenic animals expressing human proteins in their milk are numerous. For example, human serum albumin is a protein used to treat patients suffering from acute burns and over 600 tons are used each year. By removing the gene that expresses bovine serum albumin, cattle clones can be made to express human serum albumin. Another example is found at one biotech company that uses goats to produce human tissue plasminogen activator, a human protein involved in blood clotting cascades. Another biotech company has a flock that produces alpha-1-antitrypsin, a drug currently in clinical trials for the use in treating patients with cystic fibrosis. Cows can also be genetically manipulated using nuclear gene transfer to produce milk that does not have lactose for lactose-intolerant people. There are also certain proteins in milk that cause immunological reactions in certain individuals that can be removed and replaced with other important proteins.

There is currently a significant shortage of organs for patients needing transplants. Long waiting lists lead to prolonged suffering and people often die before they find the necessary matches for transplantation. Transplantation technology in terms of hearts and kidneys is commonplace, but very expensive. Xenotransplantation, or the transplantation of organs from animals into humans, is being investigated, yet graft versus host rejection remains problematic. As an alternative to xenotransplantation, stem cells can be used therapeutically, such as in blood disorders where blood stem cells are used to deliver normal blood cell types. However, the availability of adequate amount of stem cells is a limiting factor for stem cell therapy.

One solution to supersede problems associated with transplantation or stem cell therapy is to use cloning technology along with factors that induce differentiation. The process is termed, "therapeutic cloning" and might be used routinely in the near future. It entails obtaining adult cells, reprogramming them to become stem cell-like using nuclear transfer, and inducing them to proliferate but not to differentiate. Then factors that induce these proliferated cells to differentiate will be used to produce specialized cell types. These now differentiated cell types or organs can then be transplanted into the same donor that supplied the original cells for nuclear transfer.

Although many applications of cloning technology remain in developmental stages, the therapeutic value has great potential. With technological advancements that allow scientists to broaden the applications of cloning becoming available almost daily, modern medicine stands to make rapid improvements in previously difficult areas.

See also DNA hybridization; Immunogenetics; Microbial genetics; Transplantation genetics and immunology

CLOSTRIDIUM • *see* BOTULISM

COAGULASE

Coagulase is an enzyme that is produced by some types of **bacteria**. The enzyme clots the plasma component of the blood. The only significant disease-causing bacteria of humans that produces coagulase is *Staphylococcus aureus*.

In the human host, the action of coagulase produces clotting of the plasma in the immediate vicinity of the bacterium. The resulting increased effective diameter of the bacterium makes it difficult for the defense reactions of the host to deal with the infecting cell. In particular, the defensive mechanism of **phagocytosis**, where the bacterium is engulfed by a host cell and then dissolved, is rendered ineffective. This enables the bacterium to persist in the presence of a host immune response, which can lead to the establishment of n infection. Thus, coagulase can be described as a disease-causing (or virulence) factor of *Staphylococcus aureus*

A test for the presence of active coagulase distinguishes the aureus Staphylococcus from the non-aureus **Staphylococci**. *Staphylococcus aureus* is one of the major causes of hospital-acquired infection. **Antibiotic resistance** of this strain is a major concern. In the non-aureus, coagulase-negative group, *Staphylococcus epidermidis* is a particular concern. This strain is also an important disease-causing organism in hospital settings and can establish infections on artificial devices inserted into the body. The ability to quickly and simply differentiate the two different types of *Staphylococcus* from each other enables the proper treatment to be started before the infections become worse.

In the test, the sample is added to rabbit plasma and held at 37° C or a specified period of time, usually bout 12 hours. A positive test is the formation of a visible clump, which is the clotted plasma. Samples must be observed for clotting within 24 hours. This is because some strains that produce coagulase also produce an enzyme called fibrinolysin, which can dissolve the clot. Therefore, the absence of a clot after 24 hours is no guarantee that a clot never formed. The formation of a clot by 12 hours and the subsequent disappearance of the clot by 24 hours could produce a so-called false negative if the test were only observed at the 24-hour time.

See also Biochemical analysis techniques; Laboratory techniques in microbiology

COHEN, STANLEY N. (1935-   )

American geneticist

Modern biology, **biochemistry**, and genetics were fundamentally changed in 1973 when Stanley N. Cohen, **Herbert W. Boyer**, Annie C. Y. Chang, and Robert B. Helling developed a technique for transferring **DNA**, the molecular basis of heredity, between unrelated species. Not only was DNA propagation made possible among different bacterial species, but successful **gene** insertion from animal cells into bacterial cells was also accomplished. Their discovery, called recombinant DNA or genetic engineering, introduced the world to the age of modern **biotechnology**.

As with any revolutionary discovery, the benefits of this new technology were both immediate and projected. Immediate gains were made in the advancement of fundamental biology by increasing scientists' knowledge of gene structure and function. This knowledge promised new ways to overcome disease, increase food production, and preserve renewable resources. For example, the use of recombinant DNA methodology to overcome **antibiotic resistance** on the part of **bacteria** anticipated the development of better vaccines. A new source for producing insulin and other life-sustaining drugs had the potential to be realized. And, by creating new, nitrogen-fixing organisms, it was thought that food production could be increased, and the use of expensive, environmentally harmful nitrogen fertilizers eliminated. Genetic engineering also offered the promise of nonpolluting energy sources, such as hydrogen-producing algae. In the decades following the discovery of the means for propagating DNA, many assumptions regarding the benefits of genetic engineering have proved to be viable, and the inventions and technology that were by-products of genetic engineering research became marketable commodities, propelling biotechnology into a dynamic new industry.

Stanley N. Cohen was born in Perth Amboy, New Jersey, to Bernard and Ida Stolz Cohen. He received his undergraduate education at Rutgers University, and his M.D. degree from the University of Pennsylvania in 1960. Then followed medical positions at Mt. Sinai Hospital in New York City, University Hospital in Ann Arbor, Michigan, the National Institute for Arthritis and Metabolic Diseases in Bethesda, Maryland, and Duke University Hospital in Durham, North Carolina. Cohen completed postdoctoral research in 1967 at the Albert Einstein College of Medicine in the Bronx, New York. He joined the faculty at Stanford University in 1968, was appointed professor of medicine in 1975, professor of genetics in 1977, and became Kwoh-Ting Li professor of genetics in 1993.

At Stanford Cohen began the study of **plasmids**—bits of DNA that exist apart from the genetic information-carrying **chromosomes**—to determine the structure and function of plasmid genes. Unlike species ordinarily do not exchange genetic information. But Cohen found that the independent **plasmids** had the ability to transfer DNA to a related-species cell, though the phenomenon was not a commonplace occurrence. In 1973 Cohen and his colleagues successfully achieved a DNA transfer between two different sources. These functional molecules were made by joining two different plasmid segments taken from **Escherichia coli**, a bacteria found in the colon, and inserting the combined plasmid DNA back into **E. coli** cells. They found that the DNA would replicate itself and express the genetic information contained in each original plasmid segment. Next, the group tried this experiment with an unrelated bacteria, *Staphylococcus*. This, too, showed that the original *Staphylococcus* plasmid genes would transfer their biological properties into the *E. coli* host. With this experiment, the DNA barrier between species was broken. The second attempt at DNA replication between unlike species was that of animal to bacteria. This was successfully undertaken with the insertion into *E. coli* of genes taken from a frog. This experiment had great significance for human application; bacteria containing human genetic information could now be used to create the body's own means for fighting disease and birth disorders. The biological **cloning** methods used by Cohen and other scientists came to be popularly known as genetic engineering. The cloning process consisted of four steps: separating and joining DNA molecules acquired from unlike species; using a gene carrier that could replicate itself, as well as the unlike DNA segment joined to it; introducing the combined DNA molecule into another bacterial host; and selecting out the clone that carries the combined DNA.

DNA research not only added to the store of scientific knowledge about how genes function, but also had practical applications for medicine, agriculture, and industry. By 1974, there was already speculation in the media about the benefits that could accrue from gene transplant techniques. The creation of bacteria "factories" that could turn out large amounts of life-saving medicines was just one possibility. In fact, insulin made from bacteria was just seven years from becoming a reality. Still in the future at that time, but proved possible within two decades, were supermarket tomatoes hardy enough to survive cross-country trucking that taste as good as those grown in one's own garden. Using DNA technology, other plants were also bred for disease and pollution resistance. Scientists also projected that nitrogen-fixing microbes, such as those that appear in the soil near the roots of soybeans and other protein-rich plants, could be duplicated and introduced into corn and wheat fields to reduce the need for petroleum-based nitrogen fertilizer. Cohen himself said, in an article written for the July 1975 issue of *Scientific American:* "Gene manipulation opens the prospect of constructing bacterial cells, which can be grown easily and inexpensively, that will synthesize a variety of biologically produced substances such as **antibiotics** and hormones, or **enzymes** that can convert sunlight directly into food substances or usable energy."

When news of this remarkable research became widespread throughout the general population during the 1970s and 1980s, questions were raised about the dangers that might be inherent in genetic engineering technology. Some people were concerned that the potential existed for organisms altered by recombinant DNA to become hazardous and uncontrollable. Although safety guidelines had long been in place to protect both scientists and the public from disease-causing bacteria, toxic chemicals, and radioactive substances, genetic engineering seemed, to those outside the laboratory, to require measures much more restrictive. Even though, as responsible scientists, Cohen and others who were directly involved with DNA research had already placed limitations on the types of DNA experiments that could be performed, the National Academy of Sciences established a group to study these concerns and decide what restrictions should be imposed. In 1975, an international conference was held on this complicated issue, which was attended by scientists, lawyers, legislators, and journalists from seventeen countries. Throughout this period, Cohen spent much time speaking to the public and testifying to government agencies regarding

DNA technology, attempting to ease concerns regarding DNA experimentation.

Cohen contended that public outcry over the safety of DNA experiments resulted in an overly cautious approach that slowed the progress of DNA research and reinforced the public's belief that real, not conjectural, hazards existed in the field of biotechnology. In an article on this subject published in 1977 for *Science* he pointed out that during the initial recombinant DNA experiments, billions of bacteria played host to DNA molecules from many sources; these DNA molecules were grown and propagated "without hazardous consequences so far as I am aware. And the majority of these experiments were carried out prior to the strict containment procedures specified in the current federal guidelines."

The controversy over the safety of DNA technology absorbed much of Cohen's time and threatened to obscure the importance of other plasmid research with which he was involved during those years. For instance, his work with bacterial **transposons**, the "jumping genes" that carry antibiotic resistance, has yielded valuable information about how this process functions. He also developed a method of using "reporter genes" to study the behavior of genes in bacteria and eukaryotic cells. In addition, he has searched for the mechanism that triggers plasmid inheritance and **evolution**. Increased knowledge in this area offers the medical community more effective tools for fighting antibiotic resistance and better understanding of genetic controls.

Cohen has made the study of plasmid biology his life's work. An introspective, modest man, he is most at home in the laboratory and the classroom. He has been at Stanford University for more than twenty-five years, serving as chair of the Department of Genetics from 1978 to 1986. He is the author of more than two hundred papers, and has received many awards for his scientific contributions, among them the Albert Lasker Basic Medical Research Award in 1980, the Wolf Prize in Medicine in 1981, both the National Medal of Science and the LVMH Prize of the Institut de la Vie in 1988, the National Medal of Technology in 1989, the American Chemical Society Award in 1992, and the Helmut Horten Research Award in 1993. Cohen has held memberships in numerous professional societies, including the National Academy of Sciences (chairing the genetics section from 1988 to 1991), the Institute of Medicine of the National Academy, and the Genetics Society of America. In addition, he served on the board of the *Journal of Bacteriology* in the 1970s, and was associate editor of *Plasmid* from 1977 to 1986. Since 1977, he has been a member of the Committee on Genetic Experimentation for the International Council of Scientific Unions. Married in 1961 to Joanna Lucy Wolter, and the father of two children, Cohen lives mostly near Stanford University in a small, rural community. Free time away from his laboratory and his students has been spent skiing, playing five-string banjo, and sailing his aptly named boat, *Genesis.*

See also Microbial genetics

COHN, FERDINAND JULIUS (1828-1898)

German microbiologist

Ferdinand Cohn, a founder of modern microbiology, became the first to recognize and study bacteriology as a separate science. Cohn developed a system for classifying **bacteria** and discovered the importance of heat-resistant endospores. Additionally, Cohn recognized that both pathogens and non-pathogens could be found in drinking water and spoke of the importance of analyzing drinking water. Finally, Cohn worked with **Robert Koch** on the development of the etiology of the **anthrax** bacillus.

Cohn initially began his studies in botany at the University of Breslau in 1844. After being denied entry into the doctoral program in 1846 because of his Jewish heritage, Cohn moved to Berlin. There he completed his doctoral degree in 1847, at the age of 19, on the structure and germination of seeds.

After returning to Breslau in 1849, Cohn was presented with a top of the line **microscope** from his father. There he studied the cell biology of plants including the growth and division of plant cells, plasma streaming, cell differentiation, and cellular structures. In time, Cohn's studies were redirected toward algae, **protozoa**, **fungi**, and bacteria. His efforts on the developmental and sexual cycles of these **microorganisms** led to important advancements in cell biology.

At that time, bacteriology was an emerging field and although scientists knew that bacteria existed, they had failed to isolate bacteria in pure cultures. Scientists began to name bacteria without regard for someone else that had already observed and named the very same bacteria. Moreover, scientists believed bacteria to be a single species and that variations observed were due to different stages of development. Cohn recognized that bacteria could not be classified as a single species and developed a system for classifying them. He proposed that bacteria could be divided into groups based on whether they had similar development, chemical make-up, or descent. In 1875, he defined bacteria as "chlorophyll-less cells of characteristic shape that multiply by cross division and live as singe cells, filamentous cell chains, or cell aggregates." Eventually he extended his definition to include that "bacteria can be divided into distinct species with typical characteristics, which are transmitted to the following generations when bacteria multiply and that variations exist within each species."

After comprehensive studies of bacteria, Cohn believed that bacteria were related to algae and should thus be classified in the plant kingdom. Additionally, Cohn studied the growth of bacteria and found that in some bacteria organic substances were broken down in the presence of nitrogen. He also claimed that carbon dioxide could not be utilized as a carbon source in bacteria. It was not until 1890 when Sergei N. Winogradsky disproved this statement and discovered autotrophy.

Cohn's initial classification of bacteria consisted of four groups based on shape: Sphaerobacteria (sphere-shaped), Microbacteria (rod-shaped), Desmobacteria (filamentous), and Spirobacteria (screw-like shaped). Of those four groups the genus *Micrococcus* was classified as Sphaerobacteria, *Bacterium* was classified as Microbacteria, *Bacillus* and *Vibrio* were classified as Desmobacteria, and *Spirillum* and *Spirochaeta* were classified as Spirobacteria. Some of the genera could be further divided into subcategories.

Through the studies of *Bacillus subtilis* Cohn was able to disprove the earlier theory of spontaneous generation. Cohn recognized that some solutions were easily sterilized by heat, requiring only a few minutes of boiling, while other solutions required several hours of boiling. He found that still others, such as hay infusions, could not be sterilized at all. Cohn discovered heat-resistant structures called endospores, not spontaneous generation, were responsible for tainting sterilized cultures. Endospores are not killed in boiling water while the vegetative cells are. It was the heat resistant endospores from which bacteria grew, discounting the old theory of spontaneous generation.

Early on Cohn assisted in diagnosing fungal infections of crops and provided treatment options to the farmers for these plant diseases. Additionally, Cohn recognized that water sources were capable of harboring and transferring infectious diseases to humans. It was Robert Koch who first identified the pathogen that caused cholera in the drinking water; however, Cohn also analyzed the drinking water and found disease and non-disease causing microorganisms. Cohn developed a system for chemical analysis of water and claimed that drinking water should be monitored for microorganisms on a regular basis.

Later when Robert Koch was studying anthrax bacillus, Koch sought the help of Cohn. Cohn realized the importance of studying the disease causing anthrax bacillus and worked with Koch to further investigate the etiology of the bacteria. In 1875, Cohn founded the journal *Beitrage zur Biologie der Pflanzen* and published Koch's findings on anthrax bacillus in 1877.

See also Water quality; Cell cycle and cell division; History of microbiology

COLD, COMMON

Dedicated researchers have searched for a cure or even an effective treatment for the common cold (rhinitis) for years. Discovering or constructing the agent that will be universally lethal to all the cold-causing **viruses** has been fruitless. A drug that will kill only one or two of the viruses would be of little use since the patient would not know which of the viruses was the one that brought on his cold.

The common cold differs in several ways from **influenza** or the flu. Cold symptoms develop gradually and are relatively mild. The flu has a sudden onset and has more serious symptoms the usually put the sufferer to bed, and the flu lasts about twice as long as the cold. Also influenza can be fatal, especially to elderly persons, though the number of influenza viruses is more limited than the number of cold viruses, and vaccines are available against certain types of flu.

Rhinoviruses, **adenoviruses**, influenza viruses, parainfluenza viruses, syncytial viruses, echoviruses, and coxsackie viruses—all have been implicated as the agents that cause the

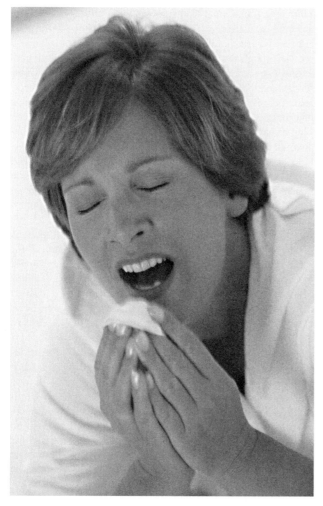

Sneezing is a symptom of the common cold.

runny nose, cough, sore throat, and sneezing that advertise that you have a cold. More than 200 viruses, each with its own favored method of being passed from one person to another, its own gestation period, each different from the others, wait patiently to invade the mucous membranes that line the nose of the next cold victim.

Passing the cold-causing virus from one person to the next can be done by sneezing onto the person, by shaking hands, or by an object handled by the infected person and picked up by the next victim. Oddly, direct contact with the infected person, as in kissing, is not an efficient way for the virus to spread. Only in about 10% of such contacts does the uninfected person get the virus. Walking around in a cold rain will not cause a cold. Viruses like warm, moist surroundings, so they thrive indoors in winter. Colds are easily passed in the winter, because people spend more time indoors then than they do outdoors. However, being outdoors in cold weather can dehydrate the mucous membranes in the nose and make them more susceptible to infection by a rhinovirus.

In addition, cold-causing viruses mutate with regularity. Each time it is passed from one person to the next, the virus

changes slightly, so it is not the virus the first person had. Viruses are obligate **parasites**, meaning that they can carry out their functions only when they invade another living cell.

The virus has a tough envelope surrounding its nucleic acids, the genetic material for any living thing. Once it invades the body, the virus waits to be placed in the location in which it can function best. Once there, it attaches to a cell by means of receptor areas on its envelope and on the cell membrane. The viral nucleic acid then is inserted into the cell **nucleus** and it takes over the functions of the nucleus, telling it to reproduce viruses.

Taking regular doses of vitamin C will not ward off a cold. However, high doses of vitamin C once a person has a cold may help to alleviate symptoms and reduce discomfort. Over-the-counter drugs to treat colds treat only the symptoms. They may dry up the patient's runny nose, but after a few days the nose will compensate and overcome the effects of the medication and begin to drip again. The runny nose is from the loss of plasma from the blood vessels in the nose. Some researchers assert the nose drip is a defensive mechanism to prevent the invasion of other viruses. **Antibiotics** such as **penicillin** are useless against the cold because they do not affect viruses.

Scientists agree that the old wives' remedy of chicken soup can help the cold victim, but so can any other hot liquid. The steam and heat produced by soup or tea helps to liquefy the mucus in the sinus cavities, allowing them to drain, reducing the pressure and making the patient feel better. The remedy is temporary and has no effect on the virus. Colds are usually self-limiting, and recovery usually occurs within a week.

See also Cold, viruses; Infection and resistance; Viruses and responses to viral infection

COLD, VIRUSES

The cold is one of the most common illnesses of humans. In the Unites States alone, there are more than one billion colds each year. Typically a cold produces sneezing, scratchy throat, and a runny nose for one or two weeks. The causes of the common **cold** are **viruses.**

More than 200 different viruses can cause a cold. Rhinoviruses account for anywhere from 35% to over half of all colds, particularly in younger and older people. This has likely been the case for millennia. Indeed, the name Rhinovirus is from the Greek word *rhin*, meaning, "nose." There are over one hundred different types of Rhinovirus, based on the different proteins that are on the surface of the virus particle. Rhinovirus belongs to the virus family Picornaviridae. The genetic material of the virus is **ribonucleic acid (RNA)** and the genome is of a very small size.

Rhinovirus is spread from one person to another by "hand to hand" contact, that is, by physical contact or from one person sneezing close by another person. The virus needs to inside the human body to be able to replicate. The internal temperature of the body, which is normally between 97–99°F (36.1–37.2° C) is perfect for Rhinovirus. If the temperature varies only a few degrees either way of the window, the virus will not replicate.

Rhinovirus has been successful in causing colds for such as long time because of the large number of antigenic types of the virus that exist. Producing a **vaccine** against the virus would require the inclusion of hundreds of antibodies to the hundreds of different possible antigens. This is not practical to achieve. Furthermore, not all the Rhinovirus antigens that are important in generating a cold are exposed at the surface. So, even if a corresponding **antibody** were present, neutralization of the **antigen** via the binding of the antibody with the antigen would not occur. Another factor against vaccine development is the difficulty in being able to grow Rhinovirus in the laboratory.

Another virus that causes colds are members of the Coronavirus family. The name of the virus derives from the distinctive flexible shape and appearance of the virus particle. Surface projections give the virus a crown-like, or corona, appearance. There are more than 30 known strains of Coronavirus. Of these, three or four from the genus *Coronavirus* can infect humans. Cattle, pigs, rodents, cats, dogs, and birds are also hosts. Members of the genus *Torovirus* can also cause **gastroenteritis**.

Coronavirus has been known since 1937, when it was isolated from chickens. It was suspected of being a cause of colds, but this could not be proven until the 1960s, when techniques to grow the virus in laboratory cultures were devised. Like Rhinovirus, Coronavirus also contains RNA. However, in contrast to the same amount of genetic material carried in Rhinoviruses, the genome of the Coronavirus is the largest of all the RNA-containing viruses.

Other viruses account for 10–15% of colds in adults. These **adenoviruses**, coxsackieviruses, echoviruses, orthomyxoviruses (including the **influenza** A and B viruses), paramyxoviruses, respiratory syncytial virus and enteroviruses can also cause other, more severe illnesses.

Aside from vaccines, various "home remedies" to the common cold exist. Larger than normal doses of Vitamin C have been claimed to lessen the symptoms or prevent the common cold. The evidence for this claim is still not definitive. Another remedy, mythologized as an example of a mother's care for her children, is chicken soup. Studies have demonstrated that chicken soup may indeed shorten the length of a cold and relieve some of the symptoms. The active ingredient(s), if any, that are responsible are not known, however. For now, the best treatment for a cold is to attempt to relieve the symptoms via such home remedies and over the counter medications. Nasal decongestants decrease the secretions from the nose and help relieve congestion. Antihistamines act to depress the **histamine** allergic response of the **immune system**. This has been claimed to help relieve cold symptoms. Analgesics relieve some of pain and fever associated with a cold.

Some so-called alternative medications may have some benefit. For example, lozenges composed of zinc can sometimes reduce the duration of the common cold, perhaps due to the need for zinc by the immune system. Echinacea is known to stimulate white blood cell activity.

See also Virology

COLIFORM BACTERIA · *see* ESCHERICHIA COLI (E. COLI)

COLONY AND COLONY FORMATION

A colony is population of a single type of microorganism that is growing on a solid or semi-solid surface. **Bacteria**, **yeast**, **fungi**, and molds are capable of forming colonies. Indeed, when a surface is available, these microbes prefer the colonial mode of growth rather than remaining in solution.

On a colonized solid surface, such as the various growth media used to **culture microorganisms**, each colony arises from a single microorganism. The cell that initially adheres to the surface divides to form a daughter cell. Both cells subsequently undergo another round of growth and division. This cycle is continually repeated. After sufficient time, the result is millions of cells piled up in close association with each other. This pile, now large enough to be easily visible to the unaided eye, represents a colony.

The appearance of a colony is governed by the characteristic of the organism that is the building block of that colony. For example, if a bacterium produces a color (the organism is described as being pigmented), then the colony can appear colored. Colonies can be smooth and glistening, rough and dry looking, have a smooth border or a border that resembles an undulating coastline, and can have filamentous appearance extensions sticking up into the air above the colony.

The visual appearance of a colony belies the biochemical complexities of the population within. For example, in a bacterial colony, the organisms buried in the colony and those near the more aged center of the colony are not as robustly growing as those bacteria at the periphery of the colony. Indeed, researchers have shown that the various phases of growth found when bacteria grow in a liquid growth medium in a flask (fast-growing and slower-growing bacteria, dying bacteria, and newly forming bacteria) all occur simultaneously in various regions of a colony. Put another way, within colonies, cells will have different phenotypes (structure) and genotypes (expression of genes).

Variations of **phenotype** and **genotype** have been elegantly demonstrated using a variant of *Escherichia coli* that differentially expresses a **gene** for the **metabolism** of a sugar called lactose depending on the growth rate of the bacteria. Growth on a specialized medium produces a blue color in those cells were the gene is active. Colonies of the variant will have blue-colored sectors and colorless sectors, corresponding to populations of bacteria that are either expressing the lactose-metabolizing gene or where the gene is silent.

The nature of the solid surface also affects the formation of a colony. For example, nutrients can diffuse deeper into a semi-solid growth medium than in a very stiff medium. Colonies of *Bacillus subtilis* bacteria tend to form more wavy, fern-like edges to their colonies in the semi-solid medium. This is because of uneven distribution of nutrients. Those bacteria in a relatively nutrient-rich zone will be able to grow

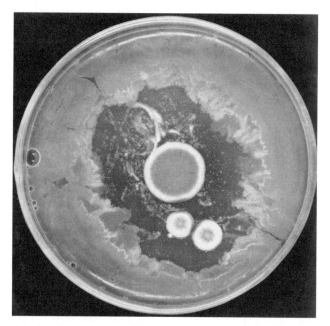

Colonies of *Penicillium notatus*, showing surrounding zone of bacterial inhibition. This is the phenomenon noted by Fleming in 1929, that led to his discovery of Penicillin. Undated.

COLWELL, RITA R. (1934-)

American marine microbiologist

Rita R. Colwell is a leader in marine **biotechnology**, the application of molecular techniques to marine biology for the harvesting of medical, industrial and aquaculture products from the sea. As a scientist and professor, Colwell has investigated the ecology, physiology, and evolutionary relationships of marine **bacteria**. As a founder and president of the University of Maryland Biotechnology Institute, she has nurtured a vision to improve the environment and human health by linking **molecular biology** and genetics to basic knowledge scientists have gleaned from life and chemistry in the oceans.

Rita Rossi was born in Beverly, Massachusetts, the seventh of eight children to parents Louis and Louise Di Palma Rossi. Her father was an Italian immigrant who established his own construction company, and her mother was an artistic woman who worked to help ensure her children would have a good education. She died when her daughter was just thirteen years old, but she had expressed pride in her success in school. In the sixth grade, after Rossi had scored higher on an IQ test than anyone previously in her school, the principal sternly stressed that Rossi had the responsibility to go to college. Eventually, Rossi received a full scholarship from Purdue University. She earned her B.S. degree with distinction in bacteriology in 1956. Although she had been accepted to medical school, Rossi chose instead to earn a master's degree so that she could remain at the same institution as graduate student Jack Colwell, whom she married on May 31, 1956. Colwell would have continued her studies in bacteriology, but the department chairman at Purdue informed her that giving fellowship money to women would have been a waste. She instead earned her master's degree in the department of genetics. The University of Washington, Seattle, granted her a Ph.D. in 1961 for work on bacteria commensal to marine animals, which is the practice of an organism obtaining food or other benefits from another without either harming or helping it. Colwell's contributions included establishing the basis for the systematics of marine bacteria.

In 1964, Georgetown University hired Colwell as an assistant professor, and gave her tenure in 1966. Colwell and her research team were the first to recognize that the bacterium that caused cholera occurred naturally in estuaries. They isolated the bacterium from Chesapeake Bay and in ensuing years sought to explain how outbreaks in human populations might be tied to the seasonal abundance of the host organisms in the sea, particularly **plankton**. In 1972, Colwell took a tenured professorship at the University of Maryland. Her studies expanded to include investigations on the impact of marine pollution at the microbial level. Among her findings was that the presence of oil in estuarine and open ocean water was associated with the numbers of bacteria able to break down oil. She studied whether some types of bacteria might be used to treat oil spills. Colwell and her colleagues also made a discovery that held promise for improving oyster yields in aquaculture—a bacterial film

faster, and often grow in the direction of the nutrient source. Even the shape of the bacteria changes from an oval to a longer form in these fast growing regions. The molecular basis of this shape **transformation** remains unresolved.

In another example of the influence of the surface on colony dynamics, the periphery of colonies grown on wet surfaces contains very motile (moveable) bacteria. Their motion is constrained by the high number of bacteria. The results is the formation of so-called "whirls and jets" that form, disappear and re-form. These motions, which appear under the light **microscope** to be very random and chaotic, are in fact very highly organized and helps drive the further formation of the colony.

Another phenomenon of colony formation is the communication between constituent cells. This is also known as "cross-talk." Cells of the amoeba *Dictyostelium discoideum*, for example, can actually signal one another when growing in a colony, especially in nutrient-poor environments. Cells that encounter nutrients emit a compound called cyclic adenosine monophosphate (cAMP). The subsequent growth of cells is in the direction of the increasing cAMP concentration. Visually, a spiraling pattern of growth results. Mounds of amoebas also form. The microbes at the top of the mounds produce spores that can become dispersed by air movement, allowing the colonization and new colony formation of other surfaces.

Chemical signalling within a colony has also been demonstrated in yeast, such as *Candida mogii* and in bacteria, such as *Escherichia coli*.

See also Agar and agarose; Biofilm formation and dynamic behavior formed on surfaces under water that attracted oyster larvae to settle and grow.

In the spirit of using knowledge gained from the sea to benefit humans and the environment, Colwell prepared a seminal paper on marine biotechnology published in the journal *Science* in 1983. It brought attention to the rich resources of the ocean that might be tapped for food, disease-curing drugs, and environmental clean-up by the applications of genetic engineering and **cloning**. In order to realize the potential of marine biotechnology as originally outlined in her 1983 paper, Colwell helped foster the concept and growth of the University of Maryland Biotechnology Institute, established in 1987. As president of the U.M.B.I., she has formed alliances between researchers and industry and has succeeded in raising funds to develop the center as a prestigious biotech research complex.

In addition, Colwell has held numerous professional and academic leadership positions throughout her career and is a widely published researcher. At the University of Maryland, Colwell was director of the Sea Grant College from 1977 to 1983. She served as president of Sigma Xi, the American Society for Microbiology, and the International Congress of Systematic and Evolutionary Biology, and was president-elect of the American Association for the Advancement of Science. Colwell has written and edited more than sixteen books and over four hundred papers and articles. She also produced an award-winning film, *Invisible Seas*. Her honors included the 1985 Fisher Award of the American Society for Microbiology, the 1990 Gold Medal Award of the International Institute of Biotechnology, and the 1993 Phi Kappa Phi National Scholar Award.

Colwell is the mother of two daughters who pursued careers in science. She is an advocate for equal rights for women, and one of her long-standing aspirations is to write a novel about a woman scientist. Her hobbies include jogging and competitive sailing.

See also Bioremediation; *E. coli* O157:H7 infection; Economic uses and benefits of microorganisms; Water purification

COMBINED IMMUNODEFICIENCY · *see* IMMUNODEFICIENCY DISEASE SYNDROMES

COMMERCIAL USES OF MICROORGANISMS
· *see* ECONOMIC USES AND BENEFITS OF MICROORGANISMS

COMMON VARIABLE IMMUNODEFICIENCY DISEASE (CVID) · *see* IMMUNODEFICIENCY DISEASE SYNDROMES

COMPETITIVE EXCLUSION OF BACTERIAL ADHESION · *see* ANTI-ADHESION METHODS

COMPLEMENT

Complement refers to a series of some 30 proteins that enhance the bacterial killing effect of antibodies. This complementation involves facilitating the engulfing of **bacteria** by immune cells in the process known as **phagocytosis**, or by the puncturing of the bacterial membrane. Additionally, complement helps dispose of antigen-antibody complexes that form in the body.

The various complement proteins circulate throughout the bloodstream in an inactive form. When one of the proteins is converted to an active form upon interaction with an antigen-antibody complex, a series of reactions is triggered. The activation step involves the cleaving, or precise cutting, of the particular complement protein. The cleavage turns the complement protein into a protease, a protein that is itself capable of cleaving other proteins. In turn, cleavage of a second complement protein makes that protein a protease. The resulting cleavage reaction generates a series of active complement proteins. These reactions, known as the complement cascade, occur in an orderly sequence and are under precise regulation.

The reactions involve two pathways. One is known as the classical complement activation pathway. The end result is an enzyme that can degrade a protein called C3. The other pathway is known as the alternative pathway. The second pathway does not require the presence of **antibody** for the activation of complement. Both pathways result in the formation of an entity that is called the membrane attack complex. The complex is actually a channel that forms in the bacterial membrane. Under the magnification of the **electron microscope**, a bacterial membrane that is a target of the complement system appears riddled with holes.

The channels that form in a membrane allow the free entry and exit of fluids and molecules. Because the concentration of various ions is higher inside the bacterium than outside, fluid will flow inward to attempt to balance the concentrations. As a result, the bacterium swells and bursts.

Other reaction products of the complement cascade trigger an inflammatory immune response. In addition, the invading bacteria are coated with an immune molecule (C3b) that makes the bacteria more recognizable to phagocytes. This process is called **opsonization**. The phagocytes then engulf the bacteria and degrade them.

Tight control over the activity of the complement system is essential. At least 12 proteins are involved in the regulation of complement activation. Defects in this control, or the operation of the pathways, result in frequent bacterial infections.

See also Immune system; Infection and control

COMPLEMENT DEFICIENCY · *see* IMMUNODEFICIENCY DISEASE SYNDROMES

COMPLETED TESTS · *see* LABORATORY TECHNIQUES IN MICROBIOLOGY

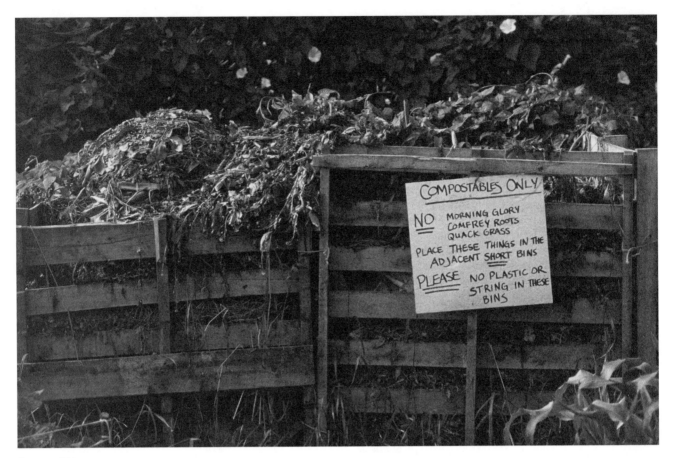

A compost bin.

COMPLEX MEDIA · *see* GROWTH AND GROWTH MEDIA

COMPOSTING, MICROBIOLOGICAL ASPECTS

Composting is the conversion of organic material, such as plant material and household foodstuffs, to a material having a soil-like consistency. This material is called compost. The composting process, which is one of decomposition, relies upon living organisms. Insects and earthworms participate. **Bacteria** and **fungi** are of fundamental importance.

Composting is a natural process and enables nutrients to be cycled back into an ecosystem. The end products of composition are compost, carbon dioxide, water and heat.

The decomposition process is achieved mainly by bacteria and fungi. Bacteria predominate, making up 80 to 90% of the **microorganisms** found in compost.

There are several phases to the composting process, which involve different microorganisms. The first phase, which lasts a few days after addition of the raw material to the compost pile, is a moderate temperature (mesophilic) phase. As microbial activity produces decomposition and by-products, including heat, a high-temperature (thermophilic) phase

takes over. The dominant microorganisms will become those that are adapted to life at higher temperature, the so-called thermophiles. The high-temperature (thermophilic) phase will last anywhere from a few days to a few months. Finally, as decomposition activity of the microbial population slows and ceases, a cooling-down phase ensues over several months.

Initially, the mesophilic microorganisms break down compounds that readily dissolve in water. This decomposition is rapid, causing the temperature inside the compost pile to rise quickly. The microbes involved at this stage tend to be those that predominate in the soil. One example is **Actinomyces**, which resemble fungi but which are actually bacteria composed of filaments. They are what give the soil its earthy smell. **Enzymes** in Actinomyces are capable of degrading grass, bark and even newspaper. Species of fungi and **protozoa** can also be active at this stage.

As the internal temperature of the pile exceeds 40° C (104° F), the mesophiles die off and are replaced by the thermophilic microbes. A decomposition temperature around 55° C (131° F) is ideal, as microbial activity is pronounced and because that temperature is lethal to most human and animal microbial pathogens. Thus, the composting process is also a sterilizing process, from an infectious point of view. However, temperatures much above this point can kill off the microbes involved in the decomposition. For this reason, compost piles are occasionally agitated or "turned over" to mix the contents, allow oxygen to diffuse throughout the material (efficient decomposition requires the presence of oxygen) and to disperse some of the heat. The ideal blend of microorganisms can be established and maintained by the addition of waste material to the compost pile so as to not let the pile become enriched in carbon or nitrogen. A proper ratio is about 30 parts carbon to one part nitrogen by weight.

Thermophilic bacteria present at this stage of decomposition include *Bacillus stearothermophilus* and bacteria of the genus Thermus. A variety of thermophilic fungi are present as well. These include *Rhizomucor pusills, Chaetomium thermophile, Humicola insolens, Humicola lanuginosus, Thermoascus aurabtiacus*, and *Aspergillus fumigatus*.

Thermophilic activity decomposes protein, fat, and carbohydrates such as the cellulose that makes up plants and grass. As this phase of decomposition ends, the temperature drops and once again the lower-temperature microbes become dominant. The decomposition of the complex materials by the thermophilic organisms provides additional nutrients for the continued decomposition by the mesophilic populations.

Microbiological composting is becoming increasingly important as space for waste disposal becomes limited. Some 30% of yard and household waste in the United States is compostable. An average household can decompose about 700 pounds of material per year. If such waste is added to landfills intact, the subsequent decomposition produces methane gas and acidic run-off, both of which are environmentally undesirable.

See also Chemoautotrophic and chemolithotrophic bacteria; Economic uses and benefits of microorganisms; Soil formation, involvement of microorganisms

COMPOUND MICROSCOPE · *see* MICROSCOPE AND MICROSCOPY

CONDITIONAL LETHAL MUTANT · *see* MICROBIAL GENETICS

CONFIRMED TESTS · *see* LABORATORY TECHNIQUES IN MICROBIOLOGY

CONFOCAL MICROSCOPY · *see* MICROSCOPE AND MICROSCOPY

CONJUGATION

Conjugation is a mechanism whereby a bacterium can transfer genetic material to an adjacent bacterium. The genetic transfer requires contact between the two **bacteria**. This contact is mediated by the bacterial appendage called a pilus.

Conjugation allows bacteria to increase their genetic diversity. Thus, an advantageous genetic trait present in a bac-

terium is capable of transfer to other bacteria. Without conjugation, the normal bacterial division process does not allow for the sharing of genetic information and, except for **mutations** that occur, does not allow for the development of genetic diversity.

A pilus is a hollow tube constructed of a particular protein. One end is anchored to the surface of a bacterium. The other end is capable of binding to specific proteins on the surface of another bacterium. A pilus can then act as a portal from the **cytoplasm** of one bacterium to the cytoplasm of the other bacterium. How the underlying membrane layers form channels to the bacterial cytoplasm is still unclear, although channel formation may involve what is termed a mating pair formation (mpf) apparatus on the bacterial surface.

Nonetheless, once a channel has been formed, transfer of **deoxyribonucleic acid** (**DNA**) from one bacterium (the donor) to the other bacterium (the recipient) can occur.

Conjugation requires a set of F (fertility) genes. Transfer of DNA from the genome of a bacterium can occur if the F set of genes is integrated in the bacterial chromosome. These F genes enter the pilus and literally drag the trailing genome along behind. Often the pilus will break before the transfer of the complete genome can occur. Thus, genes that are located in the vicinity of the F genes will tend to be successfully transferred in conjugation more often than genes located far away from the F genes. This process was originally discovered in *Escherichia coli*. Strains that exhibit a higher than usual tendency to transfer genomic DNA are known as High Frequency of **Recombination** (Hfr) strains.

Conjugation also involves transfer of DNA that is located on a plasmid. A plasmid that contains the F genes is called the F episome or F plasmid. Other genes on the episome will be transferred very efficiently, since the entire episome can typically be transferred before conjugation is terminated by pilus breakage. If one of the genes codes for a disease causing factor or **antibiotic resistance** determinant, then episomal conjugation can be a powerful means of spreading the genetic trait through a bacterial population. Indeed, conjugation is the principle means by which bacterial antibiotic resistance is spread.

Finally, conjugation can involve the transfer of only a plasmid containing the F genes. This type of conjugation is also an efficient means of spreading genetic information to other bacteria. In this case, as more bacteria acquire the F genes, the proportion of the population that is capable of genetic transfer via conjugation increases.

Joshua Lederberg discovered the process of conjugation in 1945. He experimented with so-called nutritional **mutants** (bacteria that required the addition of a specific nutrient to the growth medium). By incubating the nutritional mutants in the presence of bacteria that did not require the nutrient to be added, Lederberg demonstrated that the mutation could be eliminated. Subsequently, another bacteriologist, William Hayes, demonstrated that the acquisition of genetic information occurred in a one-way manner (e.g., information was passing from one bacterium into another), and that the basis for the information transfer was genetic (i.e., mutants were isolated in which the transfer did not occur).

Another landmark experiment in microbiology also centered on conjugation. This experiment is known as the interrupted mating experiment (or blender experiment, since a common kitchen blender was used). Donor and recipient bacteria were mixed together and left to allow conjugation to begin. Then, at various times, the population was vigorously blended. This sheared off the pili that were connected the conjugating bacteria, interrupting the mating process. By analyzing the recipient bacteria for the presence of known genes that has been transferred, the speed of conjugation could be measured.

Conjugation has been exploited in the **biotechnology** era to permit the transfer of desired genetic information. A target **gene** can be inserted into the donor bacterial DNA near the F genes. Or, an F plasmid can be constructed in the laboratory and then inserted into a bacterial strain that will function as the donor. When conjugation occurs, bacteria in the recipient population will acquire the target gene.

See also Evolution and evolutionary mechanisms; Laboratory techniques in microbiology

CONTAMINATION AND RELEASE PREVENTION PROTOCOL

Contamination is the unwanted presence of a microorganism in a particular environment. That environment can be in the laboratory setting, for example, in a medium being used for the growth of a species of **bacteria** during an experiment. Another environment can be the human body, where contamination of various niches can produce an infection. Still another environment can be the solid and liquid nutrients that sustain life. A final example, which is becoming more relevant since the burgeoning use of **biotechnology**, is the natural environment. The consequences of the release of bioengineered **microorganisms** into the natural environment to the natural microflora and to other species that depend on the environment for their welfare, are often unclear.

The recognition of the adverse effects of contamination have been recognized for a long time, and steps that are now a vital part of microbiological practice were developed to curb contamination. The prevention of microbial contamination goes hand in hand with the use of microorganisms.

Ever since the development of techniques to obtain microorganisms in pure **culture**, the susceptibility of such cultures to the unwanted growth of other microbes has been recognized. This contamination extends far beyond being merely a nuisance. Differing behaviors of different microorganisms, in terms of how nutrients are processed and the by-products of this **metabolism**, can compromise the results of an experiment, leading to erroneous conclusions.

In the medical setting, microbial contamination can be life threatening. As recognized by **Joseph Lister** in the mid-nineteenth century, such contamination can be lessened, if not prevented completely, by the observance of various hygienic practices in the hospital setting. In modern medicine and sci-

ence, the importance of hand washing and the maintenance of a sterile operating theatre is taken for granted.

Prevention of microbiological contamination begins in the laboratory. A variety of prevention procedures are a common part of an efficient microbiology laboratory. The use of sterile equipment and receptacles for liquid and solid growth media is a must. The prevention of contamination during the manipulations of microorganisms in the laboratory falls under the term asceptic technique. Examples of asceptic technique include the **disinfection** of work surfaces and the hands of the relevant lab personnel before and after contact with the microorganisms and the flaming of the metal loops or rods used to transfer bacter from one location to another.

In other areas of a laboratory, microorganisms that are known to be of particular concern, because they can easily contaminate or be contaminated, or because they represent a health threat, can be quarantined in special work areas. Examples of such areas include fume hoods and the so-called glove box. The latter is an enclosed space where the lab worker is kept physically separate from the microorganisms, but can manipulate the organisms by virtue of rubber gloves that are part of the wall of the enclosure.

In both the laboratory and other settings, such as processing areas for foods, various monitoring steps are instituted as part of a proper quality control regimen to ensure that contamination does not occur, or can be swiftly detected and dealt with. A well-established technique of contamination monitoring is the air plate technique, where a non-specific growth medium is exposed to the circulating air in the work area for a pre-determined period of time. Air-borne microorganisms can be detected in this manner. More recently, as the importance of the adherent (biofilm) mode of growth of, in particular, bacteria became recognized, contamination monitoring can also include the installation of a device that allows the fluid circulating through pipelines to be monitored. Thus, for example, water used in processing operations can be sampled to determine if **bacterial growth** on the pipeline is occurring and also whether remediation is necessary.

A necessary part of the prevention of microbiological contamination is the establishment of various quality control measures. For example, the swiping of a lab bench with a sterile cotton swab and the incubation of the swab in a nonspecific growth medium is a regular part of many microbiology laboratories quality control regimen. The performance of all equipment that is used for **sterilization** and microorganism confinement is also regularly checked.

With the advent of biotechnology and in particular the use of genetically modified microorganisms in the agricultural sector, the prevention of the unwanted release of the bioengineered microbes into the natural environment has become an important issue to address.

The experimentation with genetically engineered microorganisms in the natural environment is subject to a series of rigid controls in many countries around the world. A series of benchmarks must be met to ensure that an organism is either incapable of being spread or, if so, is incapable of prolonged survival.

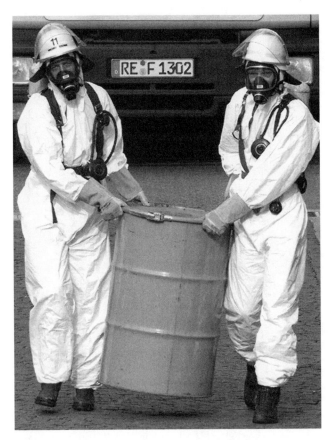

Firefighters remove barrel conaining suspected infectious agent.

CONTAMINATION, BACTERIAL AND VIRAL

Contamination by **bacteria** and **viruses** can occur on several levels. In the setting of the laboratory, the growth media, tissues and other preparations used for experimentation can support the growth of unintended and unwanted **microorganisms**. Their presence can adversely influence the results of the experiments. Outside the laboratory, bacteria and viruses can contaminate drinking water supplies, foodstuffs, and products, causing illness. Infection is another form of contamination.

Equipment and growth media used in the laboratory must often be treated to render them free of microorganisms. Bacteria and viruses can be present in the air, as aerosolized droplets, and can be present on animate surfaces, such as the skin and the mucous membranes of the nasal passage, and on inanimate surfaces, such as the workbenches in the laboratory. Without precautions and the observance of what is known as sterile technique, these microbes can contaminate laboratory growth media, solutions and equipment. This contamination can be inconvenient, necessitating the termination of an experiment. However, if the contamination escapes the notice of the researcher, then the results obtained will be unknowingly marred. Whole avenues of research could be compromised.

Contamination of drinking water by bacteria and viruses has been a concern since antiquity. Inadequate sanitation practices can introduce fecal material into the water. Enteroviruses and fecal bacteria such as *Shigella* and *Escherichia coli* O157:H7 are capable of causing debilitating, even life-threatening, diseases. Even in developed countries, contamination of drinking water remains a problem. If a treatment system is not functioning properly, water sources, especially surface sources, are vulnerable to contamination. An example occurred in the summer of 2000 in Walkerton, Ontario, Canada. Contamination of one of the town's wells by *Escherichia coli* O157:H7 run-off from a cattle operation killed seven people, and sickened over two thousand.

Other products can be contaminated as well. An example is blood and blood products. Those who donate blood might be infected, and the infectious agents can be transmitted to the recipient of the blood or blood product. In the 1970s and 1980s, the Canadian blood supply was contaminated with the viral agents of **hepatitis** and acquired **immunodeficiency** syndrome. At that time, tests for these agents were not as sophisticated and as definitive as they are now. The viruses that escaped detection sickened thousands of people. Blood supplies in Canada and elsewhere are now safeguarded from contamination by stringent monitoring programs.

Food products are also prone to contamination. The contamination can originate in the breeding environment. For example, poultry that are grown in crowded conditions are reservoirs of bacterial contamination, particularly with *Campylobacter jejuni*. Over half of all poultry entering processing plants are contaminated with this bacterium. Other food products can become contaminated during processing, via bacteria that are growing on machinery or in processing solutions. Quality control measures, which monitor critical phases of the process from raw material to finished product, are helpful in pinpointing and eliminating sources of contamination.

Prevention of genetic contamination, via the exchange of genetic material between the bioengineered microbe and the natural microbial population, is difficult to prevent. However, available evidence supports the view that the genetic traits bred into the bioengineered organism to permit its detection, such as **antibiotic resistance**, are not traits that will be maintained in the natural population. This is because of the energy cost to the microorganism to express the trait and because of the mathematical dynamics of population genetics (i.e., the altered genes are not present in numbers to become established within the greater population) and the absence of the need for the trait (the antibiotic of interest is not present in the natural environment). Hence, contamination prevention procedures have tended to focus on those aspects of contamination that are both relevant and likely to occur.

As an example of the measures currently in place, the United States has three agencies that are concerned with the regulation of biotechnology. These are the Department of Agriculture, Environmental Protection Agency, and the Food and Drug Administration. Each of these agencies oversee regulatory legislation that addresses the contamination of various natural and commercially relevant environments.

See also Asilomar conferences; Biotechnology; Hazard Analysis and Critical Point Program (HACPP); Laboratory techniques in microbiology

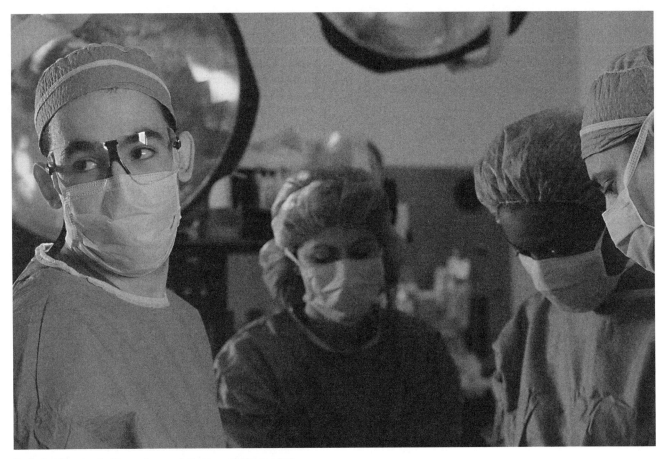

Typical anti-contamination garb worn during a surgical procedure.

With respect to contamination of food, the **hygiene** of food handlers is a key factor. In the United States, estimates are the one in five food-borne disease outbreaks is caused by the handling of foods by personnel whose hands are contaminated with bacteria or viruses. Poor hand washing following use of the bathroom is the main problem.

In the nineteenth century, similar hygiene problems created a death rate in most surgical procedures. The contamination of open wounds, incisions and entry routes of catheters killed the majority of surgical patients. With the adoption of sterile operating room technique and scrupulous personnel hygiene, the death rate from surgical procedures is now very low.

See also Blood borne infections; Hazard Analysis and Critical Point Program (HAACP); History of public health; Transmission of pathogens

CORYNEFORM BACTERIA

Coryneform **bacteria** are normal residents of the skin. They can also cause opportunistic infections. These are infections that occur as a secondary infection, when the immune response of a host has been weakened by another infection or by another insult to the **immune system**, such as **chemother-**

apy. An example is *Corynebacterium jeikeium*, whose infection can be taxing to treat as the organism is resistant to numerous **antibiotics.** Over the past two decades, the numbers of such infections have been rising. This may be an indication of an immune stress on the body.

Coryneform bacteria can stain positive in the Gram stain protocol. However, this reaction is not consistent. A characteristic feature is their tendency to arrange themselves in a V-like pattern or lined up, much like logs stacked one against the other.

While there are some consistencies among the members of the Coryneform bacteria, a hallmark of these bacteria is their diversity of habitats. This, and their inconsistent Gram stain reaction, can make identification of the microorganism tedious. More rigorous biochemical and molecular biological tools of identification are being used by organizations such as the **Centers for Disease Control** (CDC) to establish a definitive classification scheme for Coryneform bacteria. For example, CDC groups JK and D-2 in the genus *Corynebacterium* are now recognized as important human disease-causing **microorganisms.** Conversely, these rigorous techniques have resulted in the removal of some species of bacteria from the genus.

Coryneform bacteria are important medically. *Corynebacterium diphtheriae* is the organism that causes **diphtheria.** In fact, before Coryneform bacteria were known to be comprised of several species, the bacteria were referred to as diphtheroids. Diphtheria is apparent as an **inflammation** and bleeding of the throat and as a generalized toxic poisoning of the body, due to the release of a powerful toxin by the bacteria. The toxin spreads throughout the body via the bloodstream and has a particular affinity for tissues such as the heart, nerve endings and the adrenal glands. Diphtheria is treatable with antibiotics.

Other species of the genus *Corynebacterium* cause mastitis in cows (an infection and inflammation of the udder), infection of the lymph nodes of sheep, and skin rashes and ulcerations in humans. *Rhodococcus equi*, which inhabits soil, is an important pathogen of young horses. Another human pathogen is It is also a normal resident on skin surfaces, and can cause an infection in those receiving chemotherapy.

See also Gram staining

COSTERTON, JOHN WILLIAM (1934-)
Canadian microbiologist

J. William (Bill) Costerton is a Canadian microbiologist who has pioneered the recognition of bacterial **biofilms** as the dominant mode of growth of **bacteria**, and who first demonstrated their importance in the resistance of bacteria to antibacterial agents and the persistence of some chronic bacterial infections.

Costerton was born in Vernon, British Columbia. His early education was in that province. In 1955, he received a B.S. in bacteriology and **immunology** from the University of British Columbia, followed by a M.S. in the same discipline from UBC in 1956. He then studied in the laboratory of Dr. **Robert Murray** at the University of Western Ontario in London, Ontario, where he received a Ph.D. in 1960. Following post-doctoral training at Cambridge University, Costerton moved to MacDonald College of McGill University, in the Canadian province of Quebec, where he became first a Professional Associate in 1966 then an Assistant Professor in 1968. In 1970 he moved to the University of Calgary as an Associate Professor. He became a tenured Professor at Calgary in 1975. From 1985 to 1992, he held positions at Calgary as the AOS-TRA Research Professor followed by the National Sciences and Engineering Research Council Industrial Research Chair. These two appointments freed him from teaching to concentrate on his burgeoning research into bacterial biofilms.

Research on biofilms has occupied Costerton since his move to Calgary. Costerton and his colleagues demonstrated the existence of biofilms and when on to show that biofilms are the dominant mode of growth for bacteria. The elaboration of an extensive sugar network that adheres bacteria to surfaces and subsequently buries them was revealed. Research over a decade demonstrated the importance of this exopolysaccharide in enabling the bacteria to survive doses of antibacterial agents, including **antibiotics** that readily killed bacteria grown in conventional lab cultures. This research was so convincing that an initially skeptical scientific community became convinced of the importance and widespread nature of biofilms.

In 1993, Costerton left Calgary to take up the post of Director of the Center for Biofilm Engineering at Montana State University, Bozeman. Since then, he and his colleagues have used techniques such as confocal microscopy to probe intact biofilms without disrupting them. These studies have revealed the complex nature of biofilm structure and the coordinated nature of the interaction between the bacterial populations in the biofilms. As well, Costerton discovered the so-called bioelectric effect, in which an application of current makes a biofilm much more susceptible to antibiotic killing. These discoveries are having profound influence on the design of strategies to combat chronic infections, such as the *Pseudomonas aeruginosa* lung infections that occur, and can ultimately kill those afflicted with cystic fibrosis.

For these and other pioneering contributions to biofilm research, Costerton has received many awards. These include the Sir Frederick Haultain Prize for outstanding achievement in the physical sciences (1986), the Isaak Walton Killam Memorial Prize for Scientific Achievement in Canada (1990), and a Fellowship in the American Association for the Advancement of Science (1997).

Costerton continues his research at Montana State and is actively involved internationally in promoting the multidisciplinary structure of the Center's research and education curriculum.

See also Antibiotic resistance, tests for; Bacterial adaptation; Glycocalyx

COULTER COUNTER

A Coulter counter is a device that is used to measure the number of cells in a certain volume of a sample suspension. The counter achieves this enumeration by monitoring the decrease in electrical conductivity that occurs when the cells pass through a small opening in the device. While originally developed for use with blood cells, the Coulter counter has found great use in a diverse number of disciplines, including microbiology, where it is used to determine the total number of **bacteria** in samples.

Because the device operates on the physical blockage of electrical conductivity by particles in a sample, the Coulter counter cannot distinguish between living and dead bacteria. An indication of the total number of bacteria (alive, dormant, and dead) is provided. The number of living bacteria can, however, usually be easily determined using another volume from the same sample (e.g., the heterotrophic plate count).

The Coulter counter is named after its inventor. Wallace H. Coulter conceived and constructed the first counter in the basement of his home in Chicago in the early 1950s. Then as now, the device relies on a vacuum pump that draws a solution or suspension through an electrically charged tube that has a tiny hole at the other end. As particles pass through the hole the electrical field is interrupted. The pattern of the interruption can be related to the number of particles and even to particle type (e.g., red blood cell versus bacteria).

A bacterial suspension is best analyzed in the Coulter counter when the suspension has been thoroughly shaken beforehand. This step disperses the bacteria. Most bacteria tend to aggregate together in a suspension. If not dispersed, a clump of bacteria passing through the orifice of the counter could be counted as a single bacterium. This would produce an underestimate of the number of bacteria in the suspension.

The Coulter counter has been used for many applications, both biological and nonbiological. In the 1970s, the device was reconfigured to incorporate a laser beam. This allowed the use of fluorescent labeled monoclonal antibodies to detect specific types of cells (e.g., cancer cells) or to detect a specific species of bacteria. This refinement of the Coulter counter is now known as flow cytometry.

See also Bacterial growth and division; Laboratory techniques in microbiology

COWPOX

Cowpox refers to a disease that is caused by the cowpox or catpox virus. The virus is a member of the orthopoxvirus family. Other **viruses** in this family include the **smallpox** and vaccinia viruses. Cowpox is a rare disease, and is mostly noteworthy as the basis of the formulation, over 200 years ago, of an injection by **Edward Jenner** that proved successful in curing smallpox.

The use of cowpox virus as a means of combating smallpox, which is a much more threatening disease to humans, has remained popular since the time of Jenner.

Once a relatively common malady in humans, cowpox is now confined mostly to small mammals in Europe and the United Kingdom. The last recorded case of a cow with cowpox was in the United Kingdom in 1978. Occasionally the disease is transmitted from these sources to human. But this is very rare. Indeed, only some 60 cases of human cowpox have been reported in the medical literature.

The natural reservoir for the cowpox virus is believed to be small woodland animals, such as voles and wood mice. Cats and cows, which can harbor the virus, are thought to be an accidental host, perhaps because of their contact with the voles or mice.

The cowpox virus, similar to the other orthopoxvirus, is best seen using the **electron microscopic** technique of negative staining. This technique reveals surface details. The cowpox virus is slightly oval in shape and has a very ridged-appearing surface.

Human infection with the cowpox virus is thought to require direct contact with an infected animal. The virus gains entry to the bloodstream through an open cut. In centuries past, farmers regularly exposed to dairy cattle could acquire the disease from hand milking the cows, for example. Cowpox is typically evident as pus-filled sores on the hands and face that subsequently turn black before fading away. While present, the lesions are extremely painful. There can be scars left at the site of the infection. In rare instances, the virus can become more widely disseminated through the body, resulting in death.

Both males and females are equally as likely to acquire cowpox. Similarly, there no racial group is any more susceptible to infection. There is a predilection towards acquiring the infection in youth less than 18 years of age. This may be because of a closer contact with animals such as cats by this age group, or because of lack of administration of smallpox **vaccine**.

Treatment for cowpox tends to be ensuring that the patient is as comfortable as possible while waiting for the infection to run its course. Sometimes, a physician may wish to drain the pus from the skin sores to prevent the spread of the infection further over the surface of the skin. In cases where symptoms are more severe, an immune globulin known as antivaccinia gamaglobulin may be used. This immunoglobulin is reactive against all viruses of the orthopoxvirus family. The use of this treatment needs to be evaluated carefully, as there can be side effects such as kidney damage. Antibodies to the vaccinia virus may also be injected into a patient, as these antibodies also confer protection against cowpox.

See also Vaccination; Virology; Zoonoses

COXIELLA BURNETII • *see* Q FEVER

CRANBERRY JUICE AS AN ANTI-ADHESION METHOD • *see* ANTI-ADHESION METHODS

CREUTZFELDT-JAKOB DISEASE (CJD) •
see BSE AND CJD DISEASE

CRICK, FRANCIS (1916-)
English molecular biologist

Francis Crick is one half of the famous pair of molecular biologists who unraveled the mystery of the structure of **DNA** (**deoxyribonucleic acid**), the carrier of genetic information, thus ushering in the modern era of **molecular biology**. Since this fundamental discovery, Crick has made significant contributions to the understanding of the **genetic code** and **gene** action, as well as the understanding of molecular neurobiology. In Horace Judson's book *The Eighth Day of Creation,* Nobel laureate **Jacques Lucien Monod** is quoted as saying, "No one man created molecular biology. But Francis Crick dominates intellectually the whole field. He knows the most and understands the most." Crick shared the Nobel Prize in medicine in 1962 with **James Watson** and **Maurice Wilkins** for the elucidation of the structure of DNA.

The eldest of two sons, Francis Harry Compton Crick was born to Harry Crick and Anne Elizabeth Wilkins in Northampton, England. His father and uncle ran a shoe and boot factory. Crick attended grammar school in Northampton, and was an enthusiastic experimental scientist at an early age, producing the customary number of youthful chemical explo-

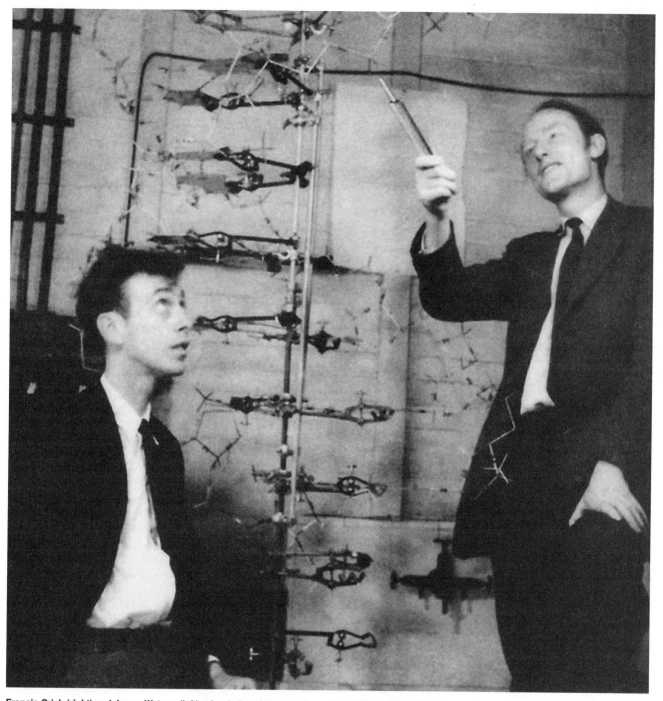

Francis Crick (right) and James Watson (left), who deduced the structure of the DNA double helix (shown between them).

sions. As a schoolboy, he won a prize for collecting wildflowers. In his autobiography, *What Mad Pursuit,* Crick describes how, along with his brother, he "was mad about tennis," but not much interested in other sports and games. At the age of fourteen, he obtained a scholarship to Mill Hill School in North London. Four years later, at eighteen, he entered University College, London. At the time of his matriculation, his parents had moved from Northampton to Mill Hill, and this

allowed Crick to live at home while attending university. Crick obtained a second-class honors degree in physics, with additional work in mathematics, in three years. In his autobiography, Crick writes of his education in a rather light-hearted way. Crick states that his background in physics and mathematics was sound, but quite classical, while he says that he learned and understood very little in the field of chemistry. Like many of the physicists who became the first molecular biologists and who began their careers around the end of World War II, Crick read and was impressed by Erwin Schrödinger's book *What Is Life?*, but later recognized its limitations in its neglect of chemistry.

Following his undergraduate studies, Crick conducted research on the viscosity of water under pressure at high temperatures, under the direction of Edward Neville da Costa Andrade, at University College. It was during this period that he was helped financially by his uncle, Arthur Crick. In 1940, Crick was given a civilian job at the Admiralty, eventually working on the design of mines used to destroy shipping. Early in the year, Crick married Ruth Doreen Dodd. Their son Michael was born during an air raid on London on November 25, 1940. By the end of the war, Crick was assigned to scientific intelligence at the British Admiralty Headquarters in Whitehall to design weapons.

Realizing that he would need additional education to satisfy his desire to do fundamental research, Crick decided to work toward an advanced degree. Crick became fascinated with two areas of biology, particularly, as he describes it in his autobiography, "the borderline between the living and the non-living, and the workings of the brain." He chose the former area as his field of study, despite the fact that he knew little about either subject. After preliminary inquiries at University College, Crick settled on a program at the Strangeways Laboratory in Cambridge under the direction of Arthur Hughes in 1947, to work on the physical properties of **cytoplasm** in cultured chick fibroblast cells. Two years later, he joined the Medical Research Council Unit at the Cavendish Laboratory, ostensibly to work on protein structure with British chemists Max Perutz and John Kendrew (both future Nobel Prize laureates), but eventually to work on the structure of DNA with Watson.

In 1947, Crick was divorced, and in 1949, married Odile Speed, an art student whom he had met during the war. Their marriage coincided with the start of Crick's Ph.D. thesis work on the x-ray diffraction of proteins. X-ray diffraction is a technique for studying the crystalline structure of molecules, permitting investigators to determine elements of three-dimensional structure. In this technique, x rays are directed at a compound, and the subsequent scattering of the x-ray beam reflects the molecule's configuration on a photographic plate.

In 1941 the Cavendish Laboratory where Crick worked was under the direction of physicist Sir William Lawrence Bragg, who had originated the x-ray diffraction technique forty years before. Perutz had come to the Cavendish to apply Bragg's methods to large molecules, particularly proteins. In 1951, Crick was joined at the Cavendish by James Watson, a visiting American who had been trained by Italian physician Salvador Edward Luria and was a member of the Phage Group, a group of physicists who studied bacterial **viruses** (known as bacteriophages, or simply phages). Like his phage colleagues, Watson was interested in discovering the fundamental substance of genes and thought that unraveling the structure of DNA was the most promising solution. The informal partnership between Crick and Watson developed, according to Crick, because of their similar "youthful arrogance" and similar thought processes. It was also clear that their experi-

ences complemented one another. By the time of their first meeting, Crick had taught himself a great deal about x-ray diffraction and protein structure, while Watson had become well informed about phage and bacterial genetics.

Both Crick and Watson were aware of the work of biochemists Maurice Wilkins and Rosalind Franklin at King's College, London, who were using x-ray diffraction to study the structure of DNA. Crick, in particular, urged the London group to build models, much as American chemist Linus Pauling had done to solve the problem of the alpha helix of proteins. Pauling, the father of the concept of the chemical bond, had demonstrated that proteins had a three-dimensional structure and were not simply linear strings of amino acids. Wilkins and Franklin, working independently, preferred a more deliberate experimental approach over the theoretical, model-building scheme used by Pauling and advocated by Crick. Thus, finding the King's College group unresponsive to their suggestions, Crick and Watson devoted portions of a two-year period discussing and arguing about the problem. In early 1953, they began to build models of DNA.

Using Franklin's x-ray diffraction data and a great deal of trial and error, they produced a model of the DNA molecule that conformed both to the London group's findings and to the data of Austrian-born American biochemist Erwin Chargaff. In 1950, Chargaff had demonstrated that the relative amounts of the four nucleotides, or bases, that make up DNA conformed to certain rules, one of which was that the amount of adenine (A) was always equal to the amount of thymine (T), and the amount of guanine (G) was always equal to the amount of cytosine (C). Such a relationship suggests pairings of A and T, and G and C, and refutes the idea that DNA is nothing more than a tetranucleotide, that is, a simple molecule consisting of all four bases.

During the spring and summer of 1953, Crick and Watson wrote four papers about the structure and the supposed function of DNA, the first of which appeared in the journal *Nature* on April 25. This paper was accompanied by papers by Wilkins, Franklin, and their colleagues, presenting experimental evidence that supported the Watson-Crick model. Watson won the coin toss that placed his name first in the authorship, thus forever institutionalizing this fundamental scientific accomplishment as "Watson-Crick."

The first paper contains one of the most remarkable sentences in scientific writing: "It has not escaped our notice that the specific pairing we have postulated immediately suggests a possible copying mechanism for the genetic material." This conservative statement (it has been described as "coy" by some observers) was followed by a more speculative paper in *Nature* about a month later that more clearly argued for the fundamental biological importance of DNA. Both papers were discussed at the 1953 Cold Spring Harbor Symposium, and the reaction of the developing community of molecular biologists was enthusiastic. Within a year, the Watson-Crick model began to generate a broad spectrum of important research in genetics.

Over the next several years, Crick began to examine the relationship between DNA and the genetic code. One of his first efforts was a collaboration with Vernon Ingram, which led to Ingram's 1956 demonstration that sickle cell hemoglobin differed from normal hemoglobin by a single amino acid. Ingram's research presented evidence that a molecular genetic disease, caused by a Mendelian mutation, could be connected to a DNA-protein relationship. The importance of this work to Crick's thinking about the function of DNA cannot be underestimated. It established the first function of "the genetic substance" in determining the specificity of proteins.

About this time, South African-born English geneticist and molecular biologist **Sydney Brenner** joined Crick at the Cavendish Laboratory. They began to work on the coding problem, that is, how the sequence of DNA bases would specify the amino acid sequence in a protein. This work was first presented in 1957, in a paper given by Crick to the Symposium of the Society for Experimental Biology and entitled "On Protein Synthesis." Judson states in *The Eighth Day of Creation* that "the paper permanently altered the logic of biology." While the events of the **transcription** of DNA and the synthesis of protein were not clearly understood, this paper succinctly states "The Sequence Hypothesis... assumes that the specificity of a piece of nucleic acid is expressed solely by the sequence of its bases, and that this sequence is a (simple) code for the amino acid sequence of a particular protein." Further, Crick articulated what he termed "The Central Dogma" of molecular biology, "that once 'information' has passed into protein, it cannot get out again. In more detail, the transfer of information from nucleic acid to nucleic acid, or from nucleic acid to protein may be possible, but transfer from protein to protein, or from protein to nucleic acid is impossible." In this important theoretical paper, Crick establishes not only the basis of the genetic code but predicts the mechanism for **protein synthesis**. The first step, transcription, would be the transfer of information in DNA to **ribonucleic acid** (**RNA**), and the second step, **translation**, would be the transfer of information from RNA to protein. Hence, the genetic message is transcribed to a messenger, and that message is eventually translated into action in the synthesis of a protein. Crick is credited with developing the term "codon" as it applies to the set of three bases that code for one specific amino acid. These codons are used as "signs" to guide protein synthesis within the cell.

A few years later, American geneticist Marshall Warren Nirenberg and others discovered that the nucleic acid sequence U-U-U (polyuracil) encodes for the amino acid phenylalanine, and thus began the construction of the DNA/RNA dictionary. By 1966, the DNA triplet code for twenty amino acids had been worked out by Nirenberg and others, along with details of protein synthesis and an elegant example of the control of protein synthesis by French geneticist **François Jacob**, Arthur Pardée, and French biochemist Jacques Lucien Monod. Brenner and Crick themselves turned to problems in developmental biology in the 1960s, eventually studying the structure and possible function of histones, the class of proteins associated with **chromosomes**.

In 1976, while on sabbatical from the Cavendish, Crick was offered a permanent position at the Salk Institute for Biological Studies in La Jolla, California. He accepted an endowed chair as Kieckhefer Professor and has been at the Salk Institute ever since. At the Salk Institute, Crick began to study the workings of the brain, a subject that he had been interested in from the beginning of his scientific career. While his primary interest was consciousness, he attempted to approach this subject through the study of vision. He published several speculative papers on the mechanisms of dreams and of attention, but, as he stated in his autobiography, "I have yet to produce any theory that is both novel and also explains many disconnected experimental facts in a convincing way."

During his career as an energetic theorist of modern biology, Francis Crick has accumulated, refined, and synthesized the experimental work of others, and has brought his unusual insights to fundamental problems in science.

See also Cell cycle (eukaryotic), genetic regulation of; Cell cycle (prokaryotic), genetic regulation of; Genetic identification of microorganisms; Genetic mapping; Genetic regulation of eukaryotic cells; Genetic regulation of prokaryotic cells; Genotype and phenotype; Immunogenetics

CRYOPROTECTION

Cryopreservation refers to the use of a very low temperature (below approximately –130° C [–202° F]) to store a living organism. Organisms (including many types of **bacteria**, **yeast**, **fungi**, and algae) can be frozen for long periods of time and then recovered for subsequent use.

This form of long-term storage minimizes the chances of change to the microorganism during storage. Even at refrigeration temperature, many **microorganisms** can grow slowly and so might become altered during storage. This behavior has been described for strains of *Pseudomonas aeruginosa* that produce an external slime layer. When grown on a solid **agar** surface, the colonies of such strains appear like mucous drops. However, when recovered from refrigeration storage, the mucoid appearance can be lost. Cryopreservation of mucoid strains maintains the mucoid characteristic.

Cryostorage of bacteria must be done at or below the temperature of –130° C [–202° F], as it is at this temperature that frozen water can form crystals. Because much of the interior of a bacterium and much of the surrounding membrane(s) are made of water, crystal formation would be disastrous to the cell. The formation of crystals would destroy structure, which would in turn destroy function.

Ultralow temperature freezers have been developed that achieve a temperature of –130° C . Another popular option for cryopreservation is to immerse the sample in a compound called liquid nitrogen. Using liquid nitrogen, a temperature of –196° C [–320.8° F] can be achieved.

Another feature of bacteria that must be taken into account during cryopreservation is called osmotic pressure. This refers to the balance of ions on the outside versus the inside of the cell. An imbalance in osmotic pressure can cause water to flow out of or into a bacterium. The resulting shrinkage or ballooning of the bacterium can be lethal.

To protect against crystal formation and osmotic pressure shock to the bacteria, bacterial suspensions are typically prepared in a so-called cryoprotectant solution. Glycerol is an effective cryoprotective agent for many bacteria. For other bacteria, such as cyanobacteria, methanol and dimethyl sulfoxide are more suitable.

The microorganisms used in the cryoprotection process should be in robust health. Bacteria, for example, should be obtained from the point in their growth cycle where they are actively growing and divided. In conventional liquid growth media, this is described as the mid-logarithmic phase of growth. In older cultures, where nutrients are becoming depleted and waste products are accumulating, the cells can deteriorate and change their characteristics.

For bacteria, the cryoprotectant solution is added directly to an agar **culture** of the bacteria of interest and bacteria are gently dislodged into the solution. Alternately, bacteria in a liquid culture can be centrifuged and the "pellet" of bacteria resuspended in the cryoprotectant solution. The resulting bacterial suspension is then added to several specially designed cryovials. These are made of plastic that can withstand the ultralow temperature.

The freezing process is done as quickly as possible to minimize crystal formation. This is also referred to as "snap freezing." Bacterial suspensions in t cryoprotectant are initially at room temperature. Each suspension is deep-frozen in a step-wise manner. First, the suspensions are chilled to refrigerator temperature. Next, they are stored for a few hours at –70° C [–94° F]. Finally, racks of cryovials are either put into the ultralow temperature freezer or plunged into liquid nitrogen. The liquid nitrogen almost instantaneously brings the samples to –196° C [–320.8° F]. Once at this point, the samples can be stored indefinitely.

Recovery from cryostorage must also be rapid to avoid crystal formation. Each suspension is warmed rapidly to room temperature. The bacteria are immediately recovered by centrifugation and the pellet of bacteria is resuspended in fresh growth medium. The suspension is allowed to adapt to the new temperature for a few days before being used.

Cryoprotection can be used for other purposes than the long-term storage of samples. For example, cryoelectron microscopy involves the rapid freezing of a sample and examination of portions of the sample in an electro **microscope** under conditions where the ultralow temperature is maintained. If done correctly, cryoelectron microscopy will revel features of microorganisms that are not otherwise evident in conventional electron microscopy. For example, the watery **glycocalyx**, which is made of chains of sugar, collapses onto the surface of a bacterium as the sample is dried out during preparation for conventional electron microscopy. But glycocalyx structure can be cryopreserved. In another example, cryoelectron microscopy has also maintained external structural order on virus particles, allowing researchers to deduce how these structures function in the viral infection of tissue.

See also Bacterial ultrastructure; Donnan equilibrium; Quality control in microbiology

CRYPTOCOCCI AND CRYPTOCOCCOSIS

Cryptococcus is a **yeast** that has a capsule surrounding the cell. In the yeast classification system, *Cryptococcus* is a member of the Phylum Basidimycota, Subphylum Basidimycotina, Order Sporidiales, and Family Sporidiobolaceae.

There are 37 species in the genus *Cryptococcus*. One of these, only one species is disease-causing, *Cryptococcus neoformans*. There are three so-called varieties of this species, based on antigenic differences in the capsule, some differences in biochemical reactions such as the use of various sugars as nutrients, and in the shape of the spores produced by the yeast cells. The varieties are *Cryptococcus neoformans* var. *gatti*, *grubii*, and *neoformans*. The latter variety causes the most cryptococcal infections in humans.

Cryptococcus neoformans has a worldwide distribution. It is normally found on plants, fruits and in birds, such as pigeons and chicken. Transmission via bird waste is a typical route of human infection.

Cryptococcus neoformans causes an infection known as cryptococcosis. Inhalation of the microorganism leads to the persistent growth in the lungs. For those whose **immune system** is compromised, such as those having Acquired **Immunodeficiency** Syndrome (**AIDS**), the pulmonary infection can be life-threatening. In addition, yeast cells may become distributed elsewhere in the body, leading to **inflammation** of nerve lining in the brain (**meningitis**). A variety of other infections and symptoms can be present, including infections of the eye (conjunctivitis), ear (otitis), heart (myocarditis), liver (**hepatitis**), and bone (arthritis).

The most common illness caused by the cryptococcal fungus is cryptococcal meningitis. Those at most risk of developing cryptococcosis are AIDS patients. Those who have received an organ, are receiving **chemotherapy** for cancer or have Hodgkin's disease are also at risk, since frequently their immune systems are suppressed. As the incidence of AIDS and the use of immunosupressant drugs have grown over the past decade, the number of cases of cryptococcosis has risen. Until then, cases of cryptococcus occurred only rarely. Even today, those with a well-functioning immune system are seldom at risk for cryptococcosis. For these individuals a slight skin infection may be the only adverse effect of exposure to Cryptococcus.

Cryptococcus begins with the inhalation of *Cryptococcus neoformans*. Likely, the inhaled yeast is weakly encapsulated and is relatively small. This allows the cells to penetrate into the alveoli of the lungs. There the production of capsule occurs. The capsule surrounding each yeast cell aids the cell in avoiding the immune response of the host, particularly the engulfing of the yeast by macrophage cells (which is called **phagocytosis**). The capsule is comprised of chains of sugars, similar to the capsule around **bacteria**. The capsule of *Cryptococcus neoformans* is very negatively charged. Because cells such as macrophages are also negatively charged, repulsive forces will further discourage interaction of macrophages with the capsular material.

Another important virulence factor of the yeast is an enzyme called phenol oxidase. The enzyme operates in the production of melanin. Current thought is that the phenol oxidase prevents the formation of charged hydroxy groups, which can be very damaging to the yeast cell. The yeast may actually recruit the body's melanin producing machinery to make the compound.

Cryptococcus neoformans also has other **enzymes** that act to degrade certain proteins and the **phospholipids** that make up cell membranes. These enzymes may help disrupt the host cell membrane, allowing the yeast cells penetrate into host tissue more easily.

Cryptococcus neoformans is able to grow at body temperature. The other Cryptococcus species cannot tolerate this elevated temperature.

Yet another virulence factor may operate. Evidence from laboratory studies has indicated that antigens from the yeast can induce a form of **T cells** that down regulates the immune response of the host. This is consistent with the knowledge that survivors of cryptococcal meningitis display a poorly operating immune system for a long time after the infection has ended. Thus, *Cryptococcus neoformans* may not only be capable of evading an immune response by the host, but may actually dampen down that response.

If the infection is treated while still confined to the lungs, especially in patients with a normally operative immune system, the prospects for full recovery are good. However, spread to the central nervous system is ominous, especially in immunocompromised patients.

The standard treatment for cryptococcal meningitis is the intravenous administration of a compound called amphotericin B. Unfortunately the compound has a raft of side effects, including fever, chills, headache, nausea with vomiting, diarrhea, kidney damage, and suppression of bone marrow. The latter can lead to a marked decrease in red blood cells. Studies are underway in which amphotericin B is enclosed in bags made of lipid material (called liposomes). The use of liposomes can allow the drug to be more specifically targeted to the site where treatment is most needed, rather than flooding the entire body with the drug. Hopefully, the use of liposome-delivered amphotericin B will lessen the side effects of therapy.

See also Fungi; Immunomodulation; Yeast, infectious

CRYPTOSPORIDIUM AND CRYPTOSPORIDIOSIS

Cryptosporidum is a protozoan, a single-celled parasite that lives in the intestines of humans and other animals. The organism causes an intestinal malady called cryptosporidiosis (which is commonly called "crypto").

The members of the genus *Cryptosporidium* infects epithelial cells, especially those that line the walls of the intestinal tract. One species, *Cryptosporidium muris*, infects laboratory tests species, such as rodents, but does not infect humans. Another species, *Cryptosporidium parvum*, infects a wide variety of mammals, including humans. Calculations

have indicated that cattle alone release some five tons of the parasite each year in the United States alone.

Non-human mammals are the reservoir of the organism for humans. Typically, the organism is ingested when in water that has been contaminated with Cryptosporidium-containing feces. Often in an environment such as water, Cryptosporidium exists in a form that is analogous to a bacterial spore. In the case of Cryptosporidium, this dormant and environmentally resilient form is called an oocyst.

An oocyst is smaller than the growing form of Cryptosporidium. The small size can allow the oocyst to pass through some types of filters used to treat water. In addition, an oocyst is also resistant to the concentrations of chlorine that are widely used to disinfect drinking water. Thus, even drinking water from a properly operating municipal treatment plant has the potential to contain Cryptosporidium.

The organism can also be spread very easily by contact with feces, such as caring with someone with diarrhea or changing a diaper. Spread of cryptosporidiosis in nursing homes and day care facilities is not uncommon.

Only a few oocytes need to be ingested to cause cryptosporidiosis. Studies using volunteers indicate that an infectious dose is anywhere from nine to 30 oocysts. When an oocyte is ingested, it associates with intestinal epithelial cells. Then, four bodies called sporozoites, which are contained inside the oocyst, are released. These burrow inside the neighbouring epithelial cells and divide to form cells that are called merozoites. Eventually, the host cell bursts, releasing the merozoites. The freed cells go on to attack neighbouring epithelial cells and reproduce. The new progeny are released and the cycle continues over and over. The damage to the intestinal cells affects the functioning of the intestinal tract.

Cryptosporidium and its oocyte form have been known since about 1910. *Cryptosporidium parvum* was first described in 1911. Cryptosporidiosis has been a veterinary problem for a long time. The disease was recognized as a human disease in the 1970s. In the 1980s, the number of human cases rose sharply along with the cases of **AIDS**.

There have been many outbreaks of cryptosporidiosis since the 1980s. In 1987, 13,000 in Carrollton, Georgia contracted cryptosporidiosis via their municipal drinking water. This incident was the first case of the spread of the disease through water that had met all state and federal standards for microbiological quality. In 1993, an outbreak of cryptosporidiosis, again via contaminated municipal drinking water that met the current standards, sickened 400,000 people and resulted in several deaths. Outbreaks such as these prompted a change in **water quality** standards in the United States.

Symptoms of cryptosporidiosis are diarrhea, weight loss, and abdominal cramping. Oocysts are released in the feces all during the illness. Even when the symptoms are gone, oocysts continue to be released in the feces for several weeks.

Even though known for a long time, detection of the organism and treatment of the malady it causes are still challenging. No **vaccine** for cryptosporidiosis exists. A well-functioning **immune system** is the best defense against the disease. Indeed, estimates are that about 30% of the population has antibodies to *Cryptosporidium parvum*, even though no symptoms of cryptosporidiosis developed. The malady is most severe in immunocompromised people, such as those infected with **HIV** (the virus that causes AIDS), or those receiving **chemotherapy** for cancer or after a transplant. For those who are diabetic, alcoholic, or pregnant, the prolonged diarrhea can be dangerous.

In another avenue of infection, some of the merozoites grow bigger inside the host epithelial cell and form two other types of cells, termed the macrogametocyte and microgametocyte. The macrogametocytes contain macrogametes. When these combine with the microgametes released from the microgametocytes, a zygote is formed. An oocyst wall forms around the zygote and the genetic process of meiosis results in the creation of four sporozoites inside the oocyst. The oocyst is released to the environment in the feces and the infectious cycle is started again.

The cycle from ingestion to the release of new infectious oocytes in the feces can take about four days. Thereafter, the production of a new generation of **parasites** takes as little as twelve to fourteen hours. Internally, this rapid division can create huge numbers of organisms, which crowd the intestinal tract. Cryptosporidiosis can spread to secondary sites, like the duodenum and the large intestine. In people whose immune systems are not functioning properly, the spread of the organism can be even more extensive, with parasites being found in the stomach, biliary tract, pancreatic ducts, and respiratory tract.

Detection of Cryptosporidium in water is complicated by the lack of a **culture** method and because large volumes of water (hundreds of gallons) need to be collected and concentrated to collect the few oocytes that may be present. Presently, oocysts are detected using a microscopic method involving the binding of a specific fluorescent probe to the oocyte wall. There are many other noninfectious species of Cryptosporidium in the environment that react with the probe used in the test. Furthermore, the test does not distinguish a living organism from one that is dead. So a positive test result is not always indicative of the presence of an infectious organism. Skilled analysts are required to perform the test and so the accuracy of detection varies widely from lab to lab.

See also Giardia and giardiasis; Water quality; Water purification

CULTURE

A culture is a single species of microorganism that is isolated and grown under controlled conditions. The German bacteriologist **Robert Koch** first developed culturing techniques in the late 1870s. Following Koch's initial discovery, medical scientists quickly sought to identify other pathogens. Today **bacteria** cultures are used as basic tools in microbiology and medicine.

The ability to separate bacteria is important because **microorganisms** exist as mixed populations. In order to study individual species, it is necessary to first isolate them. This isolation can be accomplished by introducing individual bacterial cells onto a culture medium containing the necessary

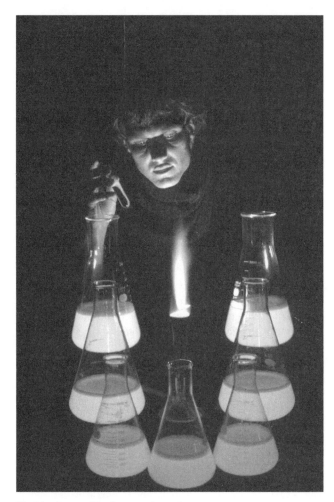

Liquid cultures of luminescent bacteria.

elements microbial growth. The medium also provides conditions favorable for growth of the desired species. These conditions may involve **pH**, osmotic pressure, atmospheric oxygen, and moisture content. Culture media may be liquids (known broths) or solids. Before the culture can be grown, the media must be sterilized to prevent growth of unwanted species. This **sterilization** process is typically done through exposure to high temperatures. Some tools like the metal loop used to introduce bacteria to the media, may be sterilized by exposure to a flame. The media itself may be sterilized by treatment with steam-generated heat through a process known as autoclaving.

To grow the culture, a number of the cells of the microorganism must be introduced to the sterilized media. This process is known as inoculation and is typically done by exposing an inoculating loop to the desired strain and then placing the loop in contact with the sterilized surface. A few of the cells will be transferred to the growth media and under the proper conditions, that species will begin to grow and form a pure **colony**. Cells in the colony can reproduce as often as every 20 minutes and under the ideal conditions, this rate of cell division could result in the production of 500,000 new cells after six hours. Such rapid growth rates help to explain the rapid development of disease, food spoilage, decay, and the speed at which certain chemical processes used in industry take place. Once the culture has been grown, a variety of observation methods can be used to record the strain's characteristics and chart its growth.

See also Agar and agarose; Agar diffusion; American type culture collection; Antibiotic resistance, tests for; Bacterial growth and division; Bacterial kingdoms; Epidemiology, tracking diseases with technology; Laboratory techniques in microbiology

CYCLOSPORIN · *see* ANTIBIOTICS

CYTOGENETICS · *see* MOLECULAR BIOLOGY AND MOLECULAR GENETICS

CYTOKINES

Cytokines are a family of small proteins that mediate an organism's response to injury or infection. Cytokines operate by transmitting signals between cells in an organism. Minute quantities of cytokines are secreted, each by a single cell type, and regulate functions in other cells by binding with specific receptors. Their interactions with the receptors produce secondary signals that inhibit or enhance the action of certain genes within the cell. Unlike endocrine hormones, which can act throughout the body, most cytokines act locally, near the cells that produced them.

Cytokines are crucial to an organism's self-defense. Cells under attack release a class of cytokines known as chemokines. Chemokines participate in a process called chemotaxis, signaling white blood cells to migrate toward the threatened region. Other cytokines induce the white blood cells to produce **inflammation**, emitting toxins to kill pathogens and **enzymes** to digest both the invaders and the injured tissue. If the inflammatory response is not enough to deal with the problem, additional **immune system** cells are also summoned by cytokines to continue the fight.

In a serious injury or infection, cytokines may call the hematopoietic, or blood-forming system into play. New white blood cells are created to augment the immune response, while additional red blood cells replace any that have been lost. Ruptured blood vessels emit chemokines to attract platelets, the element of the blood that fosters clotting. Cytokines are also responsible for signaling the nervous system to increase the organism's metabolic level, bringing on a fever that inhibits the proliferation of pathogens while boosting the action of the immune system.

Because of the central role of cytokines in fighting infection, they are being studied in an effort to find better treatments for diseases such as **AIDS**. Some have shown promise as therapeutic agents, but their usefulness is limited by the tendency of cytokines to act locally. This means that their short amino acid chains are likely either to be destroyed by enzymes in the bloodstream or tissues before reaching their destination, or to act on other cells with unintended consequences.

Other approaches to developing therapies based on research into cytokines involve studying their receptor sites on target cells. If a molecule could be developed that would bind to the receptor site of a specific cytokine, it could elicit the desired action from the cell, and might be more durable in the bloodstream or have other advantages over the native cytokine. Alternatively, a drug that blocked receptor sites could potentially prevent the uncontrolled inflammatory responses seen in certain autoimmune diseases.

See also Autoimmunity and autoimmune diseases; Immunochemistry; Immunodeficiency disease syndromes; Immunodeficiency diseases

CYTOPLASM, EUKARYOTIC

The cytoplasm, or cytosol of eukaryotic cells is the gel-like, water-based fluid that occupies the majority of the volume of the cell. Cytoplasm functions as the site of energy production, storage, and the manufacture of cellular components. The various organelles that are responsible for some of these functions in the eukaryotic cell are dispersed throughout the cytoplasm, as are the compounds that provide structural support for the cell.

The cytoplasm is the site of almost all of the chemical activity occurring in a eukaryotic cell. Indeed, the word cytoplasm means "cell substance."

Despite being comprised mainly of water (about 65% by volume), the cytoplasm has the consistency of gelatin. Unlike gelatin, however, the cytoplasm will flow. This enables **eukaryotes** such as the amoeba to adopt different shapes, and makes possible the formation of pseudopods that are used to engulf food particles. The consistency of the cytoplasm is the result of the other constituents of the cell that are floating in fluid. These constituents include salts, and organic molecules such as the many **enzymes** that catalyze the myriad of chemical reactions that occur in the cell.

When viewed using the transmission electron **microscope**, the cytoplasm appears as a three-dimensional latticework of strands. In the early days of **electron microscopy** there was doubt as to whether this appearance reflected the true nature of the cytoplasm, or was an artifact of the removal of water from the cytoplasm during the preparation steps prior to **electron microscopic examination**. However, development of techniques that do not perturb the natural structure biological specimens has confirmed that this latticework is real.

The lattice is made of various cytoplasmic proteins. They are scaffolding structures that assist in the process of cell division and in the shape of the cell. The shape-determinant is referred to as the cytoskeleton. It is a network of fibers composed of three types of proteins. The proteins form three filamentous structures known as microtubules, intermediate filaments, and microfilaments. The filaments are connected to most of organelles located in the cytoplasm and serve to hold together the organelles.

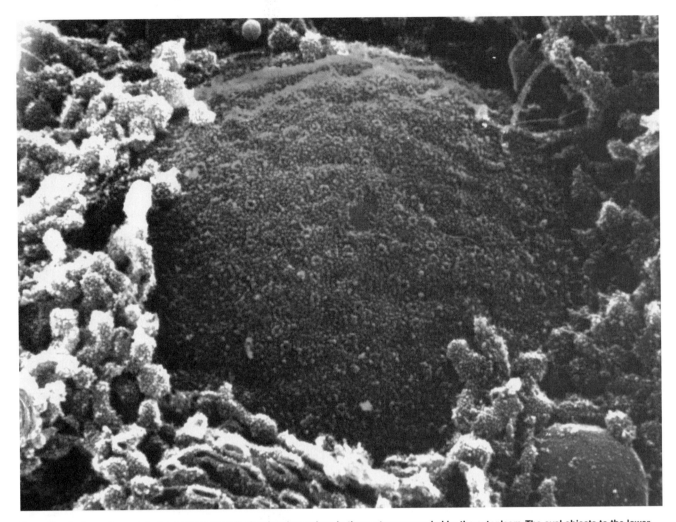

Scanning electron micrograph of an eukaryotic cell, showing the nucleus in the center surrounded by the cytoplasm. The oval objects to the lower left are ribosomes.

The microtubules are tubes that are formed by a spiral arrangement of the constituent protein. They function in the movement of the **chromosomes** to either pole of the cell during the cell division process. The microtubules are also known as the spindle apparatus. Microfilaments are a composed of two strands of protein that are twisted around one another. They function in the contraction of muscle in higher eukaryotic cells and in the change in cell shape that occurs in organisms such as the amoeba. Finally, the intermediate filaments act as more rigid scaffolding to maintain the cell shape.

The organelles of the cell are dispersed throughout the cytoplasm. The **nucleus** is bound by its own membrane to protect the genetic material from potentially damaging reactions that occur in the cytoplasm. Thus, the cytoplasm is not a part of the interior of the organelles.

The cytoplasm also contains **ribosomes**, which float around and allow protein to be synthesized all through the cell. Ribosomes are also associated with a structure called the endoplasmic reticulum. The golgi apparatus is also present, in association with the endoplasmic reticulum. Enzymes that

degrade compounds are in the cytoplasm, in organelles called lysosomes. Also present throughout the cytoplasm are the mitochondria, which are the principal energy generating structures of the cell. If the eukaryotic cell is capable of photosynthetic activity, then **chlorophyll** containing organelles known as chloroplasts are also present.

The cytoplasm of eukaryotic cells also functions to transport dissolved nutrients around the cell and move waste material out of the cell. These functions are possible because of a process dubbed cytoplasmic streaming.

See also Eukaryotes

CYTOPLASM, PROKARYOTIC

The cytoplasm of a prokaryotic cell is everything that is present inside the bacterium. In contrast to a eukaryotic cell, there is not a functional segregation inside **bacteria**. The cytoplasm houses all the chemicals and components that are used to sustain the life of a bacterium, with the exception of those components that reside in the membrane(s), and in the **periplasm** of Gram-negative bacteria.

The cytoplasm is bounded by the cytoplasmic membrane. Gram-negative bacteria contain another outer membrane. In between the two membranes lies the periplasm.

When viewed in the light **microscope**, the cytoplasm of bacteria is transparent. Only with the higher magnification available using the transmission **electron microscope** does the granular nature of the cytoplasm become apparent. The exact structure of the cytoplasm may well be different than this view, since the cytoplasm is comprised mainly of water. The dehydration necessary for conventional electron microscopy likely affect the structure of the cytoplasm.

The cytoplasm of prokaryotes and **eukaryotes** is similar in texture. Rather than being a free-flowing liquid the cytoplasm is more of a gel. The consistency has been likened to that of dessert gel, except that the bacterial gel is capable of flow. The ability of flow is vital, since the molecules that reside in the cytoplasm must be capable of movement within the bacterium as well as into and out of the cytoplasm.

The genetic material of the bacteria is dispersed throughout the cytoplasm. Sometimes, the **deoxyribonucleic acid** genome can aggregate during preparation for microscopy. Then, the genome is apparent as a more diffuse area within the granular cytoplasm. This artificial structure has been called the nucleoid. Smaller, circular arrangements of genetic material called **plasmids** can also be present. The dispersion of the bacterial genome throughout the cytoplasm is one of the fundamental distinguishing features between prokaryotic and eukaryotic cells.

Also present throughout the cytoplasm is the **ribonucleic acid**, various **enzymes**, amino acids, carbohydrates, lipids, ions, and other compounds that function in the bacterium. The constituents of the membrane(s) are manufactured in the cytoplasm and then are transported to their final destination.

Some bacteria contain specialized regions known as cytoplasmic inclusions that perform specialized functions. These inclusions can be stored products that are used for the nutrition of the bacteria. Examples of such inclusions are glycogen, poly-B-hydroxybutyrate, and sulfur granules. As well, certain bacteria contain gas-filled vesicles that act to buoy the bacterium up to a certain depth in the water, or membranous structures that contain **chlorophyll**. The latter function to harvest light for energy in photosynthetic bacteria.

The cytoplasm of prokaryotic cells also houses the **ribosomes** required for the manufacture of protein. There can be many ribosomes in the cytoplasm. For example, a rapidly growing bacterium can contain upwards of 15,000 ribosomes.

The processes of **transcription**, **translation**, protein import and export, and at least some degradation of compounds occurs in the cytoplasm. In Gram-negative bacteria, some of these functions also occur in the periplasmic fluid. The mechanisms that underlie the proper sequential orchestration of these functions are still yet to be fully determined.

See also Bacterial ultrastructure

D

D'HÉRELLE, FÉLIX (1873-1949)
Canadian bacteriologist

Félix d'Hérelle's major contribution to science was the discovery of the **bacteriophage**, a microscopic agent that appears in conjunction with and destroys disease-producing **bacteria** in a living organism. Like many researchers, d'Hérelle spent much of his life exploring the effects of his major discovery. He was also well-traveled; in the course of his life he lived for long or short periods of time in Canada, France, the Netherlands, Guatemala, Mexico, Indochina, Egypt, India, the United States, and the former Soviet Union.

D'Hérelle was born in Montreal, Quebec, Canada. His father, Félix d'Hérelle—a member of a well-established French Canadian family, died when the young Félix was six years old. After his father's death, he moved with his mother, Augustine Meert d'Hérelle, a Dutch woman, to Paris, France. In Paris, d'Hérelle received his secondary education at the Lycée Louis-le-Grand and began his medical studies. He completed his medical program at the University of Leiden in the Netherlands. He married Mary Kerr, of France, in 1893, and the couple eventually had two daughters. In 1901, d'Hérelle moved to Guatemala City, Guatemala, to become the director of the bacteriology laboratory at the general hospital and to teach microbiology at the local medical school. In 1907, he moved to Merida, Yucatan, Mexico, to study the **fermentation** of sisal hemp, and in 1908, the Mexican government sent him back to Paris to further his microbiological studies. D'Hérelle became an assistant at Paris's Pasteur Institute in 1909, became chief of its laboratory in 1914, and remained at the Institute until 1921.

During his time at the Pasteur Institute, d'Hérelle studied a bacterium called *Coccobacillus acridiorum,* which caused enteritis (**inflammation** of the intestines) in locusts and grasshoppers of the acrididae family of insects, with a view toward using the microbe to destroy locusts. In growing the bacteria on **culture** plates, d'Hérelle observed empty spots on the plates and theorized that these spots resulted from a virus

that grew along with and killed the bacteria. He surmised that this phenomenon might have great medical significance as an example of an organism fighting diseases of the digestive tract. In 1916, he extended his investigation to cultures of the bacillus that caused **dysentery** and again observed spots free of the microbe on the surface of the cultures. He was able to filter out a substance from the feces of dysentery victims that consumed in a few hours a culture broth of the bacillus. On September 10, 1917, he presented to the French Academy of Sciences a paper announcing his discovery entitled "Sur un microbe invisible, antagoniste du bacille dysentérique." He named the bacteria–destroying substance bacteriophage (literally, "eater of bacteria"). He devoted most of his research and writing for the rest of his life to the various types of bacteriophage which appeared in conjunction with specific types of bacteria. He published several books dealing with his findings.

From 1920 to the late 1930s, d'Hérelle traveled and lived in many parts of the world. In 1920, he went to French Indochina under the auspices of the Pasteur Institute to study human dysentery and septic pleuropneumonia in buffaloes. It was during the course of this expedition that he perfected his techniques for isolating bacteriophage. From 1922 to 1923, he served as an assistant professor at the University of Leiden. In 1924, he moved to Alexandria, Egypt, to direct the Bacteriological Service of the Egyptian Council on Health and Quarantine. In 1927, he went to India at the invitation of the Indian Medical Service to attempt to cure cholera through the use of the bacteriophage associated with that disease. D'Hérelle served as professor of bacteriology at Yale University from 1928 to 1933, and in 1935 the government of the Soviet Socialist Republic of Georgia requested that d'Hérelle establish institutes dedicated to the study of bacteriophage in Tiflis, Kiev, and Kharkov. However, unstable civil conditions forced d'Hérelle's departure from the Soviet Union in 1937, and he returned to Paris, where he lived, continuing his study of bacteriophage, for the remainder of his life.

D'Hérelle attempted to make use of bacteriophage in the treatment of many human and animal diseases, including dysentery, cholera, plague, and staphylococcus and strepto-coccus infections. Such treatment was widespread for a time, especially in the Soviet Union. However, use of bacteriophage for this purpose was superseded by the use of chemical drugs and **antibiotics** even within d'Hérelle's lifetime. Today bacteriophage is employed primarily as a diagnostic ultravirus. Of the many honors d'Hérelle received, his perhaps most notable is the Leeuwenhoek Medal given to him by the Amsterdam Academy of Science in 1925; before d'Hérelle, **Louis Pasteur** had been the only other French scientist to receive the award. D'Hérelle was presented with honorary degrees from the University of Leiden and from Yale, Montreal, and Laval Universities. He died after surgery in Paris at the age of 75.

See also Bacteriophage and bacteriophage typing

DARWIN, CHARLES ROBERT (1809-1882)
English naturalist

Charles Robert Darwin is credited with popularizing the concept of organic **evolution** by means of natural **selection**. Though Darwin was not the first naturalist to propose a model of biological evolution, his introduction of the mechanism of the "survival of the fittest," and discussion of the evolution of humans, marked a revolution in both science and natural philosophy.

Darwin was born in Shrewsbury, England and showed an early interest in the natural sciences, especially geology. His father, Robert Darwin, a wealthy physician, encouraged Charles to pursue studies in medicine at the University of Edinburg. Darwin soon tired of the subject, and his father sent him to Cambridge to prepare for a career in the clergy. At Cambridge, Darwin rekindled his passion for the natural sciences, often devoting more time to socializing with Cambridge scientists than to his clerical studies. With guidance from his cousin, entomologist William Darwin Fox (1805–1880), Darwin became increasingly involved in the growing circle of natural scientists at Cambridge. ox introduced Darwin to clergyman and biologist John Stevens Henslow (1796–1861). Henslow became Darwin's tutor in mathematics and theology, as well as his mentor in his personal studies of botany, geology, and zoology. Henslow profoundly influenced Darwin, and it was he who encouraged Darwin to delay seeking an appointment in the Church of England in favor of joining an expedition team and venturing overseas. After graduation, Darwin agreed to an unpaid position as naturalist aboard the *H.M.S. Beagle*. The expedition team was initially chartered for a three year voyage and survey of South America's Pacific coastline, but the ship pursued other ventures after their work was complete and Darwin remained part of H.M.S. *Beagle's* crew for five years.

Darwin used his years aboard the *Beagle* to further his study of the natural sciences. In South America, Darwin became fascinated with geology. He paid close attention to changes in the land brought about by earthquakes and volcanoes. His observations led him to reject catastrophism (a theory that land forms are the result of single, catastrophic

events), and instead espoused the geological theories of gradual development proposed by English geologist Charles Lyell (1797–1875) in his 1830 work, *Principles of Geology*. Yet, some of his observations in South America did not fit with Lyell's theories. Darwin disagreed with Lyell's assertion that coral reefs grew atop oceanic volcanoes and rises, and concluded that coral reefs built upon themselves. When Darwin returned to England in 1836, he and Lyell became good friends. Lyell welcomed Darwin's new research on coral reefs, and encouraged him to publish other studies from his voyages.

Darwin was elected a fellow of the Geological Society in 1836, and became a member of the Royal Society in 1839. That same year, he published his *Journal of Researches into the Geology and Natural History of the Various Countries Visited by H.M.S. Beagle*. Though his achievements in geology largely prompted his welcoming into Britain's scientific community, his research interests began to diverge from the discipline in the early 1840s. Discussions with other naturalists prompted Darwin's increasing interest in population diversity of fauna, extinct animals, and the presumed fixity of species. Again, he turned to notes of his observations and various specimens he gathered while on his prior expedition. The focus of his new studies was the Galápagos Islands off the Pacific coast of Ecuador. While there, Darwin was struck by the uniqueness of the island's tortoises and birds. Some neighboring islands had animal populations, which were largely similar to that of the continent, while others had seemingly different variety of species. After analyzing finch specimen from the Galápagos, Darwin concluded that species must have some means of transmutation, or ability of a species to alter over time. Darwin thus proposed that as species modified, and as old species disappeared, new varieties could be introduced. Thus, Darwin proposed an evolutionary model of animal populations.

The idea of organic evolution was not novel. French naturalist, Georges Buffon (1707–1788) had theorized that species were prone to development and change. Darwin's own grandfather, Erasmus Darwin, also published research regarding the evolution of species. Although the theoretical concept of evolution was not new, it remained undeveloped prior to Charles Darwin. Just as he had done with Lyell's geological theory, Darwin set about the further the understanding of evolution not merely as a philosophical concept, but as a practical scientific model for explaining the diversity of species and populations. His major contribution to the field was the introduction of a mechanism by which evolution was accomplished. Darwin believed that evolution was the product of an ongoing struggle of species to better adapt to their environment, with those that were best adapted surviving to reproduce and replace less-suited individuals. He called this phenomenon "survival of the fittest," or natural selection. In this way, Darwin believed that traits of maximum adaptiveness were transferred to future generations of the animal population, eventually resulting in new species.

Darwin finished an extensive draft of his theories in 1844, but lacked confidence in his abilities to convince others of the merits of his discoveries. Years later, prompted by rumors that a colleague was about to publish a theory similar to his own, Darwin decided to release his research. *On the Origin of Species by Means of Natural Selection, or The Preservation of Favoured Races in the Struggle for Life*, was published November 1859, and became an instant bestseller.

A common misconception is that *On the Origin of Species* was the introduction of the concept of human evolution. In fact, a discussion of human antiquity is relatively absent from the book. Darwin did not directly address the relationship between animal and human evolution until he published *The Descent of Man, and Selection in Relation to Sex* in 1871. Darwin introduced not only a model for the biological evolution of man, but also attempted to chart the process of man's psychological evolution. He further tried to break down the barriers between man and animals in 1872 with his work *The Expression of the Emotions in Man and Animals*. By observing facial features and voice sounds, Darwin asserted that man and non-human animals exhibited signs of emotion in similar ways. In the last years of his career, Darwin took the concept of organic evolution to its logical end by applying natural selection and specialization to the plant kingdom.

Darwin's works on evolution met with both debate from the scientific societies, and criticism from some members of the clergy. *On the Origin of Species* and *The Descent of Man* were both published at a time of heightened religious evangelicalism in England. Though willing to discuss his theories with colleagues in the sciences, Darwin refrained from participating in public debates concerning his research. In the last decade of his life, Darwin was disturbed about the application of his evolutionary models to social theory. By most accounts, he considered the emerging concept of the social and cultural evolution of men and civilizations, which later became known as Social Darwinism, to be a grievous misinterpretation of his works. Regardless of his opposition, he remained publicly taciturn about the impact his scientific theories on theology, scientific methodology, and social theory. Closely guarding his privacy, Darwin retired to his estate in Down. He died at Down House in 1882. Though his wishes were to receive an informal burial, Parliament immediately ordered a state burial for the famous naturalist at Westminster Abby. By the time of his death, the scientific community had largely accepted the arguments favoring his theories of evolution. Although the later discoveries in genetics and **molecular biology** radically reinterpreted Darwin's evolutionary mechanisms, evolutionary theory is the key and unifying theory in all biological science.

See also Evolution and evolutionary mechanisms; Evolutionary origin of bacteria and viruses

DAVIES, JULIAN E. (1932-)
Welsh bacteriologist

Julian Davies is a bacteriologist renowned for his research concerning the mechanisms of bacterial resistance to **antibiotics**, and on the use of antibiotics as research tools.

Davies was born in Casrell Nedd, Morgannwg, Cymru, Wales. He received his education in Britain. His university education was at the University of Nottingham, where he

received a B.Sc. (Chemistry, Physics, Math) in 1953 and a Ph.D. (Organic Chemistry) in 1956. From 1959 to 1962, he was Lecturer at the University of Manchester. Davies then moved to the United States where he was an Associate at the Harvard Medical School from 1962 until 1967. From 1965 to 1967, he was also a Visiting Professor at the Institute Pasteur in Paris. In 1967, Davies became an Associate Professor in the Department of **Biochemistry** at the University of Wisconsin. He attained the rank of Professor in 1970 and remained at Wisconsin until 1980. In that year, Davies took up the post of Research Director at Biogen in Geneva. In 1983, he became President of Biogen. Two years later, Davies assumed the position of Chief of Genetic Microbiology at the Institute Pasteur, where he remained until 1992. In that year, he returned to North America to become Professor and Head of the Department of Microbiology and **Immunology** at UBC. He retained this position until his retirement in 1997. Presently he remains affiliated with UBC as Emeritus Professor in the same department.

While in British Columbia, Davies returned to commercial **biotechnology**. In 1996, he founded and became President and CEO of TerraGen Diversity Inc. Davies assumed the post of Chief Scientific Officer from 1998 to 2000. From 2000 to the present, he is Executive Vice President, technology development of Cubist Pharmaceuticals, Inc.

Davies has made fundamental discoveries in the area of bacterial **antibiotic resistance**, including the origin and **evolution** of antibiotic resistance genes. He has identified bacterial **plasmids** that carry genes that carry the information that determines the resistance of **bacteria** to certain antibiotics. Furthermore, he demonstrated that this information could be transferred from one bacterium to another. These discoveries have crucial to the efforts to develop drugs that can overcome such antibiotic resistance.

Another facet of research has demonstrated how genetic information can be transferred between bacteria that are distantly related. This work has had a fundamental influence on the understanding of how bacteria can acquire genetic traits, especially those that lead to antimicrobial resistance.

Davies has also developed a technique whereby genes can be "tagged" and their path from one bacterium to another followed. This technique is now widely used to follow **gene** transfer between prokaryotic and eukaryotic cells. In another research area, Davies has explored the use of antibiotics as experimental tools to probe the mechanisms of cellular biochemistry, and the interaction between various molecules in cells.

This prodigious research output has resulted in over 200 publications in peer-reviewed journals, authorship of six books and numerous guest lectures.

Davies has also been active as an undergraduate and graduate teacher and a mentor to a number of graduate students. These research, commercial and teaching accomplishments have been recognized around the world. He is a Fellow of the Royal Society (London) and the Royal Society of Canada, and is a past President of the American Society for Microbiology. In 2000, he received a lifetime achievement award in recognition of his development of the biotechnology sector in British Columbia.

See also Microbial genetics

BROGLIE, LOUIS VICTOR DE (1892-1987)
French physicist

Louis Victor de Broglie, a theoretical physicist and member of the French nobility, is best known as the father of wave mechanics, a far-reaching achievement that significantly changed modern physics. Wave mechanics describes the behavior of matter, including subatomic particles such as electrons, with respect to their wave characteristics. For this groundbreaking work, de Broglie was awarded the 1929 Nobel Prize for physics. De Broglie's work contributed to the fledgling science of microbiology in the mid-1920s, when he suggested that electrons, as well as other particles, should exhibit wave-like properties similar to light. Experiments on electron beams a few years later confirmed de Broglie's hypothesis. Of importance to **microscope** design was the fact that the wavelength of electrons is typically much smaller than the wavelength of light. Therefore, the limitation imposed on the light microscope of 0.4 micrometers could be significantly reduced by using a beam of electrons to illuminate the specimen. This fact was exploited in the 1930s in the development of the **electron microscope**.

Louis Victor Pierre Raymond de Broglie was born on August 15, 1892, in Dieppe, France, to Duc Victor and Pauline d'Armaille Broglie. His father's family was of noble Piedmontese origin and had served French monarchs for centuries, for which it was awarded the hereditary title Duc from King Louis XIV in 1740, a title that could be held only by the head of the family.

The youngest of five children, de Broglie inherited a familial distinction for formidable scholarship. His early education was obtained at home, as befitted a great French family of the time. After the death of his father when de Broglie was fourteen, his eldest brother Maurice arranged for him to obtain his secondary education at the Lycée Janson de Sailly in Paris.

After graduating from the Sorbonne in 1909 with baccalaureates in philosophy and mathematics, de Broglie entered the University of Paris. He studied ancient history, paleography, and law before finding his niche in science, influenced by the writings of French theoretical physicist Jules Henri Poincaré. The work of his brother Maurice, who was then engaged in important, independent experimental research in x rays and radioactivity, also helped to spark de Broglie's interest in theoretical physics, particularly in basic atomic theory. In 1913, he obtained his Licencié ès Sciences from the University of Paris's Faculté des Sciences.

De Broglie's studies were interrupted by the outbreak of World War I, during which he served in the French army. Yet, even the war did not take the young scientist away from the country where he would spend his entire life; for its duration, de Broglie served with the French Engineers at the wireless station under the Eiffel Tower. In 1919, de Broglie returned to

his scientific studies at his brother's laboratory. Here he began his investigations into the nature of matter, inspired by a conundrum that had long been troubling the scientific community: the apparent physical irreconcilability of the experimentally proven dual nature of light. Radiant energy or light had been demonstrated to exhibit properties associated with particles as well as their well-documented wave-like characteristics. De Broglie was inspired to consider whether matter might not also exhibit dual properties. In his brother's laboratory, where the study of very high frequency radiation using spectroscopes was underway, de Broglie was able to bring the problem into sharper focus. In 1924, de Broglie, with over two dozen research papers on electrons, atomic structure, and x rays already to his credit, presented his conclusions in his doctoral thesis at the Sorbonne. Entitled "Investigations into the Quantum Theory," it consolidated three shorter papers he had published the previous year.

In his thesis, de Broglie postulated that all matter—including electrons, the negatively charged particles that orbit an atom's **nucleus**—behaves as both a particle and a wave. Wave characteristics, however, are detectable only at the atomic level, whereas the classical, ballistic properties of matter are apparent at larger scales. Therefore, rather than the wave and particle characteristics of light and matter being at odds with one another, de Broglie postulated that they were essentially the same behavior observed from different perspectives. Wave mechanics could then explain the behavior of all matter, even at the atomic scale, whereas classical Newtonian mechanics, which continued to accurately account for the behavior of observable matter, merely described a special, general case. Although, according to de Broglie, all objects have "matter waves," these waves are so small in relation to large objects that their effects are not observable and no departure from classical physics is detected. At the atomic level, however, matter waves are relatively larger and their effects become more obvious. De Broglie devised a mathematical formula, the matter wave relation, to summarize his findings.

American physicist Albert Einstein appreciated the significant of de Broglie's theory; de Broglie sent Einstein a copy of his thesis on the advice of his professors at the Sorbonne, who believed themselves not fully qualified to judge it. Einstein immediately pronounced that de Broglie had illuminated one of the secrets of the Universe. Austrian physicist Erwin Schrödinger also grasped the implications of de Broglie's work and used it to develop his own theory of wave mechanics, which has since become the foundation of modern physics.

De Broglie's wave matter theory remained unproven until two separate experiments conclusively demonstrated the wave properties of electrons—their ability to diffract or bend, for example. American physicists Clinton Davisson and Lester Germer and English physicist George Paget Thomson all proved that de Broglie had been correct. Later experiments would demonstrate that de Broglie's theory also explained the behavior of protons, atoms, and even molecules. These properties later found practical applications in the development of magnetic lenses, the basis for the electron microscope.

In 1928, de Broglie was appointed professor of theoretical physics at the University of Paris's Faculty of Science. De Broglie was a thorough lecturer who addressed all aspects of wave mechanics. Perhaps because he was not inclined to encourage an interactive atmosphere in his lectures, he had no noted record of guiding young research students.

During his long career, de Broglie published over twenty books and numerous research papers. His preoccupation with the practical side of physics is demonstrated in his works dealing with cybernetics, atomic energy, particle accelerators, and wave-guides. His writings also include works on x rays, gamma rays, atomic particles, optics, and a history of the development of contemporary physics. He served as honorary president of the French Association of Science Writers and, in 1952, was awarded first prize for excellence in science writing by the Kalinga Foundation. In 1953, Broglie was elected to London's Royal Society as a foreign member and, in 1958, to the French Academy of Arts and Sciences in recognition of his formidable output. With the death of his older brother Maurice two years later, de Broglie inherited the joint titles of French duke and German prince. De Broglie died of natural causes on March 19, 1987, at the age of ninety-four.

See also Electron microscope, transmission and scanning; Electron microscopic examination of microorganisms; Microscope and microscopy

DEFECTS OF CELLULAR IMMUNITY · *see* IMMUNODEFICIENCY DISEASE SYNDROMES

DEFECTS OF T CELL MEDIATED IMMUNITY · *see* IMMUNODEFICIENCY DISEASE SYNDROMES

DENGUE FEVER

Dengue fever is a debilitating and sometimes hemorrhagic fever (one that is associated with extensive internal bleeding). The disease is caused by four slightly different types of a virus from the genus *Flavivirus* that is designated as DEN. The four antigenic types are DEN-1, DEN-2, DEN-3, and DEN-4.

The dengue virus is transmitted to humans via the bite of a mosquito. The principle mosquito species is known as *Aedes aegypti*. This mosquito is found all over the world, and, throughout time, became adapted to urban environments. For example, the mosquito evolved so as to be capable of living year round in moist storage containers, rather than relying on the seasonal patterns of rainfall. Another species, *Aedes albopictus* (the "Tiger mosquito"), is widespread throughout Asia. Both mosquitoes are now well established in urban centers. Accordingly, dengue fever is now a disease of urbanized, developed areas, rather than rural, unpopulated regions.

The dengue virus is passed to humans exclusively by the bite of mosquito in search of a blood meal. This mode of transmission makes the dengue virus an arbovirus (that is, one that is transmitted by an arthropod). Studies have demonstrated that some species of monkey can harbor the virus. Thus, monkeys may serve as a reservoir of the virus. Mosquitoes who bite the monkey may acquire the virus and subsequently transfer the virus to humans.

The disease has been known for centuries. The first reported cases were in 1779–1780, occurring almost simultaneously in Asia, Africa, and North America. Since then, periodic outbreaks of the disease have occurred in all areas of the world where the mosquito resides. In particular, an outbreak that began in Asia after World War II, spread around the world, and has continued to plague southeast Asia even into 2002. As of 2001, dengue fever was the leading cause of hospitalization and death among children in southeast Asia.

Beginning in the 1980s, dengue fever began to increase in the Far East and Africa. Outbreaks were not related to economic conditions. For example, Singapore had an outbreak of dengue fever from 1990 to 1994, even after a mosquito control program that had kept the disease at minimal levels for over two decades. The example of Singapore illustrates the importance of an ongoing program of mosquito population control.

The disease is a serious problem in more than 100 countries in Africa, North and South America, the Eastern Mediterranean, South-East Asia, and the Western Pacific.

Unlike other bacterial or viral diseases, which can be controlled by **vaccination**, the four antigenic types of the dengue virus do not confer cross-protection. Thus, it is possible for an individual to be sickened with four separate bouts of dengue fever.

Following the transfer of the virus from mosquito to humans, the symptoms can be varied, ranging from nonspecific and relatively inconsequential ailments to severe and fatal hemorrhaging. The incubation period of the virus is typically 5 to 8 days, but symptoms may develop after as few as three days or as many as 15 days. The onset of symptoms is sudden and dramatic. Initially, chills tend to develop, followed by a headache. Pain with the movement of the eyes leads to more generalized and extreme pain in the legs and joints. A high fever can be produced, with temperatures reaching 104° F [40° C]. Also, a pale rash may appear transiently on the face.

These symptoms can persist for up to 96 hours. Often, the fever then rapidly eases. After a short period when symptoms disappear, the fever reappears. The temperature elevates rapidly but the fever is usually not as high as in previous episodes. The palms of the hands and soles of the feet may turn bright red and become very swollen.

In about 80% of those who are infected, recovery is complete after a convalescent period of several weeks with general weakness and lack of energy. However, in some 20% of those who are infected a severe form of dengue fever develops. This malady is characterized by the increased leakage of fluid from cells and by the abnormal clotting of the blood. These factors produce the hemorrhaging that can be a hallmark of the disease, which is called dengue hemorrhagic fever. Even then, recovery can be complete within a week. Finally, in some of those who are infected, a condition called dengue shock syndrome can result in convulsions. In addition, a failure of the circulatory system can occur, resulting in death.

The reasons for the varied degrees of severity and symptoms that the viral infection can elicit are still unclear. Not surprisingly, there is currently no cure for dengue, nor is there a **vaccine**. Treatment for those who are afflicted is palliative, that is, intended to ease the symptoms of the disease. Upon recovery, **immunity** to the particular antigenic type of the virus is in place for life. However, an infection with one antigenic type of dengue virus is not protective against the other three antigenic types. Currently, the only preventive measure that can be taken is to eradicate the mosquito vector of the virus.

See also Epidemics, viral; Zoonoses

DEOXYRIBONUCLEIC ACID · *see* DNA
(DEOXYRIBONUCLEIC ACID)

DESICCATION

Desiccation is the removal of water from a biological system. Usually this is accomplished by exposure to dry heat. Most biological systems are adversely affected by the loss of water. **Microorganisms** are no exception to this, except for those that have evolved defensive measures to escape the loss of viability typically associated with water loss.

Desiccation also results from the freezing of water, such as in the polar regions on Earth. Water is present at these regions, but is unavailable.

Microorganisms depend on water for their structure and function. Cell membranes are organized with the water-loving portions of the membrane lipids positioned towards the exterior and the water-hating portions pointing inward. The loss of water can throw this structure into disarray. Furthermore, the interior of microorganisms such as **bacteria** is almost entirely comprised of water. Extremely rapid freezing of the water can be a useful means of preserving bacteria and other microorganisms. However, the gradual loss of water will produce lethal changes in the chemistry of the interior **cytoplasm** of cells, collapse of the interior structure, and an alteration in the three-dimensional structure of **enzymes**. These drastic changes caused by desiccation are irreversible.

In the laboratory, desiccation techniques are used to help ensure that glassware is free of viable microbes. Typically, the glassware is placed in a large dry-heat oven and heated at 160° to 170° C [320° to 338° F] for up to two hours. The effectiveness of **sterilization** depends on the penetration of heat into a biological sample.

Some microorganisms have evolved means of coping with desiccation. The formation of a spore by bacteria such as Bacillus and Clostridium allows the genetic material to survive the removal of water. Cysts produced by some protozoans can also resist the destruction of desiccation for long periods of time. Bacterial biofilms might not be totally dehydrated if they are thick enough. Bacteria buried deep within the biofilm might still be capable of growth.

The fact that some microbes on Earth can resist desiccation and then resuscitate when moisture becomes available holds out the possibility of life on other bodies in our solar system, particularly Mars. The snow at the poles of Mars is proof that water is present. If liquid water becomes transiently available, then similar resuscitation of dormant Martian microorganisms could likewise occur.

See also Cryoprotection

DETECTION OF MUTANTS · *see* LABORATORY TECHNIQUES IN MICROBIOLOGY

DIATOMS

Algae are a diverse group of simple, nucleated, plant-like aquatic organisms that are primary producers. Primary producers are able to utilize **photosynthesis** to create organic molecules from sunlight, water, and carbon dioxide. Ecologically vital, algae account for roughly half of photosynthetic production of organic material on Earth in both freshwater and marine environments. Algae exist either as single cells or as multicellular organizations. Diatoms are microscopic, single-celled algae that have intricate glass-like outer cell walls partially composed of silicon. Different species of diatom can be identified based upon the structure of these walls. Many diatom species are planktonic, suspended in the water column moving at the mercy of water currents. Others remain attached to submerged surfaces. One bucketful of water may contain millions of diatoms. Their abundance makes them important food sources in aquatic ecosystems. When diatoms die, their cell walls are left behind and sink to the bottom of bodies of water. Massive accumulations of diatom-rich sediments compact and solidify over long periods of time to form rock rich in fossilized diatoms that is mined for use in abrasives and filters.

Diatoms belong to the taxonomic phylum Bacillariophyta. There are approximately 10,000 known diatom species. Of all algae phyla, diatom species are the most numerous. The diatoms are single-celled, eukaryotic organisms, having genetic information sequestered into subcellular compartments called nuclei. This characteristic distinguishes the group from other single-celled photosynthetic aquatic organisms, like the **blue-green algae** that do not possess nuclei and are more closely related to **bacteria**. Diatoms also are distinct because they secrete complex outer cell walls, sometimes called skeletons. The skeleton of a diatom is properly referred to as a frustule.

Diatom frustules are composed of pure hydrated silica within a layer of organic, carbon containing material. Frustules are really comprised of two parts: an upper and lower frustule. The larger upper portion of the frustule is called the epitheca. The smaller lower piece is the hypotheca. The epitheca fits over the hypotheca as the lid fits over a shoebox. The singular algal diatom cell lives protected inside the frustule halves like a pair of shoes snuggled within a shoebox.

Frustules are ornate, having intricate designs delineated by patterns of holes or pores. The pores that perforate the frustules allow gases, nutrients, and metabolic waste products to be exchanged between the watery environment and the algal cell. The frustules themselves may exhibit bilateral symmetry or radial symmetry. Bilaterally symmetric diatoms are like human beings, having a single plane through which halves are mirror images of one another. Bilaterally symmetric diatoms are elongated. Radially symmetric diatom frustules have many mirror image planes. No matter which diameter is used to divide the cell into two halves, each half is a mirror image of the other. The combination of symmetry and perforation patterns of diatom frustules make them beautiful biological structures that also are useful in identifying different species. Because they are composed of silica, an inert material, diatom frustules remain well preserved over vast periods of time within geologic sediments.

Diatom frustules found in sedimentary rock are microfossils. Because they are so easily preserved, diatoms have an extensive fossil record. Specimens of diatom algae extend back to the Cretaceous Period, over 135 million years ago. Some kinds of rock are formed nearly entirely of fossilized diatom frustules. Considering the fact that they are microscopic organisms, the sheer numbers of diatoms required to produce rock of any thickness is staggering. Rock that has rich concentrations of diatom fossils is known as diatomaceous earth, or diatomite. Diatomaceous earth, existing today as large deposits of chalky white material, is mined for commercial use in abrasives and in filters. The fine abrasive quality of diatomite is useful in cleansers, like bathtub scrubbing powder. Also, many toothpaste products contain fossil diatoms. The fine porosity of frustules also makes refined diatomaceous earth useful in fine water filters, acting like microscopic sieves that catch very tiny particles suspended in solution.

Fossilized diatom collections also tell scientists a lot about the environmental conditions of past eras. It is known that diatom deposits can occur in layers that correspond to environmental cycles. Certain conditions favor mass deaths of diatoms. Over many years, changes in diatom deposition rates in sediments, then, are preserved as diatomite, providing clues about prehistoric climates.

Diatom cells within frustules contain chloroplasts, the organelles in which photosynthesis occurs. Chloroplasts contain **chlorophyll**, the pigment molecule that allows plants and other photosynthetic organisms to capture solar energy and convert it into usable chemical energy in the form of simple sugars. Because of this, and because they are extremely abundant occupants of freshwater and saltwater habitats, diatoms are among the most important **microorganisms** on Earth. Some estimates calculate diatoms as contributing 20–25% of all carbon fixation on Earth. Carbon fixation is a term describing the photosynthetic process of removing atmospheric carbon in the form of carbon dioxide and converting it to organic carbon in the form of sugar. Due to this, diatoms are essential components of aquatic food chains. They are a major food source for many microorganisms, aquatic animal larvae, and grazing animals like mollusks (snails). Diatoms are even found living on land. Some species can be found in moist soil or on mosses. Contributing to the abundance of diatoms is their primary mode of reproduction, simple asexual cell division. Diatoms divide asexually by mitosis. During division, diatoms construct new frustule cell walls. After a cell divides, the epitheca and hypotheca separate, one remaining with each new daughter cell. The two cells then produce a new hypotheca. Diatoms do reproduce sexually, but not with the same frequency.

See also Autotrophic bacteria; Fossilization of bacteria; Photosynthesis; Photosynthetic microorganisms; Plankton and planktonic bacteria

DICTYOSTELIUM

Dictyostelium discoideum, also know as slime **mold**, are single-celled soil amoeba which naturally occur amongst decaying leaves on the forest floor. Their natural food sources are **bacteria** that are engulfed by **phagocytosis**. Amoeba are eukaryotic organisms, that is, they organize their genes onto **chromosomes**. *Dictyostelium* may be either haploid (the vast majority) or diploid (approximately 1 in 10,000 cells).

There is no true sexual phase of development, although two haploid cells occasionally coalesce into a diploid organism. Diploid cells may lose chromosomes one by one to transition back to a haploid state. When food sources are plentiful, *D. discoideum* reproduces by duplicating its genome and dividing into two identical diploid daughter cells. Under starvation conditions, Dictyostelium enter an extraordinary alternate life cycle in which large populations of cells spontaneously aggregate and begin to behave much like a multicellular organism. Aggregation is initiated when a small proportion of cells emit pulses of cyclic AMP drawing in cells in the immediate vicinity. In this phase of the life cycle, groups of 100,000 cells coalesce and develop a surface sheath to form well-defined slugs (pseudoplasmodia), which can migrate together as a unit. As the pseudoplasmodium phase nears its end, cells near the tip of the slug begin to produce large quantities of cellulose that aids the slug in standing erect. This new phase is called culmination. At this stage, cells from the underlying mound move upward toward the vertical tip where they are encapsulated into spores forming the fruiting body. Spores then are dispersed into the environment where they can remain dormant until favorable conditions arise to resume the primary life mode as independent organisms. Spores are resistant to heat, dehydration, and lack of food sources. When a source of amino acids is detected in the environment, spores open longitudinally, releasing a small but normal functioning amoeba.

Dictyostelium are valuable biological model organisms for studying the principals of morphological development and signaling pathways.

See also Microbial genetics

DIFFUSION · *see* CELL MEMBRANE TRANSPORT

DIGEORGE SYNDROME · *see* IMMUNODEFICIENCY
DISEASE SYNDROMES

DILUTION THEORY AND TECHNIQUES

Dilution allows the number of living **bacteria** to be determined in suspensions that contain even very large numbers of bacteria.

The number of bacteria obtained by dilution of a **culture** can involve growth of the living bacteria on a solid growth source, the so-called dilution plating technique. The objective of dilution plating is to have growth of the bacteria on the surface of the medium in a form known as a **colony**. Theoretically each colony arises from a single bacterium. So, a value called the colony-forming unit can be obtained. The acceptable range of colonies that needs to be present is between 30 and 300. If there is less than 30 colonies, the sample has been diluted too much and there is too a great variation in the number of colonies in each milliliter (ml) of the dilution examined. Confidence cannot be placed in the result. Conversely, if there are more than 300 colonies, the over-crowded colonies cannot be distinguished from one another.

To use an example, if a sample contained 100 living bacteria per ml, and if a single milliliter was added to the growth medium, then upon incubation to allow the bacteria to grow into colonies, there should be 100 colonies present. If, however, the sample contained 1,000 living bacteria per ml, then plating a single ml onto the growth medium would produce far too many colonies to count. What is needed in the second case is an intervening step. Here, a volume is withdrawn from the sample and added to a known volume of fluid. Typically either one ml or 10 ml is withdrawn. These would then be added to nine or 90 ml of fluid, respectively. The fluid used is usually something known as a **buffer**, which is fluid that does not provide nutrients to the bacteria but does provide the ions needed to maintain the bacteria in a healthy state. The original culture would thus have been diluted by 10 times. Now, if a milliliter of the diluted suspension was added to the growth medium, the number of colonies should be one-tenth of 1,000 (= 100). The number of colonies observed is then multiplied by the dilution factor to yield the number of living bacteria in the original culture. In this example, 100 colonies multiplied by the dilution factor of 10 yields 1,000 bacteria per ml of the original culture.

In practice, more than a single ten-fold dilution is required to obtain a countable number of bacterial colonies. Cultures routinely contain millions of living bacteria per milliliter. So, a culture may need to be diluted millions of times. This can be achieved in two ways. The first way is known as serial dilution. An initial 10-times dilution would be prepared as above. After making sure the bacteria are evenly dispersed throughout, for example, 10 ml of buffer, one milliliter of the dilution would be withdrawn and added to nine milliliters of buffer. This would produce a 10-times dilution of the first dilution, or a 100-times dilution of the original culture. A milliliter of the second dilution could be withdrawn and added to

another nine milliliters of buffer (1,000 dilution of the original culture) and so on. Then, one milliliter of each dilution can be added to separate plates of growth medium and the number of colonies determined after incubation. Those plates that contain between 30 and 300 colonies could be used to determine the number of living bacteria in the original culture.

The other means of dilution involves diluting the sample by 100 times each time, instead of 10 times. Taking one milliliter of culture or dilution and adding it to 99 ml of buffer accomplish this. The advantage of this dilution scheme is that dilution is obtained using fewer materials. However, the dilution steps can be so great that the countable range of 30-300 is missed, necessitating a repeat of the entire procedure.

Another dilution method is termed the "most probable number" method. Here, 10-fold dilutions of the sample are made. Then, each of these dilutions is used to inoculate tubes of growth medium. Each dilution is used to inoculate either a set of three or five tubes. After incubation the number of tubes that show growth are determined. Then, a chart is consulted and the number of positive tubes in each set of each sample dilution is used to determine the most probable number (MPN) of bacteria per milliliter of the original culture.

See also Agar and agarose; Laboratory techniques in microbiology; Qualitative and quantitative techniques in microbiology

DINOFLAGELLATES

Dinoflagellates are **microorganisms** that are regarded as algae. Their wide array of exotic shapes and, sometimes, armored appearance is distinct from other algae. The closest microorganism in appearance are the **diatoms**.

Dinoflagellates are single-celled organisms. There are nearly 2000 known living species. Some are bacterial in size, while the largest, *Noctiluca*, can be up to two millimeters in size. This is large enough to be seen by the unaided eye.

Ninety per cent of all known dinoflagellates live in the ocean, although freshwater species also exist. In fact, dinoflagellates have even been isolated from snow. In these environments, the organisms can exist as free-living and independent forms, or can take up residence in another organism. A number of photosynthetic dinoflagellates inhabit sponges, corals, jellyfish, and flatworms. The association is symbiotic. The host provides a protective environment and the growth of the dinoflagellates impart nutritive carbohydrates to the host.

As their name implies, flagella are present. Indeed, the term dinoflagellate means whirling flagella. Typically, there are two flagella. One of these circles around the body of the cell, often lying in a groove called the cingulum. The other flagellum sticks outward from the surface of the cell. Both flagella are inserted into the dinoflagellate at the same point. The arrangement of the flagella can cause the organism to move in a spiral trajectory.

The complex appearance, relative to other algae and **bacteria**, is carried onward to other aspects of dinoflagellate behavior and growth. Some dinoflagellates feed on other microorganisms, while others produce energy using photosynthesis. Still other dinoflagellates can do both. The life cycle of the organisms is also complex, involving forms that are immobile and capable of movement and forms that are capable of sexual or asexual reproduction (bacteria, for example, reproduce asexually, by the self-replication of their genetic material and other constituents). Dinoflagellates are primarily asexual in reproduction.

Some dinoflagellates contain plates of cellulose that lie between the two surface membranes that cover the organism. These plates function as protective armor.

Dinoflagellates are noteworthy for several reasons. They are one of the bedrocks of the food chain, particularly in the oceans and lakes of the world. Their numbers can be so great that they are evident as a mass of color on the surface of the water. Sometimes satellite cameras can even visualize these blooms. This abundant growth can consume so much oxygen that survival of other species in the area is threatened. As well, some dinoflagellates can produce toxins that can find their way into higher species, particularly those such as shellfish that feed by filtering water through them. Paralytic shellfish poisoning, which harms the neurological system of humans, is an example of a malady associated with the consumption of clams, mussels, and oysters that are contaminated with dinoflagellate toxins known as saxitoxin and brevitoxin. Saxitoxin is extremely potent, exerting its effect on the neurological system at concentrations 10,000 times lower than that required by cocaine. Another example of a dinoflagellate-related malady is a disease called ciguatera, which results from eating toxin-contaminated fish.

A third distinctive feature of dinoflagellates concerns their **nucleus**. The deoxyribonucleic acid shares some features with the **DNA** of **eukaryotes**, such as the presence of repeated stretches of DNA. But, other eukaryotic features, such as the supportive structures known as histones, have as yet not been detected. Also, the amount of DNA in dinoflagellates is far greater than in eukaryotes. The nucleus can occupy half the volume of the cell.

As with other microorganisms, dinoflagellates have been present on the Earth for a long time. Fossils of *Arpylorus antiquus* have been found in rock that dates back 400 million years. And, fossils that may be dinoflagellate cysts have been found in rock that is almost two billion years old. Current thought is that dinoflagellates arose when a bacterium was swallowed but not digested by another microorganism. The bacteria became symbiotic with the organism that swallowed them. This explanation is also how mitochondria are thought to have arisen.

Dinoflagellates cysts are analogous to the cysts formed by other microorganisms. They function to protect the genetic material during periods when conditions are too harsh for growth. When conditions become more favorable, resuscitation of the cyst and growth of the dinoflagellate resumes.

Dinoflagellates are sometimes referred to as Pyrrhophyta, which means fire plants. This is because of their ability to produce biological luminescence, akin to that of the firefly. Often, these luminescent dinoflagellates can be seen in the wake of ocean-going ships at night.

See also Bioluminescence; Red tide; Snow blooms

DIPHTHERIA

Diphtheria is a potentially fatal, contagious bacterial disease that usually involves the nose, throat, and air passages, but may also infect the skin. Its most striking feature is the formation of a grayish membrane covering the tonsils and upper part of the throat.

Like many other upper respiratory diseases, diphtheria is most likely to break out during the winter months. At one time it was a major childhood killer, but it is now rare in developed countries because of widespread **immunization**. Since 1988, all confirmed cases in the United States have involved visitors or immigrants. In countries that do not have routine immunization against this infection, the mortality rate varies from 1.5% to 25%.

Persons who have not been immunized may get diphtheria at any age. The disease is spread most often by droplets from the coughing or sneezing of an infected person or carrier. The incubation period is two to seven days, with an average of three days. It is vital to seek medical help at once when diphtheria is suspected, because treatment requires emergency measures for adults as well as children.

The symptoms of diphtheria are caused by toxins produced by the diphtheria bacillus, *Corynebacterium diphtheriae* (from the Greek for "rubber membrane"). In fact, toxin production is related to infections of the bacillus itself with a particular **bacteria** virus called a phage (from **bacteriophage**; a virus that infects bacteria). The intoxication destroys healthy tissue in the upper area of the throat around the tonsils, or in open wounds in the skin. Fluid from the dying cells then coagulates to form the telltale gray or grayish green membrane. Inside the membrane, the bacteria produce an exotoxin, which is a poisonous secretion that causes the life-threatening symptoms of diphtheria. The exotoxin is carried throughout the body in the bloodstream, destroying healthy tissue in other parts of the body.

The most serious complications caused by the exotoxin are inflammations of the heart muscle (myocarditis) and damage to the nervous system. The risk of serious complications is increased as the time between onset of symptoms and the administration of antitoxin increases, and as the size of the membrane formed increases. The myocarditis may cause disturbances in the heart rhythm and may culminate in heart failure. The symptoms of nervous system involvement can include seeing double (diplopia), painful or difficult swallowing, and slurred speech or loss of voice, which are all indications of the exotoxin's effect on nerve functions. The exotoxin may also cause severe swelling in the neck ("bull neck").

The signs and symptoms of diphtheria vary according to the location of the infection. Nasal diphtheria produces few symptoms other than a watery or bloody discharge. On examination, there may be a small visible membrane in the nasal passages. Nasal infection rarely causes complications by itself, but it is a **public health** problem because it spreads the disease more rapidly than other forms of diphtheria.

Pharyngeal diphtheria gets its name from the pharynx, which is the part of the upper throat that connects the mouth and nasal passages with the larynx. This is the most common form of diphtheria, causing the characteristic throat membrane. The membrane often bleeds if it is scraped or cut. It is important not to try to remove the membrane because the trauma may increase the body's absorption of the exotoxin. Other signs and symptoms of pharyngeal diphtheria include mild sore throat, fever of 101–102°F (38.3–38.9°C), a rapid pulse, and general body weakness.

Laryngeal diphtheria, which involves the voice box or larynx, is the form most likely to produce serious complications. The fever is usually higher in this form of diphtheria (103–104°F or 39.4–40°C) and the patient is very weak. Patients may have a severe cough, have difficulty breathing, or lose their voice completely. The development of a "bull neck" indicates a high level of exotoxin in the bloodstream. Obstruction of the airway may result in respiratory compromise and death.

The skin form of diphtheria, which is sometimes called cutaneous diphtheria, accounts for about 33% of diphtheria cases. It is found chiefly among people with poor **hygiene**. Any break in the skin can become infected with diphtheria. The infected tissue develops an ulcerated area and a diphtheria membrane may form over the wound but is not always present. The wound or ulcer is slow to heal and may be numb or insensitive when touched.

The diagnosis of diphtheria can be confirmed by the results of a **culture** obtained from the infected area. Material from the swab is put on a **microscope** slide and stained using a procedure called **Gram's stain**. The diphtheria bacillus is called Gram-positive because it holds the dye after the slide is rinsed with alcohol. Under the microscope, diphtheria bacilli look like beaded rod-shaped cells, grouped in patterns that resemble Chinese characters. Another laboratory test involves growing the diphtheria bacillus on Loeffler's medium.

The most important treatment is prompt administration of diphtheria antitoxin. The antitoxin is made from horse serum and works by neutralizing any circulating exotoxin. The physician must first test the patient for sensitivity to animal serum. Patients who are sensitive (about 10%) must be desensitized with diluted antitoxin, since the antitoxin is the only specific substance that will counteract diphtheria exotoxin. No human antitoxin is available for the treatment of diphtheria.

Antibiotics are given to wipe out the bacteria, to prevent the spread of the disease, and to protect the patient from developing **pneumonia**. They are not a substitute for treatment with antitoxin. Both adults and children may be given **penicillin**, ampicillin, or erythromycin. Erythromycin appears to be more effective than penicillin in treating people who are carriers because of better penetration into the infected area. Cutaneous diphtheria is usually treated by cleansing the wound thoroughly with soap and water, and giving the patient antibiotics for 10 days.

Universal immunization is the most effective means of preventing diphtheria. The standard course of immunization for healthy children is three doses of DPT (diphtheria-tetanus-pertussis) preparation given between two months and six months of age, with booster doses given at 18 months and at entry into school. Adults should be immunized at 10-year intervals with Td (tetanus-diphtheria) toxoid. A toxoid is a

bacterial toxin that is treated to make it harmless but still can induce **immunity** to the disease.

Diphtheria patients must be isolated for one to seven days or until two successive cultures show that they are no longer contagious. Because diphtheria is highly contagious and has a short incubation period, family members and other contacts of diphtheria patients must be watched for symptoms and tested to see if they are carriers. They are usually given antibiotics for seven days and a booster shot of diphtheria/tetanus toxoid.

Reporting is necessary to track potential **epidemics**, to help doctors identify the specific strain of diphtheria, and to see if resistance to penicillin or erythromycin has developed. In 1990, an outbreak of diphtheria began in Russia and spread within four years to all of the newly independent states of the former Soviet Union. By the time that the epidemic was contained, over 150,000 cases and 5000 deaths were reported. A vast public health immunization campaign largely confined the epidemic by 1999.

See also Bacteria and bacterial infection; Epidemics, bacterial; Public health, current issues

DIRECT MICROSCOPIC COUNT · *see* LABORATORY TECHNIQUES IN MICROBIOLOGY

DISEASE OUTBREAKS · *see* EPIDEMICS AND PANDEMICS

DISINFECTION AND DISINFECTANTS

Disinfection and the use of chemical disinfectants is one key strategy of **infection control**. Disinfection refers to the reduction in the number of living **microorganisms** to a level that is considered to be safe for the particular environment. Typically, this entails the destruction of those microbes that are capable of causing disease.

Disinfection is different from **sterilization**, which is the complete destruction of all microbial life on the surface or in the liquid. The steam-heat technique of autoclaving is an example of sterilization.

There are three levels of disinfection, with respect to power of the disinfection. High-level disinfection will kill all organisms, except for large concentrations of bacterial spores, using a chemical agent that has been approved as a so-called sterilant by the United States Food and Drug Administration. Intermediate level disinfection is that which kills mycobacteria, most **viruses**, and all types of **bacteria**. This type of disinfection uses a chemical agent that is approved as a tuberculocide by the United States Environmental Protection Agency (EPA). The last type of disinfection is called low-level disinfection. In this type, some viruses and bacteria are killed using a chemical compound designated by the EPA as a hospital disinfectant.

There are a variety of disinfectants that can be used to reduce the microbial load on a surface or in a solution. The disinfectant that is selected and the use of the particular disinfectant depend on a number of factors. The nature of the surface is important. A smoother surface is easier to disinfect, as there are not as many crevasses for organisms to hide. Generally, a smoother surface requires less time to disinfect than a rough surface. The surface material is also important. For example, a wooden surface can soak up liquids that can act as nutrients for the microorganisms, while a plastic surface that is more **hydrophobic** (water-hating) will tend to repel liquids and so present a more hostile environment for microbes.

Another factor in the **selection** of a disinfectant is the number of living microorganisms present. Generally, more organisms require a longer treatment time and sometimes a more potent disinfectant. The nature of the microbial growth is also a factor. Bacteria growing a slime-encased **biofilm** are hardier than bacteria that are not growing in biofilms. Other resistance mechanisms can operate. A general order of resistance, from the most to the least resistant, is: bacterial spores, mycobacteria (because of their unusual cell wall composition), viruses that repel water, **fungi**, actively growing bacteria, and viruses whose outer surface is mostly lipid.

Alcohol is a disinfectant that tends to be used on the skin to achieve a short-term disinfection. It can be used on surfaces as a spray. However, because alcohol evaporates quickly, it may not be present on a surface long enough to adequately disinfect the surface. A type of disinfectant known as tamed iodines, or iodophors, are also useful as skin disinfectants. In hospital settings, iodophors are used as a replacement for hand soap.

A better choice of disinfectant for surfaces is sodium hypochlorite. It can also be added to drinking water, where dissociation to produce free chlorine provides disinfection power. Bacteria such as *Escherichia coli* are susceptible to chlorine. **Chlorination** of drinking water is the most popular choice of water treatment in the world. If left for five minutes, sodium hypochlorite performs as an intermediate level disinfectant on surfaces. However, chlorine bleach can be corrosive to metal surfaces and irritating to mucous membranes of the eye and nose.

Another surface disinfectant is compounds that contain a phenol group. A popular commercial brand known as Lysol is a phenolic disinfectant. Phenolics are intermediate level disinfectants, derived from coal tar, that are effective on contaminated surfaces. However, certain types of viruses and some bacteria are resistant to the killing action of phenolic compounds.

Another disinfectant is chlorhexidine. It is effective against fungus and **yeast**, but is not as effective against Gram-negative bacteria. Nor will it inactivate viruses whose surfaces are water loving. In situations where the contaminant is expected to be fungi or yeast, chlorhexidine is a suitable choice of disinfectant.

Aldehyde compounds, such as formaldehyde and glutaraldehyde, are very effective disinfectants. Glutaraldehyde has other uses as well, such as preserving specimens prior to their examination by the technique of electron microscopy. Glutaraldehyde kills many microorganisms, and all known disease-causing microorganisms, after only a few minutes exposure. Another effective general disinfectant is those that contain quaternary ammonium.

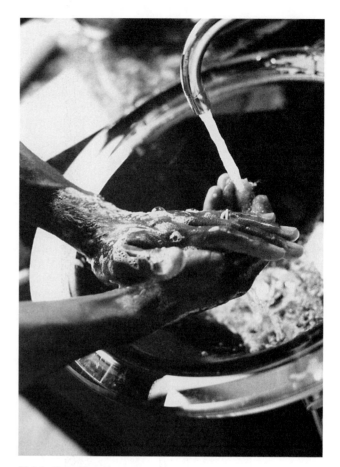

Disinfection of hands.

Many disinfectants are non-specific in their action. They will act against any biological material that is present. These are referred to as broad-spectrum disinfectants. Examples of broad-spectrum disinfectants are glutaraldehyde, sodium hypochlorite (the active ingredient in common household bleach), and hydrogen peroxide. Disinfectants such as phenolics and quaternary ammonium compounds are very specific. Other disinfectants lie in between the highly specific and broadly based categories. For example, alcohol is effective against actively growing bacteria and viruses with a lipid-based outer surface, but is not effective against bacterial spores or viruses that prefer watery environments.

The potency of a disinfectant can also be affected by the concentration that is used. For example, pure alcohol is less effective than alcohol diluted with water, because the more dilute form can penetrate farther into biological specimens than the pure form can.

Another factor that can decrease the effectiveness of disinfectants can be the presence of organic (carbon-containing) material. This can be a great problem in the chlorine disinfection of surface water. The vegetation in the water can bind the chlorine, leaving less of the disinfectant available to act on the microorganisms in the water. Proteins can also bind disinfectants. So, the presence of blood or blood products, other body fluids, and fecal waste material can compromise disinfectant performance.

Microorganisms can develop resistance to disinfectants, or can even have built-in, or intrinsic, resistance. For example, application of some disinfectants to contaminated surfaces for too short a time can promote the development of resistance in those bacteria that survive the treatment.

See also Bacteriocidal and bacteriostatic; Fungicide

DISPOSAL OF INFECTIOUS MICROORGANISMS

In research and clinical settings, the safe disposal of **microorganisms** is of paramount importance. Microbes encountered in the hospital laboratory have often been isolated from patients. These organisms can be the cause of the malady that has hospitalized the patient. Once examination of the microorganisms has ended, they must be disposed of in a way that does not harm anyone in the hospital or in the world outside of the hospital. For example, if solutions of the living microorganisms were simply dumped down the sink, the infectious organisms could find their way to the water table, or could become aerosolized and infect those who happened to inhale the infectious droplets.

A similar scenario operates in the research laboratory. Research can involve the use of hazardous microorganisms. Facilities can be constructed to minimize the risk to researchers who work with the organisms, such as fume hoods, glove boxes and, in special circumstances, whole rooms designed to contain the microbes. However, steps need to be taken to ensure that the organisms that are disposed of no longer present a risk of infection.

In addition to the cultures of microorganisms, anything that the organisms contacted must be disposed of carefully. Such items include tissues, syringes, the bedding in animal cages, **microscope** slides, razors, and pipettes. Often glassware and syringe are disposed of in sturdy plastic containers, which can be sterilized. The so-called "sharps" container prevents the sharp glass or syringe tip from poking out and cutting those handling the waste.

Depending on the material, there are several means by which items can be treated. The most common methods of treatment and disposal are **disinfection** using chemicals, **sterilization** using steam (such as in an autoclave), and burning at high temperature (which is also called incineration).

Disinfection can be done using chemicals. For example, a common practice in a microbiology laboratory is to wipe off the lab bench with alcohol both before and after a work session. Other liquid chemicals that are used as disinfectants include formaldehyde and chlorine-containing compounds (that are commonly referred to as bleach). Chemical disinfection can be achieved using a gas. The most common example is the use of ethylene oxide. Gas disinfection is advantageous when the sample is such that scrubbing of inner surfaces cannot be done, such as in tubing.

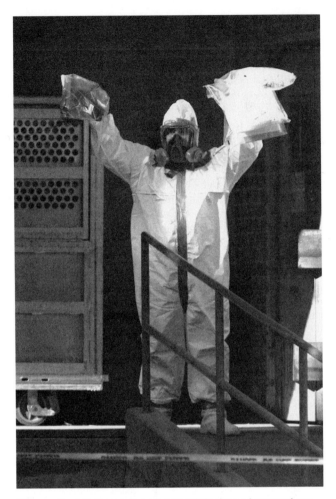

Biohazard technician handles suspected infectious microorganisms.

A second means of waste treatment is sterilization. This is the complete elimination of living organisms. A very common means of sterilization is the use of steam. The most common form of steam sterilization in laboratory settings is the autoclave. For example, in disinfection procedures and other laboratory procedures, items such as the adsorbent material used to wipe the bench and plastic gloves are usually put into a special biohazard bag. The bag is sealed when it is full and is sterilized, typically in an autoclave. The seal is typically an indicator tape that displays marking if the sterilization conditions have been achieved. The inclusion in the load being autoclaved of a solution containing spores of *Bacillus sterothermophilus* is typically done at regular intervals. Attempts to grow the contents of the solution after autoclaving should be unsuccessful if the sterilization procedure worked. After successful sterilization, the bag can be treated as normal waste.

An autoclave is essentially a large pressure cooker. Samples to be treated are placed in a chamber and a door can be tightly sealed. The seal is so tight that air cannot escape. Steam is introduced into the chamber at high pressure. At higher pressure a higher temperature can be achieved than the 100° C [212° F] possible at atmospheric pressure.

The relationship between time and temperature determines the speed of sterilization. The higher the temperature the more quickly a sample can be sterilized. Typical combinations of temperature and pressure are 115° C [239° F]–10 pounds per square inch (psi), 121° C [249.8° F]–15 psi, and 132° C [269.6° F]–27psi. Which combination is used depends on the material being sterilized. For example, a large and bulky load, or a large volume of **culture** should be kept in longer. Shorter sterilizations times are sufficient for contaminated objects such as surgical dressing, instruments, and empty glassware.

The third method of treatment of microorganisms and material contaminated with microorganisms is incineration. On a small scale incineration is practiced routinely in a microbiology laboratory to sterilize the metal loops used to transfer microorganisms from one place to another. Exposing the metal loop to a gas flame will burn up and vaporize any living microbes that are on the loop, ensuring that infectious organisms are not inadvertently transferred elsewhere. The method of incineration is also well suited to the treatment of large volumes of contaminated fluids or solids. Incineration is carried out in specially designed furnaces that achieve high temperatures and are constructed to be airtight. The use of a flame source such as a fireplace is unsuitable. The incineration needs to occur very quickly and should not leave any residual material. The process needs to be smoke-free, otherwise microbes that are still living could be wafted away in the rising smoke and hot air to cause infection elsewhere. Another factor in proper incineration is the rate at which sample is added to the flame. Too much sample can result in an incomplete burn.

Disposal of microorganisms also requires scrupulous record keeping. The ability to back track and trace the disposal of a sample is very important. Often institutions will have rules in place that dictate how samples should be treated, the packaging used for disposal, the labeling of the waste, and the records that must be maintained.

See also Laboratory techniques in microbiology; Steam pressure sterilizer

DNA (DEOXYRIBONUCLEIC ACID)

DNA, or deoxyribonucleic acid, is the genetic material that codes for the components that make life possible. Both prokaryotic and eukaryotic organisms contain DNA. An exception is a few **viruses** that contain **ribonucleic acid**, although even these viruses have the means for producing DNA.

The DNA of **bacteria** is much different from the DNA of eukaryotic cells such as human cells. Bacterial DNA is dispersed throughout the cell, while in eukaryotic cells the DNA is segregated in the **nucleus**, a membrane-bound region. In eukaryotics, structures called mitochondria also contain DNA. The dispersed bacterial DNA is much shorter than eukaryotic DNA. Hence the information is packaged more tightly in bacterial DNA. Indeed, in DNA of **microorganisms** such as

viruses, several genes can overlap with each other, providing information for several proteins in the same stretch of nucleic acid. Eukaryotic DNA contains large intervening regions between genes.

The DNA of both prokaryotes and **eukaryotes** is the basis for the transfer of genetic traits from one generation to the next. Also, alterations in the genetic material (**mutations**) can produce changes in structure, **biochemistry**, or behavior that might also be passed on to subsequent generations.

Genetics is the science of heredity that involves the study of the structure and function of genes and the methods by which genetic information contained in genes is passed from one generation to the next. The modern science of genetics can be traced to the research of Gregor Mendel (1823–1884), who was able to develop a series of laws that described mathematically the way hereditary characteristics pass from parents to offspring. These laws assume that hereditary characteristics are contained in discrete units of genetic material now known as genes.

The story of genetics during the twentieth century is, in one sense, an effort to discover the **gene** itself. An important breakthrough came in the early 1900s with the work of the American geneticist, Thomas Hunt Morgan (1866–1945). Working with fruit flies, Morgan was able to show that genes are somehow associated with the **chromosomes** that occur in the nuclei of cells. By 1912, Hunt's colleague, American geneticist A. H. Sturtevant (1891–1970) was able to construct the first chromosome map showing the relative positions of different genes on a chromosome. The gene then had a concrete, physical referent; it was a portion of a chromosome.

During the 1920s and 1930s, a small group of scientists looked for a more specific description of the gene by focusing their research on the gene's molecular composition. Most researchers of the day assumed that genes were some kind of protein molecule. Protein molecules are large and complex. They can occur in an almost infinite variety of structures. This quality is expected for a class of molecules that must be able to carry the enormous variety of genetic traits.

A smaller group of researchers looked to a second family of compounds as potential candidates as the molecules of heredity. These were the nucleic acids. The nucleic acids were first discovered in 1869 by the Swiss physician Johann Miescher (1844–1895). Miescher originally called these compounds "nuclein" because they were first obtained from the nuclei of cells. One of Miescher's students, Richard Altmann, later suggested a new name for the compounds, a name that better reflected their chemical nature: nucleic acids.

Nucleic acids seemed unlikely candidates as molecules of heredity in the 1930s. What was then known about their structure suggested that they were too simple to carry the vast array of complex information needed in a molecule of heredity. Each nucleic acid molecule consists of a long chain of alternating sugar and phosphate fragments to which are attached some sequence of four of five different nitrogen bases: adenine, cytosine, guanine, uracil and thymine (the exact bases found in a molecule depend slightly on the type of nucleic acid).

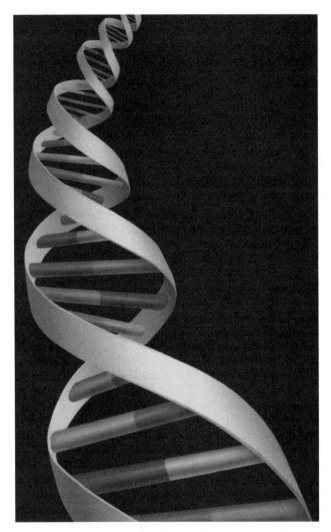

Computer-generated image of the DNA double helix, showing the deoxyribose backbone (vertical ribbons) and the linking nucloetides (horizontal bars).

It was not clear how this relatively simple structure could assume enough different conformations to "code" for hundreds of thousands of genetic traits. In comparison, a single protein molecule contains various arrangements of twenty fundamental units (amino acids) making it a much better candidate as a carrier of genetic information.

Yet, experimental evidence began to point to a possible role for nucleic acids in the transmission of hereditary characteristics. That evidence implicated a specific sub-family of the nucleic acids known as the deoxyribose nucleic acids, or DNA. DNA is characterized by the presence of the sugar deoxyribose in the sugar-phosphate backbone of the molecule and by the presence of adenine, cytosine, guanine, and thymine, but not uracil.

As far back as the 1890s, the German geneticist Albrecht Kossel (1853–1927) obtained results that pointed to the role of DNA in heredity. In fact, historian John Gribbin has suggested that the evidence was so clear that it "ought to have

been enough alone to show that the hereditary information...*must* be carried by the DNA." Yet, somehow, Kossel himself did not see this point, nor did most of his colleagues for half a century.

As more and more experiments showed the connection between DNA and genetics, a small group of researchers in the 1940s and 1950s began to ask how a DNA molecule could code for genetic information. The two who finally resolved this question were **James Watson**, a 24-year-old American trained in genetics, and **Francis Crick**, a 36-year-old Englishman, trained in physics and self-taught in chemistry. The two met at the Cavendish Laboratories of Cambridge University in 1951. They shared the view that the structure of DNA held the key to understanding how genetic information is stored in a cell and how it is transmitted from one cell to its daughter cells.

The key to lay in a technique known as x-ray crystallography. When x rays are directed at a crystal of some material, such as DNA, they are reflected and refracted by atoms that make up the crystal. The refraction pattern thus produced consists of a collection of spots and arcs. A skilled observer can determine from the refraction pattern the arrangement of atoms in the crystal.

Watson and Crick were fortunate in having access to some of the best x-ray diffraction patterns that then existed. These "photographs" were the result of work being done by **Maurice Wilkins** and Rosalind Elsie Franklin at King's College in London. Although Wilkins and Franklin were also working on the structure of DNA, they did not recognize the information their photographs contained. Indeed, it was only when Watson accidentally saw one of Franklin's photographs that he suddenly saw the solution to the DNA puzzle.

Watson and Crick experimented with tinker-toy-like models of the DNA molecule, shifting atoms around into various positions. They were looking for an arrangement that would give the kind of x-ray photograph that Watson had seen in Franklin's laboratory. On March 7, 1953, the two scientists found the answer. They built a model consisting of two helices (corkscrew-like spirals), wrapped around each other. Each helix consisted of a backbone of alternating sugar and phosphate groups. To each sugar was attached one of the four nitrogen bases, adenine, cytosine, guanine, or thymine. The sugar-phosphate backbone formed the outside of the DNA molecule, with the nitrogen bases tucked inside. Each nitrogen base on one strand of the molecule faced another nitrogen base on the opposite strand of the molecule. The base pairs were not arranged at random, however, but in such a way that each adenine was paired with a thymine, and each cytosine with a guanine.

The Watson-Crick model was a remarkable achievement, for which the two scientists won the 1954 Nobel Prize in Chemistry. The molecule had exactly the shape and dimensions needed to produce an x-ray photograph like that of Franklin's. Furthermore, Watson and Crick immediately saw how the molecule could "carry" genetic information. The sequence of nitrogen bases along the molecule, they said, could act as a **genetic code**. A sequence, such as A-T-T-C-G-C-T...etc., might tell a cell to make one kind of protein (such

DNA Replication

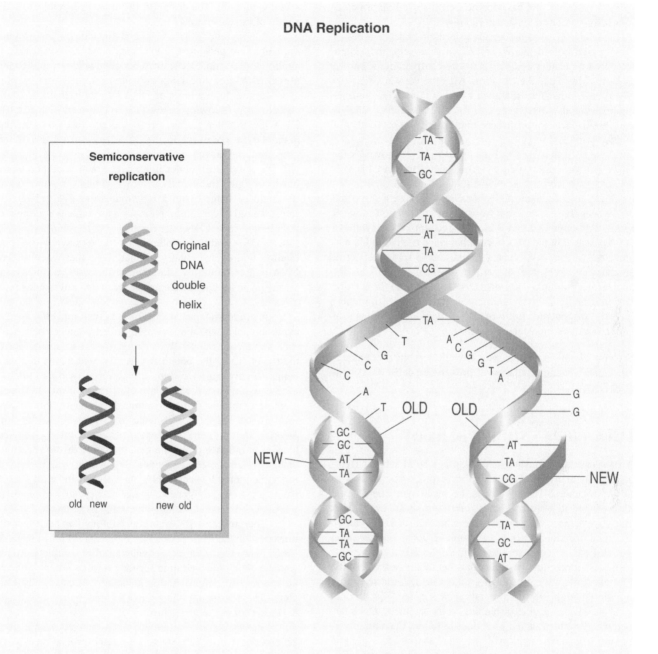

Diagram depicting semiconservative DNA replication.

as that for red hair), while another sequence, such as G-C-T-C-T-C-G...etc., might code for a different kind of protein (such as that for blonde hair). Watson and Crick themselves contributed to the deciphering of this genetic code, although that process was long and difficult and involved the efforts of dozens of researchers over the next decade.

Watson and Crick had also considered, even before their March 7th discovery, what the role of DNA might be in the manufacture of proteins in a cell. The sequence that they outlined was that DNA in the nucleus of a cell might act as a template for the formation of a second type of nucleic acid, **RNA** (ribonucleic acid). RNA would then leave the nucleus, emigrate to the **cytoplasm** and then itself act as a template for the production of protein. That theory, now known as the Central Dogma, has since been largely confirmed and has become a critical guiding principal of much research in **molecular biology**.

Scientists continue to advance their understanding of DNA. Even before the Watson-Crick discovery, they knew that DNA molecules could exist in two configurations, known as the "A" form and the "B" form. After the Watson-Crick discovery, two other forms, known as the "C" and "D" configurations were also discovered. All four of these forms of DNA are right-handed double helices that differ from each other in relatively modest ways.

In 1979, however, a fifth form of DNA known as the "Z" form was discovered by Alexander Rich and his colleagues at the Massachusetts Institute of Technology. The "Z" form was given its name partly because of its zigzag shape and partly because it is different from the more common A and B forms. Although Z-DNA was first recognized in synthetic DNA prepared in the laboratory, it has since been found in natural cells whose environment is unusual in some respect or another. The presence of certain types of proteins in the nucleus, for example, can cause DNA to shift from the B to the Z conformation. The significance and role of this most recently discovered form of DNA remains a subject of research among molecular biologists.

See also Chemical mutagenesis; Genetic regulation of eukaryotic cells; Genetic regulation of prokaryotic cells; Mitochondrial DNA

DNA CHIPS AND MICROARRAYS

A **DNA (deoxyribonucleic acid)** chip is a solid support (typically glass or nylon) onto which are fixed single strands of DNA sequences. The sequences are made synthetically and are arranged in a pattern that is referred to as an array. DNA chips are a means by which a large amount of DNA can be screened for the presence of target regions. Furthermore, samples can be compared to compare the effects of a treatment, environmental condition, or other factor on the activity. One example of the use of a DNA microarray is the screening for the development of a mutation in a **gene**. The original gene would be capable of binding to the synthetic DNA target, whereas the mutated gene does not bind. Such an experiment has been exploited in the search for genetic determinants of **antibiotic resistance**, and in the manufacture of compounds to which the resistant **microorganisms** will be susceptible.

A gene chip is wafer-like in appearance, and resembles a microtransistor chips. However, instead of transistors, a DNA chip contains an orderly and densely packed array of DNA species. Arrays are made by spotting DNA samples over the surface of the chip in a patterned manner. The spots can be applied by hand or with robotic automation. The latter can produce very small spots, which collectively is termed a microarray.

Each spot in an array is, in reality, a single-stranded piece of DNA. Depending upon the sequence of the tethered piece of DNA, a complimentary region of sample DNA can specifically bind. The design of the array is dependent on the nature of the experiment.

The synthetic DNA is constructed so that known sequences are presented to whatever sample is subsequently applied to the chip. DNA, or **ribonucleic acid** (typically messenger **RNA**) from the samples being examined are treated to as to cut the double helix of DNA into its two single strand components, following be enzymatic treatment that cuts the DNA into smaller pieces. The pieces are labeled with **fluorescent dyes**. For example, the DNA from one sample of **bacteria** could be tagged with a green fluorescent dye (dye that will fluoresce green under illumination with a certain wavelength of light) and the DNA from a second sample of bacteria could be tagged with a red fluorescent dye (which will fluoresce red under illumination with the same wavelength of light). Both sets of DNA are flooded over the chip. Where the sample DNA finds a complimentary piece of synthetic DNA, binding will occur. Finally the nature of the bound sample DNA is ascertained by illuminating the chip and observing for the presence and the pattern of green and red regions (usually dots).

A microarray can also be used to determine the level of expression of a gene. For example, an array can be constructed such that the messenger RNA of a particular gene will bind to the target. Thus, the bound RNAs represent genes that were being actively transcribed, or at least recently. By monitoring genetic expression, the response of microorganisms to a treatment or condition can be examined. As an example, DNA from a bacterial species growing in suspension can be compared with the same species growing as surface-adherent biofilm in order to probe the genetic nature of the alterations that occur in the bacteria upon association with a surface. Since the method detects DNA, the survey can be all-encompassing, assaying for genetic changes to protein, carbohydrate, lipid, and other constituents in the same experiment.

The power of DNA chip technology has been recently illustrated in the Human Genome Project. This effort began in 1990, with the goal of sequencing the complete human genome. The projected time for the project's completion was 40 years. Yet, by 2001, the sequencing was essentially complete. The reason for the project's rapid completion is the development of the gene chip.

Vast amounts of information are obtained from a single experiment. Up to 260,000 genes can be probed on a single chip. The analysis of this information has spawned a new science called **bioinformatics**, where biology and computing mesh.

Gene chips are having a profound impact on research. Pharmaceutical companies are able to screen for gene-based drugs much faster than before. In the future, DNA chip technology will extend to the office of the family physician. For example, a patient with a sore throat could be tested with a single-use, disposable, inexpensive gene chip in order to identify the source of the infection and its antibiotic susceptibility profile. Therapy could commence sooner and would be precisely targeted to the causative infectious agent.

See also DNA (Deoxyribonucleic acid); DNA chips and micro arrays; DNA hybridization; Genetic identification of microorganisms; Laboratory techniques in immunology; Laboratory techniques in microbiology; Molecular biology and molecular genetics

DNA Hybridization

Evolution deals with heritable changes in populations over time. Because **DNA** is the molecule of heredity, evolutionary changes will be reflected in changes in the base pairs in DNA. Two species that have evolved from a common ancestor will have DNA that has very similar base pair sequences. The degree of relatedness of two species can be estimated by examining how similar their base pair sequences are. One method of assessing relatedness uses hybridization of DNA.

In the molecular genetic technique of hybridization of DNA, single strands of DNA from two different species are allowed to join together to form hybrid double helices. These hybrid segments of DNA can be used to determine the evolutionary relatedness of organisms by examining how similar or dissimilar the DNA base pair sequences are.

The technique of DNA hybridization is based on two principles: the first, that double strands of DNA are held together by hydrogen bonds between complementary base pairs, and the second is that the more closely related two species are, the greater will be the number of complementary base pairs in the hybrid DNA. In other words, the degree of hybridization is proportional to the degree of similarity between the molecules of DNA from the two species.

Hybridization of DNA is accomplished by heating strands of DNA from two different species to 86° C [186.8° F]. This breaks the hydrogen bonds between all complementary base pairs. The result is many single-stranded segments of DNA. The single-stranded DNA from both species is mixed together and allowed to slowly cool. Similar strands of DNA from both species will begin to chemically join together or re-anneal at complementary base pairs by reforming hydrogen bonds.

The resulting hybrid DNA is then reheated and the temperature at which the DNA once again becomes single-stranded is noted. Because one cannot observe DNA separating, another technique must be used simultaneously with heating to show when separation has occurred. This technique employs the absorption of UV light by DNA. Single strands of DNA absorb UV light more effectively than do double strands. Therefore, the separation of the DNA strands is measured by UV light absorption; as more single strands are liberated, more UV light is absorbed.

The temperature at which hybrid DNA separation occurs is related to the number of hydrogen bonds formed between complementary base pairs. Therefore, if the two species are closely related, most base pairs will be complementary and the temperature of separation will be very close to 86° C [186.8° F]. If the two species are not closely related, they will not share many common DNA sequences and fewer complementary base pairs will form. The temperature of separation will be less than 86° C [186.8° F] because less energy is required to break fewer hydrogen bonds. Using this type of information, a tree of evo-

lutionary relationships based on the separation temperature of the hybrid helices can be generated.

See also Evolution and evolutionary mechanisms; Evolutionary origin of bacteria and viruses

DONNAN, FREDERICK GEORGE (1870-1956)
British chemist

Frederick George Donnan was a British chemist whose work in the second decade of the twentieth century established the existence of an electrochemical potential between a semipermeable membrane. The membrane allows an unequal distribution of ionic species to become established on either side of the membrane. In **bacteria**, this **Donnan equilibrium** has been demonstrated to exist across the outer membrane of Gram-negative bacteria, which separates the external environment from the **periplasm**. The energy derived from this ionic inequity is vital for the operation of the bacteria.

Donnan was born in Colombo, Ceylon (now known as Sri Lanka). He was educated at Queen's College in Belfast, Northern Ireland, at the University of Leipzig in Berlin, and at the University College, London. He taught at Liverpool University from 1904 until 1913, when he rejoined the faculty of University College as a Professor of Inorganic and Physical Chemistry. He remained there until his retirement in 1937.

In 1911, Donnan began his studies of the equilibrium between solutions separated by a semipermeable membrane that led to the establishment of the Donnan equilibrium. He also was involved in important studies in physical chemistry, which included the study of colloids and soap solutions, behavior of various gases, oxygen solubility, and the manufacture of nitric acid.

Of all his research achievements, Donnan's major accomplish was the theory of membrane equilibrium. In his productive research career, Donnan authored more than one hundred research papers.

See also Bacterial membranes and cell wall

DONNAN EQUILIBRIUM

Donnan equilibrium (which can also be referred to as the Gibbs-Donnan equilibrium) describes the equilibrium that exists between two solutions that are separated by a membrane. The membrane is constructed such that it allows the passage of certain charged components (ions) of the solutions. The membrane, however, does not allow the passage of all the ions present in the solutions and is thus a selectively permeable membrane.

Donnan equilibrium is named after **Frederick George Donnan**, who proved its existence in biological cells. J. Willard Gibbs had predicted the effect some 30 years before.

The impermeability of the membrane is typically related to the size of the particular ion. An ion can be too large to pass through the pores of the membrane to the other side. The concentration of those ions that can pass freely though the membrane is the same on both sides of the membrane. As well, the total number of charged molecules on either side of the membrane is equal.

A consequence of the selective permeability of the membrane barrier is the development of an electrical potential between the two sides of the membrane. The two solutions vary in osmotic pressure, with one solution having more of a certain type (species) or types of ion that does the other solution.

As a result, the passage of some ions across the membrane will be promoted. In **bacteria**, for example, the passage of potassium across the outer membrane of Gram-negative bacteria occurs as a result of an established Donnan equilibrium between the external environment and the **periplasm** of the bacterium. The potassium enters in an attempt to balance the large amount of negative ion inside the cell. Since potassium is freely permeable, it will tend to diffuse out again. The inward movement of sodium corrects the imbalance. In the absence of a Donnan equilibrium, the bulky sodium molecule would not normally tend to move across the membrane and an electrical potential would be created.

See also Biochemistry

DOOLITTLE, W. FORD (1942-)
American biochemist and evolutionary biologist

Ford Doolittle is a Professor in the Department of **Biochemistry** at Dalhousie University in Halifax, Nova Scotia, Canada. He is also Director of the Canadian Institute of Advanced Research Program in Evolutionary Biology. Doolittle is one of the world's premier evolutionary biologists, who has used molecular techniques to explore the similarities and disparities between the genetic material in a variety of prokaryotic and eukaryotic organisms. In particular, his pioneering studies with the evolutionarily ancient archaebacteria have led to a fundamental re-evaluation of the so-called "tree of life."

Doolittle was born in Urbana, Illinois. Following his high school education, he received a B.A. in Biological Sciences (magna cum laude) from Harvard College in 1963, and a Ph.D. in Biological Sciences from Stanford University in 1969. He was a Postdoctoral Fellow in Microbiology at the University of Illinois from 1968 to 1969, and at the National Jewish Hospital and Research Center in Denver from 1969 to 1971. From there he moved to Dalhousie University as an Assistant Professor in the Department of Biochemistry in 1971. He became an Associate Professor in 1976, and a Professor in 1982.

Doolittle and his colleagues have made fundamental contributions to the field of evolutionary biology. Specifically, Doolittle has pioneered studies examining the origin of the nuclear genetic material in eukaryotic cells, the origin of the organizing genetic material known as introns, and the genetic

organization and regulation of the archaebacteria that inhabit thermal hot springs. The latter **bacteria** are among the most ancient **microorganisms** known, and knowledge of their genetic composition and behavior has clarified the early events of **evolution**.

From Doolittle's research, it is now known that mitochondria, the so-called "powerhouse" of eukaryotic cells, were once autonomous bacteria. Mitochondria arose from the integration of the ancient bacteria and a eukaryote and the establishment of a symbiotic relationship between the two. In addition, prokaryotic cells may well have evolved by acquiring genes from other species, even **eukaryotes**. This concept, which Doolittle has dubbed lateral **gene** transfer, challenges a fundamental pillar of evolution, which is the separateness of the kingdoms of life. For example, a fundamental scientific opposition to genetically modified organisms is that the acquisition of eukaryotic genes by the altered bacteria violates evolutionary laws.

Doolittle has received numerous awards and honors for his research, including the Award of Excellence from the Genetics Society of Canada and a fellowship in the Royal Society of Canada.

See also Archaeobacteria; Bacterial kingdoms; Evolutionary origin of bacteria and viruses

DUBOS, RENÉ (1901-1982)
French-born American microbiologist

René Dubos was a distinguished microbiologist whose pioneering work with soil-dwelling **bacteria** paved the way for the development of life-saving antibiotic drugs. Widely acclaimed for his discovery of tyrothricin, a chemical substance capable of destroying dangerous staphylococcus, pneumococcus, and streptococcus bacteria in both humans and animals, Dubos later turned to the study of **tuberculosis** and the role of physiological, social, and environmental factors in an individual's susceptibility to infection. In the 1960s, Dubos's interest in the effects of the total environment on human health and well-being prompted him to give up his laboratory work at New York's Rockefeller Institute for Medical Research to concentrate on writing and lecturing on ecological and humanitarian issues.

Over the years, Dubos produced a number of popular books on scientific subjects, including *So Human an Animal,* the 1968 Pulitzer-Prize winner for general nonfiction, and *Only One Earth: The Care and Maintenance of a Small Planet,* which formed the basis for the United Nations Conference on the Human Environment in 1992. Dubos's greatest concern was not man's inability to adapt to pollution, noise, overcrowding, and the other problems of highly industrialized societies, but rather the ease with which this adaptation could occur and its ensuing cost to humanity. "It is not man the ecological crisis threatens to destroy, but the quality of human life," Dubos wrote in *Life* magazine. "What we call humanness is the expression of the interplay between man's nature and the environment, an interplay which is as old as life itself and which is the mechanism for creation on Earth."

Dubos was born in Saint-Brice-sous-Foret, France, the only child of Georges Alexandre and Adeline Madeleine de Bloedt Dubos. Young Dubos spent his early years in the farming villages of Ile-de-France, north of Paris. Amongst the rolling hills and agricultural fields, Dubos developed a keen appreciation for the influence of landscape on the human spirit, a subject that would come to dominate his thoughts in later years. A bout with rheumatic fever at the age of ten both restricted Dubos's physical activity and enhanced his contemplative nature. When Dubos was 13, his father moved the family to Paris to open a butcher shop; a few months later, Georges Dubos was called to military service in World War I, leaving his wife and young son in charge of the business. Despite the best efforts of mother and son, the shop did poorly and the family had a difficult time getting by. Upon completing high school at the College Chaptal in 1919, Dubos had hoped to study history at the university, but the death of his father from head injuries suffered at the front forced him to stay closer to home to look after his mother. Dubos was granted a scholarship to study agricultural science at the Institut National Agronomique in Paris, receiving his bachelor of science degree in 1921. He spent part of the next year as an officer trainee in the French Army, but was soon discharged because of heart problems.

In 1922, Dubos was offered the job of assistant editor at a scholarly journal called *International Agriculture Intelligence,* published by the International Institute of Agriculture, then part of the League of Nations in Rome. Not long after he arrived in Italy, Dubos came across an article on soil microbes written by the Russian bacteriologist Sergei Winogradsky, who was then associated with the Pasteur Institute in Paris. Winogradsky's contention that microbes should be studied in their own environment rather than in pure, laboratory-grown cultures so intrigued Dubos that he resolved to become a bacteriologist. "This is really where my scholarly life began," he told John Culhane in an interview for the *New York Times Magazine.* "I have been restating that idea in all forms ever since." Soon after, Dubos happened to meet the American delegate to the International Institute of Agriculture, who convinced him to pursue graduate studies in the United States.

In order to finance his trip, Dubos translated books on forestry and agriculture and gave guided tours of Rome to foreign visitors. He eventually set sail for New York in 1924. During the crossing, Dubos ran into **Selman Waksman**, head of the soil microbiology division of the State Agricultural Experiment Station at Rutgers University in New Jersey (a man the aspiring scientist had guided around Rome some months before). After the ship docked in New York, Waksman introduced Dubos to his colleagues at Rutgers University, helping the young man secure a research assistantship in soil microbiology. While serving as an instructor in bacteriology over the next three years, Dubos completed work on his doctorate. His thesis, published in 1927, focused on the ways in which various soil **microorganisms** work to decompose cellulose in paper.

Upon completing his work at Rutgers, Dubos left for the University of North Dakota at Fargo to accept a teaching position in the department of microbiology. Soon after he arrived, however, Dubos received a telegram from the Rockefeller Institute for Medical Research in New York City offering him a fellowship in the department of pathology and bacteriology. Dubos immediately packed his bags, in part because the offer involved work on a project begun by Rockefeller bacteriologist **Oswald T. Avery**. Avery and his colleagues had been searching for a substance that could break down the semi-cellulose envelope which protects pneumococci bacteria, the microorganisms responsible for lobar **pneumonia** in human beings, from attack by the body's defense mechanisms. Dubos's bold assertion that he could identify an enzyme capable of decomposing this complex polysaccharide capsule with minimal damage to the host had evidently impressed Avery. With the exception of a two-year period in the early 1940s when he served on the faculty at Harvard Medical School, Dubos remained at the Rockefeller Institute, renamed Rockefeller University in 1965, for the next 44 years.

Guided by the studies of renowned bacteriologist **Louis Pasteur**, who maintained that any organic substance that accumulated could be broken down by natural energy, Dubos spent his first two years at the Institute searching fields, bogs, and swamps for a bacterium or fungus that could attack and decompose the tough polysaccharide coat surrounding pneumococci bacteria. Unlike other scientific investigators, who used enriched laboratory solutions to cultivate bacteria and force them to produce **enzymes**, Dubos concocted a solution rich in capsular polysaccharide, which he spread over a variety of soils. In 1929, he succeeded in isolating a swamp-dwelling bacillus which, because of its need for nourishment in an energy-starved environment, had been compelled to produce an enzyme capable of decomposing the polysaccharide capsule and digesting the pneumococci within. The following year Dubos was able to demonstrate the value of this particular enzyme in fighting pneumococcal infections in both animals and humans. The discovery confirmed Dubos's belief that soil bacteria were an important source of anti-infectious agents, inspiring him to search for other disease-fighting microbes.

In 1939, Dubos announced the discovery of a substance called tyrothricin, which had proved effective in fighting staphylococcus, pneumococcus, and streptococcus infections. Produced by the soil microorganism *Bacillus brevis,* tyrothricin was later found to contain two powerful chemicals, gramicidin and tyrocidine, which, though too toxic for ingestion, found widespread application in the treatment of external conditions, such as infectious lesions in humans and udder infections in cows. Dubos's groundbreaking work prompted scientists from around the world to conduct a wide-ranging search for antibiotic substances in natural environments. This ultimately resulted in a reexamination of the therapeutic properties of penicillin—first discovered in a bread **mold** ten years earlier by Alexander Fleming—and led to the isolation of a variety of new **antibiotics**, including streptomycin and the tetracyclines.

The death of Dubos's first wife, Marie Louise Bonnet, from tuberculosis in 1942 had a profound effect upon the scientist's career. "There seemed no reason," he recalled for Culhane. "Why should she get [tuberculosis] in this environment?" After spending two years as a professor of tropical medicine at Harvard Medical School, Dubos returned to the Rockefeller Institute to begin a full-scale investigation of tuberculosis and its causes. Until that time, scientists attempting to study tuberculosis bacilli had been hindered by the fact that laboratory methods of cultivation often modified the organisms to such an extent that they no longer resembled or behaved like the strains that infected humans. By 1947, however, Dubos had discovered that by adding a common detergent to the **culture** medium, he could raise bacilli so quickly and in such large quantities that they had little chance to mutate. This enabled researchers to study the microorganism more closely and develop the highly effective Bacillus Calmette-GuÉrin, or BCG, **vaccine.**

During the course of his research with tuberculosis, Dubos focused on the importance of heredity, nutrition, physiology, and social and emotional trauma on an individual's vulnerability to infection. He used his wife's case as his first example. A careful examination of her early health records revealed that she had suffered from tuberculosis as a child. Although his wife recovered from the acute attack, Dubos became convinced that the emotional upheaval of World War II and her concern for her family's safety in France had served to weaken her and reawaken the dormant germ. Some years later, Dubos's second wife's battle with tuberculosis and her subsequent recovery prompted the couple to collaborate on *The White Plague: Tuberculosis, Man, and Society,* a non-technical account of the disease. Published in 1952, the book provided additional evidence linking tuberculosis with certain environmental conditions, such as inadequate nourishment and sudden economic or social disturbances.

Later, Dubos's interest in the effects of the total environment on human health encouraged him to become involved with the sociomedical problems of poor communities and to speak out on the dangers of pollution, as well as social, economic, and spiritual deprivation. By 1964, he had become a leading spokesman for the fledgling environmental movement and an outspoken critic of what he viewed as the narrow, short-range approach used by most biologists.

According to Dubos, the problems of technologically advanced societies posed an equal, if not greater, threat to human survival. Two of Dubos's most popular books, *Man Adapting* and *So Human an Animal,* examine the close relationship between environmental conditions and man's physical, mental, and spiritual development, emphasizing the dangers inherent in adapting to a polluted, highly mechanized, highly stressful environment. "Wild animals can survive in zoos, but only at the cost of losing the physical and behavioral splendor they possess in their natural habitat," he wrote in *Life.* "Similarly, human beings can survive in the polluted cage of technological civilization, but in adapting to such conditions, we may sacrifice much of our humanness." Dubos also warned against introducing new substances, such as laundry detergents containing potentially dangerous enzymes, into the American marketplace without thorough testing. Unlike many environmentalists, however, Dubos maintained an enormous faith in

both the ability of nature to recover from man's abuses and man's own capacity to recognize and learn from mistakes.

Dubos became a naturalized American citizen in 1938. Although he maintained a laboratory and an apartment in New York City, Dubos spent most weekends at his large estate in Garrison, New York. There, he and his wife planted trees, raised vegetables, and enjoyed long walks in the scenic Hudson River Valley. Over the years, Dubos earned numerous awards for his work, including the Modern Medicine Award, 1961, the Phi Beta Kappa Award, 1963, and the Tyler Ecology Award, 1976; he also received more than thirty honorary degrees from various colleges and universities. A member of professional organizations such the National Academy of Sciences, Dubos was also appointed by President Richard M. Nixon in 1970 to serve on the Citizens' Advisory Committee on Environmental Quality. Always eager to make his scientific and philosophical ideas accessible to people from all walks of life, Dubos continued to write and lecture until shortly before his death from heart failure at age 82 in New York City.

See also History of microbiology; History of public health; History of the development of antibiotics

DYSENTERY

Dysentery is an infectious disease that has ravaged armies, refugee camps, and prisoner-of-war camps throughout history. The disease still is a major problem in developing countries with primitive sanitary facilities.

The acute form of dysentery, called shigellosis or bacillary dysentery, is caused by the bacillus (bacterium) of the genus *Shigella,* which is divided into four subgroups and distributed worldwide. Type A, *Shigella dysenteriae,* is a particularly virulent species. Infection begins from the solid waste from someone infected with the bacterium. Contaminated soil or water that gets on the hands of an individual often is conveyed to the mouth, where the person contracts the infection. Flies help to spread the bacillus.

Young children living in primitive conditions of overcrowded populations are especially vulnerable to the disease. Adults, though susceptible, usually will have less severe disease because they have gained a limited resistance. **Immunity** as such is not gained by infection, however, and an infected person can become reinfected by the same species of **Shigella.**

Once the bacterium has gained entrance through the mouth, it travels to the lower intestine (colon) where it penetrates the mucosa (lining) of the intestine. In severe cases, the entire colon may be involved, but usually only the lower half of the colon is involved. The incubation period is one to four days, that is the time from infection until symptoms appear.

Symptoms may be sudden and severe in children. They experience abdominal pain or distension, fever, loss of appetite, nausea, vomiting, and diarrhea. Blood and pus will appear in the stool, and the child may pass 20 or more bowel movements a day. Left untreated, he will become dehydrated from loss of water and will lose weight rapidly. If untreated, death may occur within 12 days of infection. If treated or if the

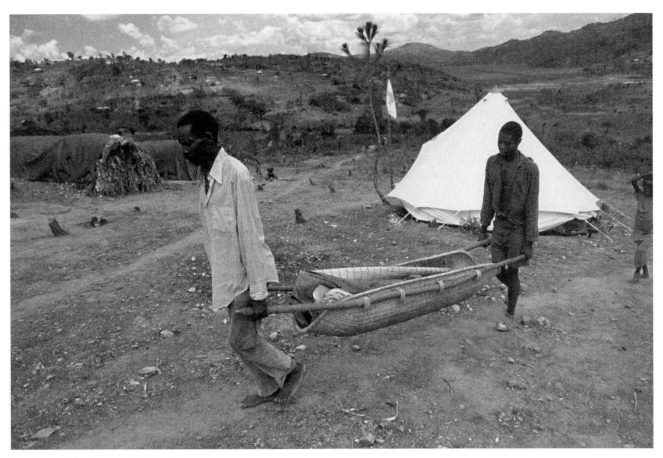

Dysentery epidemic amongst Hutu refugees.

infection is weathered, the symptoms will subside within approximately two weeks.

Adults experience a less severe course of disease. They will initially feel a griping pain in the abdomen, develop diarrhea, though without any blood in the stool at first. Blood and pus will appear soon, however, as episodes of diarrhea recur with increasing frequency. Dysentery usually ends in the adult within four to eight days in mild cases, and up to six weeks in severe infections.

Shigella dysenteriae brings about a particularly virulent infection that can be fatal within 12 to 24 hours. The patient has little or no diarrhea, but experiences delirium, convulsions, and lapses into a coma. Fortunately, infection with this species is uncommon.

Treatment of the patient with dysentery usually is by fluid therapy to replace the liquid and electrolytes lost in sweating and diarrhea. **Antibiotics** may be used, but some Shigella species have developed resistance to them, and in these cases, antibiotics may be relatively ineffective.

Some individuals harbor the bacterium without having symptoms. Like those who are convalescent from the disease, the carriers without symptoms can spread the disease. This may occur by someone with improperly washed hands preparing food, which becomes infected with the organism.

Another form of dysentery called **amebic dysentery** or intestinal amebiasis is spread by a protozoan, *Entamoeba histolytica*. The protozoan occurs in an active form, which infects the bowel, and an encysted form, which forms the source of infection. If the patient develops diarrhea, the active form of amoeba will pass from the bowel and rapidly die. If no diarrhea is present, the amoeba will form a hard cyst about itself and pass from the bowel to be picked up by another victim. Once ingested, it will lose its shell and begin the infectious cycle. Amebic dysentery can be waterborne, so anyone drinking infested water that is not purified is susceptible to infection.

Amebic dysentery is common in the tropics and relatively rare in temperate climates. Infection may be so subtle as to be practically unnoticed. Intermittent bouts of diarrhea, abdominal pain, flatulence, and cramping mark the onset of infection. Spread of infection may occur with the organisms entering the liver, so abdominal tenderness may occur over the area of the liver. Because the amoeba invades the lining of the colon, some bleeding may occur, and in severe infections, the patient may require blood transfusions to replace lost blood.

Treatment, again, is aimed at replacement of lost fluids and the relief of symptoms. Microscopic examination of the stool will reveal the active protozoan or its cysts. Special medications aimed at eradicating the infectious organism may be needed.

An outbreak of amebic dysentery can occur seemingly mysteriously because the carrier of the amoeba may be without symptoms, especially in a temperate zone. A person with inadequate sanitation can spread the disease through food that he has handled. Often, health officials can trace a disease outbreak back to a single kitchen and then test the cooks for evidence of amebic dysentery.

Before the idea of the spread of infectious agents was understood, dysentery often was responsible for more casualties among the ranks of armies than was actual combat. It also was a constant presence among prisoners, who often died because little or no medical assistance was available to them. Dysentery remains a condition present throughout the world that requires vigilance. Prevention is the most effective means to maintain the health of populations living in close quarters. Hand washing, especially among food preparation personnel, and water purification are the most effective means of prevention.

See also Waste water treatment; Water pollution and purification; Water quality

E

E.COLI O157:H7 INFECTION

Escherichia coli, commonly shortened to *E. coli*, is a Gram-negative bacterium that lives in the intestinal tract of humans and other warm-blooded animals. There are many sub-types, or strains of the organism. One strain is designated as O157:H7, based on two antigens that are present on the surface of the bacterium and of the locomotive appendage called the flagella.

In contrast to many of the other strains, *E. coli* O157:H7 is not a normal resident of the humans intestinal tract. When present in the intestinal tract, via the ingestion of contaminated food or water, O157:H7 causes a severe, even life-threatening malady known as hemorrhagic colitis.

E. coli O157:H7 is a strain of enterohemorrhagic *E. coli* that was initially isolated in Argentina in 1977. The strain is thought to have arisen from a genetic **recombination** between another *E. coli* strain and a toxin-producing strain of *Shigella dysenterae* in the intestinal tract of someone. The resulting genetically altered *E. coli* now carried the genetic information for the toxins.

Strain O157:H7 was recognized as a cause of illness in 1982. Then, an outbreak of severe diarrhea was microbiologically traced to a batch of undercooked hamburgers. Most cases are stilled associated with improperly cooked contaminated meat. For this reason, the infection has acquired the cache of "hamburger disease." However, numerous other foods can deliver the **bacteria**, including alfalfa sprouts, unpasteurized fruits juices such as apple juice, lettuce and cheese curds, and raw milk. **Contamination** of vegetables can occur when they are sprayed in the filed with sewage-containing water and then inadequately washed prior to eating. For example, organically grown produce might not be adequately washed, given the perception that the absence of **antibiotics** negates the need for washing.

Meat can become contaminated with fecal material during slaughter. The bacteria are subsequently distributed throughout the meat when the meat is ground. Thorough cooking is necessary to kill the bacteria buried in the ground meat. Although not clear yet, indications are that the ingestion of as few as 10 surviving bacteria can be sufficient to trigger the infection.

E. coli O157:H7 is also passed onto humans via water that has been contaminated with fecal material, typically from cattle who are a reservoir of the bacterium. For example, the contamination of the water supply of Walkerton, Ontario, Canada, by run-off from a neighbouring cattle farm in the summer of 2000 caused thousands of illnesses and killed seven people.

The damage of the infection results from two potent toxins produced by the bacteria. The toxins are known as verotoxin and shiga-like toxin. These toxins are very similar in structure and action as those produced by another bacteria of health concern, *Shigella dysenteriae*, the agent of bacterial **dysentery**. The toxins exert their effect by both physically damaging the host epithelial cell and by preventing repair of the damage, because of the shutdown of the host cell's ability to manufacture new protein. The toxins bind to a specific receptor called Gb3, which is found on the surface of epithelial cells in blood vessels, smooth muscle cells, kidney cells, and red blood cells. The bound toxins inhibit **protein synthesis**, thus killing the cells.

The toxic damage occurs following the tight association of the bacteria with the surface of the intestinal epithelial cells. Research has proven that this association relies on the manufacture and extrusion of a specific protein by the bacteria that acts as an anchor to which the bacteria bind. As binding occurs, the host cells change their configuration, becoming so-called pedestals on which each bacterium sits. At this point the binding of the bacteria with the host cells is tenacious and the infection is established.

Hemorrhagic colitis begins as a severe abdominal pain accompanied by watery diarrhea. As damage to the epithelial cells lining the intestinal tract occurs, the diarrhea becomes bloody. Vomiting can also occur. These symptoms, as severe and debilitating as they are, usually last only between one and two weeks, and terminate naturally as the body's immune defenses successfully cope with the infection. Usually no permanent damage results from the infection. However in those who are immunocompromised and in children, the disease can become more disseminated. Damage to the kidney can be so devastating that complete loss of kidney function occurs. If not treated the death rate from hemolytic anemia is high. Even with rapid diagnoses and treatment that includes antibiotics, blood transfusions and kidney dialysis, the death rate is still three to five percent.

Approximately ten to fifteen per cent of those infected with strain O157:H7 develop hemolytic anemia. The syndrome is the leading cause of sudden-onset kidney failure in children in the world. As well, the elderly can develop a condition known as thrombocytopenic purpura, which consists of a fever and nerve damage. In the elderly, this malady can kill almost half of those who become infected.

The chances of infection from *E. coli* O157:H7 are greatly lessened by proper food preparation, washing of food surfaces that have been exposed to raw ground meat, and proper personal **hygiene**, especially hand washing. Also, since the bacterium is very sensitive to heat, boiling suspect water prior to drinking the water is a sure way to eliminate the risk of infection from the bacteria and to inactivate the toxins.

Also, a **vaccine** for cattle is in the final testing stages prior to being approved for sale. Approval is expected in 2002. The vaccine blocks the binding and pedestal formation by the bacteria in cattle. The bacteria remain free in the intestinal tract and so are washed out of the cow. Eliminating the reservoir of the organism lessens the spread of O157:H7 infection to humans.

See also Anti-adhesion mechanisms; *Escherichia coli*; Food safety; Vaccination

EAR INFECTIONS, CHRONIC

Chronic ear infection, which is also referred to as chronic otitis media, is a recurring infection of the middle ear that occurs in animals and in humans. In humans, children between a few months of age and about six years of age are the most susceptible. The infection can be caused by **bacteria** and, occasionally, by **viruses**.

The ear consists of outer, middle, and inner regions. The outer ear is the visible portion that channels sound vibrations to the middle ear. The middle ear contains three small bones that pass on the vibration to the nerve endings housed in the inner ear. The middle ear is connected to the nasal cavity and the throat by a drainage tube known as the Eustachian tube. Improper drainage from the Eustachian tubes result in a retention of fluid in the middle ear, which can become infected by bacteria.

Such infections are common in children. Each year in the United States, over 10 million children are treated for ear infections. However, ear infections tend to be infrequent and disappear as the construction of the ear changes with age. Specifically, the Eustachian tube becomes more slanted in

orientation, which promotes drainage that is more efficient. However, in some children the normally short-term (or acute) middle ear infections begin to recur. For these children, many ear infections can occur in the first six or so years of life. Chronic ear infections affects about two out of every 10,000 people.

In some cases, surgical intervention is necessary to install a plastic drainage tube (a procedure called myringotomy) or to remove infected adenoids or tonsils, which can swell and block the eustachian tube. Myringotomy is one of the most common operations that are performed in the United States. As the ear matures structurally and the eustachian tube acquires the ability to drain more freely, the tube is removed.

As with other chronic bacterial infections, the symptoms associated with chronic ear infections can be less severe and uncomfortable than those of the acute form of the infection. Chronic infections may thus escape detection for long periods of time.

Usually a chronic ear infection is more inconvenient and uncomfortable than a health threat. However, in some cases, the chronic bacterial or viral ear infections can lead to complications that are much more serious. The infection can spread into the bones of the ear. Also, the increased pressure from the build-up of fluid can rupture the eardrum. Such damage can produce permanent impairment of hearing.

Another damaging aspect of chronic ear infections, which is shared with other chronic bacterial infections, is the damage to tissues that results from a prolonged immune response to the infection. The failure to clear the infection can produce a prolonged immune response. This response, particularly **inflammation**, can be damaging to tissue.

Treatment consists of decongestants or antihistamines to promote drainage through the Eustachian tube, and of **antibiotics** in the case of a **bacterial infection**. Even with treatment a chronic infection can take weeks or months to completely clear. Adherence to the treatment schedule is critical, especially since the symptoms of chronic ear infections can pass before the infection is fully cleared. Stopping therapy when the symptoms fade may allow the bacteria that are still surviving to become re-established as another infection. Moreover, because the bacteria were exposed to an antibacterial agent, resistance to that agent can develop, making the recurrent infection harder to eradicate.

See also Bacteria and bacterial infection

EBOLA VIRUS

The Ebola virus is one of two members of a family of **viruses** that is designated as the Filoviridae. The name of the virus comes from a river located in the Democratic Republic of the Congo, where the virus was discovered.

The species of Ebola virus are among a number of viruses that cause a disease that is typified by copious internal bleeding and bleeding from various orifices of the body, including the eyes. The disease can be swiftly devastating and results in death in over 90% of cases.

To date, four species of Ebola virus have been identified, based on differences in their genetic sequences and in the immun reaction they elicit in infected individuals. Three of the species cause disease in humans. These are Ebola-Zaire (isolated in 1976), Ebola-Sudan (also isolated in 1976), and Ebola–Ivory Coast (isolated in 1994). The fourth species, called Ebola-Reston, causes disease in primates. The latter species is capable of infecting humans but so far has not caused disease in humans. Ebola-Reston is named for the United States military primate research facility where the virus was isolated, during a 1989 outbreak of the disease caused by infected monkeys that had been imported from the Philippines. Until the non-human involvement of the disease was proven, the outbreak was thought to be the first outside of Africa.

The appearance of the Ebola virus only dates back to 1976. The explosive onset of the illness and the under-developed and wild nature of the African region of the virus's appearance, has complicated the definitive determinations of the origin and natural habitat of Ebola. The source of the Ebola virus is still unknown. However, given that filovirus, which produce similar effects, establish a latent infection in African monkeys, macaques, and chimpanzees, scientists consider the possibility that the Ebola virus likewise normally resides in an animal that lives in Africa. A search for Ebola virus in such primates has so far not revealed evidence of the virus.

Almost all confirmed cases of Ebola from 1976 to 2002 have been in Africa. In the latest outbreak, which has been ongoing since late in 2001, 54 people have died in the Gabon as of February of 2002. In the past, one individual in Liberia presented immunological evidence of exposure to Ebola, but had no symptoms. As well, a laboratory worker in England developed Ebola fever as a result of a laboratory accident in which the worker was punctured by an Ebola-containing needle.

The Ebola virus produces a high fever, headache, muscle aches, abdominal pain, tiredness and diarrhea within a few days after infecting a person. Some people will also display bloody diarrhea and vomit blood. At this stage of the disease some people recover. But, for most of those who are infected, the disease progresses within days to produce copious internal bleeding, shock and death.

Outbreaks of infection with the Ebola virus appear sporadically and suddenly. The outbreak rapidly moves through the local population and often just as quickly ends. The initial infection is presumable by contact between the person and the animal that harbors the virus. Subsequent person-to-person spread likely occurs by **contamination** with the infected blood or body tissues of an infected person in the home or hospital setting, or via contaminated needles. The fact that infected people tend to be in more under-developed regions, where even the health care facilities are not as likely to be equipped with isolation wards, furthers the risk of spread. The person-to-person passage is immediate; unlike the animal host, people do not harbor the virus for lengthy periods of time.

The possibility of air-borne transmission of the virus is debatable. Ebola-Reston may well have been transmitted from monkey to monkey in the Reston military facility via the air distribution system, since some of the monkeys that were

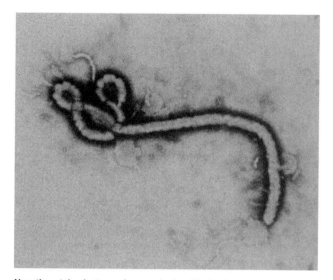

Negative stain electron micrograph of an Ebola virus.

infected were never in physical contact with the other infected monkeys. However, if the other species of the virus are capable of similar transmission, this has not yet been documented. Laboratory studies have shown that Ebola virus can remain infectious when aerosolized. But the current consensus is that airborne transmission is possible but plays a minor role in the spread of the virus.

In the intervening years between the sporadic outbreaks, the Ebola virus probably is resident in the natural reservoir.

Currently there is no cure for the infection caused by the Ebola virus. However, near the end of an outbreak of the virus in 1995 in Kikwit, Africa, blood products from survivors of the infection were transfused into those actively experiencing the disease. Of those eight people who received the blood, only one person died. Whether or not the transfused blood conveyed protective factor was not ascertained. A detailed examination of this possibility awaits another outbreak.

The molecular basis for the establishment of an infection by the Ebola virus is still also more in the realm of proposal than fact. One clue has been the finding of a glycoprotein that is a shortened version of the viral constituent in the in the circulating fluid of humans and monkeys. This protein has been suggested to function as a decoy for the **immune system**, diverting the immune defenses from the actual site of viral infection. Another immunosuppressive mechanism may be the selective invasion and damage of the spleen and the lymph nodes, which are vital in the functioning of the immune system.

The devastating infection caused by the Ebola virus is all the more remarkable given the very small size of the viral genome, or **complement** of genetic material. Fewer than a dozen genes have been detected. How the virus establishes an infection and evades the host immune system with only the capacity to code for less than twelve proteins is unknown.

See also Hemorrhagic fevers and diseases; Zoonoses

ECOLOGY OF THE ORAL CAVITY · *see*
MICROBIAL FLORA OF THE ORAL CAVITY, DENTAL CARIES

ECOLOGY OF THE STOMACH AND GASTROINTESTINAL TRACT · *see* MICROBIAL
FLORA OF THE STOMACH AND GASTROINTESTINAL TRACT

ECONOMIC USES AND BENEFITS OF MICROORGANISMS

Microorganisms have been used as tools for the production of products for millennia. Even in ancient times, the ability to produce vinegar by allowing water to percolate through wood shavings was known and widely practiced. Likewise, the **transformation** of a **yeast** suspension into beer or a suspension of crushed grapes into wine was common knowledge. The basis of these events may not have been known, but that did not impede the sale or trade of such products.

These economic uses of microorganisms are the earliest examples of **biotechnology**. As the knowledge of **bacteria** and yeast-chemical behaviors grew, other biotechnological uses for the microbes were found. A few examples include the use of the bacterium *Lactobacillus acidophilus* to produce yogurt, the exploitation of a number of different bacteria to produce a variety of cheeses, and the **fermentation** of cabbage to produce sauerkraut. In the agricultural sector, the discovery of the ability of *Rhizobium spp.* to convert elemental nitrogen to a form that was useable by a growing plant, led to the use of the microorganism as a living fertilizer that grew in association with the plant species.

In more modern times, the use of microorganisms as biotechnological agents of profit has not only continued but has explosively increased. Indeed the biotechnology sector as it is recognized today, is already a multi-billion dollar sector worldwide.

The unraveling of the structure of **DNA (deoxyribonucleic acid)**, various species of **ribonucleic acid (RNA)**, and the various processes whereby the manufacture of protein from the nucleic acid templates occurs was pivotal in advancing the use of microorganisms as factories. As important was the discovery of how to remove DNA from one region of the genome and move the DNA in a controlled way to another region of the same DNA, or DNA in a completely different organism (prokaryotic or eukaryotic). These **gene** splicing technologies, which can be accomplished by various splicing and reannealing **enzymes**, or by the use of **viruses** or mobile regions of viral DNA (such as **transposons**) as vectors have allowed biotechnologists to create what are termed "designer genes," which are designed for a specific purpose. This ability has fueled the use of microorganisms for economic gain and/or benefit.

The gene for the production of human insulin has been transferred into the genome of the common intestinal tract bacterium *Escherichia coli*. Successful expression and excretion of human insulin by the bacteria allows the production of a large amount of insulin. Additionally, because the insulin is

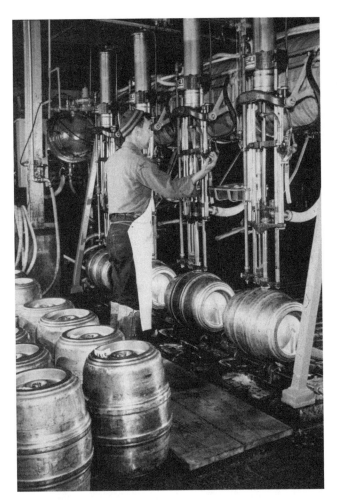

Dispensing beer into kegs.

identical to that produced in a human being, the chance of immune reaction against the protein is virtually nonexistent. The example of insulin reflects both the health benefit of the use of microbes and the economic benefit to be realized, since the mass production of insulin that is possible using bacteria lowers the cost of the product.

Other medical uses of microorganisms, particularly in the production of **antibiotics**, have been the greatest boon to humans and other animals. The list of maladies that can now be treated using microbiologically derived compounds is lengthy, and includes cystic fibrosis, hemophilia, **hepatitis** B, Karposi's sarcoma, rejection of transplanted organs, growth hormone deficiency, and cancer. The worldwide sales of medical and pharmaceutical drugs of microbial origin now exceeds U.S. $13 billion annually.

Microorganisms have also been harnessed as factories to produce compounds that are used in areas as divers as textile manufacture, agriculture, and nutrition. Enzymes discovered in bacteria that can exist at very elevated temperatures (thermophilic, or "heat loving" bacteria) cab be used to age denim to produce a "pre-washed" look. Similar enzymes are being exploited in laundry detergent that operates in hot water.

Microorganisms are used to enhance the nutritional content of plants and other food sources. The growing nutraceutical sector relies in part on the nutritional enhancements afforded by microbes. Bacteria are also useful in providing a degree of resistance to plants. An example is the use of *Bacillus thuringensis* to supply a protein that is lethal to insect when they consume it. The use of bacterial insecticides has reduced the use of chemical insecticides, which is both a cost savings to the producer and less stressful on the environment. Other bacterial enzymes and constituents of the organisms are utilized to produce materials such as plastic.

A process known as DNA fingerprinting, which relies upon enzymes that are produced and operate in bacteria, has enabled the tracing of the fate of genes in plant and animal populations, and enhanced gathering of evidence at crime scenes.

The mode of growth of bacterial populations has also proved to be exploitable as a production tool. A prime example is the surface-adherent mode of **bacterial growth** that is termed a **biofilm**. Although not known at the time, the production of vinegar hundreds of years ago was, as now, based on the percolation of water through biofilms growing on wood shavings. Immobilized bacteria can produce all manner of compounds. As well, the cells can provide a physical barrier to the flow of fluid. This dynamic aspect has been utilized in a so far small-scale way to increase the production of oil from fields oil thought to be depleted. Bacteria can plug up the zones were water and oil flows most easily. Subsequent pumping of water through the field forces the oil still resident in lower permeability areas to the surface.

With the passing of time, the realized and potential benefits of microorganisms and the implementation of strict standards of microbe use, is lessening the concern over the use of engineered microorganisms for economic and social benefit. The use of microorganisms can only increase.

See also Bioremediation; Composting, microbiological aspects; DNA chips and micro arrays

EDELMAN, GERALD M. (1929-   )

American biochemist

For his "discoveries concerning the chemical structure of antibodies," Gerald M. Edelman and his associate Rodney Porter received the 1972 Nobel Prize in physiology or medicine. During a lecture Edelman gave upon acceptance of the prize, he stated that **immunology** "provokes unusual ideas, some of which are not easily come upon through other fields of study.... For this reason, immunology will have a great impact on other branches of biology and medicine." He was to prove his own prediction correct by using his discoveries to draw conclusions not only about the **immune system** but about the nature of consciousness as well.

Born in New York City to Edward Edelman, a physician, and Anna Freedman Edelman, Gerald Maurice Edelman attended New York City public schools through high school. After graduating, he entered Ursinus College, in Collegeville, Pennsylvania, where he received his B.S. in chemistry in

1950. Four years later, he earned an M.D. degree from the University of Pennsylvania's Medical School, spending a year as medical house officer at Massachusetts General Hospital.

In 1955, Edelman joined the United States Army Medical Corps, practicing general medicine while stationed at a hospital in Paris. There, Edelman benefited from the heady atmosphere surrounding the Sorbonne, where future Nobel laureates **Jacques Lucien Monod** and **François Jacob** were originating a new study, **molecular biology**. Following his 1957 discharge from the Army, Edelman returned to New York City to take a position at Rockefeller University studying under Henry Kunkel. Kunkel, with whom Edelman would conduct his Ph.D. research, and who was examining the unique flexibility of antibodies at the time.

Antibodies are produced in response to infection in order to work against diseases in diverse ways. They form a class of large blood proteins called globulins—more specifically, immunoglobulins—made in the body's lymph tissues. Each immunoglobulin is specifically directed to recognize and incapacitate one **antigen**, the chemical signal of an infection. Yet they all share a very similar structure.

Through the 1960s and 1970s, a debate raged between two schools of scientists to explain the situation whereby antibodies share so many characteristics yet are able to perform many different functions. In one camp, George Wells Beadle and **Edward Lawrie Tatum** argued that despite the remarkable diversity displayed by each **antibody**, each immunoglobulin, must be coded for by a single **gene**. This has been referred to as the "one gene, one protein" theory. But, argued the opposing camp, led by the Australian physician Sir **Frank Macfarlane Burnet**, if each antibody required its own code within the **DNA** (**deoxyribonucleic acid**), the body's master plan of protein structure, the immune system alone would take up all the possible codes offered by the human DNA.

Both camps generated theories, but Edelman eventually disagreed with both sides of the debate, offering a third possibility for antibody synthesis in 1967. Though not recognized at the time because of its radical nature, the theory he and his associate, Joseph Gally, proposed would later be confirmed as essentially correct. It depended on the vast diversity that can come from chance in a system as complex as the living organism. Each time a cell divided, they theorized, tiny errors in the transcription—or reading of the code—could occur, yielding slightly different proteins upon each misreading. Edelman and Gally proposed that the human body turns the advantage of this variability in **immunoglobulins** to its own ends. Many strains of antigens when introduced into the body modify the shape of the various immunoglobulins in order to prevent the recurrence of disease. This is why many illnesses provide for their own cure—why humans can only get chicken pox once, for instance.

But the proof of their theory would require advances in the state of biochemical techniques. Research in the 1950s and 1960s was hampered by the difficulty in isolating immunoglobulins. The molecules themselves are comparatively large, too large to be investigated by the chemical means then available. Edelman and Rodney Porter, with whom Edelman was to be honored with the Nobel Prize, sought methods of breaking immunoglobulins into smaller units that could more profitably be studied. Their hope was that these fragments would retain enough of their properties to provide insight into the functioning of the whole.

Porter became the first to split an immunoglobulin, obtaining an "active fragment" from rabbit blood as early as 1950. Porter believed the immunoglobulin to be one long continuous molecule made up of 1,300 amino acids—the building blocks of proteins. However, Edelman could not accept this conclusion, noting that even insulin, with its 51 amino acids, was made up of two shorter strings of amino acid chains working as a unit. His doctoral thesis investigated several methods of splitting immunoglobulin molecules, and, after receiving his Ph.D. in 1960 he remained at Rockefeller as a faculty member, continuing his research.

Porter's method of splitting the molecules used **enzymes** that acted as chemical knives, breaking apart amino acids. In 1961 Edelman and his colleague, M. D. Poulik succeeded in splitting IgG—one of the most studied varieties of immunoglobulin in the blood—into two components by using a method known as "reductive cleavage." The technique allowed them to divide IgG into what are known as light and heavy chains. Data from their experiments and from those of the Czech researcher, Frantisek Franek, established the intricate nature of the antibody's "active sight." The sight occurs at the folding of the two chains, which forms a unique pocket to trap the antigen. Porter combined these findings with his, and, in 1962, announced that the basic structure of IgG had been determined. Their experiments set off a flurry of research into the nature of antibodies in the 1960s. Information was shared throughout the scientific community in a series of informal meetings referred to as "Antibody Workshops," taking place across the globe. Edelman and Porter dominated the discussions, and their work led the way to a wave of discoveries.

Still, a key drawback to research remained. In any naturally obtained immunoglobulin sample a mixture of ever so slightly different molecules would reduce the overall purity. Based on a crucial finding by Kunkel in the 1950s, Porter and Edelman concentrated their study on myelomas, cancers of the immunoglobulin-producing cells, exploiting the unique nature of these cancers. Kunkel had determined that since all the cells produced by these cancerous myelomas were descended from a common ancestor they would produce a homogeneous series of antibodies. A pure sample could be isolated for experimentation. Porter and Edelman studied the amino acid sequence in subsections of different myelomas, and in 1965, as Edelman would later describe it: "Mad as we were, [we] started on the whole molecule." The project, completed in 1969, determined the order of all 1,300 amino acids present in the protein, the longest sequence determined at that time.

Throughout the 1970s, Edelman continued his research, expanding it to include other substances that stimulate the immune system, but by the end of the decade the principle he and Poulik uncovered led him to conceive a radical theory of how the brain works. Just as the structurally limited immune system must deal with myriad invading organisms, the brain must process vastly complex sensory data with a theoretically limited number of switches, or neurons.

Rather than an incoming sensory signal triggering a predetermined pathway through the nervous system, Edelman theorized that it leads to a **selection** from among several choices. That is, rather than seeing the nervous system as a relatively fixed biological structure, Edelman envisioned it as a fluid system based on three interrelated stages of functioning.

In the formation of the nervous system, cells receiving signals from others surrounding them fan out like spreading ivy—not to predetermined locations, but rather to regions determined by the concert of these local signals. The signals regulate the ultimate position of each cell by controlling the production of a cellular glue in the form of cell-adhesion molecules. They anchor neighboring groups of cells together. Once established, these cellular connections are fixed, but the exact pattern is different for each individual.

The second feature of Edelman's theory allows for an individual response to any incoming signal. A specific pattern of neurons must be made to recognize the face of one's grandmother, for instance, but the pattern is different in every brain. While the vast complexity of these connections allows for some of the variability in the brain, it is in the third feature of the theory that Edelman made the connection to immunology. The neural networks are linked to each other in layers. An incoming signal passes through and between these sheets in a specific pathway. The pathway, in this theory, ultimately determines what the brain experiences, but just as the immune system modifies itself with each new incoming virus, Edelman theorized that the brain modifies itself in response to each new incoming signal. In this way, Edelman sees all the systems of the body being guided in one unified process, a process that depends on organization but that accommodates the world's natural randomness.

Dr. Edelman has received honorary degrees from a number of universities, including the University of Pennsylvania, Ursinus College, Williams College, and others. Besides his Nobel Prize, his other academic awards include the Spenser Morris Award, the Eli Lilly Prize of the American Chemical Society, Albert Einstein Commemorative Award, California Institute of Technology's Buchman Memorial Award, and the Rabbi Shai Schaknai Memorial Prize.

A member of many academic organizations, including New York and National Academy of Sciences, American Society of Cell Biologists, Genetics Society, American Academy of Arts and Sciences, and the American Philosophical Society, Dr. Edelman is also one of the few international members of the Academy of Sciences, Institute of France. In 1974, he became a Vincent Astor Distinguished Professor, serving on the board of governors of the Weizmann Institute of Science and is also a trustee of the Salk Institute for Biological Studies. Dr. Edelman married Maxine Morrison on June 11, 1950; the couple have two sons and one daughter.

See also Antibody and antigen; Antibody formation and kinetics; Antibody, monoclonal; Antibody-antigen, biochemical and molecular reactions; Antigenic mimicry

EHRLICH, PAUL (1854-1915)

German physician

Paul Ehrlich's pioneering experiments with cells and body tissue revealed the fundamental principles of the **immune system** and established the legitimacy of chemotherapy—the use of chemical drugs to treat disease. His discovery of a drug that cured **syphilis** saved many lives and demonstrated the potential of systematic drug research. Ehrlich's studies of dye reactions in blood cells helped establish hematology, the scientific field concerned with blood and blood-forming organs, as a recognized discipline. Many of the new terms he coined as a way to describe his innovative research, including "chemotherapy," are still in use. From 1877 to 1914, Ehrlich published 232 papers and books, won numerous awards, and received five honorary degrees. In 1908, Ehrlich received the Nobel Prize in medicine or physiology.

Ehrlich was born on March 14, 1854, in Strehlen, Silesia, once a part of Germany, but now a part of Poland known as Strzelin. He was the fourth child after three sisters in a Jewish family. His father, Ismar Ehrlich, and mother, Rosa Weigert, were both innkeepers. As a boy, Ehrlich was influenced by several relatives who studied science. His paternal grandfather, Heimann Ehrlich, made a living as a liquor merchant but kept a private laboratory and gave lectures on science to the citizens of Strehlen. Karl Weigert, cousin of Ehrlich's mother, became a well-known pathologist. Ehrlich, who was close friends with Weigert, often joined his cousin in his lab, where he learned how to stain cells with dye in order to see them better under the **microscope**. Ehrlich's research into the dye reactions of cells continued during his time as a university student. He studied science and medicine at the universities of Breslau, Strasbourg, Freiburg, and Leipzig. Although Ehrlich conducted most of his course work at Breslau, he submitted his final dissertation to the University of Leipzig, which awarded him a medical degree in 1878.

Ehrlich's 1878 doctoral thesis, "Contributions to the Theory and Practice of Histological Staining," suggests that even at this early stage in his career he recognized the depth of possibility and discovery in his chosen research field. In his experiments with many dyes, Ehrlich had learned how to manipulate chemicals in order to obtain specific effects: Methylene blue dye, for example, stained nerve cells without discoloring the tissue around them. These experiments with dye reactions formed the backbone of Ehrlich's career and led to two important contributions to science. First, improvements in staining permitted scientists to examine cells, healthy or unhealthy, and **microorganisms**, including those that caused disease. Ehrlich's work ushered in a new era of medical diagnosis and histology (the study of cells), which alone would have guaranteed Ehrlich a place in scientific history. Secondly, and more significantly from a scientific standpoint, Ehrlich's early experiments revealed that certain cells have an affinity to certain dyes. To Ehrlich, it was clear that chemical and physical reactions were taking place in the stained tissue. He theorized that chemical reactions governed all biological life processes. If this were true, Ehrlich reasoned, then chemicals could perhaps be used to heal diseased cells and to attack harmful microorganisms. Ehrlich began studying the chemical structure of the dyes he used and postulated theories for what chemical reactions might be taking place in the body in the presence of dyes and other chemical agents. These efforts would eventually lead Ehrlich to study the immune system.

Upon Ehrlich's graduation, medical clinic director Friedrich von Frerichs immediately offered the young scientist a position as head physician at the Charite Hospital in Berlin. Von Frerichs recognized that Ehrlich, with his penchant for strong cigars and mineral water, was a unique talent, one that should be excused from clinical work and be allowed to pursue his research uninterrupted. The late nineteenth century was a time when infectious diseases like cholera and **typhoid fever** were incurable and fatal. Syphilis, a sexually transmitted disease caused by a then unidentified microorganism, was an epidemic, as was **tuberculosis**, another disease whose cause had yet to be named. To treat human disease, medical scientists knew they needed a better understanding of harmful microorganisms.

At the Charite Hospital, Ehrlich studied blood cells under the microscope. Although blood cells can be found in a perplexing multiplicity of forms, Ehrlich was with his dyes able to begin identifying them. His systematic cataloging of the cells laid the groundwork for what would become the field of hematology. Ehrlich also furthered his understanding of chemistry by meeting with professionals from the chemical industry. These contacts gave him information about the structure and preparation of new chemicals and kept him supplied with new dyes and chemicals.

Ehrlich's slow and steady work with stains resulted in a sudden and spectacular achievement. On March 24, 1882, Ehrlich had heard **Robert Koch** announce to the Berlin Physiological Society that he had identified the bacillus causing tuberculosis under the microscope. Koch's method of staining the bacillus for study, however, was less than ideal. Ehrlich immediately began experimenting and was soon able to show Koch an improved method of staining the tubercle bacillus. The technique has since remained in use.

On April 14, 1883, Ehrlich married 19-year-old Hedwig Pinkus in the Neustadt Synagogue. Ehrlich had met Pinkus, the daughter of an affluent textile manufacturer of Neustadt, while visiting relatives in Berlin. The marriage brought two daughters. In March, 1885, von Frerichs committed suicide and Ehrlich suddenly found himself without a mentor. Von Frerichs's successor as director of Charite Hospital, Karl Gerhardt, was far less impressed with Ehrlich and forced him to focus on clinical work rather than research. Though complying, Ehrlich was highly dissatisfied with the change. Two years later, Ehrlich resigned from the Charite Hospital, ostensibly because he wished to relocate to a dry climate to cure himself of tuberculosis. The mild case of the disease, which Ehrlich had diagnosed using his staining techniques, was almost certainly contracted from cultures in his lab. In September of 1888, Ehrlich and his wife embarked on an extended journey to southern Europe and Egypt and returned to Berlin in the spring of 1889 with Ehrlich's health improved.

In Berlin, Ehrlich set up a small private laboratory with financial help from his father-in-law, and in 1890, he was hon-

•

ored with an appointment as Extraordinary Professor at the University of Berlin. In 1891, Ehrlich accepted Robert Koch's invitation to join him at the Institute for Infectious Diseases, newly created for Koch by the Prussian government. At the institute, Koch began his immunological research by demonstrating that mice fed or injected with the toxins ricin and abrin developed antitoxins. He also proved that antibodies were passed from mother to offspring through breast milk. Ehrlich joined forces with Koch and **Emil Adolf von Behring** to find a cure for **diphtheria**, a deadly childhood disease. Although von Behring had identified the antibodies to diphtheria, he still faced great difficulties transforming the discovery into a potent yet safe cure for humans. Using blood drawn from horses and goats infected with the disease, the scientists worked together to concentrate and purify an effective antitoxin. Ehrlich's particular contribution to the cure was his method of measuring an effective dose.

The commercialization of a diphtheria antitoxin began in 1892 and was manufactured by Höchst Chemical Works. Royalties from the drug profits promised to make Ehrlich and von Behring wealthy men. But Ehrlich, possibly at von Behring's urging, accepted a government position in 1885 to monitor the production of the diphtheria serum. Conflict-of-interest clauses obligated Ehrlich to withdraw from his profit-sharing agreement. Forced to stand by as the diphtheria antitoxin made von Behring a wealthy man, he and von Behring quarreled and eventually parted. Although it is unclear whether bitterness over the royalty agreement sparked the quarrel, it certainly couldn't have helped a relationship that was often tumultuous. Although the two scientists continued to exchange news in letters, both scientific and personal, the two scientists never met again.

In June of 1896, the Prussian government invited Ehrlich to direct its newly created Royal Institute for Serum Research and Testing in Steglitz, a suburb of Berlin. For the first time, Ehrlich had his own institute. In 1896, Ehrlich was invited by Franz Adickes, the mayor of Frankfurt, and by Friedrich Althoff, the Prussian Minister of Educational and Medical Affairs, to move his research to Frankfurt. Ehrlich accepted and the Royal Institute for Experimental Therapy opened on November 8, 1899. Ehrlich was to remain as its director until his death sixteen years later. The years in Frankfurt would prove to be among Ehrlich's most productive.

In his speech at the opening of the Institute for Experimental Therapy, Ehrlich seized the opportunity to describe in detail his "side-chain theory" of how antibodies worked. "Side-chain" is the name given to the appendages on benzene molecules that allow it to react with other chemicals. Ehrlich believed all molecules had similar side-chains that allowed them to link with molecules, nutrients, infectious toxins and other substances. Although Ehrlich's theory is false, his efforts to prove it led to a host of new discoveries and guided much of his future research.

The move to Frankfurt marked the dawn of **chemotherapy** as Ehrlich erected various chemical agents against a host of dangerous microorganisms. In 1903, scientists had discovered that the cause of **sleeping sickness**, a deadly disease

prevalent in Africa, was a species of trypanosomes (parasitic protozoans). With help from Japanese scientist Kiyoshi Shiga, Ehrlich worked to find a dye that destroyed trypanosomes in infected mice. In 1904, he discovered such a dye, which was dubbed "trypan red."

Success with trypan red spurred Ehrlich to begin testing other chemicals against disease. To conduct his methodical and painstaking experiments with an enormous range of chemicals, Ehrlich relied heavily on his assistants. To direct their work, he made up a series of instructions on colored cards in the evening and handed them out each morning. Although such a management strategy did not endear him to his lab associates, and did not allow them opportunity for their own research, Ehrlich's approach was often successful. In one famous instance, Ehrlich ordered his staff to disregard the accepted notion of the chemical structure of atoxyl and to instead proceed in their work based on his specifications of the chemical. Two of the three medical scientists working with Ehrlich were appalled at his scientific heresy and ended their employment at the laboratory. Ehrlich's hypothesis concerning atoxyl turned out to have been correct and would eventually lead to the discovery of a chemical cure for syphilis.

In September of 1906, Ehrlich's laboratory became a division of the new Georg Speyer Haus for Chemotherapeutical Research. The research institute, endowed by the wealthy widow of Georg Speyer for the exclusive purpose of continuing Ehrlich's work in chemotherapy, was built next to Ehrlich's existing laboratory. In a speech at the opening of the new institute, Ehrlich used the phrase "magic bullets" to illustrate his hope of finding chemical compounds that would enter the body, attack only the offending microorganisms or malignant cells, and leave healthy tissue untouched. In 1908, Ehrlich's work on **immunity**, particularly his contribution to the diphtheria antitoxin, was honored with the Nobel Prize in medicine or physiology. He shared the prize with Russian bacteriologist **Élie Metchnikoff**.

By the time Ehrlich's lab formally joined the Speyer Haus, he had already tested over 300 chemical compounds against trypanosomes and the syphilis spirochete (distinguished as slender and spirally undulating **bacteria**). With each test given a laboratory number, Ehrlich was testing compounds numbering in the nine hundreds before realizing that "compound 606" was a highly potent drug effective against relapsing fever and syphilis. Due to an assistant's error, the potential of compound 606 had been overlooked for nearly two years until Ehrlich's associate, Sahashiro Hata, experimented with it again. On June 10, 1909, Ehrlich and Hata filed a patent for 606 for its use against relapsing fever.

The first favorable results of 606 against syphilis were announced at the Congress for Internal Medicine held at Wiesbaden in April 1910. Although Ehrlich emphasized he was reporting only preliminary results, news of a cure for the devastating and widespread disease swept through the European and American medical communities and Ehrlich was besieged with requests for the drug. Physicians and victims of the disease clamored at his doors. Ehrlich, painfully aware that mishandled dosages could blind or even kill patients, begged physicians to wait until he could test 606 on ten or twenty thousand more patients. There was no halting the demand, however, and the Georg Speyer Haus ultimately manufactured and distributed 65,000 units of 606 to physicians all over the globe free of charge. Eventually, the large-scale production of 606, under the commercial name "Salvarsan," was taken over by Höchst Chemical Works. The next four years, although largely triumphant, were also filled with reports of patients' deaths and maiming at the hands of doctors who failed to administer Salvarsan properly.

In 1913, in an address to the International Medical Congress in London, Ehrlich cited trypan red and Salvarsan as examples of the power of chemotherapy and described his vision of chemotherapy's future. The City of Frankfurt honored Ehrlich by renaming the street in front of the Georg Speyer Haus "Paul Ehrlichstrasse." Yet in 1914, Ehrlich was forced to defend himself against claims made by a Frankfurt newspaper, *Die Wahrheit* (The Truth), that Ehrlich was testing Salvarsan on prostitutes against their will, that the drug was a fraud, and that Ehrlich's motivation for promoting it was personal monetary gain. In June 1914, Frankfurt city authorities took action against the newspaper and Ehrlich testified in court as an expert witness. Ehrlich's name was finally cleared and the newspaper's publisher sentenced to a year in jail, but the trial left Ehrlich deeply depressed. In December, 1914, he suffered a mild stroke.

Ehrlich's health failed to improve and the start of World War I had further discouraged him. Afflicted with arteriosclerosis, his health deteriorated rapidly. He died in Bad Homburg, Prussia (now Germany), on August 20, 1915, after a second stroke. Ehrlich was buried in Frankfurt. Following the German Nazi era, during which time Ehrlich's widow and daughters were persecuted as Jews before fleeing the country and the sign marking Paul Ehrlichstrasse was torn down, Frankfurt once again honored its famous resident. The Institute for Experimental Therapy changed its name to the Paul Ehrlich Institute and began offering the biennial Paul Ehrlich Prize in one of Ehrlich's fields of research as a memorial to its founder.

See also History of immunology; History of microbiology; History of public health; History of the development of antibiotics; Infection and resistance

ELECTRON MICROSCOPE, TRANSMISSION AND SCANNING

Described by the Nobel Society as "one of the most important inventions of the century," the electron **microscope** is a valuable and versatile research tool. The first working models were constructed by German engineers **Ernst Ruska** and Max Knoll in 1932, and since that time, the electron microscope has found numerous applications in chemistry, engineering, medicine, **molecular biology** and genetics.

Electron microscopes allow molecular biologists to study small structural details related to cellular function. Using an electron microscope, it is possible to observe and

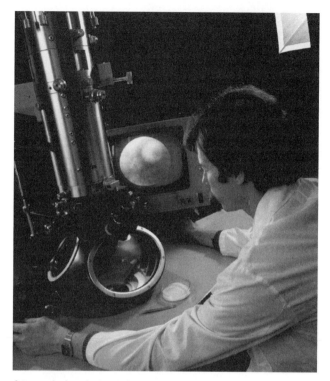

A transmission electron microscope.

study many internal cellular structures (organelles). Electron microscopy can also be used to visualize proteins, virus particles, and other microbiological materials.

At the turn of the twentieth century, the science of microscopy had reached an impasse: because all optical microscopes relied upon visible light, even the most powerful could not detect an image smaller than the wavelength of light used. This was tremendously frustrating for physicists, who were anxious to study the structure of matter on an atomic level. Around this time, French physicist **Louis de Broglie** theorized that subatomic particles sometimes act like waves, but with much shorter wavelengths. Ruska, then a student at the University of Berlin, wondered why a microscope couldn't be designed that was similar in function to a normal microscope but used a beam of electrons instead of a beam of light. Such a microscope could resolve images thousands of times smaller than the wavelength of visible light.

There was one major obstacle to Ruska's plan, however. In a compound microscope, a series of lenses are used to focus, magnify, and refocus the image. In order for an electron-based instrument to perform as a microscope, some device was required to focus the electron beam. Ruska knew that electrons could be manipulated within a magnetic field, and in the late 1920s, he designed a magnetic coil that acted as an electron lens. With this breakthrough, Ruska and Knoll constructed their first electron microscope. Though the prototype model was capable of magnification of only a few hundred power (about that of an average laboratory microscope), it proved that electrons could indeed be used in microscopy.

The microscope built by Ruska and Knoll is similar in principle to a compound microscope. A beam of electrons is directed at a specimen sliced thin enough to allow the beam to pass through. As they travel through, the electrons are deflected according to the atomic structure of the specimen. The beam is then focused by the magnetic coil onto a photographic plate; when developed, the image on the plate shows the specimen at very high magnification.

Scientists worldwide immediately embraced Ruska's invention as a major breakthrough in microscopy, and they directed their own efforts toward improving upon its precision and flexibility. A Canadian-American physicist, James Hillier, constructed a microscope from Ruska's design that was nearly 20 times more powerful. In 1939, modifications made by Vladimir Kosma Zworykin enabled the electron microscope to be used for studying **viruses** and protein molecules. Eventually, electron microscopy was greatly improved, with microscopes able to magnify an image 2,000,000 times. One particularly interesting outcome of such research was the invention of holography and the hologram by Hungarian-born engineer Dennis Gabor in 1947. Gabor's work with this three-dimensional photography found numerous applications upon development of the laser in 1960.

There are now two distinct types of electron microscopes: the transmission variety (such as Ruska's), and the scanning variety. The Transmission Electron Microscope (TEM), developed in the 1930's, operates on the same physical principles as the light microscope but provides enhanced resolution due to the shorter wavelengths of electron beams. TEM offers resolutions to approximately 0.2 nanometers as opposed to 200 nanometers for the best light microscopes. The TEM has been used in all areas of biological and biomedical investigations because of its ability to view the finest cell structures. Scanning electron microscopes (SEM), instead of being focused by the scanner to peer through the specimen, are used to observe electrons that are scattered from the surface of the specimen as the beam contacts it. The beam is moved along the surface, scanning for any irregularities. The scanning electron microscope yields an extremely detailed three-dimensional image of a specimen but can only be used at low resolution; used in tandem, the scanning and transmission electron microscopes are powerful research tools.

Today, electron microscopes can be found in most hospital and medical research laboratories.

The advances made by Ruska, Knoll, and Hillier have contributed directly to the development of the field ion microscope (invented by Erwin Wilhelm Muller) and the scanning tunneling microscope (invented by Heinrich Rohrer and Gerd Binnig), now considered the most powerful optical tools in the world. For his work, Ruska shared the 1986 Nobel Prize for physics with Binnig and Rohrer.

See also Biotechnology; Laboratory techniques in immunology; Laboratory techniques in microbiology; Microscope and microscopy; Molecular biology and molecular genetics

ELECTRON MICROSCOPIC EXAMINATION OF MICROORGANISMS

Depending upon the **microscope** used and the preparation technique, an entire intact organism, or thin slices through the interior of the sample can be examined by electron microscopy. The electron beam can pass through very thin sections of a sample (transmission electron microscopy) or bounced off of the surface of an intact sample (scanning electron microscopy). Samples must be prepared prior to insertion into the microscope because the microscope operates in a vacuum. Biological material is comprised mainly of water and so would not be preserved, making meaningful interpretation of the resulting images impossible. For transmission electron microscopy, where very thin samples are required, the sample must also be embedded in a resin that can be sliced.

For scanning electron microscopy, a sample is coated with a metal (typically, gold) from which the incoming electrons will bounce. The deflected electrons are detected and converted to a visual image. This simple-sounding procedure requires much experience to execute properly.

Samples for transmission electron microscopy are processed differently. The sample can be treated, or fixed, with one or more chemicals to maintain the structure of the specimen. Chemicals such as glutaraldehyde or formaldehyde act to cross-link the various constituents. Osmium tetroxide and uranyl acetate can be added to increase the contrast under the electron beam. Depending on the embedding resin to be used, the water might then need to be removed from the chemically fixed specimen. In this case, the water is gradually replaced with ethanol or acetone and then the dehydrating fluid is gradually replaced with the resin, which has a consistency much like that of honey. The resin is then hardened, producing a block containing the sample. Other resins, such as Lowicryl, mix easily with water. In this case, the hydrated sample is exposed to gradually increasing concentrations of the resins, to replace the water with resin. The resin is then hardened.

Sections a few millionths of a meter in thickness are often examined by electron microscopy. The sections are sliced off from a prepared specimen in a device called a microtome, where the sample is passed by the sharp edge of a glass or diamond knife and the slice is floated off onto the surface of a volume of water positioned behind the knife-edge. The slice is gathered onto a special supporting grid. Often the section is exposed to solutions of uranyl acetate and lead citrate to further increase contrast. Then, the grid can be inserted into the microscope for examination.

Samples can also be rapidly frozen instead of being chemically fixed. This cryopreservation is so rapid that the internal water does not form structurally disruptive crystals. Frozen thin sections are then obtained using a special knife in a procedure called cryosectioning. These are inserted into the microscope using a special holder that maintains the very cold temperature.

Thin sections (both chemically fixed and frozen) and whole samples can also be exposed to antibodies in order to reveal the location of the target **antigen** within the thin section.

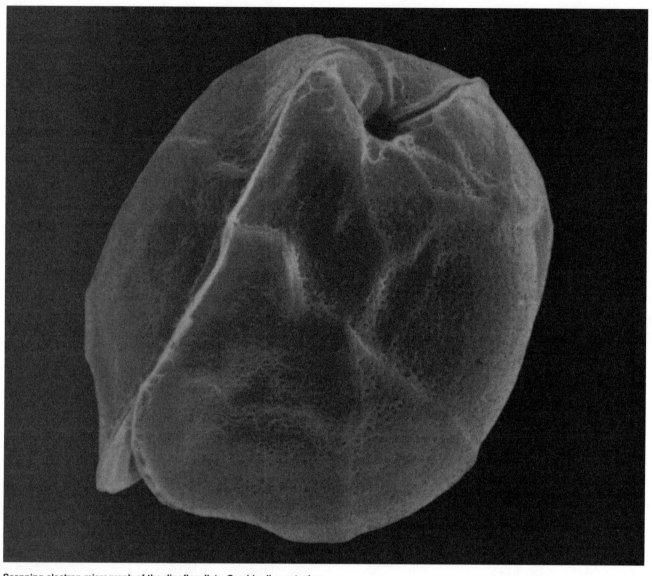

Scanning electron micrograph of the dinoflagellate *Gambierdiscus toxicus*.

This technique is known as immunoelectron microscopy. Care is required during the fixation and other preparation steps to ensure that the antigenic sites are not changed so that **antibody** is still capable of binding to the antigen.

Frozen samples can also be cracked open by allowing the sample to strike the sharp edge of a frozen block. The crack, along the path of least chemical resistance, can reveal internal details of the specimen. This technique is called freeze-fracture. Frozen water can be removed from the fracture (freeze-etching) to allow the structural details of the specimen to appear more prominent.

Samples such as **viruses** are often examined in the transmission **electron microscope** using a technique called negative staining. Here, sample is collected on the surface of a thin plastic support film. Then, a solution of stain is flowed over the surface. When the excess stain is carefully removed, stain will pool in the surface irregularities. Once in the microscope, electrons will not pass through the puddles of stain, producing a darker appearing region in the processed image of the specimen. Negative staining is also useful to reveal surface details of **bacteria** and appendages such as pili, flagella and spinae. A specialized form of the staining technique can also be used to visualize genetic material.

Electron microscopes exist that allow specimens to be examined in their natural, water-containing, state. Examination of living specimens has also been achieved. The so-called high-vacuum environmental microscope is finding an increasing application in the examination of microbiological samples such as **biofilms**.

See also Bacterial ultrastructure; Microscope and microscopy

•

ELECTRON TRANSPORT SYSTEM

The electron transport system is a coordinated series of reactions that operate in eukaryotic organisms and in prokaryotic **microorganisms**, which enables electrons to be passed from one protein to another. The purpose of the electron transport system is to pump hydrogen ions to an enzyme that utilizes the energy from the ions to manufacture the molecule known as adenine triphosphate (ATP). ATP is essentially the fuel or energy source for cellular reactions, providing the power to accomplish the many varied reactions necessary for life.

The reactions of the electron transport system can also be termed oxidative phosphorylation.

In microorganisms such as **bacteria** the machinery of the electron transport complex is housed in the single membrane of Gram-positive bacteria or in the outer membrane of Gram-negative bacteria. The electron transport process is initiated by the active, energy-requiring movement of protons (which are hydrogen ions) from the interior gel-like **cytoplasm** of the bacterium to a protein designated NADH. This protein accepts the hydrogen ion and shuttles the ion to the exterior. In doing so, the NADH is converted to NAD, with the consequent release of an electron. The released electron then begins a journey that moves it sequentially to a series of electron acceptors positioned in the membrane. Each component of the chain is able to first accept and then release an electron. Upon the electron release, the protein is ready to accept another electron. The electron transport chain can be envisioned as a coordinated and continual series of switches of its constituents from electron acceptance to electron release mode.

The energy of the electron transport system decreases as the electrons move "down" the chain. The effect is somewhat analogous to water running down a slope from a higher energy state to a lower energy state. The flow of electrons ends at the final compound in the chain, which is called ATP synthase.

The movement of electrons through the series of reactions causes the release of hydrogen to the exterior, and an increased concentration of OH- ions (hydroxyl ions) in the interior of the bacterium.

The proteins that participate in the flow of electrons are the flavoproteins and the cytochromes. These proteins are ubiquitous to virtually all prokaryotes and **eukaryotes** that have been studied.

The ATP synthase attempts to restore the equilibrium of the hydrogen and hydronium ions by pumping a hydrogen ion back into the cell for each electron that is accepted. The energy supplied by the hydrogen ion is used to add a phosphate group to a molecule called adenine diphosphate (ADP), generating ATP.

In aerobic bacteria, which require the presence of oxygen for survival, the final electron acceptor is an atom of oxygen. If oxygen is absent, the electron transport process halts. Some bacteria have an alternate process by which energy can be generated. But, for many aerobic bacteria, the energy produced in the absence of oxygen cannot sustain bacterial survival for an extended period of time. Besides the lack of oxygen, compounds such as cyanide block the electron transport chain. Cyanide accomplishes this by binding to one of the cytochrome components of the chain. The blockage halts ATP production.

The flow of hydrogen atoms back through the membrane of bacteria and the mitochondrial membrane of eukaryotic cells acts to couple the electron transport system with the formation of ATP. Peter Mitchell, English chemist (1920–1992), proposed this linkage in 1961. He termed this the chemiosmotic theory. The verification of the mechanism proposed in the chemiosmotic theory earned Mitchell a 1978 Nobel Prize.

See also Bacterial membranes and cell wall; Bacterial ultrastructure; Biochemistry; Cell membrane transport

ELECTROPHORESIS

Protein electrophoresis is a sensitive analytical form of chromatography that allows the separation of charged molecules in a solution medium under the influence of an electric field. A wide range of molecules may be separated by electrophoresis, including, but not limited to **DNA**, **RNA,** and protein molecules.

The degree of separation and rate of molecular migration of mixtures of molecules depends upon the size and shape of the molecules, the respective molecular charges, the strength of the electric field, the type of medium used (e.g., cellulose acetate, starch gels, paper, agarose, polyacrylamide gel, etc.) and the conditions of the medium (e.g., electrolyte concentration, **pH**, ionic strength, viscosity, temperature, etc.).

Some mediums (also known as support matrices) are porous gels that can also act as a physical sieve for macromolecules.

In general, the medium is mixed with buffers needed to carry the electric charge applied to the system. The medium/buffer matrix is placed in a tray. Samples of molecules to be separated are loaded into wells at one end of the matrix. As electrical current is applied to the tray, the matrix takes on this charge and develops positively and negatively charged ends. As a result, molecules such as DNA and RNA that are negatively charged, are pulled toward the positive end of the gel.

Because molecules have differing shapes, sizes, and charges they are pulled through the matrix at different rates and this, in turn, causes a separation of the molecules. Generally, the smaller and more charged a molecule, the faster the molecule moves through the matrix.

When DNA is subjected to electrophoresis, the DNA is first broken by what are termed **restriction enzymes** that act to cut the DNA is selected places. After being subjected to restriction **enzymes**, DNA molecules appear as bands (composed of similar length DNA molecules) in the electrophoresis matrix. Because nucleic acids always carry a negative charge, separation of nucleic acids occurs strictly by molecular size.

Proteins have net charges determined by charged groups of amino acids from which they are constructed. Proteins can also be amphoteric compounds, meaning they can take on a negative or positive charge depending on the surrounding conditions. A protein in one solution might carry a positive charge in a particular medium and thus migrate toward the negative end of the matrix. In another solution, the same protein might carry a negative charge and migrate toward the positive end of the matrix. For each protein there is an isoelectric point related to a pH characteristic for that protein where the protein molecule has no net charge. Thus, by varying pH in the matrix, additional refinements in separation are possible.

The advent of electrophoresis revolutionized the methods of protein analysis. Swedish biochemist Arne Tiselius was awarded the 1948 Nobel Prize in chemistry for his pioneering research in electrophoretic analysis. Tiselius studied the separation of serum proteins in a tube (subsequently named a Tiselius tube) that contained a solution subjected to an electric field.

Sodium dodecyl sulfate (SDS) polyacrylamide gel electrophoresis techniques pioneered in the 1960s provided a powerful means of protein fractionation (separation). Because the protein bands did not always clearly separate (i.e., there was often a great deal of overlap in the protein bands) only small numbers of molecules could be separated. The subsequent development in the 1970s of a two-dimensional electrophoresis technique allowed greater numbers of molecules to be separated.

Two-dimensional electrophoresis is actually the fusion of two separate separation procedures. The first separation (dimension) is achieved by isoelectric focusing (IEF) that separates protein polypeptide chains according to amino acid composition. IEF is based on the fact that proteins will, when subjected to a pH gradient, move to their isoelectric point. The second separation is achieved via SDS slab gel electrophoresis that separates the molecule by molecular size. Instead of broad, overlapping bands, the result of this two-step process is the formation of a two-dimensional pattern of spots, each comprised of a unique protein or protein fragment. These spots are subsequently subjected to staining and further analysis.

Some techniques involve the application of radioactive labels to the proteins. Protein fragments subsequently obtained from radioactively labels proteins may be studied my radiographic measures.

There are many variations on gel electrophoresis with wide-ranging applications. These specialized techniques include Southern, Northern, and Western blotting. Blots are named according to the molecule under study. In Southern blots, DNA is cut with restriction enzymes then probed with radioactive DNA. In Northern blotting, RNA is probed with radioactive DNA or RNA. Western blots target proteins with radioactive or enzymatically tagged antibodies.

Modern electrophoresis techniques now allow the identification of homologous DNA sequences and have become an integral part of research into **gene** structure, gene expression, and the diagnosis of heritable and autoimmune diseases. Electrophoretic analysis also allows the identification of bacterial and viral strains and is finding increasing acceptance as a powerful forensic tool.

See also Autoimmunity and autoimmune diseases; Biochemical analysis techniques; Immunoelectrophoresis

ELION, GERTRUDE BELLE (1918-1999)
American biochemist

Gertrude Belle Elion's innovative approach to drug discovery advanced the understanding of cellular **metabolism** and led to the development of medications for leukemia, gout, **herpes**, **malaria**, and the rejection of transplanted organs. Azidothymidine (AZT), the first drug approved for the treatment of **AIDS**, came out of her laboratory shortly after her retirement in 1983. One of the few women who held a top post at a major pharmaceutical company, Elion worked at Wellcome Research Laboratories for nearly five decades. Her work, with colleague George H. Hitchings, was recognized with the Nobel Prize for physiology or medicine in 1988. Her Nobel Prize was notable for several reasons: few winners have been women, few have lacked the Ph.D., and few have been industrial researchers.

Elion was born on January 23, 1918, in New York City, the first of two children, to Robert Elion and Bertha Cohen. Her father, a dentist, immigrated to the United States from Lithuania as a small boy. Her mother came to the United States from Russia at the age of fourteen. Elion, an excellent student who was accelerated two years by her teachers, graduated from high school at the height of the Great Depression. As a senior in high school, she had witnessed the painful death of her grandfather from stomach cancer and vowed to become a cancer researcher. She was able to attend college only because several New York City schools, including Hunter College, offered free tuition to students with good grades. In college, she majored in chemistry.

In 1937, Elion graduated Phi Beta Kappa from Hunter College with a B.A. at the age of nineteen. Despite her outstanding academic record, Elion's early efforts to find a job as a chemist failed. One laboratory after another told her that they had never employed a woman chemist. Her self-confidence shaken, Elion began secretarial school. That lasted only six weeks, until she landed a one-semester stint teaching **biochemistry** to nurses, and then took a position in a friend's laboratory. With the money she earned from these jobs, Elion began graduate school. To pay for her tuition, she continued to live with her parents and to work as a substitute science teacher in the New York public schools system. In 1941, she graduated summa cum laude from New York University with a M.S. degree in chemistry.

Upon her graduation, Elion again faced difficulties finding work appropriate to her experience and abilities. The only job available to her was as a quality control chemist in a food laboratory, checking the color of mayonnaise and the acidity of pickles for the Quaker Maid Company. After a year and a half, she was finally offered a job as a research chemist at Johnson & Johnson. Unfortunately, her division closed six months after she arrived. The company offered Elion a new job testing the tensile strength of sutures, but she declined.

As it did for many women of her generation, the start of World War II ushered in a new era of opportunity for Elion. As men left their jobs to fight the war, women were encouraged to join the workforce. "It was only when men weren't available that women were invited into the lab," Elion told the *Washington Post.*

For Elion, the war created an opening in the research lab of biochemist George Herbert Hitchings at Wellcome Research Laboratories in Tuckahoe, New York, a subsidiary of Burroughs Wellcome Company, a British firm. When they met, Elion was 26 years old and Hitchings was 39. Their working relationship began on June 14, 1944, and lasted for the rest of their careers. Each time Hitchings was promoted, Elion filled the spot he had just vacated, until she became head of the Department of Experimental Therapy in 1967, where she was to remain until her retirement 16 years later. Hitchings became vice president for research. During that period, they wrote many scientific papers together.

Settled in her job and encouraged by the breakthroughs occurring in the field of biochemistry, Elion took steps to earn a Ph.D., the degree that all serious scientists are expected to attain as evidence that they are capable of doing independent research. Only one school offered night classes in chemistry, the Brooklyn Polytechnic Institute (now Polytechnic University), and that is where Elion enrolled. Attending classes meant taking the train from Tuckahoe into Grand Central Station and transferring to the subway to Brooklyn. Although the hour-and-a-half commute each way was exhausting, Elion persevered for two years, until the school accused her of not being a serious student and pressed her to attend full-time. Forced to choose between school and her job, Elion had no choice but to continue working. Her relinquishment of the Ph.D. haunted her, until her lab developed its first successful drug, 6-mercaptopurine (6MP).

In the 1940s, Elion and Hitchings employed a novel approach in fighting the agents of disease. By studying the biochemistry of cancer cells, and of harmful **bacteria** and **viruses**, they hoped to understand the differences between the metabolism of those cells and normal cells. In particular, they wondered whether there were differences in how the disease-causing cells used nucleic acids, the chemicals involved in the replication of **DNA**, to stay alive and to grow. Any dissimilarity discovered might serve as a target point for a drug that could destroy the abnormal cells without harming healthy, normal cells. By disrupting one crucial link in a cell's biochemistry, the cell itself would be damaged. In this manner, cancers and harmful bacteria might be eradicated.

Elion's work focused on purines, one of two main categories of nucleic acids. Their strategy, for which Elion and Hitchings would be honored by the Nobel Prize forty years later, steered a radical middle course between chemists who randomly screened compounds to find effective drugs and scientists who engaged in basic cellular research without a thought of drug therapy. The difficulties of such an approach were immense. Very little was known about nucleic acid biosynthesis. Discovery of the double helical structure of DNA still lay ahead, and many of the instruments and methods that make **molecular biology** possible had not yet been invented. But Elion and her colleagues persisted with the tools at hand and their own ingenuity. By observing the microbiological results of various experiments, they could make knowledgeable deductions about the biochemistry involved.

To the same ends, they worked with various species of lab animals and examined varying responses. Still, the lack of advanced instrumentation and computerization made for slow and tedious work. Elion told *Scientific American,* "if we were starting now, we would probably do what we did in ten years."

By 1951, as a senior research chemist, Elion discovered the first effective compound against childhood leukemia. The compound, 6-mercaptopurine (6MP; trade name Purinethol), interfered with the synthesis of leukemia cells. In clinical trials run by the Sloan-Kettering Institute (now the Memorial Sloan-Kettering Cancer Center), it increased life expectancy from a few months to a year. The compound was approved by the Food and Drug Administration (FDA) in 1953. Eventually 6MP, used in combination with other drugs and radiation treatment, made leukemia one of the most curable of cancers.

In the following two decades, the potency of 6MP prompted Elion and other scientists to look for more uses for the drug. Robert Schwartz, at Tufts Medical School in Boston, and Roy Calne, at Harvard Medical School, successfully used 6MP to suppress the immune systems in dogs with transplanted kidneys. Motivated by Schwartz and Calne's work, Elion and Hitchings began searching for other immunosuppressants. They carefully studied the drug's course of action in the body, an endeavor known as pharmacokinetics. This additional work with 6MP led to the discovery of the derivative azathioprine (Imuran), which prevents rejection of transplanted human organs and treats rheumatoid arthritis. Other experiments in Elion's lab intended to improve 6MP's effectiveness led to the discovery of allopurinol (Zyloprim) for gout, a disease in which excess uric acid builds up in the joints. Allopurinol was approved by the FDA in 1966. In the 1950s, Elion and Hitchings's lab also discovered pyrimethamine (Daraprim and Fansidar) a treatment for malaria, and trimethoprim, for urinary and respiratory tract infections. Trimethoprim is also used to treat Pneumocystis carinii **pneumonia**, the leading killer of people with AIDS.

In 1968, Elion heard that a compound called adenine arabinoside appeared to have an effect against DNA viruses. This compound was similar in structure to a chemical in her lab, 2,6-diaminopurine. Although her own lab was not equipped to screen antiviral compounds, she immediately began synthesizing new compounds to send to a Wellcome Research lab in Britain for testing. In 1969, she received notice by telegram that one of the compounds was effective against herpes simplex viruses. Further derivatives of that compound yielded acyclovir (Zovirax), an effective drug against herpes, shingles, and chickenpox. An exhibit of the success of acyclovir, presented in 1978 at the Interscience Conference on Microbial Agents and **Chemotherapy**, demonstrated to other scientists that it was possible to find drugs that exploited the differences between viral and cellular **enzymes**. Acyclovir (Zovirax), approved by the FDA in 1982, became one of Burroughs Wellcome's most profitable drugs. In 1984, at Wellcome Research Laboratories, researchers trained by Elion and Hitchings developed azidothymidine (AZT), the first drug used to treat AIDS.

Although Elion retired in 1983, she continued at Wellcome Research Laboratories as scientist emeritus and kept an office there as a consultant. She also accepted a position as a research professor of medicine and pharmacology at Duke University. Following her retirement, Elion has served as president of the American Association for Cancer Research and as a member of the National Cancer Advisory Board, among other positions.

In 1988, Elion and Hitchings shared the Nobel Prize for physiology or medicine with Sir James Black, a British biochemist. Although Elion had been honored for her work before, beginning with the prestigious Garvan Medal of the American Chemical Society in 1968, a host of tributes followed the Nobel Prize. She received a number of honorary doctorates and was elected to the National Inventors' Hall of Fame, the National Academy of Sciences, and the National Women's Hall of Fame. Elion maintained that it was important to keep such awards in perspective. "The Nobel Prize is fine, but the drugs I've developed are rewards in themselves," she told the *New York Times Magazine.*

Elion never married. Engaged once, Elion dismissed the idea of marriage after her fiancé became ill and died. She was close to her brother's children and grandchildren, however, and on the trip to Stockholm to receive the Nobel Prize, she brought with her 11 family members. Elion once said that she never found it necessary to have women role models. "I never considered that I was a woman and then a scientist," Elion told the *Washington Post.* "My role models didn't have to be women—they could be scientists." Her other interests were photography, travel, and music, especially opera. Elion, whose name appears on 45 patents, died on February 21, 1999.

See also AIDS, recent advances in research and treatment; Antiviral drugs; Autoimmunity and autoimmune diseases; Immunosuppressant drugs; Transplantation genetics and immunology

ELISA · *see* ENZYME-LINKED IMMUNOSORBANT ASSAY (ELISA)

ENDERS, JOHN F. (1897-1985)

American virologist

John F. Enders' research on **viruses** and his advances in tissue **culture** enabled microbiologists **Albert Sabin** and **Jonas Salk** to develop vaccines against polio, a major crippler of children in the first half of the twentieth century. Enders' work also served as a catalyst in the development of vaccines against **measles, mumps** and chicken pox. As a result of this work, Enders was awarded the 1954 Nobel Prize in medicine or physiology.

John Franklin Enders was born February 10, 1897, in West Hartford, Connecticut. His parents were John Enders, a wealthy banker, and Harriet Whitmore Enders. Entering Yale in 1914, Enders left during his junior year to enlist in the U.S. Naval Reserve Flying Corps following America's entry into World War I in 1917. After serving as a flight instructor and rising to the rank of lieutenant, he returned to Yale, graduating

in 1920. After a brief venture as a real estate agent, Enders entered Harvard in 1922 as a graduate student in English literature. His plans were sidetracked in his second year when, after seeing a roommate perform scientific experiments, he changed his major to medicine. He enrolled in Harvard Medical School, where he studied under the noted microbiologist and author Hans Zinsser. Zinsser's influence led Enders to the study of microbiology, the field in which he received his Ph.D. in 1930. His dissertation was on **anaphylaxis**, a serious allergic condition that can develop after a foreign protein enters the body. Enders became an assistant at Harvard's Department of Bacteriology in 1929, eventually rising to assistant professor in 1935, and associate professor in 1942.

Following the Japanese attack on Pearl Harbor, Enders came to the service of his country again, this time as a member of the Armed Forces **Epidemiology** Board. Serving as a consultant to the Department of War, he helped develop diagnostic tests and immunizations for a variety of diseases. Enders continued to work with the military after the war, offering his counsel to the U.S. Army's Civilian Commission on Virus and Rickettsial Disease, and the Secretary of Defense's Research and Development Board. Enders left his position at Harvard in 1946 to set up the Infectious Diseases Laboratory at Boston Children's Hospital, believing this would give him greater freedom to conduct his research. Once at the hospital, he began to concentrate on studying those viruses affecting his young patients. By 1948, he had two assistants, Frederick Robbins and **Thomas Weller**, who, like him, were graduates of Harvard Medical School. Although Enders and his colleagues did their research primarily on measles, mumps, and chicken pox, their lab was partially funded by the National Foundation for Infantile Paralysis, an organization set up to help the victims of polio and find a **vaccine** or cure for the disease. Infantile paralysis, a virus affecting the brain and nervous system was, at that time, a much-feared disease with no known prevention or cure. Although it could strike anyone, children were its primary victims during the periodic **epidemics** that swept through communities. The disease often crippled and, in severe cases, killed those afflicted.

During an experiment on chicken pox, Weller produced too many cultures of human embryonic tissue. So as not to let them go to waste, Enders suggested putting polio viruses in the cultures. To their surprise, the virus began growing in the test tubes. The publication of these results in a 1949 *Science* magazine article caused major excitement in the medical community. Previous experiments in the 1930s had indicated that the polio virus could only grow in nervous system tissues. As a result, researchers had to import monkeys in large numbers from India, infect them with polio, then kill the animals and remove the virus from their nervous system. This was extremely expensive and time-consuming, as a single monkey could provide only two or three virus samples, and it was difficult to keep the animals alive and in good health during transport to the laboratories.

The use of nervous system tissue created another problem for those working on a vaccine. Tissue from that system often stimulate allergic reactions in the brain, sometimes fatally, when injected into another body, and there was always the danger some tissue might remain in the vaccine serum after the virus had been harvested from the culture. The discovery that the polio virus could grow outside the nervous system provided a revolutionary breakthrough in the search for a vaccine. As many as 20 specimens could be taken from a single monkey, enabling the virus to be cultivated in far larger quantities. Because no nervous system tissue had to be used, there was no danger of an allergic reaction through inadvertent transmission of the tissue. In addition, the technique of cultivating the virus and studying its effects also represented a new development in viral research. Enders and his assistants placed parts of the tissues around the inside walls of the test tubes, then closed the tubes and placed the cultures in a horizontal position within a revolving drum. Because this method made it easier to observe reaction within the culture, Enders was able to discover a means of distinguishing between the different viruses in human cells. In the case of polio, the virus killed the cell, whereas the measles virus made the cells fuse together and grow larger.

Because his breakthrough made it possible to develop a vaccine against polio, Enders, Robbins, and Weller were awarded the Nobel Prize for medicine or physiology in 1954. Interestingly enough, Enders originally opposed Salk's proposal to vaccinate against polio by injecting killed viruses into an uninfected person to produce **immunity**. He feared that this would actually weaken the immunity of the general population by interfering with the way the disease developed. In spite of their disagreements, Salk expressed gratitude to Enders by stating that he could not have developed his vaccine without the help of Enders' discoveries.

Enders' work in the field of **immunology** did not stop with his polio research. Even before he won the Nobel Prize, he was working on a vaccine against measles, again winning the acclaim of the medical world when he announced the creation of a successful vaccine against this disease in 1957. Utilizing the same techniques he had developed researching polio, he created a weakened measles virus that produced the necessary antibodies to prevent infection. Other researchers used Enders' methodology to develop vaccines against German measles and chicken pox.

In spite of his accomplishments and hard work, Enders' progress in academia was slow for many years. Still an assistant professor when he won the Nobel Prize, he did not become a full professor until two years later. This may have resulted in his dislike for university life—he once said that he preferred practical research to the "arid scholarship" of academia. Yet, by the mid-fifties, Enders began receiving his due recognition. He was given the Kyle Award from the United States Public Health Service in 1955 and, in 1962, became a university professor at Harvard, the highest honor the school could grant. Enders received the Presidential Medal of Freedom in 1963, the same year he was awarded the American Medical Association's Science Achievement Award, making him one of the few non-physicians to receive this honor.

Enders married his first wife in 1927, and in 1943, she passed away. The couple had two children. He married again in 1951. Affectionately known as "The Chief" to students and colleagues, Enders took a special interest in those he taught,

keeping on the walls of his lab portraits of those who became scientists. When speaking to visitors, he was able to identify each student's philosophy and personality. Enders wrote some 190 published papers between 1929 and 1970. Towards the end of his life, he sought to apply his knowledge of immunology to the fight against **AIDS**, especially in trying to halt the progress of the disease during its incubation period in the human body. Enders died September 8, 1985, of heart failure, while at his summer home in Waterford, Connecticut.

See also Antibody and antigen; Antibody formation and kinetics; Immunity, active, passive and delayed; Immunity, cell mediated; Immunity, humoral regulation; Immunization; Immunochemistry; Poliomyelitis and polio

ENTAMOEBA HISTOLYTICA

Entamoeba histolytica is a eukaryotic microorganism; that is, the nuclear genetic material is enclosed within a specialized membrane. Furthermore, the microbe is a protozoan parasite. It requires a host for the completion of its life cycle, and its survival comes at the expense of the host organism. *Entamoeba histolytica* causes disease in humans. Indeed, after **malaria** and schistosomiasis, the **dysentery** caused by the amoeba is the third leading cause of death in the world. One-tenth of the world's population, some 500 million people, are infected by *Entamoeba histolytica*, with between 50,000 and 100,000 people dying of the infection each year.

The bulk of these deaths occurs in underdeveloped areas of the world, where sanitation and personal **hygiene** is lacking. In developed regions, where sanitation is established and where water treatment systems are in routine use, the dysentery caused by *Entamoeba histolytica* is almost nonexistent.

A characteristic feature of *Entamoeba histolytica* is the invasion of host tissue. Another species, *Entamoeba dispar* does not invade tissue and so does not cause disease. This non-pathogenic species does appear similar to the disease-causing species, however, which can complicate the diagnosis of the dysentery caused by *Entamoeba histolytica*.

Both **microorganisms** have been known for a long time, having been originally described in 1903. Even at that time the existence of two forms of the microorganisms were known. The two forms are called the cyst and the trophozoite. A cyst is an environmentally hardy form, designed to protect the genetic material when conditions are harsh and unfavorable for the growth of the organism. For example, cysts are found in food and water, and are the means whereby the organism is transmitted to humans. Often, the cysts are ingested in water or food that has been contaminated with the fecal material of an infected human. Within the small intestine, the cyst undergoes division of the nuclear material and then resuscitation and division of the remaining material to form eight trophozoites.

Some of the trophozoites go on to adhere to the intestinal wall and reproduce, so as to colonize the intestinal surface. The adherent trophozoites can feed on **bacteria** and cell debris that are present in the area. Some of the trophozoites are able to break down the membrane barrier of the intestinal cells and kill these cells. The resulting abdominal pain and tenderness, with sudden and explosive bloody diarrhea, is called dysentery. Other symptoms of the dysentery include dehydration, fever, and sometimes the establishment of a bowel malfunction that can become chronic. The damage can be so extensive that a complete perforation of the intestinal wall can occur. Leakage of intestinal contents into the abdominal cavity can be a result, as can a thickening of the abdominal wall.

Other trophozoites form cysts and are shed into the external environment via the feces. These can spread the infection to another human.

Drugs are available to treat the symptomatic and asymptomatic forms of the infection.

In about 10 percent of people who are infected, some of the trophozoites can enter the circulatory system and invade other parts of the body, such as the liver, colon, and infrequently the brain. The reasons for the ability of the trophozoites to establish infections in widespread areas of the body are still not understood. The current consensus is that these trophozoites must somehow be better equipped to evade the immune responses of the host, and have more potent virulence factors capable of damaging host tissue.

Infection can occur with no obvious symptoms being shown by the infected person. However, these people will still excrete the cysts in their feces and so can spread the infection to others. In others, infection could produce no symptoms, or symptoms ranging from mild to fatal.

Although the molecular mechanisms of infection of *Entamoeba histolytica* are still unclear, it is clear that infection is a multi-stage process. In the first step the amoeba recognizes the presence of a number of surface receptors on host cells. This likely involves a reaction between the particular host receptor and a complimentary molecule on the surface of the amoeba that is known as an adhesion. Once the association between the parasite and the host intestinal cell is firm, other molecules of the parasite, which may already be present or which may be produced after adhesion, are responsible for the damage to the intestinal wall. These virulence factors include a protein that can form a hole in the intestinal wall of the host, a protein-dissolving enzyme (protease), a **glycocalyx** that covers the surface of the protozoan, and a toxin.

Comparison of pathogenic strains of *Entamoeba histolytica* with strains that look the same but which do not cause disease has revealed some differences. For example, the non-pathogenic forms have much less of two so-called glycolipids that are anchored in the microbe membrane and protrude out from the surface. Their function is not known, although they must be important to the establishment of an infection.

Completion of the sequencing of the genome of *Entamoeba histolytica*, expected by 2005, should help identify the function of the suspected virulence factors, and other, yet unknown, virulence factors. Currently, little is known of the genetic organization and regulation of expression of the genetic material in the protozoan. For example, the reasons for the variation in the infection and the symptoms are unclear.

See also Amebic dysentery; Parasites

ENTEROBACTERIACEAE

Enterobacteria are **bacteria** from the family Enterobacteriaceae, which are primarily known for their ability to cause intestinal upset. Enterobacteria are responsible for a variety of human illnesses, including urinary tract infections, wound infections, **gastroenteritis**, **meningitis**, septicemia, and **pneumonia**. Some are true intestinal pathogens; whereas others are merely opportunistic pests which attack weakened victims.

Most enterobacteria reside normally in the large intestine, but others are introduced in contaminated or improperly prepared foods or beverages. Several enterobacterial diseases are spread by fecal-oral transmission and are associated with poor hygienic conditions. Countries with poor water decontamination have more illness and death from enterobacterial infection. Harmless bacteria, though, can cause diarrhea in tourists who are not used to a geographically specific bacterial strain. Enterobacterial gastroenteritis can cause extensive fluid loss through vomiting and diarrhea, leading to dehydration.

Enterobacteria are a family of rod-shaped, aerobic, facultatively anaerobic bacteria. This means that while these bacteria can survive in the presence of oxygen, they prefer to live in an anaerobic (oxygen-free) environment. The Enterobacteriaceae family is subdivided into eight tribes including: Escherichieae, Edwardsielleae, Salmonelleae, Citrobactereae, Klebsielleae, Proteeae, Yersineae, and Erwineae. These tribes are further divided into genera, each with a number of species.

Enterobacteria can cause disease by attacking their host in a number of ways. The most important factors are motility, colonization factors, endotoxin, and **enterotoxin**. Those enterobacteria that are motile have several flagella all around their perimeter (peritrichous). This allows them to move swiftly through their host fluid. Enterobacterial colonization factors are filamentous appendages, called fimbriae, which are shorter than flagella and bind tightly to the tissue under attack, thus keeping hold of its host. Endotoxins are the cell wall components, which trigger high fevers in infected individuals. Enterotoxins are bacterial toxins which act in the small intestines and lead to extreme water loss in vomiting and diarrhea.

A number of tests exist for rapid identification of enterobacteria. Most will ferment glucose to acid, reduce nitrate to nitrite, and test negative for cytochrome oxidase. These biochemical tests are used to pin-point specific intestinal pathogens. *Escherichia coli (E. coli), Shigella species, Salmonella*, and several *Yersinia* strains are some of these intestinal pathogens.

E. coli is indigenous to the gastrointestinal tract and generally benign. However, it is associated with most hospital-acquired infections as well as nursery and travelers diarrhea. *E. coli* pathogenicity is closely related to the presence or absence of fimbriae on individual strains. Although most *E. coli* infections are not treated with **antibiotics**, severe urinary tract infections usually are.

The *Shigella* genus of the Escherichieae tribe can produce serious disease when its toxins act in the small intestine. *Shigella* infections can be entirely asymptomatic, or lead to severe **dysentery**. *Shigella* bacteria cause about 15% of pediatric diarrheal cases in the United States. However, they are a leading cause of infant mortality in developing countries. Only a few organisms are need to cause this fecal-orally transmitted infection. Prevention of the disease is achieved by proper sewage disposal and water **chlorination**, as well as personal **hygiene** such as handwashing. Antibiotics are only used in more severe cases.

Salmonella infections are classified as nontyphoidal or typhoidal. Nontyphoidal infections can cause gastroenteritis, and are usually due to contaminated food or water and can be transmitted by animals or humans. These infections cause one of the largest communicable bacterial diseases in the United States. They are found in contaminated animal products such as beef, pork, poultry, and raw chicken eggs. As a result, any food product that uses raw eggs, such as mayonnaise, homemade ice cream, or Caesar salad, could carry these bacteria. The best prevention when serving these dishes is to adhere strictly to refrigeration guidelines.

Typhoid *Salmonella* infections are also found in contaminated food and water. Typhoid Mary was a cook in New York from 1868 to 1914. She was typhoid carrier who contaminated much of the food she handled and was responsible for hundreds of typhoid cases. **Typhoid fever** is characterized by septicemia (blood poisoning), accompanied by a very high fever and intestinal lesions. Typhoid fever is treated with the drugs Ampicillin and Chloramphenicol.

Certain *Yersinia* bacteria cause one of the most notorious and fatal infections known to man. *Yersinia pestis* is the agent of **bubonic plague** and is highly fatal without treatment. The bubonic plague is carried by a rat flea and is thought to have killed at least 100 million people in the sixth century as well as 25% of the fourteenth century European population. This plague was also known as the "black death," because it caused darkened hemorrhagic skin patches. The last widespread epidemic of *Y. pestis* began in Hong Kong in 1892 and spread to India and eventually San Francisco in 1900. The bacteria can reside in squirrels, prairie dogs, mice, and other rodents, and are mainly found (in the U.S.) in the Southwest. Since 1960, fewer than 400 cases have resulted in only a few deaths, due to rapid antibiotic treatment.

Two less severe *Yersinia* strains are *Y. pseudotuberculosis* and *Y. enterocolotica*. *Y. pseudotuberculosis* is transmitted to humans by wild or domestic animals and causes a non-fatal disease which resembles appendicitis. *Y. enterocolotica* can be transmitted from animals or humans via a fecal-oral route and causes severe diarrhea.

See also Colony and colony formation; Enterobacterial infections; Infection and resistance; Microbial flora of the stomach and gastrointestinal tract

ENTEROBACTERIAL INFECTIONS

Enterobacterial infections are caused by a group of **bacteria** that dwell in the intestinal tract of humans and other warm-blooded animals. The bacteria are all Gram-negative and rod-shaped. As a group they are termed **Enterobacteriaceae**. A prominent member of this group is ***Escherichia coli***. Other members are the various species in the genera ***Salmonella, Shigella***, *Klebsiella*, *Enterobacter*, *Serratia*, *Proteus*, and *Yersinia*.

The various enterobacteria cause intestinal maladies. As well, if they infect regions of the body other than their normal intestinal habitat, infections can arise. Often, the **bacterial infection** arises during the course of a hospital stay. Such infections are described as being nosocomial, or hospital acquired, infections. For example, both *Klebsiella* and *Proteus* are capable of establishing infections in the lung, ear, sinuses, and the urinary tract if they gain entry to these niches. As another example, both *Enterobacter* and *Serratia* can cause an infection of the blood, particularly in people whose immune systems are compromised as a result of therapy or other illness.

A common aspect of enterobacterial infections is the presence of diarrhea. Indeed, the diarrhea caused by enterobacteria is a common problem even in countries like the United States, which has an excellent medical infrastructure. In the United States is has been estimated that each person in the country experiences 1.5 episodes of diarrhea each year. While for most of those afflicted the diarrhea is a temporary inconvenience, those who are young, old, or whose immune systems are malfunctioning can be killed by the infection. Moreover, in other countries where the medical facilities are less advanced, enterobacterial infections remain a serious health problem.

Even in the intestinal tract, where they normally reside, enterobacteria can cause problems. Typically, intestinal maladies arise from types of the enterobacteria that are not part of the normal flora. An example is *E. coli* **O157:H7**. While this bacterial strain is a normal resident in the intestinal tract of cattle, its presence in the human intestinal tract is abnormal and problematic.

The O157:H7 strain establishes an infection by invading host tissue. Other bacteria, including other strains of *Escherichia coli*, do not invade host cells. Rather, they adhere to the intestinal surface of the cells and can exert their destructive effect by means of toxins they elaborate. Both types of infections can produce diarrhea. Bloody diarrhea (which is also known as **dysentery**) can result when host cells are damaged. Some types of *Escherichia coli*, *Salmonella*, and *Shigella* produce dysentery.

Escherichia coli O157:H7 can also become disseminated in the blood and cause destruction of red blood cells and impaired or complete loss of function of the kidneys. This debilitating and even life-threatening infection is known as hemolytic-uremic syndrome.

Another intestinal upset that occurs in prematurely born infants is called necrotizing enterocolitis. Likely the result of a bacterial (or perhaps a viral) infection, the cells lining the bowel is killed. In any person such an infection is serious. But in a prematurely borne infant, whose **immune system** is not able to deal with an infection, necrotizing enterocolitis can be lethal. The enterobacteria that have been associated with the disease are *Salmonella*, *Escherichia coli*, *Klebsiella*, and *Enterobacter*.

The diagnosis of enterobacterial infections can be complicated by the fact that **viruses**, **protozoa**, and other kinds of bacteria can also cause similar symptoms. The location of some of the symptoms can help determine the nature of the infection. For example, if nausea and vomiting is involved, then the enterobacterial infection could well be centered in the small intestine. If a fever is present, then dysentery is more likely.

The treatment for many enterobacterial infections is the administration of the suitable antibiotic or combination of **antibiotics** that the isolated organism is determined to be susceptible to. As well, and every bit as important, is the administration of fluids to prevent dehydration because of the copious loss of fluids during diarrhea. The dehydration can be extremely debilitating to infants and the elderly.

See also E. coli O157:H7 infection; Invasiveness and intracellular infections

ENTEROTOXIN AND EXOTOXIN

Enterotoxin and exotoxin are two classes of toxin that are produced by **bacteria**.

An exotoxin is a toxin that is produced by a bacterium and then released from the cell into the surrounding environment. The damage caused by an exotoxin can only occur upon release. As a general rule, enterotoxins tend to be produced by Gram-positive bacteria rather than by Gram-negative bacteria. There are exceptions, such as the potent enterotoxin produced by *Vibrio cholerae*. In contrast to Gram-positive bacteria, many Gram-negative species posses a molecule called lipopolysaccharide. A portion of the lipopolysaccharide, called the lipid A, is a cell-associated toxin, or an endotoxin.

An enterotoxin is a type of exotoxin that acts on the intestinal wall. Another type of exotoxin is a neurotoxin. This type of toxin disrupts nerve cells.

Many kinds of bacterial enterotoxins and exotoxins exist. For example, an exotoxin produced by *Staphylococcus aureus* is the cause of **toxic shock syndrome**, which can produce symptoms ranging from nausea, fever and sore throat, to collapse of the central nervous and circulatory systems. As another example, *Staphylococcus aureus* also produces enterotoxin B, which is associated with food-borne illness. Growth of the bacteria in improperly handled foods leads to the excretion of the enterotoxin. Ingestion of the toxin-contaminated food produces fever, chills, headache, chest pain and a persistent cough. This type of illness is known as a food intoxication, to distinguish it from bacterial food-borne illness that results from growth of the bacteria following ingestion of the food (food poisoning).

Enterotoxins have three different basis of activity. One type of enterotoxin, which is exemplified by **diphtheria** toxin, causes the destruction of the host cell to which it binds. Typically, the binding of the toxin causes the formation of a hole, or pore, in the host cell membrane. Another example of a pore-forming exotoxin is the aerolysin produced by *Aeromonas hydrophila*.

A second type of enterotoxin is known as a superantigen toxin. Superantigen exotoxins work by overstimulating the immune response, particularly with respect to the T-cells. Examples of superantigen exotoxins include that from *Staphylococcus aureus* and from the "flesh-eating" bacterium *Streptococcus pyogenes*.

A third type of enterotoxin is known as an A-B toxin. An A-B toxin consists of two or more toxin subunits that work together as a team to exert their destructive effect. Typically, the A subunit binds to the host cell wall and forms a channel through the membrane. The channel allows the B subunit to get into the cell. An example of an A-B toxin is the enterotoxin that is produced by *Vibrio cholerae*.

The cholera toxin disrupts the ionic balance of the host's intestinal cell membranes. As a result, the cells of the small intestine exude a large amount of water into the intestine. Dehydration results, which can be lethal if not treated.

In contrast to the destructive effect of some exotoxins, the A-B exotoxin (an enterotoxin of *Vibrio cholerae* does not damage the structure of the affected host cells. Therefore, in the case of the cholera toxin, treatment can led to a full resumption of host cell activity.

See also Anthrax, terrorist use of as a biological weapon; Bacteria and bacterial infection

ENTEROVIRUS INFECTIONS

Enteroviruses are a group of **viruses** that contain **ribonucleic acid** as their genetic material. They are members of the picornavirus family. The various types of enteroviruses that infect humans are referred to as serotypes, in recognition of their different antigenic patterns. The different immune response is important, as infection with one type of enterovirus does not necessarily confer protection to infection by a different type of enterovirus. There are 64 different enterovirus serotypes. The serotypes include polio viruses, coxsackie A and B viruses, echoviruses and a large number of what are referred to as non-polio enteroviruses.

The genetic material is enclosed in a shell that has 20 equilateral triangles (an icosahedral virus). The shell is made up of four proteins.

Despite the diversity in the antigenic types of enterovirus, the majority of enterovirus cases in the United States is due to echoviruses and Coxsackie B viruses. The infections that are caused by these viruses are varied. The paralytic debilitation of polio is one infection. The importance of polio on a global scale is diminished now, because of the advent and worldwide use of polio vaccines. Far more common are the **cold**-like or flu-like symptoms caused by various enteroviruses. Indeed, the non-polio enteroviruses rival the cause of the "common cold," the rhinovirus, as the most common infectious agent in humans. In the United States, estimates from the **Centers for Disease Control** are that at least ten to fifteen million people in the United States develop an enterovirus infection each year.

Enterovirus infection is spread easily, as the virus is found in saliva, sputum or nasal secretions, and also in the feces of those who are infected. Humans are the only known reservoir of enteroviruses. Following spread to water via feces, enteroviruses can persist in the environment. Thus, surface and ground water can be a source of enterovirus.

Spread of an enterovirus occurs by direct contact with the fluids from an infected person, by use of utensils that have been handled by an infected person, or by the ingestion of contaminated food or water. For example, coughing into someone's face is an easy way to spread enterovirus, just as the cold-causing rhinoviruses are spread from person to person. Fecal contact is most common in day care facilities or in households where there is a newborn, where diapers are changed and soiled babies cleaned up.

The spread of enterovirus infections is made even easier because some of those who are infected do not display any symptoms of illness. Yet such people are still able to transfer the infectious virus to someone else.

The common respiratory infection can strike anyone, from infants to the elderly. The young are infected more frequently, however, and may indeed be the most important transmitters of the virus. Common symptoms of infection include a runny nose, fever with chills, muscle aches and sometimes a rash. In addition, but more rarely, an infection of the heart (endocarditis), meninges (**meningitis**) or the brain (encephalitis) can develop. In newborns, enterovirus infection may be related to the development of juvenile-onset diabetes, and, in rare instances, can lead to an overwhelming infection of the body that proves to be lethal.

Although enterovirus-induced meningitis is relatively rare, it afflicts between 30,000 and 50,000 people each year in the United States alone.

Evidence is accumulating that suggests that enterovirus infections may not only be short in duration (also referred as acute) but may also become chronic. Diseases such as chronic heart disease and chronic fatigue syndrome may well have an enterovirus origin. Moreover, juvenile diabetes may involve an autoimmune response.

The climate affects the prevalence of the infections. In tropical climates, where warm temperatures are experienced throughout the year, enterovirus infections occur with similar frequency year-round. But, in more temperate climates, where a shift in seasons is pronounced, enterovirus infections peak in the late summer and fall.

Another factor in the spread of enterovirus infections is the socio-economic conditions. Poor sanitation that is often coincident with lower economic standing is often associated with the spread of enterovirus infections.

Following inhalation or ingestion of enterovirus, viral replication is thought to occur mainly in lymphoid tissues of the respiratory and gastrointestinal tract that are in the immediate vicinity of the virus. Examples of tissues include the tonsils and the cells lining the respiratory and intestinal tracts. The virus may continue to replicate in these tissues, or can spread to secondary sites including the spinal cord and brain, heart or the skin.

As with other viruses, enteroviruses recognize a receptor molecule on the surface of host cells and attach to the receptor via a surface molecule on the virus particle. Several viral molecules have been shown to function in this way. The virus then enters the host cell and the genetic material is released into the **cytoplasm** (the interior gel-like region) of the host cell. The various steps in viral replication cause, initially, the host cell **nucleus** to shrink, followed by shrinkage of the entire. Other changes cause the host cell to lose its ability to function and finally to explode, which releases newly made virus.

Currently, no **vaccine** exists for the maladies other than polio. One key course of action to minimize the chances of infection is the observance of proper **hygiene**. Handwashing is a key factor in reducing the spread of many microbial infections, including those caused by enteroviruses. Spread of enteroviruses is also minimized by covering the mouth when coughing and the nose when sneezing.

See also Cold, common; Viruses and responses to viral infection

ENZYME-LINKED IMMUNOSORBANT ASSAY (ELISA)

The enzyme-linked immunosorbant assay, which is commonly abbreviated to ELISA, is a technique that promotes the binding of the target antigen or **antibody** to a substrate, followed by the binding of an enzyme-linked molecule to the bound antigen or antibody. The presence of the antigen or antibody is revealed by color development in a reaction that is catalyzed by the enzyme which is bound to the antigen or antibody.

Typically, an ELISA is performed using a plastic plate which contains an 8 x 12 arrangement of 96 wells. Each well permits a sample to be tested against a whole battery of antigens.

There are several different variations on the ELISA theme. In the so-called direct ELISA, the antigen that is fixed to the surface of the test surface is the target for the binding of a complimentary antibody to which has been linked an enzyme such as horseradish peroxidase. When the substrate of the enzyme is added, the conversion of the substrate to a colored product produces a darkening in whatever well an antigen-antibody reaction occurred.

Another ELISA variation is known as the indirect technique. In this technique a specific antibody recognizes the antigen that is bound to the bottom of the wells on the plastic plate. Binding between the antigen and the antibody occurs. The bound antibody can then be recognized by a second antibody, to which is fixed the enzyme that produces the color change. For example, in this scheme the first, or primary, antibody could be a rabbit antibody to the particular antigen. The so-called secondary antibody could be a goat-antirabbit antibody. That is, the primary antibody has acted as an antigen to produce an antibody in a second animal. Once again, the darkening of a well indicates the formation of a complex between the antigen and the antibodies.

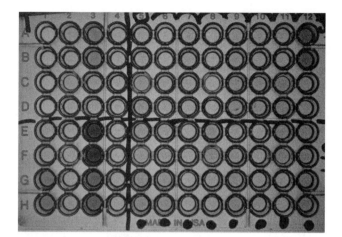

ELISA assay 96 well test plate.

The third variation of the ELISA is known as the capture or sandwich ELISA. As the names imply, the antigen is sandwiched between the primary and secondary antibodies. In this technique, the primary antibody is bound to the bottom of the wells, rather than the antigen. Then, the antigen is added. Where the bound antibody recognizes the antigen, binding occurs. A so-called blocking solution is added, which occupies the vacant antibody sites. Then, an enzyme-labeled secondary antibody is added. The secondary antibody also recognizes the antigen, but the antigenic recognition site is different than that recognized by the primary antibody. The result is that the antigen is sandwiched in between two bound antibodies. Again, a color reaction reveals the complex.

The ELISA procedure has many applications. The procedure can provide qualitative ("yes or no") and quantitative ("how much") information on a myriad of prokaryotic and eukaryotic antibodies. Serum can be screened against a battery of antigens in order to rapidly assess the range of antibodies that might be present. For example, ELISA has proven very useful in the scrutiny of serum for the presence of antibodies to the **Human immunodeficiency virus**.

See also Laboratory techniques in immunology

ENZYME INDUCTION AND REPRESSION

Microorganisms have many **enzymes** that function in the myriad of activities that produce a growing and dividing cell. From a health standpoint, some enzymes are vital for the establishment of an infection by the microbes. Some enzymes are active all the time. These are known as constitutive enzymes. However, other enzymes are active only periodically, when their product is required. Such enzymes are known as inducible enzymes.

The ability of microorganisms such as **bacteria** to control the activity of inducible enzymes is vital for their survival. The constant activity of such enzymes could result in the overproduction of a compound, which would be an energy drain on

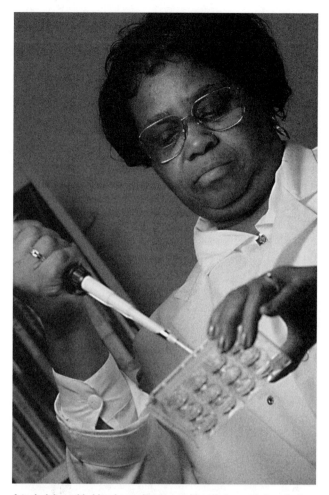

A technician adds blood samples to a multi-welled sample tray during an Enzyme-linked ImmunoSorbent Assay (ELISA) test for viral diseases such as AIDS and Hepatitis B and C. Blood serum of the patient is added to burst T cells of blood that have been infected with disease. A color change occurrs if viral antibodies are present.

the microorganism. At the same time, inducible enzymes must be capable of a rapid response to whatever condition they are geared to respond.

The twin goals of control of activity and speed of response are achieved by the processes of induction and repression.

Induction and repression are related in that they both focus on the binding of a molecule known as **RNA** polymerase to **DNA**. Specifically, the RNA polymerase binds to a region that is immediately "upstream" from the region of DNA that codes for a protein. The binding region is termed the operator. The operator acts to position the polymerase correctly, so that the molecule can then begin to move along the DNA, interpreting the genetic information as it moves along.

The three-dimensional shape of the operator region influences the binding of the RNA polymerase. The configuration of the operator can be altered by the presence of molecules called effectors. An effector can alter the shape of the polymerase-binding region so that the polymerase is more easily and efficiently able to bind. This effect is called induction. Conversely, effectors can associate with the operator and alter the configuration so that the binding of the polymerase occurs less efficiently or not at all. This effect is known as repression.

Enzyme induction is a process where an enzyme is manufactured in response to the presence of a specific molecule. This molecule is termed an inducer. Typically, an inducer molecule is a compound that the enzyme acts upon. In the induction process, the inducer molecule combines with another molecule, which is called the repressor. The binding of the inducer to the repressor blocks the function of the repressor, which is to bind to a specific region called an operator. The operator is the site to which another molecule, known as **ribonucleic acid** (RNA) polymerase, binds and begins the **transcription** of the **gene** to produce the so-called messenger RNA that acts as a template for the subsequent production of protein. Thus, the binding of the inducer to the repressor keeps the repressor from preventing transcription, and so the gene coding for the inducible enzyme is transcribed. Repression of transcription is essentially the default behavior, which is overridden once the inducing molecule is present.

In bacteria, the lactose (lac) **operon** is a very well characterized system that operates on the basis of induction.

Enzyme repression is when the repressor molecules prevent the manufacture of an enzyme. Repression typically operates by feedback inhibition. For example, if the end product of a series of enzyme-catalyzed reactions is a particular amino acid, that amino acid acts as the repressor molecule to further production. Often the repressor will combine with another molecule and the duo is able to block the operation of the operator. This blockage can occur when the repressor duo outcompetes with the polymerase for the binding site on the operator. Alternately, the repressor duo can bind directly to the polymerase and, by stimulating a change in the shape of the polymerase, prevent the subsequent binding to the operator region. Either way, the result is the blockage of the transcription of the particular gene.

The gene that is blocked in enzyme repression tends to be the first enzyme in the pathway leading to the manufacture of the repressor. Thus, repression acts to inhibit the production of all the enzymes involved in the metabolic pathway. This saves the bacterium energy. Otherwise, enzymes would be made—at a high metabolic cost—for which there would be no role in cellular processes.

Induction and repression mechanisms tend to cycle back and forth in response to the level of effector, and in response to nutrient concentration, **pH**, or other conditions for which the particular effector is sensitive.

See also Metabolism; Microbial genetics

ENZYMES

Enzymes are molecules that act as critical catalysts in biological systems. Catalysts are substances that increase the rate of chemical reactions without being consumed in the reaction. Without enzymes, many reactions would require higher levels of energy and higher temperatures than exist in biological systems. Enzymes are proteins that possess specific binding sites for other molecules (substrates). A series of weak binding interactions allow enzymes to accelerate reaction rates. Enzyme kinetics is the study of enzymatic reactions and mechanisms. Enzyme inhibitor studies have allowed researchers to develop therapies for the treatment of diseases, including **AIDS**.

French chemist **Louis Pasteur** (1822–1895) was an early investigator of enzyme action. Pasteur hypothesized that the conversion of sugar into alcohol by **yeast** was catalyzed by "ferments," which he thought could not be separated from living cells. In 1897, German biochemist Eduard Buchner (1860–1917) isolated the enzymes that catalyze the **fermentation** of alcohol from living yeast cells. In 1909, English physician Sir Archibald Garrod (1857–1936) first characterized enzymes genetically through the one gene-one enzyme hypothesis. Garrod studied the human disease alkaptonuria, a hereditary disease characterized by the darkening of excreted urine after exposure to air. He hypothesized that alkaptonurics lack an enzyme that breaks down alkaptans to normal excretion products, that alkaptonurics inherit this inability to produce a specific enzyme, and that they inherit a mutant form of a **gene** from each of their parents and have two mutant forms of the same gene. Thus, he hypothesized, some genes contain information to specify particular enzymes.

The early twentieth century saw dramatic advancement in enzyme studies. German chemist Emil Fischer (1852–1919) recognized the importance of substrate shape for binding by enzymes. German-American biochemist Leonor Michaelis (1875–1949) and Canadian biologist Maud Menten (1879–1960) introduced a mathematical approach for quantifying enzyme-catalyzed reactions. American chemists James Sumner (1887–1955) and John Northrop (1891–1987) were among the first to produce highly ordered enzyme crystals and firmly establish the proteinaceous nature of these biological catalysts. In 1937, German-born British biochemist **Hans Krebs** (1900–1981) postulated how a series of enzymatic reactions were coordinated in the citric acid cycle for the production of ATP from glucose metabolites. Today, enzymology is a central part of biochemical study, and the fields of industrial microbiology and genetics employ enzymes in numerous ways, from food production to gene **cloning**, to advanced therapeutic techniques.

Enzymes are proteins that encompass a large range of molecular size and mass. They may be composed of more than one polypeptide chain. Each polypeptide chain is called a subunit and may have a separate catalytic function. Some enzymes require non-protein groups for enzymatic activity. These components include metal ions and organic molecules called coenzymes. Coenzymes that are tightly or covalently attached to enzymes are termed prosthetic groups. Prosthetic groups contain critical chemical groups which allow the overall catalytic event to occur.

Enzymes bind their substrates at special folds and clefts in their structures called active sites. Because active sites have chemical groups precisely located and oriented for binding the substrate, they generally display a high degree of substrate specificity. The active site of an enzyme consists of two key regions, the catalytic site, which interacts with the substrate during the reaction, and the binding site, the chemical groups of the enzyme that bind the substrate, allowing the interactions at the catalytic site to occur. The crevice of the active site creates a microenvironment whose properties are critical for catalysis. Environmental factors influencing enzyme activity include **pH**, polarity and hydrophobicity of amino acids in the active site, and a precise arrangement of the chemical groups of the enzyme and its substrate.

Enzymes have high catalytic power, high substrate specificity, and are generally most active in aqueous solvents at mild temperature and physiological pH. Most enzymes catalyze the transfer of electrons, atoms, or groups of atoms. There are thousands of known enzymes, but most can be categorized according to their biological activities into six major classes: oxidoreductases, transferases, hydrolases, lyases, isomerases, and ligases.

Enzymes generally have an optimum pH range in which they are most active. The pH of the environment will affect the ionization state of catalytic groups at the active site and the ionization of the substrate. Electrostatic interactions are therefore controlled by pH. The pH of a reaction may also control the conformation of the enzyme by influencing amino acids critical for the three-dimensional shape of the macromolecule.

Inhibitors can diminish the activity of an enzyme by altering the binding of substrates. Inhibitors may resemble the structure of the substrate, thereby binding the enzyme and competing for the correct substrate. Inhibitors may be large organic molecules, small molecules, or ions. They can be used for chemotherapeutic treatment of diseases.

Regulatory enzymes are characterized by increased or decreased activity in response to chemical signals. Metabolic pathways are regulated by controlling the activity of one or more enzymatic steps along that path. Regulatory control allows cells to meet changing demands for energy and metabolites.

See also Biochemical analysis techniques; Biotechnology; Bioremediation; Cloning, application of cloning to biological problems; Enzyme induction and repression; Enzyme-linked immunosorbant assay (ELISA); Food preservation; Food safety; Immunologic therapies; Immunological analysis techniques

EPIDEMICS AND PANDEMICS

Epidemics are outbreaks of disease of bacterial or viral origin that involve many people in a localized area at the same time. An example of an epidemic is the hemorrhagic fever outbreak caused by the **Ebola virus** in Zaire in 1976. When Ebola fever occurs, it tends to be confined to a localized area, and can involve many people. If an outbreak is worldwide in scope, it is referred to as a pandemic. The periodic outbreaks of **influenza** can be pandemic.

Some maladies can be both epidemic and pandemic. This can be a function of time. An example is Acquired Immunodeficiency Syndrome (**AIDS**). Initially, the acknowledged viral agent of AIDS, the **Human Immunodeficiency Virus (HIV)**, was prevalent in a few geographic regions, such as Haiti, and among certain groups, such as homosexual men in the United States. In these regions and populations, the infection was epidemic in scope. Since these early days, AIDS has expanded to become a worldwide disease that cuts across all racial, cultural, economic and geographic categories. AIDS is now a pandemic.

Influenza can also be epidemic or pandemic. In this case, the antigenic composition of the viral agent of the disease determines whether the virus becomes global in its distribution or not. Antigenic variants of the virus that are quite different from varieties that have preceded it, and so require an adaptive response by the **immune system** before the infection can be successfully coped with, tend to become pandemic.

Pandemics of influenza can be devastating. The huge number of people who become ill can tax the capability of a regions' or countries' health infrastructure. The preparation to attempt to thwart an influenza pandemic is immense. For example, the preparation and distribution of the required **vaccine**, and the subsequent inoculation of those who might be at risk, is a huge undertaking. In human terms, influenza pandemics exact a huge toll in loss of life. Even thought the death rate from influenza is typically less than one percent of those who are infected, a pandemic involving hundreds of millions of people will result in a great many deaths.

Epidemics and pandemics have been a part of human history for millennia. An example of this long-standing presence is cholera. Cholera is an infection that is caused by a bacterium called *Vibrio cholerae*. The bacterium is present in the feces, and can be spread directly to drinking water, and to food via handling of the food in an unhygienic manner. The resulting watery diarrhea and dehydration, which can lead to collapse of body functions and death if treatment is not prompt, has devastated populations all over the world since the beginning of recorded history. The first reports that can be identified as cholera date back to 1563 in India. This and other epidemics in that part of the world lead to the spread of the infection. By 1817 cholera had become pandemic. The latest cholera pandemic began in 1961 in Indonesia. The outbreak spread through Europe, Asia, Africa, and finally reached South America in the early 1990s. In Latin America, cholera still causes 400,000 cases of illness and over 4000 deaths each year.

Influenza is another example of am illness that has been present since antiquity. Indeed, the philosopher Hippocrates first described an influenza outbreak in 412 B.C. There were three major outbreaks of influenza in the sixteenth century (the one occurring in 1580 being a pandemic), and at least three pandemics in the eighteenth century. In the twentieth century there were pandemics in 1918, 1957, and 1968. These were caused by different antigenic types of the influenza virus. The 1918 pandemic is thought to have killed some 30 million people, more than were killed in World War I.

A common theme of epidemics and pandemics throughout history has been the association of outbreaks and sanitary

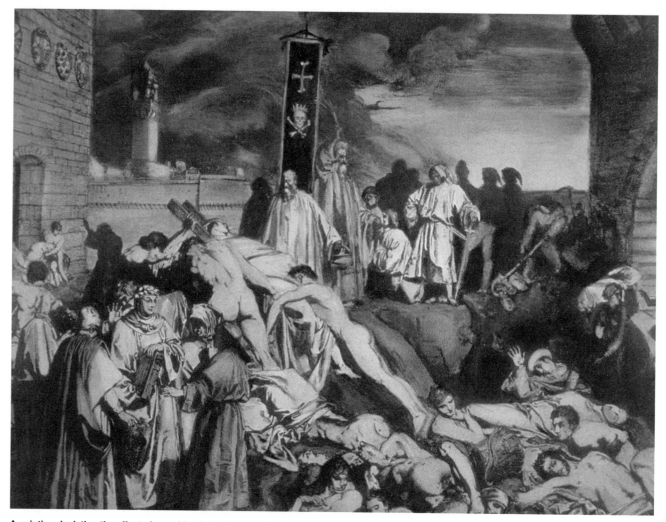

A painting depicting the effect of an epidemic (in this case, the plague in Florence, Italy).

conditions. Inadequate sanitation has and continues to be the breeding ground for the **bacteria** and **viruses** that can sweep through populations. The gathering of people in the burgeoning cities of seventeenth and eighteenth century Europe lead to a series of epidemics. These included **typhus**, **typhoid fever**, plague, **smallpox**, **dysentery**, and cholera. Outbreaks are less of a problem in modern day cities, due to better sanitation conditions and standards of housing. However, in underdeveloped areas of the world, or even in the developed world where sanitation and housing conditions are deficient, such diseases are still present.

Epidemics and pandemics can be so devastating that they can alter the course of history. An example is the Black Plague that spread through Europe and Britain in the seventeenth century. An estimated one-third of the population of Europe was killed, and cities such as London became nearly deserted, as those who could afford to do so fled the city. In the Crimean War (1853–1856), more than 50,000 soldiers died of typhus, while only 2,000 soldiers were actually killed in battle. As a final example, the spread of the plague to the New

World by contaminated blankets aboard French sailboats that docked at Halifax, Nova Scotia, in 1746, lead to the decimation of the aboriginal inhabitants of North America.

Within the past several decades, there has been an increasing recognition that disease that were previously assumed to be of genetic or other, nonbacterial or nonviral origin are in fact caused by **microorganisms** has lead to the recognition that there may be an epidemic or pandemic or maladies such as stomach ulcers and heart disease. These diseases differ from other bacterial and viral epidemics and pandemics, because they do not appear and fade over a relatively short time. Rather, the stomach ulcers caused by the bacterium *Helicobacter pylori* and the heart disease caused by the reaction of the immune system to infection by the bacterium *Chlamydia* are so-called chronic infections. These infections are present for a long time, essentially causing a non-stop pandemic of the particular malady.

See also Bacteria and bacterial infections; Bubonic plague; Flu, Great flu epidemic of 1918

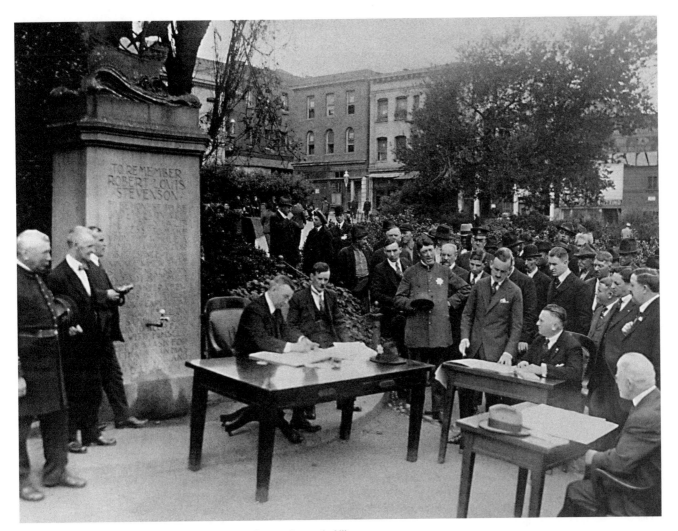

Court held outside during an epidemic, to lessen the chance of spread of illness.

EPIDEMICS, BACTERIAL

An epidemic is the occurrence of an illness among a large number of people in the same geographical area at the same time. Bacterial **epidemics** have probably been part of the lives of humans since the species evolved millions of years ago. Certainly by the time humans were present, **bacteria** were well established.

On example of a bacterial epidemic is the plague. Plague is caused by the bacterium *Yersinia pestis*. The bacterium lives in a type of rodent flea and is transmitted to people typically via the bite of the flea. People who come into contact with an infected animal or a flea-infested animals such as a rat can also contract the disease.

Plague has been a scourge on human populations for centuries. In the Middle Ages, the so-called Black Plague (**Bubonic plague**) killed millions of people in Europe. The crowded living conditions and poor sanitation that were typical of the disadvantaged populations of the large European cities of that time were breeding grounds for the spread of plague.

While often thought of as an epidemic of the past, plague remains today. Indeed, in the United States the last epidemic of plague occurred as recently as 1924–1925 in Los Angeles. The widespread use of **antibiotics** has greatly reduced the incidence of plague. Nonetheless, the potential for an epidemic remains.

As for plague, the use of antibiotics has reduced bacterial epidemics. However, this reduction generally tends to be a feature of developed regions of the world and regions that have ready access to health care. In other less advantaged areas of the globe, bacterial epidemics that have been largely conquered in North America and Europe, for example, still claim many lives.

An example is bacterial **meningitis**. The bacterial form of meningitis (an infection of the fluid in the spinal cord and surrounding the brain) is caused by *Haemophilus influenzae* type b, *Neisseria meningitides*, and *Streptococcus pneumoniae*. Antibiotics that are routinely given to children as part of the series of inoculations to establish **immunity** to the infection readily kill all three types of bacteria. But, in regions where such preventative measures are not practiced, meningitis epidemics are a problem. In 1996, the largest meningitis epidemic ever recorded, in terms of the numbers of affected people, occurred in West Africa. An estimated 250,000 people contracted meningitis and 25,000 people died of the infection.

Leprosy is an example of a bacterial epidemic that used to be common and which is now on the way to being eliminated. The disease is caused by *Mycobacterium leprae*. The bacterium was discovered by G.A. Hansen in 1873, and was the first bacterium to be identified as a cause of human disease.

Epidemics of leprosy were common in ancient times; indeed, During the first century A.D., millions of people were afflicted with the disease. Nowadays, the number of leprosy patients in the entire world has been reduced some ninety percent over earlier times through a concerted campaign of diagnosis and treatment that began in the 1990s. Still, leprosy remains at epidemic proportions in six countries: Brazil, India, Madagascar, Mozambique, Myanmar, and Nepal. In these countries an estimated half million new cases of leprosy appear every year.

In contrast to leprosy, **tuberculosis** is an epidemic that is increasing in prevalence with time. Tuberculosis is caused by another mycobacterium called *Mycobacterium tuberculosis*. The lung infections caused by epidemics of tuberculosis kill two million people each year around the world. The number of cases of tuberculosis is growing because of the difficulty in supplying health care to some underdeveloped areas, the increase of immunocompromising diseases such as Human **Immunodeficiency** Syndrome, and the appearance and spread of a strain of the bacterium that is resistant to many of the drugs used to treat the infection. Estimates from the **World Health Organization** indicate that if the tuberculosis epidemic continues nearly one billion people will become infected by 2020. Of those, some 35 million people will die of tuberculosis.

The re-emergence of tuberculosis is paradoxical. Whereas other bacterial epidemics have and are being controlled by modern methods of treatment, such methods are exacerbating the tuberculosis epidemic. Part of this is also due to the target of the **bacterial infection**. Lung infections are harder to conquer than infections of the skin, such as occurs in leprosy. Moreover, when the **immune system** is not functioning properly, due to the presence of another infection, the lung infection can become deadly. Thus, tuberculosis is an example of a bacterial epidemic whose scope is changing with the emergence of other infections and treatments.

The tuberculosis epidemic also underscores the danger of ineffective treatment and the effect of modern life on the spread of disease. Poorly supervised and incomplete treatment has caused the emergence of the drug-resistant strains of the bacteria. The bacteria can remain in the lungs and so can infect others. With the greater movement of people around the globe, the spread of the disease by carriers increases.

A final example of a bacterial epidemic is cholera. The disease caused by *Vibrio cholerae* is an example of an ancient bacterial epidemic that continues today. The intestinal infection produces a watery diarrhea that can lead to a fatal dehy-

dration. An epidemic of cholera caused by an antigenic version of *Vibrio cholerae* known as El Tor has been in progress since 1961. Indeed, the various epidemics are so widespread geographically that the disease can be considered pandemic (a simultaneously outbreak of illness on a worldwide scale). The latest epidemics have included countries in West Africa and Latin America that had been free of cholera for over a century.

Cholera is spread by contaminated food or water. Thus, the sanitary condition of a region is important to the presence of the epidemic. As with other bacterial epidemics of the past and present, underdeveloped regions are the focus of epidemic outbreaks of cholera.

See also Bacteria and bacterial infection; Biological warfare; Vaccination; Water quality

EPIDEMICS, VIRAL

An epidemic is an outbreak of a disease that involves a large number of people in a contained area (e.g., village, city, country). An epidemic that is worldwide in scope is referred to as a pandemic. A number of **viruses** have been responsible for **epidemics**. Some of these have been present since antiquity, while others have emerged only recently.

Smallpox is an example of an ancient viral epidemic. Outbreaks of smallpox were described in 1122 B.C. in China. In A.D. 165, Roman Legionnaires returning from military conquests in Asia and Africa spread the virus to Europe. One third of Europe's population died of smallpox during the 15-year epidemic. Smallpox remained a scourge until the late eighteenth century. Then, **Edward Jenner** devised a **vaccine** for the smallpox virus, based on the use of infected material from **cowpox** lesions. Less than a century later, naturally occurring smallpox epidemics had been ended.

Influenza is an example of a viral epidemic that also has its origins in ancient history. In contrast to smallpox, influenza epidemics remain a part of life today, even with the sophisticated medical care and vaccine development programs that can be brought to bear on infections.

Epidemics of influenza occurred in Europe during the Middle Ages. By the fifteenth century, epidemics began with regularity. A devastating epidemic swept through Spain, France, the Netherlands, and the British Isles in 1426–1427. Major outbreaks occurred in 1510, 1557, and 1580. In the eighteenth century there were three to five epidemics in Europe. Three more epidemics occurred in the nineteenth century. Another worldwide epidemic began in Europe in 1918. American soldiers returning home after World War I brought the virus to North America. In the United States alone almost 200,000 people died. The influenza epidemic of 1918 ranks as one of the worst natural disasters in history. In order to put the effects of the epidemic into perspective, the loss of life due to the four years of conflict of World War I was 10 million. The death toll from influenza during 5 months of the 1918 epidemic was 20 million.

Epidemics of influenza continue to occur. Examples include epidemics of the Asian flu (1957), and the Hong Kong

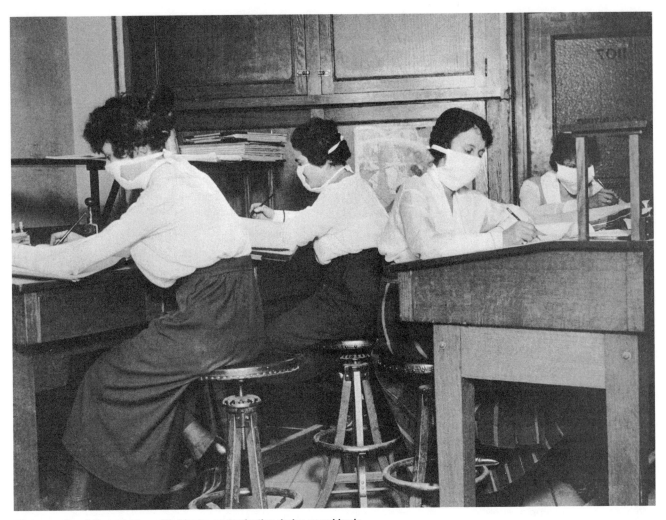

Clerks wearing cloth masks to avoid airborne contamination during an epidemic.

flu (1968). Potential epidemics due to the emergence of new forms of the virus in 1976 (the Swine flu) and 1977 (Russian flu) failed to materialize.

The continuing series of influenza epidemics is due to the ability of the various types of the influenza virus to alter the protein composition of their outer surface. Thus, the antibodies that result from an influenza epidemic in one year may be inadequate against the immunologically distinct influenza virus that occurs just a few years later. Advances in vaccine design and the use of agents that lessen the spread of the virus are contributing to a decreased scope of epidemics. Still, the threat of large scale influenza epidemics remains.

In the twentieth century, new viral epidemics have emerged. A number of different viruses have been grouped together under the designation of **hemorrhagic fevers**. These viruses are extremely contagious and sweep rapidly through the affected population. A hallmark of such infections is the copious internal bleeding that results from the viral destruction of host tissue. Death frequently occurs. The high death rate in fact limits the scope of these epidemics. Essentially the virus runs out of hosts to infect. The origin of hemorrhagic

viruses such as the **Ebola virus** is unclear. A developing consensus is that the virus periodically crosses the species barrier from its natural pool in primates.

Another viral epidemic associated with the latter half of the twentieth century is acquired **immunodeficiency** syndrome. This debilitating and destructive disease of the **immune system** is almost certainly caused by several types of a virus referred to as the **Human Immunodeficiency Virus** (**HIV**). The first known death due to HIV infection was a man in the Congo in 1959. The virus was detected in the United States only in 1981. Subsequent examination of stored blood sample dating back 40 years earlier revealed the presence of HIV.

HIV may have arisen in Africa, either from a previously unknown virus, or by the mutation of a virus resident in a non-human population (e.g., primates). The tendency of the virus to establish a latent infection in the human host before the appearance of the symptoms of an active infection make it difficult to pinpoint the origin of the virus. Moreover, this aspect of latency, combined with the ready ability of man to travel the globe, contributes to the spread of the epidemic. Indeed, the epidemic may now be more accurately considered to be a pandemic.

A final example of a twentieth century viral epidemic is that caused by the Hanta virus. The virus causes a respiratory malady that can swiftly overwhelm and kill the patient. The virus is normally resident on certain species of mouse. In the mid-1990s, an epidemic of Hanta virus syndrome occurred in native populations in the Arizona and New Mexico areas of the United States west. As with other viral epidemics, the epidemic faded away as quickly as it had emerged. However, exposure of someone to the mouse host or to dried material containing the virus particles can just as quickly fuel another epidemic.

Given their history, it seems unlikely viral epidemics will be eliminated. While certain types of viral agents will be defeated, mainly by the development of effective vaccines and the undertaking of a worldwide **vaccination** program (e.g., smallpox), other viral diseases will continue to plague mankind.

See also AIDS; Hemorrhagic fevers and diseases; Virology

EPIDEMIOLOGY

Epidemiology is the study of the various factors that influence the occurrence, distribution, prevention, and control of disease, injury, and other health-related events in a defined human population. By the application of various analytical techniques including mathematical analysis of the data, the probable cause of an infectious outbreak can be pinpointed. This connection between epidemiology and infection makes **microorganisms** an important facet of epidemiology.

Epidemiology and genetics are two distinct disciplines that converge into a new field of human science. Genetic epidemiology, a broad term used for the study of genetics and inheritance of disease, is a science that deals with origin, distribution, and control of disease in groups of related individuals, as well as inherited causes of diseases in populations. In particular, genetic epidemiology focuses on the role of genetic factors and their interaction with environmental factors in the occurrence of disease. This area of epidemiology is also known as molecular epidemiology.

Much information can come from molecular epidemiology even in the exact genetic cause of the malady is not known. For example, the identification of a malady in generations of related people can trace the genetic characteristic, and even help identify the original source of the trait. This approach is commonly referred to as genetic screening. The knowledge of why a particular malady appears in certain people, or why such people are more prone to a microbial infection than other members of the population, can reveal much about the nature of the disease in the absence of the actual **gene** whose defect causes the disease.

Molecular epidemiology has been used to trace the cause of bacterial, viral, and parasitic diseases. This knowledge is valuable in developing a strategy to prevent further outbreaks of the microbial illness, since the probable source of a disease can be identified.

Furthermore, in the era of the use of biological weapons by individuals, organizations, and governments, epidemiological studies of the effect of exposure to infectious microbes has become more urgently important. Knowledge of the effect of a bioweapon on the battlefield may not extend to the civilian population that might also be secondarily affected by the weapons. Thus, epidemiology is an important tool in identifying and tracing the course of an infection.

The origin of a genetic disease, or the genetic defect that renders someone more susceptible to an infection (e.g., cystic fibrosis), can involve a single gene or can be more complex, involving more than one gene. The ability to sort through the information and the interplay of various environmental and genetic factors to approach an answer to the source of a disease outbreak, for example, requires sophisticated analytical tools and personnel.

Aided by advances in computer technology, scientists develop complex mathematical formulas for the analysis of genetic models, the description of the transmission of the disease, and genetic-environmental interactions. Sophisticated mathematical techniques are now used for assessing classification, diagnosis, prognosis and treatment of many genetic disorders. Strategies of analysis include population study and family study. Population study must be considered as a broad and reliable study with an impact on **public health** programs. They evaluate the distribution and the determinants of genetic traits. Family study approaches are more specific, and are usually confirmed by other independent observations. By means of several statistical tools, genetic epidemiologic studies evaluate risk factors, inheritance and possible models of inheritance. Different kinds of studies are based upon the number of people who participate and the method of sample collection (i.e., at the time of an outbreak or after an outbreak has occurred). A challenge for the investigator is to achieve a result able to be applied with as low a bias as possible to the general population. In other words, the goal of an epidemiological study of an infectious outbreak is to make the results from a few individuals applicable to the whole population.

Such analytical tools and trained personnel are associated more with the developed world, in the sense that expensive analytical equipment and chemicals, and highly trained personnel are required. However, efforts from the developed world have made such resources available to under-developed regions. For example, the response of agencies such as the **World Health Organization** to outbreaks of **hemorrhagic fevers** that occur in underdeveloped regions of Africa can include molecular epidemiologists.

A fundamental underpinning of infectious epidemiology is the confirmation that a disease outbreak has occurred. Once this is done, the disease is followed with time. The pattern of appearance of cases of the disease can be tracked by developing what is known as an epidemic curve. This information is vital in distinguishing a natural outbreak from a deliberate and hostile act, for example. In a natural outbreak the number of cases increases over time to a peak, after which the cases subside as **immunity** develops in the population. A deliberate release of organisms will be evident as a sudden appearance of a large number of cases at the same time.

Analysis of a proper sample size, as well as study type are techniques belonging to epidemiology and statistics. They were developed in order to produce reliable information from a study regarding the association of genetic and environmental factors. Studies that are more descriptive consider genetic trait frequency, geographic distribution differences, and prevalence of certain conditions in different populations. On the other hand, studies that analyze numerical data consider factors like association, probability of occurrence, inheritance, and identification of specific groups of individuals.

Thus, molecular epidemiology arises from varied scientific disciplines, including genetics, epidemiology, and statistics. The strategies involved in genetic epidemiology encompass population studies and family studies. Sophisticated mathematical tools are now involved, and computer technology is playing a predominant role in the development of the discipline. Multidisciplinary collaboration is crucial to understanding the role of genetic and environmental factors in disease processes.

See also Bacteria and bacterial infection; Genetic identification of microorganisms; History of microbiology; History of public health; Infection control; Public health, current issues; Transmission of pathogens

EPIDEMIOLOGY, TRACKING DISEASES WITH TECHNOLOGY

Epidemiology is a term that refers to the techniques and analysis methods that are used to pinpoint the source of an illness. As well, epidemiologists (those who conduct the epidemiological investigations) are concerned with the distribution of the infection.

Typically, epidemiology is concerned with an illness outbreak involving the sudden appearance of a disease or other malady among a group of people. Examples of situations where epidemiology would be of use are an outbreak of food poisoning among patrons of a restaurant, or a disease outbreak in a geographically confined area.

Many illnesses of epidemiological concern are caused by **microorganisms**. Examples include **hemorrhagic fevers** such as that caused by the **Ebola virus, toxic shock syndrome, Lyme disease** caused by the Norwalk virus, and Acquired **Immunodeficiency** Syndrome caused by the **Human Immunodeficiency Virus**. The determination of the nature of illness outbreaks due to these and other microorganisms involve microbiological and immunological techniques.

Various routes can spread infections (i.e., on contact, air borne, insect borne, food, water). Some microorganisms are spread via a certain route. For example, *Coxiella burnetii*, the cause of **Q fever**, is spread from animals to humans via the air. Knowledge of how an infection was spread can suggest possible causes of the infection. This saves time, since the elimination of the many infectious microorganisms requires a lot of laboratory analysis.

Likewise, the route of entry of an infectious microbe can also vary from microbe to microbe. Hepatitis viruses are transmitted via direct contact (e.g., sharing of needles). Thus, a water-borne illness is likely not due to a **hepatitis** virus.

If an outbreak is recognized early enough, samples of the suspected cause (i.e., food, in the case of a food poisoning incident) as well as samples from the afflicted (i.e., feces) can be gathered for analysis. The analysis will depend on the symptoms. For example, in the case of a food poisoning, symptoms such as the rapid development of cramping, nausea with vomiting, and diarrhea after eating a hamburger would be grounds to consider *Escherichia coli* O157:H7 as the culprit. Analyses would likely include the examination for other known microbes associated with food poisoning (i.e., *Salmonella*) in order to save time in identifying the organism.

Analysis can involve the use of conventional laboratory techniques (e.g., use of nonselective and selective growth media to detect **bacteria**). As well, more recent technological innovations can be employed. An example is the use of antibodies to a known microorganism that are complexed with a fluorescent particle. The binding of the **antibody** to the microbes can be detected by the examination of a sample using fluorescence microscopy or flow cytometry. Molecular techniques such as the **polymerase chain reaction** are employed to detect genetic material from a target organism. However, the expense of the techniques such as **PCR** tend to limit its use to more of a confirmatory role, rather than as an initial tool of an investigation.

Another epidemiological tool is the determination of the antibiotic susceptibility and resistance of bacteria. This is especially true in the hospital setting, where **antibiotic resistance** bacteria are a problem in nosocomial (hospital acquired) infections. An outbreak of illness in a hospital should result in a pre-determined series of steps designed to rapidly determine the cause of the infection, to isolate the infection to as small an area of the hospital as possible, and to eliminate the infection. Knowing what **antibiotics** will be effective is a vital part of this strategy.

Such laboratory techniques can be combined with other techniques to provide information related to the spread of an outbreak. For example, microbiological data can be combined with geographic information systems (GIS). GIS information has helped pinpoint the source of outbreaks of Lyme disease. As well, the outbreak patterns can be used in the future to identify areas that will be high-risk areas for another outbreak. Besides geographic information, epidemiologists will use information including the weather on the days preceding an outbreak, mass transit travel schedules and schedules of mass-participation events that occurred around the time of an outbreak to try an establish a pattern of movement or behavior to those who have been affected by the outbreak. Use of credit cards and bank debit cards can also help piece together the movements of those who subsequently became infected.

The spread of **AIDS** in North America provides an example of the result of an epidemiological study of an illness. Analysis of the pattern of outbreaks and tracing the behavioral patterns of those who became infected led to the conclusion that the likely originator of the epidemic was a flight attendant. Because of his work, he was well traveled. His sexual behavior helped spread the virus to sexual partners all over North America, and they subsequently passed the virus on to other partners. Without the techniques and investigative protocols of epidemiology, the source of the AIDS epidemic would not have been resolved.

Reconstructing the movements of people is especially important when the outbreak is of an infectious disease. The occurrence of the disease over time can yield information as to the source of an outbreak. For example, the appearance of a few cases at first with the number of cases increasing over time to a peak is indicative of a natural outbreak. The number of cases usually begins to subside as the population develops **immunity** to the infection (e.g., **influenza**). However, if a large number of cases occur in the same area at the same time, the source of the infection might not be natural. Examples include a food poisoning or a bioterrorist action.

The ultimate aim of the various steps taken in an epidemiological investigation is to prevent infections by the use of prudent **public health** measures, rather than having to rely on reactive steps such as **vaccination** to defeat ongoing infections. Indeed, for some infections (i.e., **HIV**, hepatitis B and C) vaccination may not ultimately prove to be as effective as the identification of the factors that promote the diseases, and addressing those factors.

See also Bacteria and bacterial infection; Epidemics and pandemics; Laboratory techniques in immunology; Laboratory techniques in microbiology

EPIDERMAL INFECTIONS • *see* SKIN INFECTIONS

EPISOMES, PLASMIDS, INSERTION SEQUENCES, AND TRANSPOSONS

Episomes, **plasmids**, insertion sequences, and transposons are elements of **DNA (deoxyribonucleic acid)** that can exist independent of the main, or genomic, DNA.

An episome is a non-essential genetic element. In addition to its independent existence, an episome can also exist as an integrated part of the host genome of **bacteria**. It originates outside the host, in a virus or another bacterium. When integrated, a new copy of the episome will be made as the host chromosome undergoes replication. As an autonomous unit, the viral episome genetic material destroys the host cell as it utilizes the cellular replication machinery to make new copies of itself. But, when integrated into the bacterial chromosome they multiply in cell division and are transferred to the daughter cells. Another type of episome is called the F factor. The F factor is the best studied of the incompatibility groups that have the property of **conjugation** (the transfer of genetic material from one bacterial cell to another). The F factor can exist in three states. F+ is the autonomous, extrachromosomal state. Hfr (or high frequency **recombination**) refers to a factor, which has integrated into the host chromosome. Finally, F, or

F prime, state refers to the factor when it exists outside the chromosome, but with a section of chromosomal DNA attached to it. An episome is distinguished from other pieces of extrachromosomal DNA, such as plasmids, on the basis of their size. Episomes are large, having a molecular weight of at least 62 kilobases.

In contrast to episomes, a plasmid exists only as an independent piece of DNA. It is not capable of integration with the chromosomal DNA; it carries all the information necessary for its own replication. In order to maintain itself, a plasmid must divide at the same rate as the host bacterium. A plasmid is typically smaller than an episome, and exists as a closed circular piece of double stranded DNA. A plasmid can be readily distinguished from the chromosomal DNA by the techniques of gel **electrophoresis** or cesium chloride buoyant density gradient centrifugation. In addition to the information necessary for their replication, a plasmid can carry virtually any other **gene**. While not necessary for bacterial survival, plasmids can convey a selective advantage on the host bacterium. For example, some plasmids carry genes encoding resistance to certain **antibiotics**. Such plasmids are termed resistance or R factors. Other traits carried on plasmids include degradation of complex macromolecules, production of bacteriocins (molecules that inhibit **bacterial growth** or kill the bacteria), resistance to various heavy metals, or disease-causing factors necessary for infection of animal or plant hosts. Such traits can then be passed on to other bacteria, as some (but not all) plasmids also have the ability to promote transfer of their genetic material, in a process called conjugation. Conjugation is a one-way event—the DNA is transferred from one bacterium (the donor) to another bacterium (the recipient). All plasmids belong to one of the 30 or more incompatibility groups. The groups determine which plasmids can co-exist in a bacterial cell and help ensure that the optimum number of copies of each plasmid is maintained.

Plasmids have been exploited in **molecular biology** research. The incorporation of genes into plasmids, which maintain large numbers of copies in a cell (so-called multi-copy plasmids), allows higher levels of the gene product to be expressed. Such plasmids are also a good source of DNA for **cloning**.

Transposons and insertion sequences are known as mobile genetic elements. While they can also exist outside of the chromosome, they prefer and are designed to integrate into the chromosome following their movement from one cell to another. The are of interest to researchers for the insight they provide into basic molecular biology and **evolution**, as well as for their use as basic genetic tools. Transposons contain genes unrelated to the **transposition** of the genetic material from one cell to another. For example, Class 1 transposons encode drug resistance genes. In contrast, insertion sequences encode only the functions involved in their insertion into chromosomal DNA. Both transposons and insertion sequences can induce changes in chromosomal DNA upon their exiting and insertions, and so can generate **mutations**.

See also Bacteria; DNA (deoxyribonucleic acid); Electro-phoresis; Microbial genetics

EPSTEIN-BARR VIRUS

Epstein-Barr virus (EBV) is part of the family of human **herpes viruses**. Infectious **mononucleosis** (IM) is the most common disease manifestation of this virus, which once established in the host, can never be completely eradicated. Very little can be done to treat EBV; most methods can only alleviate resultant symptoms.

In addition to infectious mononucleosis, EBV has also been identified in association with—although not necessarily believed to cause—as many as 50 different illnesses and diseases, including chronic fatigue syndrome, rheumatoid arthritis, arthralgia (joint pain without **inflammation**), and myalgia (muscle pain). While studying aplastic anemia (failure of bone marrow to produce sufficient red blood cells), researchers identified EBV in bone marrow cells of some patients, suggesting the virus may be one causative agent in the disease. Also, several types of cancer can be linked to presence of EBV, particularly in those with suppressed immune systems, for example, suffering from **AIDS** or having recently undergone kidney or liver transplantation. The diseases include hairy cell leukemia, Hodgkin's and non-Hodgkin lymphoma, Burkitt's lymphoma (cancer of the lymphatic system endemic to populations in Africa), and nasopharyngeal carcinoma (cancers of the nose, throat, and thymus gland, particularly prevalent in East Asia). Recently, EBV has been associated with malignant smooth-muscle tissue tumors in immunocompromised children. Such tumors were found in several children with AIDS and some who had received liver transplants. Conversely, it appears that immunosuppressed adults show no elevated rates of these tumors.

Epstein-Barr virus was first discovered in 1964 by three researchers—Epstein, Achong, and Barr—while studying a form of cancer prevalent in Africa called Burkitt's lymphoma. Later, its role in IM was identified. A surge of interest in the virus has now determined that up to 95% of all adults have been infected with EBV at some stage of their lives. In seriously immunocompromised individuals and those with inherited **immune system** deficiencies, the virus can become chronic, resulting in "chronic Epstein-Barr virus" which can be fatal.

EBV is restricted to a very few cells in the host. Initially, the infection begins with its occupation and replication in the thin layer of tissue lining the mouth, throat, and cervix, which allow viral replication. The virus then invades the **B cells**, which do not facilitate the virus's replication but do permit its occupation. Infected B cells may lie dormant for long periods or start rapidly producing new cells. Once activated in this way, the B cells often produce antibodies against the virus residing in them. EBV is controlled and contained by killer cells and suppressor cells known as CD4 T lymphocytes in the immune system. Later, certain cytotoxic (destructive) CD8 T lymphocytes with specific action against EBV also come into play. These cells normally defend the host against the spread of EBV for the life of the host.

A healthy body usually provides effective **immunity** to EBV in the form of several different antibodies, but when this natural defense mechanism is weakened by factors that suppress its normal functioning—factors such as AIDS, organ transplantation, bone marrow failure, **chemotherapy** and other drugs used to treat malignancies, or even extended periods of lack of sleep and overexertion—EBV escape from their homes in the B cells, disseminate to other bodily tissue, and manifest in disease.

Infection is determined by testing for the antibodies produced by the immune system to fight the virus. The level of a particular antibody—the heterophile antibody—in the blood stream is a good indicator of the intensity and stage of EBV infection. Even though EBV proliferates in the mouth and throat, cultures taken from that area to determine infection are time-consuming, cumbersome, and usually not accurate.

Spread of the virus from one person to another requires close contact. Because of viral proliferation and replication in the lining of the mouth, infectious mononucleosis is often dubbed "the kissing disease." Also, because it inhabits cervical cells, researchers now suspect EBV may be sexually transmitted. Rarely is EBV transmitted via blood transfusion.

EBV is one of the latent viruses, which means it may be present in the body, lying dormant often for many years and manifesting no symptoms of disease. The percentage of shedding (transmission) of the virus from the mouth is highest in people with active IM or who have become immunocompromised for other reasons. A person with active IM can prevent transmission of the disease by avoiding direct contact—such as kissing—with uninfected people. However, shedding has been found to occur in 15% of adults who test positive for antibodies but who show no other signs of infection, thus allowing the virus to be transmitted. Research efforts are directed at finding a suitable **vaccine**.

The prevalence of antibodies against EBV in the general population is high in developing countries and lower socioeconomic groups where individuals become exposed to the virus at a very young age. In developed countries, such as the United States, only 50% of the population shows traces of **antibody** by the age of five years, with an additional 12% in college-aged adolescents, half of whom will actually develop IM. This situation indicates that children and young persons between the ages of 10 and 21 years are highly susceptible to IM in developed countries, making it a significant health problem among students.

See also Latent viruses and diseases; Mononucleosis, infectious; Viruses and responses to viral infection

ERYTHROMYCINS · *see* ANTIBIOTICS

ESCHERICHIA COLI

Escherichia coli is a bacterium, which inhabits the intestinal tract of humans and other warm-blooded mammals. It constitutes approximately 0.1% of the total **bacteria** in the adult intestinal tract. Its name comes from the name of the person, Escherich, who in 1885 first isolated and characterized the bacterium.

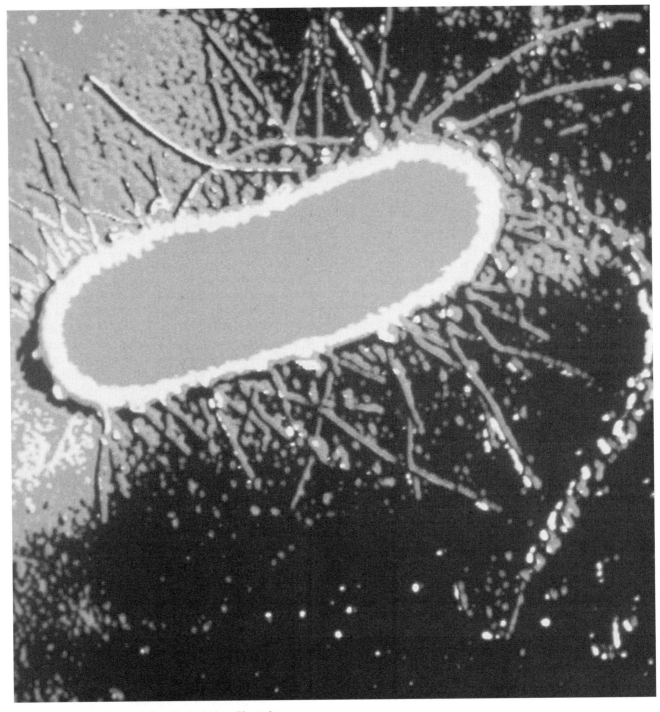

Scanning electron micrograph of an *Escherichia coli* bacterium.

The bacterium, particularly one type called strain K–12, is one of the most widely studied organisms in modern research. Its biochemical behavior and structure are well known, having been studied for much of this century. This plethora of information has made *E. coli* indispensable as the bacterial model system for biochemical, behavioral and structural studies. *E. coli* is also the most encountered bacterium in clinical laboratories, being the primary cause of human urinary tract infections. Pathogenic (diseases causing) strains of *E. coli* are responsible for **pneumonia**, **meningitis** and traveler's diarrhea.

As part of the normal flora of the intestinal tract, *E. coli* is beneficial. It is crucial in the digestion of food, and is our principle source of vitamin K and B-complex vitamins.

Outside of the intestinal tract, *E. coli* dies quickly. This trait has been exploited, and *E. coli* is a popular indicator of drinking **water quality**, as its presence indicates the recent **contamination** of the water with feces.

One of the most harmful types of *E. coli* is a strain called O157:H7. Researchers surmise that O157:H7 arose when an innocuous *E. coli* bacterium was infected by a virus carrying the genes coding for a powerful toxin called Shiga-like toxin. The toxin can destroy cells in the intestinal tract and, if they enter the bloodstream, can impair or destroy the kidneys and the liver. The intestinal damage causes a lot of bleeding. In children and elderly people, this hemorrhaging can be lethal. In other people, damage to the kidney and liver can be permanent or even lethal. In the summer of 2000, more than 2,000 people in Walkerton, Ontario, Canada were sickened and seven people died from drinking water which had been contaminated with O157:H7.

Strain O157:H7 was first linked to human disease in 1983, when it was shown to have been the cause of two outbreaks of an unusual and severe gastrointestinal ailment in the Unites States. Since then, the number of documented human illnesses and deaths caused by O157:H7 has increased steadily worldwide. Disease caused by *E. coli* is preventable, by proper hand washing after bowel movements, avoidance of unpasteurized milk or apple cider, washing of raw foods before consumption and thorough cooking of ground meat.

Modern genetics techniques have been successful in obtaining the sequence of the genetic material of *E. coli.* Frederick Blattner and his colleagues published the genome sequence of strain K–12 in 1997. The genome was discovered to have approximately 4300 protein coding regions making up about 88 per cent of the bacterial chromosome. The most numerous types of proteins were transport and binding proteins—those necessary for the intake of nutrients. A fairly large portion of the genome is reserved for metabolism—the processing of the acquired nutrients into useable chemicals. In 2000, Nicole Perna and her colleagues published the genome sequence of O157:H7. The O157:H7 genome shows similarity to tat of k12, reflecting a common ancestry. But, in contrast to K12, much of the genome of O157:H7 codes for unique proteins, over 1,300, some of which may be involved in disease causing traits. Many of these genes appear to have been acquired from other **microorganisms**, in a process called lateral transfer. Thus, strain O157:H7 appears to be designed to undergo rapid genetic change. This distinction is important; indicating that strategies to combat problems caused by one strain of *E. coli* might not be universally successful. Knowledge of the genetic organization of these strains will enable more selective strategies to be developed to combat *E.coli* infections.

See also Food safety; Microbial flora of the stomach and gastrointestinal tract; Microbial genetics; Waste water treatment; Water purification; Water quality

ESCHERICHIA COLI (E. COLI) INFECTION

• *see* E. COLI O157:H7 INFECTION

ESCHERICHIA COLI, ENTEROHEMOR-RHAGIC • *see* ESCHERICHIA COLI (E. COLI)

EUBACTERIA

The Eubacteria are the largest and most diverse taxonomic group of **bacteria**. Some scientists regard the Eubacteria group as an artificial assemblage, merely a group of convenience rather than a natural grouping. Other scientists regard eubacteria as comprising their own kingdom. Another recent classification holds Eubacteria and Archaebacteria as domains or major groupings, classified above the kingdom level. The Eubacteria are all easily stained, rod-shaped or spherical bacteria. They are generally unicellular, but a small number of multicellular forms do occur. They can be motile or non-motile and the motile forms are frequently characterized by the presence of numerous flagellae. Many of the ecologically important bacteria responsible for the fixation of nitrogen, such as *Azotobacter* and *Rhizobium,* are found in this group.

The cell walls of all of these species are relatively thick and unchanging, thus shape is generally constant within groups found in the Eubacteria. Thick cell walls are an evolutionary adaptation that allows survival in extreme situations where thinner walled bacteria would dry out. Some of the bacteria are gram positive while others are gram negative. One commonality that can be found within the group is that they all reproduce by transverse binary fission, although not all bacteria that reproduce in this manner are members of this group.

Eubacteria are often classified according to the manner in which they gain energy. Photoautotrophic Eubacteria manufacture their own energy through **photosynthesis**. Cyanobacteria, often called **blue-green algae**, are common photoautotrophic Eubacteria that are found in ponds and wetlands. Although not true algae, Cyanobacteria grow in chain-like colonies and contain chloroplasts as do aquatic algae. Cyanobacteria fossils are among the oldest-known fossils on Earth, some more than 3.5 billion years old.

Heterotrphic Eubacteria depend upon organic molecules to provide a source of energy. Heterotrophic Eubacteria are among the most abundant and diverse bacteria on Earth, and include bacteria that live as **parasites**, decomposers of organic material (saprophytes), as well as many pathogens (disease-causing bacteria). Chemoautotrophic Eubacteria bacteria obtain their own energy by the oxidation of inorganic molecules. **Chemoautotrophic bacteria** are responsible for releasing the sulfur resulting in a sulfur taste of freshwater near many beaches (such as in Florida), and for supplying nitrogen in a form able to be used by plants.

See also Autotrophic bacteria; Heterotrophic bacteria; Nitrogen cycle in microorganisms; Oxidation-reduction reaction; Photosynthetic microorganisms

EUKARYOTES

Eukaryotic organisms encompass a range of organisms, from humans to single-celled **microorganisms** such as **protozoa**. Eukaryotes are fundamentally different from prokaryotic microorganisms, such as **bacteria**, in their size, structure and functional organization.

The oldest known eukaryote fossil is about 1.5 billion years old. Prokaryote fossils that are over 3 billion years old are known. Thus, prokaryotic cells appeared first on Earth. The appearance of eukaryotic cells some 1.5 billion years ago became possible when cellular function was organized into regions within the cell called organelles.

The eukaryotes are organized into a division of life that is designated as the Eukaryota. The Eukaryota are one of the three branches of living organisms. The other two branches are the Prokaryota and the Archae.

The evolutionary divergence of life into these three groups has been deduced in the pasts several decades. Techniques of molecular analysis have been used, in particular the analysis of the sequence of a component of ribosomal **ribonucleic acid** (**RNA**), which is known as 16S RNA. This RNA species is highly conserved in life forms. Thus, great differences in the sequence of 16 S RNA between a eukaryotic and a prokaryotic microorganism, for example, indicate that the two organisms diverged evolutionarily a very long time ago. A similar 16 S RNA indicates the converse; that evolutionary branching is a relatively recent event.

Eukaryotic cells are about 10 times the size of all but a few prokaryotes. This translates to an internal volume which is very much larger, some 1000 times, that the internal volume of a bacterium. In order to survive, eukaryotes evolved a highly organized internal structure, in order that all the tasks necessary for life can be accomplished in the large internal volume. This internal structure is the fundamental distinguishing aspect of a eukaryote versus a prokaryote.

Functional specialization is the fundamental hallmark of eukaryotes. In larger organisms, such as humans, this specialization gives rise to organs such as the heart, lover, and brain, and to functional organizations such as the **immune system**. But organization is also evident in microscopic, even single-celled, eukaryotes.

In a eukaryote, the nuclear material is segregated within a specialized region called the **nucleus**. This feature is a key constituent of eukaryotic cells. Indeed, the word eukaryote means "true nuclei." The nucleus exists because of the presence of the so-called nuclear membrane, which encloses the nuclear material. The nuclear membrane contains pores, through which material can enter and leave the nuclear region. Prokaryotes lack an organized nucleus. Indeed, for many years the presence of a nucleus was the sole key feature that distinguished a eukaryote from a prokaryote.

Most of the eukaryotic **DNA** (**deoxyribonucleic acid**) is present in the nucleus. The remainder is contained within the energy-generating structures known as the mitochondria. The organization of the eukaryotic DNA is very different from bacterial DNA. In the latter, the genetic material is usually dispersed as a large circle throughout the interior of the

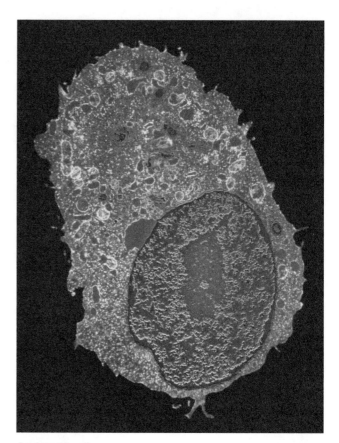

A eukaryotic cell.

bacterium, in a gel-like mixture termed the **cytoplasm**. In contrast, eukaryotic DNA is organized into discrete limb-like structures called **chromosomes**.

The replication of eukaryotic DNA is also different from that of prokaryotes. The latter is essentially an unwinding of the double helix of DNA, with ongoing complementary copies of daughter DNA strands made from each unwinding parental strand. The result is two double helices. The replication process in eukaryotes is more complex, involving several phases of chromosome replication, segregation to areas of the cell, collection together, and enclosure in a nuclear membrane.

Eukaryotic cells, including microorganisms, contain a specialized functional region known as the endoplasmic reticulum. This network of tubular structures is involved in the manufacture of protein from the template of RNA. In many eukaryotes a region called the Golgi apparatus or Golgi body is associated with the endoplasmic reticulum. The Golgi body is involved with the transport of compounds into and out of the cell.

Another distinctive feature of eukaryotic cells is the aforementioned mitochondria. These are the energy factories of the cell. Additionally, some eukaryotes possess structures called chloroplasts, which use the energy available in light to change carbon dioxide and water into carbohydrates. The carbohydrates provide a ready source of energy for cellular functions. This photosynthetic process is a feature of the microscopic eukaryotes called algae.

Other internal organization of eukaryotes includes lysosomes, which contain enzyme that digest food that is taken into the eukaryote. The **lysosome** represents a primitive stomach.

Eukaryotic cells such as amoeba possess an internal scaffolding that helps provide the shape and support to the cell. The scaffolding consists of filaments that are made of protein. Depending on the protein the filaments are designated as actin filaments, microtubules, and intermediate filaments.

Eukaryotes such as amoebae and algae are part of a group that is called Protista. More commonly, members of the group are referred to as **protists.**

The evolutionary branching of eukaryotes from prokaryotes involved the acquisition of regions specialized function within the eukaryotic cell. One of these regions, the mitochondria, was likely derived from the habitation of a eukaryote by a bacterium. Evidence from ultrastructural and molecular studies for a symbiosis between a bacterium and a eukaryote is convincing. Over time, the bacterium became truly a component of the eukaryotic cell. Today, however, the DNA of the mitochondria remains unique, with respect to eukaryotic nuclear DNA.

Likewise, chloroplasts may have had the origin in a symbiotic relationship between a cyanobacterium and a eukaryotic cell. Current evidence does not support the development of any other eukaryotic organelle from a prokaryotic ancestor.

See also Bacterial ultrastructure; Cell cycle and cell division; Mitochondrial DNA

EUKARYOTIC CELLS, GENETIC REGULATION OF • *see* GENETIC REGULATION OF EUKARYOTIC CELLS

EULER-CHELPIN, HANS VON (1873-1964)
Swedish biochemist

Hans von Euler-Chelpin described the role of **enzymes** in the process of **fermentation** and also researched vitamins, tumors, enzymes, and coenzymes. He was an important contributor in the discovery of the structure of certain vitamins. In 1929, he shared the Nobel Prize in chemistry with Arthur Harden for their research on the fermentation of sugar and enzymes. Euler-Chelpin's research has far-reaching implications in the fields of nutrition and medicine.

Hans Karl Simon August von Euler-Chelpin was born in Augsburg in the Bavarian region of Germany on February 15, 1873, to Rigas, a captain in the Royal Bavarian Regiment, and Gabrielle (Furtner) von Euler-Chelpin. His mother was related to the Swiss mathematician Leonhard Euler. Shortly after his birth, Euler-Chelpin's father was transferred to Munich and Euler-Chelpin lived with his grandmother in Wasserburg for a time. After his early education in Munich, Würzburg, and

Ulm, he entered the Munich Academy of Painting in 1891 intending to become an artist. Eventually, he changed his professional interest to science.

In 1893, Euler-Chelpin enrolled at the University of Munich to study physics with Max Planck and Emil Warburg. He also studied organic chemistry with Emil Fischer and A. Rosenheim, after which he worked with Walther Nernst at the University of Göttingen on problems in physical chemistry. This post-doctoral work in the years 1896 to 1897 was undertaken after Euler-Chelpin received his doctorate in 1895 from the University of Berlin.

The summer of 1897 was the first of several that Euler-Chelpin spent in apprentice roles in Stockholm and in Berlin. He served as an assistant to **Svante Arrhenius** in his laboratory at the University of Stockholm, becoming a privatdocent (unpaid tutor) there in 1899. Returning to Germany that summer, he studied with Eduard Buchner and Jacobus Van't Hoff in Berlin until 1900. His studies during this period centered on physical chemistry, which was receiving a great deal of attention at that time in both Germany and Sweden. Recognition came early to Euler-Chelpin for his work. He received the Lindblom Prize from Germany in 1898.

It was evident during this time that there were new opportunities in organic chemistry. The new equipment used to measure properties could be applied to the complexities of chemical changes that took place in organisms. Euler-Chelpin's interests, therefore, shifted to organic chemistry. He visited the laboratories of others working in the field, such as Arthur Hantzsch and Johannes Thiele in Germany and G. Bertrand in Paris. These contacts contributed to his developing interest in fermentation.

In 1902, Euler-Chelpin became a Swedish citizen and in 1906, he was appointed professor of general and organic chemistry at the University of Stockholm, where he remained until his retirement in 1941. By 1910, Euler-Chelpin was able to present the fermentation process and enzyme chemistry into a systematic relationship with existing chemical knowledge. His book, *The Chemistry of Enzymes,* was first published in 1910 and again in several later editions.

In spite of being a Swedish citizen, Euler-Chelpin served in the German army during World War I, fulfilling his teaching obligations for six months of the year and military service for the remaining six. In the winter of 1916–1917, he took part in a mission to Turkey, a German ally during World War I, to accelerate the production of munitions and alcohol. He also commanded a bomber squadron at the end of the war.

After the war, Euler-Chelpin began his research into the chemistry of enzymes, particularly in the role they played in the fermentation process. This study was important because enzymes are the catalysts for biochemical reactions in plant and animal organisms. An integral aspect of Euler-Chelpin's work with enzymes was to identify each substrate (the molecule upon which an enzyme acted) in the reaction. He succeeded in demonstrating that two fragments that split from the sugar molecule were disparate in energy. He further illustrated that the less energetic fragment, which is attached to the phosphate, is destroyed in the process. Apart from tracing the phosphate through the fermentation sequence, Euler-Chelpin detailed the chemical makeup of cozymase, a non-protein constituent involved in cellular **respiration**.

In 1929, Euler-Chelpin was awarded the Nobel Prize in chemistry, which he shared with Arthur Harden "for their investigations on the fermentation of sugar and of fermentative enzymes." The presenter of the award noted that fermentation was "one of the most complicated and difficult problems of chemical research." The solution to the problem made it possible, the presenter continued, "to draw important conclusions concerning carbohydrate **metabolism** in general in both the vegetable and the animal organism."

In 1929, Euler-Chelpin became the director of the Vitamin Institute and Institute of **Biochemistry** at the University of Stockholm, which was founded jointly by the Wallenburg Foundation and the Rockefeller Foundation. Although he retired from teaching in 1941, he continued research for the remainder of his life. In 1935, he had turned his attention to the biochemistry of tumors and developed, through his collaboration with George de Hevesy, a technique for labeling the nucleic acids present in tumors, which subsequently made it possible to trace their behavior. He also helped elucidate the function of nicotinamide and thiamine in compounds which are metabolically active.

Euler-Chelpin was twice married, each time to a woman who assisted him in his research. His first wife, Astrid Cleve, was the daughter of P. T. Cleve, a professor of chemistry at the University of Uppsala. She helped him in his early research in fermentation. They married in 1902, had five children, and divorced in 1912. Euler-Chelpin married Elisabeth, Baroness Ugglas in 1913, with whom he had four children. This marriage lasted for fifty-one years. A son by his first wife, Ulf Euler, later also won a Nobel Prize. His award was made in 1970 in the field of medicine or physiology for his work on neurotransmitters and the nervous system.

Euler-Chelpin was awarded the Grand Cross for Federal Services with Star from Germany in 1959. He also received numerous honorary degrees from universities in Europe and America. He held memberships in Swedish science associations, as well as many foreign professional societies. He is the author of more than eleven hundred research papers and over half a dozen books. Euler-Chelpin died on November 6, 1964, in Stockholm, Sweden.

EVANS, ALICE (1881-1975)

American microbiologist

The bacteriologist Alice Evans was a pioneer both as a scientist and as a woman. Evans discovered that the *Brucella* **bacteria**, contracted from farm animals and their milk, was the cause of undulant fever in humans, and responded by fighting persistently for the routine, improved **pasteurization** of milk, eventually achieving success. She was the first woman president of the Society of American Bacteriologists (now American Society of Microbiology). Although marginalized early in her career, Evans overcame many obstacles and lived to see her discoveries repeatedly confirmed. She had a major impact on

microbiology in the United States and the world, and received belated honors for her numerous achievements in the field.

Alice Catherine Evans was born on January 29, 1881, in the predominantly Welsh town of Neath, Pennsylvania, the second of William Howell and Anne Evans' two children. William Howell, the son of a Welshman, was a surveyor, teacher, farmer, and Civil War veteran. Anne Evans, also Welsh, emigrated from Wales at the age of 14. Evans received her primary education at the local district school. She went on to study at the Susquehanna Institute at Towanda, Pennsylvania. She wished to go to college but, unable to afford tuition, took a post as a grade school teacher. After teaching for four years, she enrolled in a tuition-free, two-year course in nature study at the Cornell University College of Agriculture. The course was designed to help teachers in rural areas inspire an appreciation of nature in their students. It changed the path of Evans' life, however, and she never returned to the schoolroom.

At Cornell, Evans discovered her love of science and received a B.S. degree in agriculture. She chose to pursue an advanced degree in bacteriology and was recommended by her professor at Cornell for a scholarship at the University of Wisconsin. She was the first woman to receive the scholarship, and under the supervision of E. G. Hastings, Evans studied bacteriology with a focus on chemistry. In 1910, she received a Master of Science degree in bacteriology from Wisconsin. Although encouraged to pursue a Ph.D., Evans accepted a research position with the University of Wisconsin Agriculture Department's Dairy Division and began researching cheese-making methods in 1911. In 1913, she moved with the division to Washington, D.C., and served as bacteriological technician in a team effort to isolate the sources of **contamination** of raw cow's milk, which were then assumed to be external.

On her own, Evans began to focus on the intrinsic bacteria in raw cow's milk. By 1917, she had found that the bacterium responsible for undulant or "Malta" fever (later called **brucellosis**, after the responsible pathogen) was similar in important respects to one associated with spontaneous abortions in cows, and that the two bacteria produced similar clinical effects in guinea pigs. Prevailing wisdom at the time held that many bovine diseases could not be transmitted to humans. That year she presented her findings to the Society of American Bacteriologists; her ideas were received with skepticism that may have been more due to her gender and level of education than her data.

In 1918, Evans was asked to join the staff of the United States Public Health Service by director George McCoy. There, she was absorbed in the study of **meningitis**. Although she was unable to continue her milk studies during this time, support for Evans' findings was trickling in from all over the world. By the early 1920s, it was recognized that undulant fever and Malta fever were due to the same bacteria, but there was still resistance to the idea that humans could contract brucellosis by drinking the milk of infected cows. Because the symptoms of brucellosis were so similar to those of **influenza**, **typhoid fever**, **tuberculosis**, **malaria**, and rheumatism, it was not often correctly diagnosed. Evans began documenting cases of the disease among humans in the U.S. and South Africa, but it was not until 1930, after brucellosis had claimed the lives of a number of farmers' children in the U.S., that **public health** officials began to recognize the need for pasteurization.

In 1922, Evans, like many others who researched these organisms, became ill with brucellosis. Her condition was chronic, plaguing her on and off for almost 23 years, and perhaps providing her with new insight into the disease. As the problem of chronic illness became widespread, Evans began surveying different parts of the U.S. to determine the numbers of infected cows from whom raw milk was sold, and the numbers of chronic cases resulting from the milk.

In 1925, Evans was asked to serve on the National Research Council's Committee on Infectious Abortion. In this capacity, Evans argued for the pasteurization of milk, a practice that later became an industry standard. In recognition of her achievements, Evans was in 1928 elected the first woman president of the American Society of Bacteriologists. In 1930, she was chosen, along with Robert E. Buchanan of Iowa State University, as an American delegate to the First International Congress of Bacteriology in Paris. She attended the second Congress in London in 1936 and was again able to travel widely in Europe. She returned to the United States and eventually was promoted to senior bacteriologist at the Public Health Service, by then called the National Institute of Health. By 1939, Evans had changed her focus to **immunity** to streptococcal infections and in 1945, she retired. Evans, who never married, died at the age of 94 on September 5, 1975, in Alexandria, Virginia.

EVOLUTION AND EVOLUTIONARY MECHANISMS

Evolution is the process of biological change over time. Such changes, especially at the genetic level are accomplished by a complex set of evolutionary mechanisms that act to increase or decrease genetic variation. Because of their rapid development and reproduction (i.e., high generation rate), evidence of the fundamental molecular mechanisms of evolution are especially apparent in studies of **bacteria** and viral **microorganisms**. Immunological adaptation has a profound effect on fitness and survivability.

Evolutionary theory is the cornerstone of modern biology, and unites all the fields of biology under one theoretical umbrella to explain the changes in any given **gene** pool of a population over time. Evolutionary theory is theory in the scientific usage of the word. It is more than a hypothesis; there is an abundance of observational and experimental data to support the theory and its subtle variations. These variations in the interpretation of the role of various evolutionary mechanisms are because all theories, no matter how highly useful or cherished, are subject to being discarded or modified when verifiable data demand such revision. Biological evolutionary theory is compatible with nucleosynthesis (the evolution of the elements) and current cosmological theories in physics regarding the origin and evolution of the Universe. There is no currently accepted scientific data that is incompatible with the general postulates of evolutionary theory, and the mechanisms of evolution.

Fundamental to the concept of evolutionary mechanism is the concept of the syngameon, the set of all genes. By definition, a gene is a hereditary unit in the syngameon that carries information that can be used to construct proteins via the processes of **transcription** and **translation**. A gene pool is the set of all genes in a species or population.

Another essential concept, important to understanding evolutionary mechanisms, is an understanding that there are no existing (extant) primitive organisms that can be used to study evolutionary mechanism. For example, all **eukaryotes** derived from a primitive, common prokaryotic ancestral bacterium. Accordingly, all living eukaryotes have evolved as eukaryotes for the same amount of time. Additionally, no eukaryote plant or animal cell is more primitive with regard to the amount of time they have been subjected to evolutionary mechanisms. Seemingly primitive characteristics are simply highly efficient and conserved characteristics that have changed little over time.

Evolution requires genetic variation, and these variations or changes (**mutations**) can be beneficial, neutral or deleterious. In general, there are two major types of evolutionary mechanisms, those that act to increase genetic variation, and mechanisms that operate to decrease genetic mechanisms.

Mechanisms that increase genetic variation include mutation, **recombination** and gene flow.

Mutations generally occur via chromosomal mutations, point mutations, frame shifts, and breakdowns in **DNA** repair mechanisms. Chromosomal mutations include translocations, inversions, deletions, and chromosome non-disjunction. Point mutations may be nonsense mutations leading to the early termination of **protein synthesis**, missense mutations (a that results an a substitution of one amino acid for another in a protein), or silent mutations that cause no detectable change.

Recombination involves the re-assortment of genes through new chromosome combinations. Recombination occurs via an exchange of DNA between homologous **chromosomes** (crossing over) during meiosis. Recombination also includes linkage disequilibrium. With linkage disequilibrium, variations of the same gene (alleles) occur in combinations in the gametes (sexual reproductive cells) than should occur according to the rules of probability.

Gene flow occurs when gene carriers (e.g., people, bacteria, **viruses**) change their local genetic group by moving—or being transported—from one place to another. These migrations allow the introduction of new variations of the same gene (alleles) when they mate and produce offspring with members of their new group. In effect, gene flow acts to increase the gene pool in the new group. Because genes are usually carried by many members of a large population that has undergone random mating for several generations, random migrations of individuals away from the population or group usually do not significantly decrease the gene pool of the group left behind.

In contrast to mechanisms that operate to increase genetic variation, there are fewer mechanisms that operate to decrease genetic variation. Mechanisms that decrease genetic variation include genetic drift and natural **selection**.

Genetic drift, important to studies of Immunological differences between population groups, results form the changes in the numbers of different forms of a gene (allelic frequency) that result from sexual reproduction. Genetic drift can occur as a result of random mating (random genetic drift) or be profoundly affected by geographical barriers, catastrophic events (e.g., natural disasters or wars that significantly affect the reproductive availability of selected members of a population), and other political-social factors.

Natural selection is based upon the differences in the viability and reproductive success of different genotypes with a population (differential reproductive success). Natural selection can only act on those differences in **genotype** that appear as phenotypic differences that affect the ability to attract a mate and produce viable offspring that are, in turn, able to live, mate and continue the species. Evolutionary fitness is the success of an entity in reproducing (i.e., contributing alleles to the next generation).

There are three basic types of natural selection. With directional selection, an extreme **phenotype** is favored (e.g., for height or length of neck in giraffe). Stabilizing selection occurs when intermediate **phenotype** is fittest (e.g., neither too high or low a body weight) and for this reason it is often referred to a normalizing selection. Disruptive selection occurs when two extreme phenotypes are fitter that an intermediate phenotype.

Natural selection does not act with foresight. Rapidly changing environmental conditions can, and often do, impose new challenges for a species that result in extinction. In addition, evolutionary mechanisms, including natural selection, do not always act to favor the fittest in any population, but instead may act to favor the more numerous but tolerably fit.

The operation of natural evolutionary mechanisms exhibited in microorganisms is complicated in humans by geographic, ethnic, religious, and social groups and customs. Accordingly, the effects of various evolution mechanisms on human populations are not as easy to predict. Increasingly sophisticated statistical studies are carried out by population geneticists to characterize changes in the human genome, especially with regard to immunological differences between populations.

See also Antibiotic resistance, tests for; Evolutionary origin of bacteria and viruses; Extraterrestrial microbiology; Immunogenetics; Miller-Urey experiment; Molecular biology and molecular genetics; Molecular biology, central dogma of; Mutants, enhanced tolerance or sensitivity to temperature and pH ranges; Mutations and mutagenesis; Radiation mutagenesis; Radiation resistant bacteria; Rare genotype advantage; Viral genetics

EVOLUTIONARY ORIGIN OF BACTERIA AND VIRUSES

Earth formed between 4.5 and 6 billion years ago. Conditions initially remained inhospitable for the potential development of life. By about 3.0 billion years ago, however, an atmosphere that contained the appropriate blend of nitrogen, oxygen, car-

bon, and hydrogen allowed life to commence. The formation of proteins and nucleic acids led to the generation of the **genetic code**, contained in deoxyribonucleic and ribonucleic acids, and the protein machinery to translate the information into a tangible product.

Fossil evidence indicates that one of the first life forms to arise were **bacteria**. The planetary conditions that were the norm four to six billion years ago were much different from now. Oxygen was scarce, and extremes of factors such as temperature and atmospheric radiation were more common than now. Although the exact origin of bacteria will likely never be known, the present-day bacteria that variously tolerate extremes of temperature, salt concentration, radiation, **pH** and other such environmental factors may be examples of the original bacteria.

Such "**extremophiles**" are part of the division of life known as the Archae, specifically the archaebacteria.

Whether bacteria originated in the sea or on land remains a mystery. The available evidence, however, supports the origin of bacteria in the sea. With the advent of molecular means of comparing the relatedness of bacteria, it has been shown that most of the bacteria known to exist on land bear some resemblance to one another. But, only some 10% of the bacteria from the ocean are in any way related to their terrestrial counterparts. In support of the origin of bacteria in the ancient seas is the discovery of the vast quantities and variety of **viruses** in seawater.

The discovery in the 1970s of bacteria thriving at **hydrothermal vents** deep beneath the surface of the ocean suggests that bacterial life in the ancient oceans was at least certainly possible. Such bacteria would derive their energy from chemical compounds present in their environment. It is also likely that bacterial life was also developing concurrently in response to another energy source, the sun. Indeed, the evolutionarily ancient cyanobacteria are **photosynthetic microorganisms**, which derive their energy from sunlight.

One type of bacteria that is definitely known to have been among the first to appear on Earth is the cyanobacteria. Fossils of cyanobacteria have been uncovered that date back almost 4 billion years. These bacteria are suited to the low oxygen levels that were present in the planet's atmosphere at that time. The cyanobacteria produced oxygen as a waste gas of their metabolic processes and so helped to create an atmosphere containing a greater amount of oxygen. Other, oxygen-requiring bacteria could then develop, along with other life forms.

In contrast to bacteria, scientists debate if viruses are alive. They are not capable of their own reproduction. Instead, they require the presence of a host in which they can introduce their genetic material. Through the formation of products encoded by the viral genetic material and by the use of aspects of the host's replication machinery, viruses are able to direct the manufacture and assembly of components to produce new virus.

The nature of viral replication requires the prior presence of a host. It remains unclear whether the first virus arose from a prokaryotic host, such as a bacterium, or a eukaryotic host. However, the appearance of prokaryotic life prior to eukaryotic life argues for the origin of viruses as an evolutionary offshoot of prokaryotes.

Scientists are in general agreement that the first virus was a fragment of **DNA** or **ribonucleic acid** (**RNA**) from a eventual prokaryotic or eukaryotic host. The genetic fragment somehow was incorporated into a eukaryotic and became replicated along with the host's genetic material. Over evolutionary time, different viruses developed, having differing specificities for the various bacteria and eukaryotic cells that were arising.

The evolutionary origin of viruses will likely remain conjectural. No fossilized virus has been detected. Indeed, the minute size of viruses makes any distinction of their structure against the background of the rock virtually impossible. Likewise, bacterial fossilization results in the destruction of internal detail. If a virus were to be present in a fossilizing bacterium, any evidence would be obliterated over time.

Some details as to the evolutionary divergence of viruses from a common ancestor are being realized by the comparison of the sequence of evolutionarily maintained sequences of genetic material. This area of investigation is known as virus molecular systematics.

The comparison of a number of **gene** sequences of viral significance, for example the enzyme reverse transcriptase that is possessed by **retroviruses** and pararetroviruses, is consistent with the evolutionary emergence of not one specific type of virus, but rather of several different **types of viruses**. The present day plethora of viruses subsequently evolved from these initial few viral types (or "supergroups" as they have been dubbed). So, in contrast to an evolutionary "tree." viral evolutionary origin resembles more of a bush. Each of the several branches of the bush developed independently of one another. Furthermore, the consensus among virologists (scientists who study viruses) is that this independent **evolution** did not occur at the same time or progress at the same rate. In scientific terms, the viral evolution is described as being "polyphyletic."

The evolution of viruses with life forms, including bacteria, likely occurred together. On other words, as bacteria increased in diversity and in the complexity of their surfaces, new viruses evolved to be able to utilize the bacteria as a replication factory. Similarly, as more complex eukaryotic life forms appeared, such as plants, insects, birds, and mammals, viruses evolved that were capable of utilizing these as hosts.

See also Bacterial kingdoms; Evolution and evolutionary mechanisms; Mitochondrial DNA

EXOTOXIN • *see* ENTEROTOXIN AND EXOTOXIN

EXTRATERRESTRIAL MICROBIOLOGY

Extraterrestrial microbiology is the study of microbiological processes that could occur outside of the boundaries of Earth, or on other bodies in the solar system. While such **microor-**ganisms** have not yet been found, recent findings of living **bacteria** in very inhospitable environments on Earth, combined with the existence of water on planets such as Mars, have buttressed the possibility that life in similar conditions on other planets is not inconceivable.

The scientific search for extraterrestrial life began in 1860, when the microbiologist **Louis Pasteur** attempted and failed to **culture** bacteria from the Orgueil meteorite.

The search for extraterrestrial life has always been one of the curiosities that has pulled man into the exploration of space. As the chemistries of the planets in our solar system became clearer, the possibilities for human-like life faded. However, at about the same time, the diversity of microbial life on Earth became more apparent. In particular, a type of evolutionarily ancient microorganism known as archaebacteria was isolated from extremely harsh environments, such as hot springs, thermal hot vents on the ocean floor, and from deep in the subsurface of the planet. In contrast to life forms that require oxygen and organic carbon, archaebacteria live on hydrogen and carbon dioxide. Planetary bodies such as Mars and Europa contain atmospheres of hydrogen and carbon dioxide. Thus, theoretically, archaebacteria could find such planets hospitable. Moreover, the finding of bacterial life below the Earth's surface makes the probability of similar life elsewhere greater. Other worlds are more likely to have, or have had, hot and oxygen-limited conditions similar to thermal vents or the subsurface, rather than the sunlight, oxygen-rich atmosphere of Earth's surface. Furthermore, the now prevailing view that archaebacteria are very ancient indicates that life on Earth may have arisen from environments now considered inhospitable. The environment on other solar bodies may be similar to what Earth experienced when microbial life first arose.

Unmanned probes have explored a variety of bodies in our solar system. One such stellar body, Europa, has so far not proved to be a source of life. Probes sent to scan the planet's surface found only lifeless slush. However, two of the moons, which orbit the gas planet Saturn, are of interest. Enceladus has visual signs and chemical signals consistent with the presence of liquid water. The other moon, Titan, is icy and spectral monitoring of the surface has detected signals indicative of organic compounds.

By far the bulk of interest in extraterrestrial microbiology has centered on the planet Mars. Interest in Mars as a potential supporter of microbiological life prompted the *Viking* mission that occurred in 1976. The, in two separate missions, proves landed on different regions of the planet ad conducted experiments designed to detect signature molecules of microbiological activity. One experiment, the gas exchange experiment, sought to detect alterations in the composition of gases in a test chamber. The alterations would presumable be due to microbial decomposition of nutrients, with the consumption of some gases and the release of others. The results were equivocal at first, but with examination were thought to be the result of abiological activity, specifically solar ultraviolet radiation. In a second experiment, radioactive nutrient was released into wetted Martian soil. Bacterial **metabolism** would be evident by the appearance of different radioactive com-

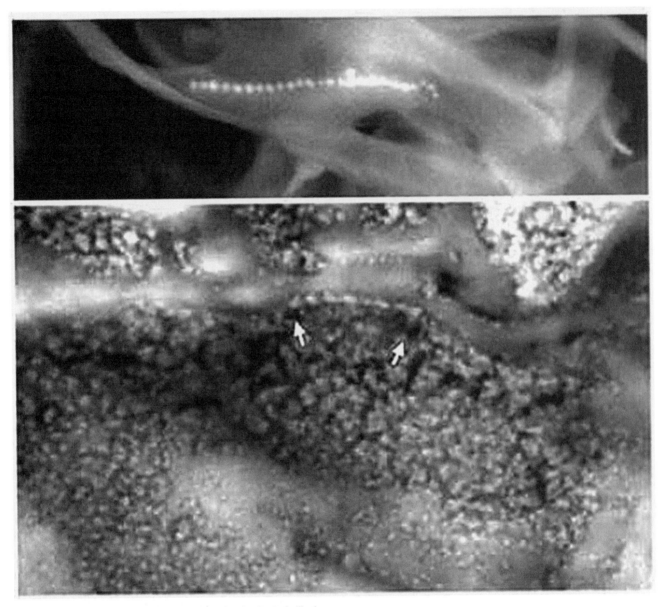

Electron microscopic view of Martian meteorite showing bacteria-like forms.

pounds. Again the results were equivocal, and may have indicated microbiological activity. A third experiment that looked for the presence of organic compounds in the soil was negative. In the final experiment, soil was examined using an instrument called a gas chromatograph-mass spectrometer for chemical signatures of biological activity. The test revealed a great deal of water but little else.

These results have been the subject of debate, and have not proven to be conclusive for the absence of microbiological life. For example, at the time of the *Viking* missions, the full extent of the diversity of microbiological life on Earth, specifically the existence of living bacteria far below the surface in regions where organic material was virtually absent, was not known. With the discovery of archaebacteria, the possibility that microbiological life could exist in the subsurface layers of a planet like Mars has warranted a reassessment of the possibility of Martian life. Furthermore, high resolution photographic surveys of the planet by orbiting probes in the 1990s revealed geological features that are the same as dried rive valleys and floodplains on the Earth. These observations have bolstered the view that Mars was once an abundantly moist planet, capable of sustaining microbiological life.

To definitively address the issue of microbiological life on Mars, the European Space Agency is scheduled to launch the so-called Mars Express in June 2003. The mission will have a two-fold purpose. An orbiting satellite will analyze the planet from high altitude, while a surface probe will sample the planet's surface. The analytical equipment aboard the probe is designed to detect minute amounts of carbon, and all metabolic forms of the atom. For example, experiments will look for the presence of methane, such as would be produced by methanogenic bacteria.

In addition to extraterrestrial microbial life, interest has arisen over the possibility that extraterrestrial microorganisms could find their way to Earth. Transport of microorganisms via meteorites and on material ejected from the solar body by a meteorite impact has been proposed. In the 1990s, the **electron microscopic examination** of meteorite ALH84001, which originated from Mars, found bacteria-like objects. Their shape, size and chemistry were at the time consistent with a biological origin. However, further study negated this possibility and no other such observations have been made.

See also Anaerobes and anaerobic infections; Biogeochemical cycles; Extremophiles

EXTREMOPHILES

Extremophiles is a term that refers to **bacteria** that are able to exist and thrive in environments that are extremely harsh, in terms of those environments classically envisioned as hospitable to the growth of bacteria.

The discovery of extremophiles, beginning in the 1970s, has had three major influences on microbiology and the **biotechnology** industry. Firstly, the discovery of bacteria growing in environments such as the hot springs of Yellowstone National Park and around the **hydrothermal vents** located on the ocean floor (where the bacteria are in fact the fundamental basis of the specialized ecosystem that is fueled by the vents) has greatly increased the awareness of the possibilities for bacterial life on Earth and elsewhere. Indeed, the growth of some extremophiles occurs in environments that by all indications could exist on planets such as Mars and other stellar bodies. Thus, extremophilic bacteria might conceivably not be confined to Earth.

The second major influence of extremophiles has been the broadening of the classification of the evolutionary development of life on Earth. With the advent of molecular means of comparing the genetic sequences of highly conserved regions from various life forms, it became clear that extremophiles were not simply offshoots of bacteria, but rather had diverged from both bacteria and eukaryotic cells early in evolutionary history. Extremophilic bacteria are grouped together in a domain called **archaea**. Archae share similarities with bacteria and with **eukaryotes**.

Thirdly, extremophiles are continuing to prove to be a rich trove of **enzymes** that are useful in biotechnological processes. The hardiness of the enzymes, such as their ability to maintain function at high temperatures, has been crucial to the development of biotechnology. A particularly well-known example is the so-called tag polymerase enzyme isolated from the extremophile *Thermus aquaticus*. This enzyme is fundamental to the procedures of the **polymerase chain reaction** (**PCR**) procedure that has revolutionized biotechnology.

There are several environments that are inhospitable to all but those extremophilic bacteria that have adapted to live in them. The best studied is elevated temperature. Heat-loving bacteria are referred to as thermophiles. More than 50 species of thermophiles have been discovered to date. Such bacteria tolerate temperatures far above the tolerable limits known for any animal, plant, or other bacteria. Some thermophiles, such as *Sulfolobus acidocaldarius*, are capable of growth and reproduction in water temperatures that exceed 212° F [100° C] (the boiling point of water at sea level). The most heat-tolerant thermophile known so far is *Pyrolobus fumarii*, that grows in the walls of the hydrothermal vents where temperatures exceed 200° F [93.33° C]. In fact, the bacterium requires a temperature above 194° F [90° C] to sustain growth. The basis of the thermophile's ability to prevent dissolution of cell wall constituents and genetic material at such high temperatures is unknown.

Other examples of extreme environments include elevated salt, pressure, and extreme acid or base concentrations.

Salt-loving, or halophilic, bacteria grow in environments where the sodium concentration is extremely high, such as in the Dead Sea or Great Salt Lake. In such an environment, a bacterium such as *Escherichia coli* would compensate for the discrepancy in sodium concentration between the bacterium's interior and exterior by shunting all the internal fluid to the exterior. The result would be the collapse and death of the bacterium. However, salt-loving bacteria such as *Halobacterium salinarum* content with the sodium discrepancy by increasing the internal concentration of potassium chloride. The enzymes of the bacterium operate only in a potassium chloride-rich environment. Yet the proteins produced by the action of these enzymes need to be tolerant of high sodium chloride levels. How the enzymes are able to accommodate both demands is not clear.

Acid-loving extremophiles prefer environments where the **pH** is below pH=5, while alkaline-loving bacteria require pHs above pH=9. Thriving populations of acid-loving bacteria have been isolated in the runoff from acidic mine drainage, where the pH is below one, which is more acidic than the contents of the stomach. Interestingly, these bacteria are similar to other bacteria in the near neutral pH of their interior. Very acidic pHs would irreversibly damage the genetic material. Acid-loving bacteria thus survive by actively excluding acid. The enzymes necessary to achieve this function at very acidic pH levels.

Similarly, alkaline-loving bacteria maintain a near neutral interior pH. The enzymes that function at such alkaline conditions are of interest to manufacturers of laundry detergents, which operate better at alkaline pHs.

Some extremophiles grow and thrive at very low temperatures. For example, *Polaromonas vacuolata* has an ideal growth temperature of just slightly above the freezing point of water. These bacteria are finding commercial applications in enzymatic processes that operate at refrigeration temperatures or in the cold cycle of a washing machine.

The discovery of bacteria in environments that were previously disregarded as being completely inhospitable for bacterial life argues that more extremophiles are yet to be

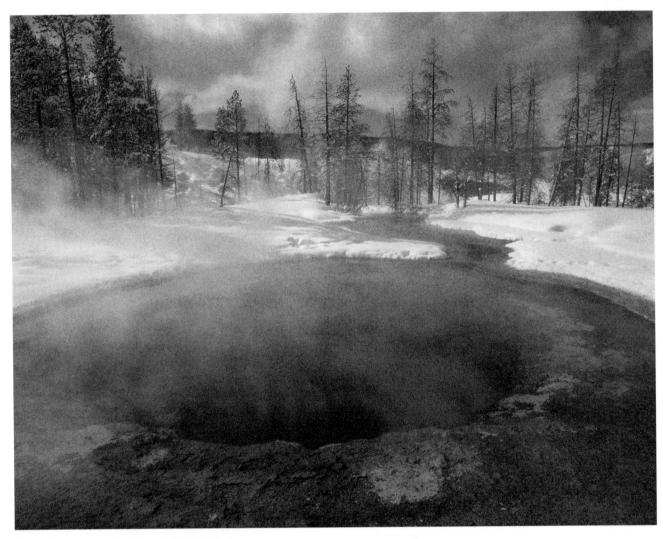

A steaming hot spring in Yellowstone National Park.

found, as other environments are explored. For example, in 2001, living bacteria were recovered from drill samples kilometers beneath the Earth's crust, in an environment where virtually no nutrients were present other than the solid rock surrounding the bacteria. By as yet unknown enzymatic mechanisms, these bacteria are able to extract elemental components including sulfur from the rocks and utilize them as nutrients.

See also Chemoautotrophic and chemolithotrophic bacteria; Economic uses and benefits of microorganisms; Extraterrestrial microbiology

EYE INFECTIONS

Eye infections can be caused by viral, bacterial, and fungal **microorganisms**. These organisms do not cause infections solely in the eye. In reality, eye infections tend to occur as infections disseminate, or spread, in the body.

Microbiological infections of the eye involve the conjunctiva, which is the membrane of the inner eyelid and corner of the eye. This infection is termed conjunctivitis. Depending on the microbial agent, infection can also occur on the eyelid (blepharitis), the cornea (keratitis), the retina and its associated blood vessels (chorioretinitis), the optic nerve (neuroritinitis), and even the fluid inside the eyeball (vitritis).

A virus associated with eye infections is the **Herpes** Zoster virus. This virus is the reactivated form of the chicken pox virus that had previously established an infection, often in childhood. A hallmark of reactivation is the dissemination of the virus throughout the body via nerve fibers. The eye can become infected through the optic nerve fibers.

Typically, the viral infection will be a rash or **inflammation** on the upper or lower eyelid and the conjunctiva. The inside of the eye and the optic nerve leading from the retina to the brain can also become infected. Herpes Zoster eye infections can produce redness, swelling, pain, light sensitivity, and blurred vision.

The cornea of the eye is prone to infection by the type of **fungi** known as molds, and by **yeast**. Such an infection is termed mycotic keratitis. Infections can arise following eye surgery, from the use of contaminated contact lens (or the **contamination** of the contact lens cleaning solution), or due to a malfunction of the **immune system**. A common fungal cause of eye infections are species of *Aspergillus*. A common yeast source of infection are species of *Candida*. The eye infection may be a secondary result of the spread of a fungal or yeast infection elsewhere in the body. For example, those

afflicted with acquired **immunodeficiency** syndrome can develop eye infections in addition to other fungal or yeast maladies.

Bacterial eye infections are often caused by *Chlamydia*, *Neiserria*, and *Pseudomonas*. The latter **bacteria**, which can infect the fluid used to clean contact lenses, can cause the rapid development of an infection that can so severe that blindness can result. Removal of the infected eye is sometimes necessary to stop the infection.

Less drastic solutions to infections include the use of antimicrobial eye drops.

See also Immune system

F

FACILITATED DIFFUSION • *see* CELL MEMBRANE
TRANSPORT

FAUCI, ANTHONY S. (1940-   )
American immunologist

Early in his career, Anthony S. Fauci carried out both basic and clinical research in **immunology** and infectious diseases. Since 1981, Fauci's research has been focused on the mechanisms of the **Human Immunodeficiency Virus** (**HIV**), which causes acquired **immunodeficiency** syndrome (**AIDS**). His work has lead to breakthroughs in understanding the virus's progress, especially during the latency period between infection and fulminant AIDS. As director of both the National Institute of Allergy and Infectious Diseases (NIAID) and the Office of AIDS Research at the National Institutes of Health (NIH), Fauci is involved with much of the AIDS research performed in the United States and is responsible for supervising the investigation of the disease mechanism and the development of vaccines and drug therapy.

Anthony Stephen Fauci was born on December 24, 1940, in Brooklyn, New York, to Stephen A. Fauci, a pharmacist, and Eugenia A. Fauci, a homemaker. He attended a Jesuit high school in Manhattan where he had a successful academic and athletic career. After high school, Fauci entered Holy Cross College in Worcester, Massachusetts, as a premedical student, graduating with a B.A. in 1962. He then attended Cornell University Medical School, from which he received his medical degree in 1966, and where he completed both his internship and residency.

In 1968, Fauci became a clinical associate in the Laboratory of Clinical Investigation of NIAID, one of the eleven institutes that comprise the NIH. Except for one year spent at the New York Hospital Cornell Medical Center as chief resident, he has remained at the NIH throughout his career. His earliest studies focused on the functioning of the human **immune system** and how infectious diseases impact the system. As a senior staff fellow at NIAID, Fauci and two other researchers delineated the mechanism of Wegener's granulomatosis, a relatively rare and fatal immune disease involving the **inflammation** of blood vessels and organs. By 1971, Fauci had developed a drug regimen for Wegener's granulomatosis that is 95% percent effective. He also found effective treatments for lymphomatoid granulomatosis and polyarteritis nodosa, two other immune diseases.

In 1972, Fauci became a senior investigator at NIAID and two years later he was named head of the Clinical Physiology Section. In 1977, Fauci was appointed deputy clinical director of NIAID. Fauci shifted the focus of the Laboratory of Clinical Infection at NIAID towards investigating the nature of AIDS in the early 1980s. It was in Fauci's lab the type of defect that occurs in the T4 helper cells (the immune cells) and enables AIDS to be fatal was demonstrated. Fauci also orchestrated early therapeutic techniques, including bone-marrow transplants, in an attempt to save AIDS patients. In 1984, Fauci became the director of NIAID, and the following year the coordinator of all AIDS research at NIH. He has worked not only against the disease but also against governmental indifference to AIDS, winning larger and larger budgets for AIDS research. When the Office of AIDS Research at NIH was founded in 1988, Fauci was made director; he also decided to remain the director of NIAID. Fauci and his research teams have developed a three-fold battle plan against AIDS: researching the mechanism of HIV, developing and testing drug therapies, and creating an AIDS **vaccine**.

In 1993, Fauci and his team at NIH disproved the theory that HIV remains dormant for approximately ten years after the initial infection, showing instead that the virus attacks the lymph nodes and reproduces itself in white blood cells known as CD4 cells. This discovery could lead to new and radical approaches in the early treatment of HIV-positive patients. Earlier discoveries that Fauci and his lab are responsible for include the 1987 finding that a protein substance known as cytokine may be responsible for triggering full-blown AIDS and the realization that the macrophage, a type of immune system cell, is the virus's means of transmission. Fauci demonstrated that HIV actually hides from the body's immune system in these macrophages and is thus more easily transmitted. In an interview with Dennis L. Breo published in the *Journal of the American Medical Association,* Fauci summed up his research to date: "We've learned that AIDS is a multiphasic, multifactorial disease of overlapping phases, progressing from infection to viral replication to chronic smoldering disease to profound depression of the immune system."

In drug therapy work, Fauci and his laboratory have run hundreds of clinical tests on medications such as azidothymidine (AZT), and Fauci has pushed for the early use of such drugs by terminally ill AIDS patients. Though no completely effective antiviral drug yet exists, drug therapies have been developed that can prolong the life of AIDS victims. Potential AIDS vaccines are still being investigated, a process complicated by the difficulty of conducting possible clinical trials, and the fact that animals do not develop AIDS as humans do, which further limits available research subjects. No viable vaccine is expected before the year 2005.

As chief government infectious disease specialist, Fauci was presented with an immediate **public health** challenge in October, 2001—bioterrorism. Coordinating with the **Centers for Disease Control**, Fauci directed the effort to not only contain the outbreak of **anthrax** resulting from *Bacillus anthracis*–contaminated letters mailed to United States Post Offices, but also to initiate the necessary research to manage the continuing threat of the disease. Fauci also labeled **smallpox** as a logical **bioterrorism** agent, and has concentrated his efforts to ensure an available adequate supply of smallpox vaccine in the U.S.

Fauci married Christine Grady, a clinical nurse and medical ethicist, in 1985. The couple has three daughters. Fauci is an avid jogger, a former marathon runner, and enjoys fishing. Widely recognized for his research, he is the recipient of numerous prizes and awards, including a 1979 Arthur S. Flemming Award, the 1984 U.S. Public Health Service Distinguished Service Medal, the 1989 National Medical Research Award from the National Health Council, and the 1992 Dr. Nathan Davis Award for Outstanding Public Service from the American Medical Association. Fauci is also a fellow of the American Academy of Arts and Sciences and holds a number of honorary degrees. He is the author or coauthor of over 800 scientific articles, and has edited several medical textbooks.

See also AIDS, recent advances in research and treatment; Anthrax, terrorist use of as a biological weapon; Bioterrorism, protective measures; Epidemiology, tracking diseases with technology; Infection and resistance

FELDMAN, HARRY ALFRED (1914-1985)

American physician and epidemiologist

Harry A. Feldman's research in **epidemiology**, **immunology**, infectious disease control, preventive medicine, **toxoplasmosis**,

bacterial chemotherapeutic and sero-therapeutic agents, respiratory diseases, and **meningitis** was internationally recognized in the scientific community of microbiology and medicine.

Feldman was born in Newark, New Jersey on May, 30, 1914, the son of Joseph Feldman, a construction contractor, and his wife Sarah. After attending public schools in Newark and graduating from Weequahic High School in 1931, he received his A.B. in zoology in 1935 and his M.D. in 1939, both from George Washington University. He completed an internship and residency at Gallinger Municipal Hospital, Washington, D.C., held a brief research fellowship at George Washington, then in 1942, became a research fellow at Harvard Medical School and an assistant resident physician at the Boston City Hospital's Thorndike Memorial Laboratory. Among his colleagues at Thorndike was Maxwell A. Finland (1902–1987), who at the time was among the nation's premier investigators of infectious diseases. From 1942 to 1946, Feldman served to the rank of lieutenant colonel in the United States Army Medical Corps.

As senior fellow in virus diseases for the National Research Council at the Children's Hospital Research Foundation, Cincinnati, Ohio, Feldman collaborated with Albert B. Sabin (1906–1993) on **poliomyelitis** and toxoplasmosis from 1946 to 1948. Together they developed the Sabin-Feldman dye test, which uses methylene blue to detect toxoplasmosis in blood serum by identifying immunoglobulin-G (IgG) antibodies against the parasitic intracellular protozoan, *toxoplasma gondii*.

In 1948, Feldman was appointed associate professor of medicine at the Syracuse University College of Medicine, which in 1950 became the State University of New York Upstate Medical Center College of Medicine. From 1949 to 1956, he also served in Syracuse as director of research at the Wieting-Johnson Hospital for Rheumatic Diseases. In 1955, Upstate named him associate professor of preventive medicine. The following year he was promoted to full professor and in 1957, became chair of the Department of Preventive Medicine, the position he held until his death. Between 1938 and 1983, he published 216 research papers, both in scientific journals and as book chapters. With Alfred S. Evans (1917-1996), he co-edited *Bacterial Infections of Humans* (1982).

Besides his groundbreaking work on toxoplasmosis, both with Sabin in Cincinnati and later as head of his own team in Syracuse, Feldman regarded his work on meningococcus and on parasitic **protozoa** such as acanthamoeba as his greatest contributions to science. Among the diseases he studied were **malaria, pneumonia,** rubella, **measles, influenza,** streptococcal infections, and **AIDS.** He conducted extensive clinical pharmaceutical trials and served enthusiastically as a member of many scientific organizations, commissions, and committees, including the **World Health Organization (WHO)** expert advisory panels on bacterial diseases, venereal diseases, treponematoses, and neisseria infections. He was president of the American Epidemiological Society (AES), the Infectious Diseases Society of America (IDSA), and the Association of Teachers of Preventive Medicine. The AES established the Harry A. Feldman Lectureship and the Harry

A. Feldman Award in his honor, and the IDSA also created its own Harry A. Feldman Award.

See also Antibody and antigen; Bacteria and bacterial infection; Chemotherapy; Epidemiology; Infection and resistance; Meningitis, bacterial and viral; Microbiology, clinical; Parasites; Poliomyelitis and polio; Protozoa; Serology

FERMENTATION

In its broadest sense, fermentation refers to any process by which large organic molecules are broken down to simpler molecules as the result of the action of **microorganisms**. The most familiar type of fermentation is the conversion of sugars and starches to alcohol by **enzymes** in **yeast**. To distinguish this reaction from other kinds of fermentation, the process is sometimes known as alcoholic or ethanolic fermentation.

Ethanolic fermentation was one of the first chemical reactions observed by humans. In nature, various types of spoil decompose because of bacterial action. Early in history, humans discovered that this kind of change could result in the formation of products that were enjoyable to consume. The spoilage (fermentation) of fruit juices, for example, resulted in the formation of primitive forms of wine.

The mechanism by which fermentation occurs was the subject of extensive debate in the early 1800s. It was a key issue among those arguing over the concept of vitalism, the notion that living organisms are in some way inherently different from non-living objects. One aspect in this debate centered on the role of so-called "ferments" in the conversion of sugars and starches to alcohol. Vitalists argued that ferments (now known as enzymes) are inextricably linked to a living cell; destroy a cell and ferments can no longer cause fermentation, they argued.

A crucial experiment on this issue was carried out in 1896 by the German chemist Eduard Buchner. Buchner ground up a group of cells with sand until they were totally destroyed. He then extracted the liquid that remained and added it to a sugar solution. His assumption was that fermentation could no longer occur because the cells that had held the ferments were dead, so they no longer carried the "life-force" needed to bring about fermentation. He was amazed to discover that the cell-free liquid did indeed cause fermentation. It was obvious that the ferments themselves, distinct from any living organism, could cause fermentation.

The chemical reaction that occurs in fermentation can be described easily. Starch is converted to simple sugars such as sucrose and glucose. Those sugars are then converted to alcohol (ethyl alcohol) and carbon dioxide. This description does not adequately convey the complexity of the fermentation process itself. During the 1930s, two German biochemists, G. Embden and O. Meyerhof, worked out the sequence of reactions by which glucose ferments. In a sequence of twelve reactions, glucose is converted to ethyl alcohol and carbon dioxide. A number of enzymes are needed to carry out this sequence of reactions, the most important of which is zymase, found in yeast cells. These enzymes are sen-

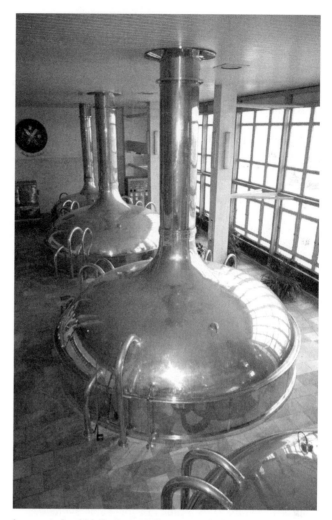

Large vats in which the fermentation process in the brewing of beer occurs.

sitive to environmental conditions in which they live. When the concentration of alcohol reaches about 14%, they are inactivated. For this reason, no fermentation product (such as wine) can have an alcoholic concentration of more than about fourteen percent.

The alcoholic beverages that can be produced by fermentation vary widely, depending primarily on two factors— the plant that is fermented and the enzymes used for fermentation. Human societies use, of course, the materials that are available to them. Thus, various peoples have used grapes, berries, corn, rice, wheat, honey, potatoes, barley, hops, cactus juice, cassava roots, and other plant materials for fermentation. The products of such reactions are various forms of beer, wine or distilled liquors, which may be given specific names depending on the source from which they come. In Japan, for example, rice wine is known as sake. Wine prepared from honey is known as mead. Beer is the fermentation product of barley, hops, and/or malt sugar.

Early in human history, people used naturally occurring yeast for fermentation. The products of such reactions depended on whatever enzymes might occur in "wild" yeast. Today, wine-makers are able to select from a variety of specially cultured yeast that control the precise direction that fermentation will take.

Ethyl alcohol is not the only useful product of fermentation. The carbon dioxide generated during fermentation is also an important component of many baked goods. When the batter for bread is mixed, for example, a small amount of sugar and yeast is added. During the rising period, sugar is fermented by enzymes in the yeast, with the formation of carbon dioxide gas. The carbon dioxide gives the batter bulkiness and texture that would be lacking without the fermentation process. Fermentation has a number of commercial applications beyond those described thus far. Many occur in the food preparation and processing industry. A variety of **bacteria** are used in the production of olives, cucumber pickles, and sauerkraut from the raw olives, cucumbers, and cabbage, respectively. The **selection** of exactly the right bacteria and the right conditions (for example, acidity and salt concentration) is an art in producing food products with exactly the desired flavors. An interesting line of research in the food sciences is aimed at the production of edible food products by the fermentation of petroleum.

In some cases, **antibiotics** and other drugs can be prepared by fermentation if no other commercially efficient method is available. For example, the important drug cortisone can be prepared by the fermentation of a plant steroid known as diosgenin. The enzymes used in the reaction are provided by the **mold** *Rhizopus nigricans.*

One of the most successful commercial applications of fermentation has been the production of ethyl alcohol for use in gasohol. Gasohol is a mixture of about 90% gasoline and 10% alcohol. The alcohol needed for this product can be obtained from the fermentation of agricultural and municipal wastes. The use of gasohol provides a promising method for using renewable resources (plant material) to extend the availability of a nonrenewable resource (gasoline).

Another application of the fermentation process is in the treatment of wastewater. In the activated sludge process, aerobic bacteria are used to ferment organic material in wastewater. Solid wastes are converted to carbon dioxide, water, and mineral salts.

See also History of microbiology; Winemaking

FERTILITY • *see* REPRODUCTIVE IMMUNOLOGY

FILOVIRUSES • *see* HEMORRHAGIC FEVERS AND DISEASES

FIMBRIA • *see* BACTERIAL APPENDAGES

FLAGELLA • *see* BACTERIAL APPENDAGES

FLAVIVIRUSES • *see* HEMORRHAGIC FEVERS AND DISEASES

FLEMING, ALEXANDER (1881-1955)
Scottish bacteriologist

With the experienced eye of a scientist, Alexander Fleming turned what appeared to be a spoiled experiment into the discovery of **penicillin**.

Fleming was born in 1881 to a farming family in Lochfield, Scotland. Following school, he worked as a shipping clerk in London and enlisted in the London Scottish Regiment. In 1901, he began his medical career, entering St. Mary's Hospital Medical School, where he was a prizewinning student. After graduation in 1906, he began working at that institution with Sir **Almroth Edward Wright**, a pathologist. From the start, Fleming was innovative and became one of the first to use **Paul Ehrlich**'s arsenic compound, Salvarsan, to treat **syphilis** in Great Britain.

Wright and Fleming joined the Royal Army Medical Corps during World War I and they studied wounds and infection-causing **bacteria** at a hospital in Boulogne, France. At that time, **antiseptics** were used to treat bacterial infections, but Wright and Fleming showed that, especially in deep wounds, bacteria survive treatment by antiseptics while the protective white blood cells in the wound are destroyed. This creates an even worse situation in which infection can spread rapidly. Forever affected by the suffering he saw during the war, Fleming decided to focus his efforts on the search for safe antibacterial substances. He studied the antibacterial power of the body's own leukocytes contained in pus. In 1921, he discovered that a sample of his own nasal mucus destroyed bacteria in a petri dish. He isolated the compound responsible for the antibacterial action, which he called lysozyme, in saliva, blood, tears, pus, milk, and in egg whites.

Fleming made his greatest discovery in 1928. While he was growing cultures of bacteria in petri dishes for experiments, he accidentally left certain dishes uncovered for several days. Fleming found a **mold** growing in the dishes and began to discard them, when he noticed, to his astonishment, that bacteria near the molds were being destroyed. He preserved the mold, a strain of Penicillium and made a **culture** of it in a test tube for further investigation. He deduced an antibacterial compound was being produced by the mold, and named it penicillin. Through further study, Fleming found that penicillin was nontoxic in laboratory animals. He described his findings in research journals but was unable to purify and concentrate the substance. Little did he realize that the substance produced by his mold would save millions of lives during the twentieth century.

Fleming dropped his investigation of penicillin and his discovery remained unnoticed until 1940. It was then that Oxford University-based bacteriologists Howard Florey and Ernst Chain stumbled upon a paper by Fleming while researching antibacterial agents. They had better fortune than Fleming, for they were able to purify penicillin and test it on humans with outstanding results. During World War II, the drug was rushed into mass-production in England and the United States and saved thousands of injured soldiers from infections that might otherwise have been fatal.

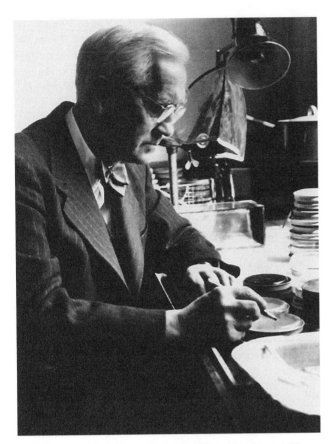

Sir Alexander Flemming, the discoverer of lysozyme and penicillin.

Accolades followed for Fleming. He was elected to fellowship in the Royal Society in 1943, knighted in 1944, and shared the Nobel Prize with Florey and Chain in 1945. Fleming continued working at St. Mary's Hospital until 1948, when he moved to the Wright-Fleming Institute. Fleming died in London in 1955.

See also Antibiotic resistance, tests for; Antibiotics; Bacteria and bacterial infection; History of the development of antibiotics; History of microbiology; History of public health

FLOREY, HOWARD WALTER (1898-1968)

English pathologist

The work of Howard Walter Florey gave the world one of its most valuable disease-fighting drugs, **penicillin. Alexander Fleming** discovered, in 1929, the **mold** that produced an antibacterial substance, but was unable to isolate it. Nearly a decade later, Florey and his colleague, biochemist **Ernst Chain**, set out to isolate the active ingredient in Fleming's mold and then conduct the clinical tests that demonstrated penicillin's remarkable therapeutic value. Florey and Chain reported the initial success of their clinical trials in 1940, and the drug's value was quickly recognized. In 1945, Florey

shared the Nobel Prize in medicine or physiology with Fleming and Chain.

Howard Walter Florey was born in Adelaide, Australia. He was one of three children and the only son born to Joseph Florey, a boot manufacturer, and Bertha Mary Wadham Florey, Joseph's second wife. Florey expressed an interest in science early in life. Rather than follow his father's career path, he decided to pursue a degree in medicine. Scholarships afforded him an education at St. Peter's Collegiate School and Adelaide University, the latter of which awarded him a Bachelor of Science degree in 1921. An impressive academic career earned Florey a Rhodes scholarship to Oxford University in England. There he enrolled in Magdalen College in January 1922. His academic prowess continued at Oxford, where he became an excellent student of physiology under the tutelage of renowned neurophysiologist Sir Charles Scott Sherrington. Placing first in his class in the physiology examination, he was appointed to a teaching position by Sherrington in 1923.

Florey's education continued at Cambridge University as a John Lucas Walker Student. Already fortunate enough to have learned under a master such as Sherrington, he now came under the influence of Sir Frederick Gowland Hopkins, who taught Florey the importance of studying biochemical reactions in cells. A Rockefeller Traveling Scholarship sent Florey to the United States in 1925, to work with physiologist Alfred Newton Richards at the University of Pennsylvania, a collaboration that would later prove beneficial to Florey's own research. On his return to England and Cambridge in 1926, Florey received a research fellowship in pathology at London Hospital. That same year, he married Mary Ethel Hayter Reed, an Australian whom he'd met during medical school at Adelaide University. The couple eventually had two children.

Florey received his Ph.D. from Cambridge in 1927, and remained there as Huddersfield Lecturer in Special Pathology. Equipped with a firm background in physiology, he was now in a position to pursue experimental research using an approach new to the field of pathology. Instead of describing diseased tissues and organs, Florey applied physiologic concepts to the study of healthy biological systems as a means of better recognizing the nature of disease. It was during this period in which Florey first became familiar with the work of Alexander Fleming. His own work on mucus secretion led him to investigate the intestine's resistance to **bacterial infection**. As he became more engrossed in antibacterial substances, Florey came across Fleming's report of 1921 describing the enzyme lysozyme, which possessed antibacterial properties. The enzyme, found in the tears, nasal secretions, and saliva of humans, piqued Florey's interest, and convinced him that collaboration with a chemist would benefit his research. His work with lysozyme showed that extracts from natural substances, such as plants, **fungi** and certain types of **bacteria**, had the ability to destroy harmful bacteria.

Florey left Cambridge in 1931 to become professor of pathology at the University of Sheffield, returning to Oxford in 1935 as director of the new Sir William Dunn School of Pathology. There, at the recommendation of Hopkins, his productive collaboration began with the German biochemist Ernst Chain. Florey remained interested in antibacterial substances even as he expanded his research projects into new areas, such as cancer studies. During the mid 1930s, sulfonamides, or **sulfa drugs**, had been introduced as clinically effective against streptococcal infections, an announcement which boosted Florey's interest in the field. At Florey's suggestion, Chain undertook biochemical studies of lysozyme. He read much of the scientific literature on antibacterial substances, including Fleming's 1929 report on the antibacterial properties of a substance extracted from a Penicillium mold, which he called penicillin. Chain discovered that lysozyme acted against certain bacteria by catalyzing the breakdown of polysaccharides in them, and thought that penicillin might also be an enzyme with the ability to disrupt some bacterial component. Chain and Florey began to study this hypothesis, with Chain concentrating on isolating and characterizing the enzyme, and Florey studying its biological properties.

To his surprise, Chain discovered that penicillin was not a protein, therefore it could not be an enzyme. His challenge now was to determine the chemical nature of penicillin, made all the more difficult because it was so unstable in the laboratory. It was, in part, for this very reason that Fleming eventually abandoned a focused pursuit of the active ingredient in Penicillium mold. Eventually, work by Chain and others led to a protocol for keeping penicillin stable in solution. By the end of 1938, Florey began to seek funds to support more vigorous research into penicillin. He was becoming convinced that this antibacterial substance could have great practical clinical value. Florey was successful in obtaining two major grants, one from the Medical Research Council in England, the other from the Rockefeller Foundation in the United States.

By March of 1940, Chain had finally isolated about one hundred milligrams of penicillin from broth cultures. Employing a freeze-drying technique, he extracted the yellowish-brown powder in a form that was yet only ten percent pure. It was non-toxic when injected into mice and retained antibacterial properties against many different pathogens. In May of 1940, Florey conducted an important experiment to test this promising new drug. He infected eight mice with lethal doses of **streptococci** bacteria, then treated four of them with penicillin. The following day, the four untreated mice were dead, while three of the four mice treated with penicillin had survived. Though one of the mice that had been given a smaller dose died two days later, Florey showed that penicillin had excellent prospects, and began additional tests. In 1941, enough penicillin had been produced to run the first clinical trial on humans. Patients suffering from severe staphylococcal and streptococcal infections recovered at a remarkable rate, bearing out the earlier success of the drugs in animals. At the outset of World War II, however, the facilities needed to produce large quantities of penicillin were not available. Florey went to the United States where, with the help of his former colleague, Alfred Richards, he was able to arrange for a U.S. government lab to begin large-scale penicillin production. By 1943, penicillin was being used to treat infections suffered by wounded soldiers on the battlefront.

Recognition for Florey's work came quickly. In 1942, he was elected a fellow in the prestigious British scientific organization, the Royal Society, even before the importance of penicillin was fully realized. Two years later, Florey was knighted. In 1945, Florey, Chain and Fleming shared the Nobel Prize in medicine or physiology for the discovery of penicillin.

Penicillin prevents bacteria from synthesizing intact cell walls. Without the rigid, protective cell wall, a bacterium usually bursts and dies. Penicillin does not kill resting bacteria, only prevents their proliferation. Penicillin is active against many of the gram positive and a few gram negative bacteria. (The gram negative/positive designation refers to a staining technique used in identification of microbes.) Penicillin has been used in the treatment of **pneumonia, meningitis,** many throat and ear infections, Scarlet Fever, endocarditis (heart infection), **gonorrhea,** and **syphilis**.

Following his work with penicillin, Florey retained an interest in antibacterial substances, including the cephalosporins, a group of drugs that produced effects similar to penicillin. He also returned to his study of capillaries, which he had begun under Sherrington, but would now be aided by the recently developed **electron microscope**. Florey remained interested in Australia, as well. In 1944, the prime minister of Australia asked Florey to conduct a review of the country's medical research. During his trip, Florey found laboratories and research facilities to be far below the quality he expected. The trip inspired efforts to establish graduate-level research programs at the Australian National University. For a while, it looked as if Florey might even return to Australia to head a new medical institute at the University. That never occurred, although Florey did do much to help plan the institute and recruit scientists to it. During the late 1940s and 1950s, Florey made trips almost every year to Australia to provide consultation to the new Australian National University, to which he was appointed Chancellor in 1965.

Florey's stature as a scientist earned him many honors in addition to the Nobel Prize. In 1960, he became president of the Royal Society, a position he held until 1965. Tapping his experience as an administrator, Florey invigorated this prestigious scientific organization by boosting its membership and increasing its role in society. In 1962, he was elected Provost of Queen's College, Oxford University, the first scientist to hold that position. He accepted the presidency of the British Family Planning Association in 1965, and used the post to promote more research on contraception and the legalization of abortion. That same year, he was granted a peerage, becoming Baron Florey of Adelaide and Marston.

See also Bacteria and bacterial infection; History of the development of antibiotics; Infection and resistance

FLU: THE GREAT FLU EPIDEMIC OF 1918

From 1918 to 1919, an outbreak of **influenza** ravaged Europe and North America. The outbreak was a pandemic; that is, individuals in a vast geographic area were affected. In the case of this particular influenza outbreak, people were infected around the world.

The pandemic killed more people, some 20 to 40 million, than had been killed in the just-ending Great War (now known as World War I). Indeed, the pandemic is still the most devastating microbiological event in the recorded history of the world. At the height of the epidemic, fully one-fifth of the world's population was infected with the virus.

The disease first arose in the fall of 1918, as World War I was nearing its end. The genesis of the disease caused by the strain of influenza virus may have been the deplorable conditions experienced by soldiers in the trenches that were dug at battlegrounds throughout Europe. The horrible conditions rendered many soldiers weak and immunologically impaired. As solders returned to their home countries, such as the United States, the disease began to spread. As the disease spread, however, even healthy people fell victim to the infection. The reason why so many apparently healthy people would suddenly become ill and even die was unknown at the time. Indeed, the viral cause of disease had yet to be discovered.

Recent research has demonstrated that the particular strain of virus was one that even an efficiently functioning **immune system** was not well equipped to cope with. A mutation produced a surface protein on the virus that was not immediately recognized by the immune system, and which contributed to the ability of the virus to cause an infection.

The influenza outbreak has also been called the "Spanish Flu" or "La Grippe." The moniker came from the some 8 million influenza deaths that occurred in Spain in one month at the height of the outbreak. Ironically, more recent research has demonstrated that the strain of influenza that ravaged Spain was different from that which spread influenza around the world.

The influenza swept across Europe and elsewhere around the globe. In the United States, some 675,000 Americans perished from the infection, which was brought to the continent by returning war veterans. The outbreaks in the United States began in military camps. Unfortunately, the significance of the illness was not recognized by authorities and few steps were taken to curtail the illnesses, which soon spread to the general population.

The resulting carnage in the United States reduced the statistical average life span of an American by 10 years. In the age range of 15 to 34 years, the death rate in 1918 due to **pneumonia** and influenza was 20 times higher than the normal rate. The large number of deaths in many of the young generation had an economic effect for decades to come. South America, Asia, and the South Pacific were also devastated by the infection.

In the United States the influenza outbreak greatly affected daily life. Gatherings of people, such as at funerals, parades, or even sales at commercial establishments were either banned or were of very short duration. The medical system was taxed tremendously.

The influenza outbreak of 1918 was characterized by a high mortality rate. Previous influenza outbreaks had displayed a mortality rate of far less than 1%. However, the 1918 pandemic had a much higher mortality rate of 2.5%. Also, the ill-

ness progressed very quickly once the symptoms of infections appeared. In many cases, an individual went from a healthy state to serious illness or death with 24 hours.

At the time of the outbreak, the case of the illness was not known. Speculations as to the source of the illness included an unknown weapon of war unleashed by the German army. Only later was the viral origin of the disease determined. In the 1970s, a study that involved a genetic characterization of viral material recovered from the time of the pandemic indicated that the strain of the influenza virus likely arose in China, and represented a substantial genetic alteration from hitherto known viral types.

In November of 1919, the influenza outbreak began to disappear as rapidly as it had appeared. With the hindsight of present day knowledge of viral epidemics, it is clear that the number of susceptible hosts for the virus became exhausted. The result was the rapid end to the epidemic.

See also Epidemics, viral; History of public health

FLUORESCENCE *IN SITU* HYBRIDIZATION (FISH)

Fluorescent *in situ* hybridization (FISH) is a technique in which single-stranded nucleic acids (usually **DNA**, but **RNA** may also be used) are permitted to interact so that complexes, or hybrids, are formed by molecules with sufficiently similar, complementary sequences. Through nucleic acid hybridization, the degree of sequence identity can be determined, and specific sequences can be detected and located on a given chromosome. It is a powerful technique for detecting RNA or DNA sequences in cells, tissues, and tumors. FISH provides a unique link among the studies of cell biology, cytogenetics, and **molecular genetics**.

The method is comprised of three basic steps: fixation of a specimen on a **microscope** slide, hybridization of labeled probe to homologous fragments of genomic DNA, and enzymatic detection of the tagged probe-target hybrids. While probe sequences were initially detected with isotopic reagents, nonisotopic hybridization has become increasingly popular, with fluorescent hybridization now a common choice. Protocols involving nonisotopic probes are considerably faster, with greater signal resolution, and provide options to visualize different targets simultaneously by combining various detection methods.

The detection of sequences on the target **chromosomes** is performed indirectly, commonly with biotinylated or digoxigenin-labeled probes detected via a fluorochrome-conjugated detection reagent, such as an **antibody** conjugated with fluorescein. As a result, the direct visualization of the relative position of the probes is possible. Increasingly, nucleic acid probes labeled directly with fluorochromes are used for the detection of large target sequences. This method takes less time and results in lower background; however, lower signal intensity is generated. Higher sensitivity can be obtained by building layers of detection reagents, resulting in amplification of the signal. Using such means, it is possible to detect single-copy sequences on chromosome with probes shorter than 0.8 kb.

Probes can vary in length from a few base pairs for synthetic oligonucleotides to larger than one Mbp. Probes of different types can be used to detect distinct DNA types. PCR-amplified repeated DNA sequences, oligonucleotides specific for repeat elements, or cloned repeat elements can be used to detect clusters of repetitive DNA in heterochromatin blocks or centromeric regions of individual chromosomes. These are useful in determining aberrations in the number of chromosomes present in a cell. In contrast, for detecting single locus targets, cDNAs or pieces of cloned genomic DNA, from 100 bp to 1 Mbp in size, can be used.

To detect specific chromosomes or chromosomal regions, chromosome-specific DNA libraries can be used as probes to delineate individual chromosomes from the full chromosomal **complement**. Specific probes have been commercially available for each of the human chromosomes since 1991.

Any given tissue or cell source, such as sections of frozen tumors, imprinted cells, cultured cells, or embedded sections, may be hybridized. The DNA probes are hybridized to chromosomes from dividing (metaphase) or non-dividing (interphase) cells.

The observation of the hybridized sequences is done using epifluorescence microscopy. White light from a source lamp is filtered so that only the relevant wavelengths for excitation of the fluorescent molecules reach the sample. The light emitted by fluorochromes is generally of larger wavelengths, which allows the distinction between excitation and emission light by means of a second optical filter. Therefore, it is possible to see bright-colored signals on a dark background. It is also possible to distinguish between several excitation and emission bands, thus between several fluorochromes, which allows the observation of many different probes on the same target.

FISH has a large number of applications in **molecular biology** and medical science, including **gene** mapping, diagnosis of chromosomal abnormalities, and studies of cellular structure and function. Chromosomes in three-dimensionally preserved nuclei can be "painted" using FISH. In clinical research, FISH can be used for prenatal diagnosis of inherited chromosomal aberrations, postnatal diagnosis of carriers of genetic disease, diagnosis of infectious disease, viral and bacterial disease, tumor cytogenetic diagnosis, and detection of aberrant gene expression. In laboratory research, FISH can be used for mapping chromosomal genes, to study the **evolution** of genomes (Zoo FISH), analyzing nuclear organization, visualization of chromosomal territories and chromatin in interphase cells, to analyze dynamic nuclear processes, somatic hybrid cells, replication, chromosome sorting, and to study tumor biology. It can also be used in developmental biology to study the temporal expression of genes during differentiation and development. Recently, high resolution FISH has become a popular method for ordering genes or DNA markers within chromosomal regions of interest.

See also Biochemical analysis techniques; Biotechnology; Laboratory techniques in immunology; Laboratory techniques in microbiology; Molecular biology and molecular genetics

FLUORESCENCE MICROSCOPY · *see*

MICROSCOPE AND MICROSCOPY

FLUORESCENT DYES

The use of fluorescent dyes is the most popular tool for measuring ion properties in living cells. Calcium, magnesium, sodium, and similar species that do not naturally fluoresce can be measured indirectly by complexing them with fluorescent molecules. The use of probes, which fluoresce at one wavelength when unbound, and at a different wavelength when bound to an ion, allows the quantification of the ion level.

Fluorescence has also become popular as an alternative to radiolabeling of peptides. Whereas labeling of peptides with a radioactive compound relies on the introduction of a radiolabeled amino acid as part of the natural structure of the peptide, fluorescent tags are introduced as an additional group to the molecule.

The use of fluorescent dyes allows the detection of minute amounts of the target molecule within a mixture of many other molecules. In combination with light microscopic techniques like confocal laser microscopy, the use of fluorescent dyes allows three-dimensional image constructs to be complied, to provide precise spatial information on the target location. Finally, fluorescence can be used to gain information about phenomena such as blood flow and organelle movement in real time.

The basis of fluorescent dyes relies on the absorption of light at a specific wavelength and, in turn, the excitation of the electrons in the dye to higher energy levels. As the electrons fall back to their lower pre-excited energy levels, they re-emit light at longer wavelengths and so at lower energy levels. The lower-energy light emissions are called spectral shifts. The process can be repeated.

Proper use of a fluorescent dye requires 1) that its use does not alter the shape or function of the target cell, 2) that the dye localizes at the desired location within or on the cell, 3) that the dye maintains its specificity in the presence of competing molecules, and 4) that they operate at near visible wavelengths. Although none of the dyes in use today meets all of these criteria, fluorescent dyes are still useful for staining and observation to a considerable degree.

See also Biochemical analysis techniques; Biotechnology; Electron microscope, transmission and scanning; Electron microscopic examination of microorganisms; Immunofluorescence; Microscope and microscopy

FOOD PRESERVATION

The term food preservation refers to any one of a number of techniques used to prevent food from spoiling. It includes methods such as canning, pickling, drying and freeze-drying, irradiation, **pasteurization**, smoking, and the addition of chemical additives. Food preservation has become an increasingly important component of the food industry as fewer people eat foods produced on their own lands, and as consumers expect to be able to purchase and consume foods that are out of season.

The vast majority of instances of food spoilage can be attributed to one of two major causes: (1) the attack by pathogens (disease-causing **microorganisms**) such as **bacteria** and molds, or (2) oxidation that causes the destruction of essential biochemical compounds and/or the destruction of plant and animal cells. The various methods that have been devised for preserving foods are all designed to reduce or eliminate one or the other (or both) of these causative agents.

For example, a simple and common method of preserving food is by heating it to some minimum temperature. This process prevents or retards spoilage because high temperatures kill or inactivate most kinds of pathogens. The addition of compounds known as BHA and BHT to foods also prevents spoilage in another different way. These compounds are known to act as antioxidants, preventing chemical reactions that cause the oxidation of food that results in its spoilage. Almost all techniques of preservation are designed to extend the life of food by acting in one of these two ways.

The search for methods of food preservation probably can be traced to the dawn of human civilization. People who lived through harsh winters found it necessary to find some means of insuring a food supply during seasons when no fresh fruits and vegetables were available. Evidence for the use of dehydration (drying) as a method of food preservation, for example, goes back at least 5,000 years. Among the most primitive forms of food preservation that are still in use today are such methods as smoking, drying, salting, freezing, and fermenting.

Early humans probably discovered by accident that certain foods exposed to smoke seem to last longer than those that are not. Meats, fish, fowl, and cheese were among such foods. It appears that compounds present in wood smoke have anti-microbial actions that prevent the growth of organisms that cause spoilage. Today, the process of smoking has become a sophisticated method of food preservation with both hot and cold forms in use. Hot smoking is used primarily with fresh or frozen foods, while cold smoking is used most often with salted products. The most advantageous conditions for each kind of smoking—air velocity, relative humidity, length of exposure, and salt content, for example—are now generally understood and applied during the smoking process. For example, electro-static precipitators can be employed to attract smoke particles and improve the penetration of the particles into meat or fish. So many alternative forms of preservation are now available that smoking no longer holds the position of importance it once did with ancient peoples. More frequently, the process is used to add interesting and distinctive flavors to foods.

Because most disease-causing organisms require a moist environment in which to survive and multiply, drying is a natural technique for preventing spoilage. Indeed, the act of simply leaving foods out in the sun and wind to dry out is probably one of the earliest forms of food preservation. Evidence for the drying of meats, fish, fruits, and vegetables go back to the earliest recorded human history. At some point, humans also learned that the drying process could be hastened and improved by various mechanical techniques. For example, the Arabs learned early on that apricots could be preserved almost indefinitely by macerating them, boiling them, and then leaving them to dry on broad sheets. The product of this technique, quamaradeen, is still made by the same process in modern Muslim countries.

Today, a host of dehydrating techniques are known and used. The specific technique adopted depends on the properties of the food being preserved. For example, a traditional method for preserving rice is to allow it to dry naturally in the fields or on drying racks in barns for about two weeks. After this period of time, the native rice is threshed and then dried again by allowing it to sit on straw mats in the sun for about three days. Modern drying techniques make use of fans and heaters in controlled environments. Such methods avoid the uncertainties that arise from leaving crops in the field to dry under natural conditions. Controlled temperature air drying is especially popular for the preservation of grains such as maize, barley, and bulgur.

Vacuum drying is a form of preservation in which a food is placed in a large container from which air is removed. Water vapor pressure within the food is greater than that outside of it, and water evaporates more quickly from the food than in a normal atmosphere. Vacuum drying is biologically desirable since some **enzymes** that cause oxidation of foods become active during normal air drying. These enzymes do not appear to be as active under vacuum drying conditions, however. Two of the special advantages of vacuum drying are that the process is more efficient at removing water from a food product, and it takes place more quickly than air drying. In one study, for example, the drying time of a fish fillet was reduced from about 16 hours by air drying to six hours as a result of vacuum drying.

Coffee drinkers are familiar with the process of dehydration known as spray drying. In this process, a concentrated solution of coffee in water is sprayed though a disk with many small holes in it. The surface area of the original coffee grounds is increased many times, making dehydration of the dry product much more efficient. Freeze-drying is a method of preservation that makes use of the physical principle known as sublimation. Sublimation is the process by which a solid passes directly to the gaseous phase without first melting. Freeze-drying is a desirable way of preserving food because at low temperatures (commonly around 14°F to –13°F [–10°C to –25°C]) chemical reactions take place very slowly and pathogens have difficulty surviving. The food to be preserved by this method is first frozen and then placed into a vacuum chamber. Water in the food first freezes and then sublimes, leaving a moisture content in the final product of as low as 0.5%.

The precise mechanism by which salting preserves food is not entirely understood. It is known that salt binds with water molecules and thus acts as a dehydrating agent in foods. A high level of salinity may also impair the conditions under which pathogens can survive. In any case, the value of adding salt to foods for preservation has been well known for centuries. Sugar appears to have effects similar to those of salt in preventing spoilage of food. The use of either compound (and of certain other natural materials) is known as curing. A desirable side effect of using salt or sugar as a food preservative is, of course, the pleasant flavor each compound adds to the final product.

Curing can be accomplished in a variety of ways. Meats can be submerged in a salt solution known as brine, for example, or the salt can be rubbed on the meat by hand. The injection of salt solutions into meats has also become popular. Food scientists have now learned that a number of factors relating to the food product and to the preservative conditions affect the efficiency of curing. Some of the food factors include the type of food being preserved, the fat content, and the size of treated pieces. Preservative factors include brine temperature and concentration, and the presence of impurities.

Curing is used with certain fruits and vegetables, such as cabbage (in the making of sauerkraut), cucumbers (in the making of pickles), and olives. It is probably most popular, however, in the preservation of meats and fish. Honey-cured hams, bacon, and corned beef ("corn" is a term for a form of salt crystals) are common examples.

Freezing is an effective form of food preservation because the pathogens that cause food spoilage are killed or do not grow very rapidly at reduced temperatures. The process is less effective in food preservation than are thermal techniques such as boiling because pathogens are more likely to be able to survive cold temperatures than hot temperatures. In fact, one of the problems surrounding the use of freezing as a method of food preservation is the danger that pathogens deactivated (but not killed) by the process will once again become active when the frozen food thaws.

A number of factors are involved in the **selection** of the best approach to the freezing of foods, including the temperature to be used, the rate at which freezing is to take place, and the actual method used to freeze the food. Because of differences in cellular composition, foods actually begin to freeze at different temperatures ranging from about 31°F (–0.6°C) for some kinds of fish to 19°F (–7°C) for some kinds of fruits.

The rate at which food is frozen is also a factor, primarily because of aesthetic reasons. The more slowly food is frozen, the larger the ice crystals that are formed. Large ice crystals have the tendency to cause rupture of cells and the destruction of texture in meats, fish, vegetables, and fruits. In order to deal with this problem, the technique of quick-freezing has been developed. In quick-freezing, a food is cooled to or below its freezing point as quickly as possible. The product thus obtained, when thawed, tends to have a firm, more natural texture than is the case with most slow-frozen foods.

About a half dozen methods for the freezing of foods have been developed. One, described as the plate, or contact, freezing technique, was invented by the American inventor Charles Birdseye in 1929. In this method, food to be frozen is placed on a refrigerated plate and cooled to a temperature less than its freezing point. Alternatively, the food may be placed between two parallel refrigerated plates and frozen. Another technique for freezing foods is by immersion in very cold liquids. At one time, sodium chloride brine solutions were widely used for this purpose. A 10% brine solution, for example, has a freezing point of about 21°F (–6°C), well within the desired freezing range for many foods. More recently, liquid nitrogen

has been used for immersion freezing. The temperature of liquid nitrogen is about –320°F (–195.5°C), so that foods immersed in this substance freeze very quickly.

As with most methods of food preservation, freezing works better with some foods than with others. Fish, meat, poultry, and citrus fruit juices (such as frozen orange juice concentrate) are among the foods most commonly preserved by this method.

Fermentation is a naturally occurring chemical reaction by which a natural food is converted into another form by pathogens. It is a process in which food spoils, but results in the formation of an edible product. Perhaps the best example of such a food is cheese. Fresh milk does not remain in edible condition for a very long period of time. Its **pH** is such that harmful pathogens begin to grow in it very rapidly. Early humans discovered, however, that the spoilage of milk can be controlled in such a way as to produce a new product, cheese.

Bread is another food product made by the process of fermentation. Flour, water, sugar, milk, and other raw materials are mixed together with yeasts and then baked. The addition of yeasts brings about the fermentation of sugars present in the mixture, resulting in the formation of a product that will remain edible much longer than will the original raw materials used in the bread-making process.

Heating food is an effective way of preserving it because the great majority of harmful pathogens are killed at temperatures close to the boiling point of water. In this respect, heating foods is a form of food preservation comparable to that of freezing but much superior to it in its effectiveness. A preliminary step in many other forms of food preservation, especially forms that make use of packaging, is to heat the foods to temperatures sufficiently high to destroy pathogens.

In many cases, foods are actually cooked prior to their being packaged and stored. In other cases, cooking is neither appropriate nor necessary. The most familiar example of the latter situation is pasteurization. During the 1860s, the French bacteriologist **Louis Pasteur** discovered that pathogens in foods could be destroyed by heating those foods to a certain minimum temperature. The process was particularly appealing for the preservation of milk since preserving milk by boiling is not a practical approach. Conventional methods of pasteurization called for the heating of milk to a temperature between 145 and 149°F (63 and 65°C) for a period of about 30 minutes, and then cooling it to room temperature. In a more recent revision of that process, milk can also be "flash-pasteurized" by raising its temperature to about 160°F (71°C) for a minimum of 15 seconds, with equally successful results. A process known as ultra-high-pasteurization uses even higher temperatures, of the order of 194–266°F (90–130°C), for periods of a second or more.

One of the most common methods for preserving foods today is to enclose them in a sterile container. The term "canning" refers to this method although the specific container can be glass, plastic, or some other material as well as a metal can, from which the procedure originally obtained its name. The basic principle behind canning is that a food is sterilized, usually by heating, and then placed within an air-tight container. In the absence of air, no new pathogens can gain access to the sterilized food. In most canning operations, the food to be packaged is first prepared in some way—cleaned, peeled, sliced, chopped, or treated in some other way—and then placed directly into the container. The container is then placed in hot water or some other environment where its temperature is raised above the boiling point of water for some period of time. This heating process achieves two goals at once. First, it kills the vast majority of pathogens that may be present in the container. Second, it forces out most of the air above the food in the container.

After heating has been completed, the top of the container is sealed. In home canning procedures, one way of sealing the (usually glass) container is to place a layer of melted paraffin directly on top of the food. As the paraffin cools, it forms a tight solid seal on top of the food. Instead of or in addition to the paraffin seal, the container is also sealed with a metal screw top containing a rubber gasket. The first glass jar designed for this type of home canning operation, the Mason jar, was patented in 1858.

The commercial packaging of foods frequently makes use of tin, aluminum, or other kinds of metallic cans. The technology for this kind of canning was first developed in the mid-1800s, when individual workers hand-sealed cans after foods had been cooked within them. At this stage, a single worker could seldom produce more than 100 "canisters" (from which the word "can" later came) of food a day. With the development of far more efficient canning machines in the late nineteenth century, the mass production of canned foods became a reality.

As with home canning, the process of preserving foods in metal cans is simple in concept. The foods are prepared and the empty cans are sterilized. The prepared foods are then added to the sterile metal can, the filled can is heated to a sterilizing temperature, and the cans are then sealed by a machine. Modern machines are capable of moving a minimum of 1,000 cans per minute through the sealing operation.

The majority of food preservation operations used today also employ some kind of chemical additive to reduce spoilage. Of the many dozens of chemical additives available, all are designed either to kill or retard the growth of pathogens or to prevent or retard chemical reactions that result in the oxidation of foods. Some familiar examples of the former class of food additives are sodium benzoate and benzoic acid; calcium, sodium propionate, and propionic acid; calcium, potassium, sodium sorbate, and sorbic acid; and sodium and potassium sulfite. Examples of the latter class of additives include calcium, sodium ascorbate, and ascorbic acid (vitamin C); butylated hydroxyanisole (BHA) and butylated hydroxytoluene (BHT); lecithin; and sodium and potassium sulfite and sulfur dioxide.

A special class of additives that reduce oxidation is known as the sequestrants. Sequestrants are compounds that "capture" metallic ions, such as those of copper, iron, and nickel, and remove them from contact with foods. The removal of these ions helps preserve foods because in their free state they increase the rate at which oxidation of foods takes place. Some examples of sequestrants used as food preservatives are ethylenediamine-tetraacetic acid (EDTA), citric acid, sorbitol, and tartaric acid.

The lethal effects of radiation on pathogens has been known for many years. Since the 1950s, research in the United States has been directed at the use of this technique for preserving certain kinds of food. The radiation used for food preservation is normally gamma radiation from radioactive isotopes or machine-generated x rays or electron beams. One of the first applications of radiation for food preservation was in the treatment of various kinds of herbs and spices, an application approved by the U.S. Food and Drug Administration (FDA) in 1983. In 1985, the FDA extended its approval to the use of radiation for the treatment of pork as a means of destroying the pathogens that cause trichinosis. Experts predict that the ease and efficiency of food preservation by means of radiation will develop considerably in the future. That future is somewhat clouded, however, by fears expressed by some scientists and members of the general public about the dangers that irradiated foods may have for humans. In addition to a generalized concern about the possibilities of being exposed to additional levels of radiation in irradiated foods (not a possibility), critics have raised questions about the creation of new and possibly harmful compounds in food that has been exposed to radiation.

See also Biotechnology; Botulism; Food safety; History of microbiology; History of public health; Salmonella food poisoning; Winemaking

FOOD SAFETY

Food is a source of nutrients not only to humans but to **microorganisms** as well. The organic compounds and moisture that are often present in foods present an ideal environment for the growth of various microorganisms. The monitoring of the raw food and of any processing steps required prior to the consumption of the food are necessary to prevent transmission of disease-causing microorganisms from the food to humans.

Bacteria, **viruses**, **parasites**, and toxin by-products of microorganisms, chemicals, and heavy metals can cause foodborne maladies. These agents are responsible for over 200 different foodborne diseases. In the United States alone, foodborne diseases cause an estimated 75 million illnesses every year, and 7,000 to 9,000 deaths.

Aside from the human toll, the economic consequences of foodborne illnesses are considerable. In 1988, for example, human foodborne diarrheal disease in the United States cost the U.S. economy an estimated five to seven billion dollars in medical care and lost productivity.

The threat from foodborne disease causing agents is not equal. For example, the Norwalk-like viruses cause approximately 9 million illnesses each year, but the fatality rate is only 0.001%. *Vibrio vulnificus* causes fewer than 50 cases each year but almost 40% of those people die. Finally, the bacteria *Salmonella*, *Listeria monocytogenes*, and *Toxoplasma gondii* cause only about 20% of the total cases but are responsible for almost 80% of the total deaths from foodborne illnesses.

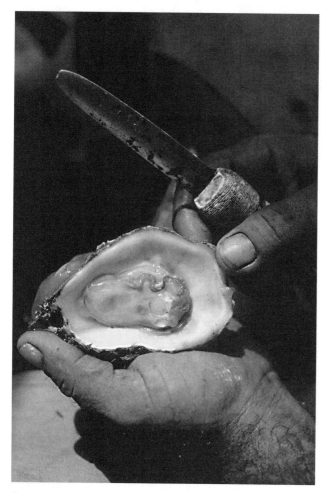

Raw oysters can harbor microbial toxins.

The **Centers for Disease Control** data has demonstrated that *Campylobacter jejuni* is the leading cause of foodborne illness in the United States. Another bacteria, *Salmonella* is the next leading cause. The third cause of foodborne illness is the bacterium *Escherichia coli* O157:H7. Poultry and ground meat are prime targets for bacterial **contamination**. Indeed, monitoring studies have demonstrated that some 70–90% of poultry carry *Campylobacter jejuni*.

Food safety needs to consider the influences of the microbial pathogen, the human host and the exposure of the food to the environment that promotes contamination. The environment can include the physical parameters such as the temperature, moisture, or other such factors. As well the environment can be the site of the foodstuff, such as the farmyard or the processing plant. Ensuring safety of food from microbial threat must consider all three of the influences. For example, reducing the length of time that a food is exposed to a questionable environment, but doing nothing to remove microbes from the environment only slightly reduces the risk of food contamination. Significant protection of foods depends on reducing the risk from the environment, microorganism of interest and of the human host.

The treatment of foods prior to consumption is a vital factor in ensuring food safety. Some of these treatments have been known for a long time. Salting of meats and drying of foods on long sea voyages was practiced several centuries ago, for example. The canning of foods began in the eighteenth century. Within the last 150 years, the link between hygienic conditions and the quality and safety of foods was recognized. Some of the advances in food safety arose from the need for foods on long military campaigns, such as those undertaken by Napoleon in the nineteenth century. Also, advances were spurred by the demands of the nascent food industry. As the distance between the farm and the market began to grow larger, and the shipping of food became more commonplace, the problems of food contamination became evident. Practices to render food safe for shipping, storage and subsequent consumption were necessary if the food industry was to grow and flourish.

The heat treatment of milk known as **pasteurization** began in the 1890s. Pasteurization is the transient exposure of milk to temperatures high enough to kill microbes, while preserving the taste and visual quality of the milk. Milk is now routinely pasteurized before sale to kill any bacteria that would otherwise growth in the wonderful growth medium that the liquid provides. Within the past thirty years the use of radiation to kill microbes in food has been utilized. While a very effective method to ensure food safety, irradiation is still subject to consumer uncertainty, which has to date limited its usefulness. As a final example, within the past two decades, the danger posed by intestinal bacterial pathogens, particularly *Escherichia coli* O157:H7 has resulted in the heightened recognition of the need for proper food preparation and personal **hygiene**.

Food safety is also dependent on the development and enforcement of standards of food preparation, handling and inspection. Often the mandated inspection of foods requires the food to be examined in certain ways and to achieve set benchmarks of quality (such as the total absence of fecal coliform bacteria). Violation of the quality standards can result in the immediate shut down of the food processing operation until the problem is located and rectified.

Most of the food safety legislation and inspection efforts are aimed at the processing of food. It is difficult to monitor the home environment and to enforce codes of hygiene there. Yet, food safety in the home is of paramount importance. The improper storage of foods prepared with raw or undercooked eggs, for example, can lead to the growth of microorganisms in the food. Depending on the microbe and whether toxins are produced, food poisoning or food intoxication can result from eating the food dish. Additionally, improper cleaning of cutting and other preparation surfaces can lead to the cross-contamination of one food by another. Good hygienic practices are as important in the home as on the farm, in the feedlot, and in the processing plant.

See also BSE and CJD disease; BSE and CJD disease, advances in research; BSE and CJD disease, ethical issues and socio-economic impact; Enterotoxin and exotoxin; Food preservation; Transmission of pathogens

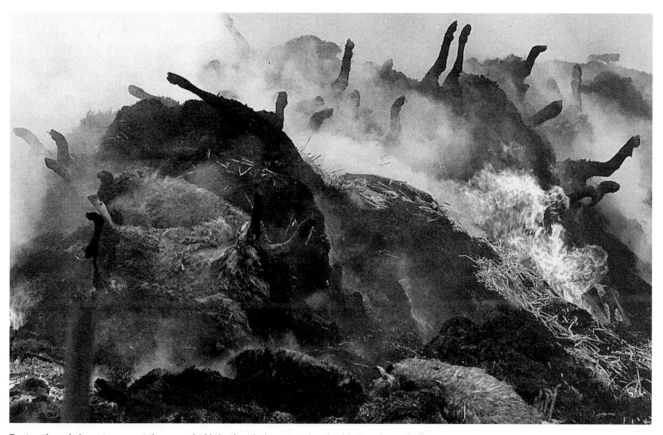

Destruction of sheep to prevent the spread of infection during an outbreak of foot-and-mouth disease.

FOOT-AND-MOUTH DISEASE

Often inaccurately called hoof-and-mouth disease, this highly contagious virus causes blisters in the mouth and on the feet surrounding hoofs of animals with cleft, or divided hoofs, such as sheep, cattle and hogs. The disease was first noted in Europe in 1809; the first outbreak in the United States came in 1870. Although it seldom spreads to humans, it can be transmitted through contaminated milk or the handling of infected animals.

Outbreaks are expensive for the animal owners who must kill the infected animals and incinerate or bury or them in quicklime. Then the animals' living quarters are disinfected, while feed and litter are burned. The farm is quarantined by state and federal officials who can decide to extend the quarantine to the general area or the whole state. Friedrich August Löffler (1852–1915), a German bacteriologist who discovered the bacillus of **diphtheria** in 1884, also demonstrated in 1898 that a virus causes hoof-and-mouth disease. It was the first time a virus was reported to be the cause of an animal disease.

An infected animal can take up to four days to begin showing symptoms of fever, smacking of lips and drooling. Eventually, blisters appear on the mouth, tongue and inside of the lips and the animal becomes lame just before blisters appear in the hoof area.

Löffler, working with Dr. Paul Frosch (1860–1928), a veterinary bacteriologist, extracted lymph from the blisters on the mouths and udders of diseased cattle. The lymph was diluted in sterile water and passed through filters. The researchers expected the filtrate to be an antitoxin of foot-and-mouth disease similar to the one for **smallpox**.

But Löffler and Frosch were wrong; when the filtrates were injected into healthy animals, they became sick. Therefore, they concluded the causative agent was not a bacterial toxin, but instead was a non-toxin producing bacterium too small to be seen under the **microscope**, yet small enough to pass through the filters. It wasn't until 1957 that scientists were able to get their first look at the causative agent, one of the smallest **viruses** to cause an animal disease.

In February, 2001, a devastating outbreak of foot-and-mouth disease began among the stock of England's pig, sheep, and cattle ranchers. Epidemiologists (investigators in infectious disease) determined that the outbreak began in a swill (garbage) feeding farm in one county, and spread first by the wind to a nearby sheep farm, then by sheep markets to farms across the English countryside. Even before the outbreak was detected, the virus had infected livestock in 43 farms. Despite massive quarantining and culling of herds (over 4 million animals were destroyed), by the time the outbreak was contained almost a year later, the disease had spread to areas of Ireland, France, and the Netherlands.

English citizens lost billions of dollars worth of income as markets for English meat and dairy products evaporated, animals were decimated, and tourists avoided the English countryside. Use of an available **vaccine** to attempt to curb the epidemic was rejected by most scientists, as the virus incubation time was short (often less than 72 hours), and the **immunity** gained from the vaccine was short-lived. Meanwhile, the Unites States and other countries adopted inclusive measures to prevent the importation of the foot-and-mouth virus, from carefully restricting the importation of animal products, to the sanitizing of shoes of airplane passengers arriving in the U.S. from England. As of April 2002, the outbreak continued to be contained, with the last confirmed foot-and-mouth case in England occurring six months prior at a farm in Northumberland, and the restoration of "Foot-and-mouth-Free" status restored to livestock herds of the United Kingdom by the World Organization for Animal Health (Office Internationale des Epizooties).

See also Animal models of infection; Epidemics, viral; Epidemiology, tracking diseases with technology; Epidemiology; Veterinary microbiology

FORENSIC IDENTIFICATION OF MICRO-ORGANISMS • *see* GENETIC IDENTIFICATION OF MICRO-ORGANISMS

FORENSIC IMMUNOLOGY AND BACTERI-OLOGY • *see* GENETIC IDENTIFICATION OF MICRO-ORGANISMS

FOSSILIZATION OF BACTERIA

Studies of fossilization of **bacteria** provide an indication of the age of ancient bacteria. Fossils of cyanobacteria or "blue-green algae" have been recovered from rocks that are nearly 3.5 million years old. Bacteria known as magnetobacteria form very small crystals of a magnetic compound inside the cells. These crystals have been found inside rock that is two billion years old.

The fossilization process in cyanobacteria and other bacteria appears to depend on the ability of the bacteria to trap sediment and metals from the surrounding solution. Cyanobacteria tend to grow as mats in their aquatic environment. The mats can retain sediment. Over time and under pressure the sediment entraps the bacteria in rock. As with other living organisms, the internal structure of such bacteria is replaced by minerals, notably pyrite or siderite (iron carbonate). The result, after thousands to millions of years, is a replica of the once-living cell.

Other bacteria that elaborate a carbohydrate network around themselves also can become fossilized. The evidence for this type of fossilization rests with laboratory experiments where bacteria are incubated in a metal-containing solution under conditions of temperature and pressure that attempt to mimic the forces found in geological formations. Experiments

with *Bacillus subtilis* demonstrated that the bacteria act as a site of precipitation for silica, the ferric form of iron, and of elemental gold. The binding of some of the metal ions to available sites within the carbohydrate network then acts to drive the precipitation of unstable metals out of solution and onto the previously deposited metal. The resulting cascade of precipitation can encase the entire bacterium in metallic species. On primordial Earth, this metal binding may have been the beginning of the fossilization process.

The deposition of metals inside carbohydrate networks like the capsule or exopolysaccharide surrounding bacteria is a normal feature of **bacterial growth**. Indeed, metal deposition can change the three-dimensional arrangement of the carbohydrate strands so as to make the penetration of antibacterial agents through the matrix more difficult. In an environment—such as occurs in the lungs of a cystic fibrosis patient— this micro-fossilization of bacteria confers a survival advantage to the cells.

In contrast to fossils of organisms such as dinosaurs, the preservation of internal detail of **microorganisms** seldom occurs. Prokaryotes have little internal structure to preserve. However, the mere presence of the microfossils is valuable, as they can indicate the presence of microbial life at that point in geological time.

Bacteria have been fossilized in amber, which is fossilized tree resin. Several reports have described the resuscitation of bacteria recovered from amber as well as bacteria recovered from a crystal in rock that is millions of years old. Although these claims have been disputed, a number of microbiologists assert that the care exercised by the experimenters lends increases the validity of their studies.

In the late 1990s a meteorite from the planet Mars was shown to contain bodies that appeared similar to bacterial fossils that have been found in rocks on Earth. Since then, further studies have indicated that the bodies may have arisen by inorganic (non-living) processes. Nonetheless, the possibility that these bodies are the first extraterrestrial bacterial fossils has not been definitively ruled out.

See also Bacterial surface layers; Biogeochemical cycles; Glycocalyx

FRIEND, CHARLOTTE (1921-1987)
American microbiologist

As the first scientist to discover a direct link between **viruses** and cancer, Charlotte Friend made important breakthroughs in cancer research, particularly that of leukemia. She was successful in immunizing mice against leukemia and in pointing a way toward new methods of treating the disease. Because of Friend's work, medical researchers developed a greater understanding of cancer and how it can be fought.

Friend was born on March 11, 1921, in New York City to Russian immigrants. Her father died of endocarditis (heart **inflammation**) when Charlotte was three, a factor that may have influenced her early decision to enter the medical field; at age ten she wrote a school composition entitled, "Why I Want to Become a Bacteriologist." Her mother's job as a pharmacist also exposed Friend to medicine. After graduating from Hunter College in 1944, she immediately enlisted in the U.S. Navy during World War II, rising to the rank of lieutenant junior grade.

After the war, Friend entered graduate school at Yale University, obtaining her Ph.D. in bacteriology in 1950. Soon afterward, she was hired by the Memorial Sloan-Kettering Institute for Cancer Research, and in 1952, became an associate professor in microbiology at Cornell University, which had just set up a joint program with the institute. During that time, Friend became interested in cancer, particularly leukemia, a cancer of blood-forming organs that was a leading killer of children. Her research on the cause of this disease led her to believe that, contrary to the prevailing medical opinion, leukemia in mice is caused by a virus. To confirm her theory, Friend took samples of leukemia tissue from mice and, after putting the material through a filter to remove cells, injected it into healthy mice. These animals developed leukemia, indicating that the cause of the disease was a substance smaller than a cell. Using an **electron microscope**, Friend was able to discover and photograph the virus she believed responsible for leukemia.

However, when Friend presented her findings at the April 1956, annual meeting of the American Association for Cancer Research, she was denounced by many other researchers, who refused to believe that a virus was responsible for leukemia. Over the next year support for Friend's theory mounted, first as Dr. Jacob Furth declared that his experiments had confirmed the existence of such a virus in mice with leukemia. Even more importantly, Friend was successful in vaccinating mice against leukemia by injecting a weakened form of the virus (now called the "Friend virus") into healthy mice, so they could develop antibodies to fight off the normal virus. Friend's presentation of a paper on this **vaccine** at the cancer research association's 1957 meeting succeeded in laying to rest the skepticism that had greeted her the previous year.

In 1962, Friend was honored with the Alfred P. Sloan Award for Cancer Research and another award from the American Cancer Society for her work. The next year she became a member of the New York Academy of Sciences, an organization that has members from all fifty states and more than eighty countries. In 1966, Friend left Sloan-Kettering to become a professor and director at the Center for Experimental Cell Biology at the newly formed medical school of New York's Mount Sinai Hospital. During this time, she continued her research on leukemia, and in 1972, she announced the discovery of a method of altering a leukemia mouse cell in a test tube so that it would no longer multiply. Through chemical treatment, the malignant red blood cell could be made to produce hemoglobin, as do normal cells.

Although the virus responsible for leukemia in mice has been discovered, there is no confirmation that a virus causes leukemia in humans. Likewise, her treatment for malignant red blood cells has limited application, because it will not work outside of test tubes. Nonetheless, Friend had pointed out a possible cause of cancer and developed a first step toward fighting leukemia (and possibly other cancers) by targeting specific cells.

In 1976, Friend was elected president of the American Association for Cancer Research, the same organization

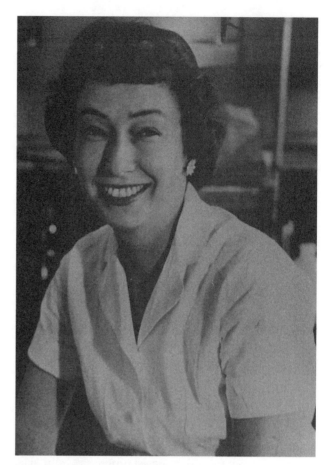

Charlotte Friend, an important cancer researcher.

whose members had so strongly criticized her twenty years earlier. Two years later, she was chosen the first woman president of the New York Academy of Sciences. Friend was long active in supporting other women scientists and in speaking out on women's issues. During her later years, she expressed concern over the tendency to emphasize patient care over basic research, feeling that without sufficient funding for research, new breakthroughs in patient care would be impossible. Friend died on January 13, 1987, of lymphoma.

See also Viral vectors in gene therapy; Virology; Virus replication; Viruses and responses to viral infection

FUME HOOD

A fume hood is an enclosed work space in a laboratory that prevents the outward flow of air. Fume hoods cab be designed for work with inorganic or radioactive materials, or with biological materials. Biological fume hoods can be equipped with filters, to ensure that the air entering and exiting the cabinet is sterile. This minimizes the risk of exposure of laboratory personnel to biological agents that could be a health threat. Also, the work surfaces and materials inside the fume hood are protected from

contamination from airborne **bacteria** or **viruses**. The latter is of particular relevance in some viral research, where the tissue surfaces used to grow the virus are prone to contamination.

The design of fume hoods differs, depending on the intended purpose (general purpose, chemical, radioisotope, biological). But all fume hoods share the feature of an inward flow of air. In biological fume hoods the flow of sterile air is typically from the back of the cabinet toward the laboratory worker, and from the top of the fume hood downward across the opening at the front of the hood. This pattern of airflow ensures that any **microorganisms** residing on the laboratory worker are not carried into the work surface, and that no air from inside the cabinet escapes to the outside of the cabinet. Any air that is exhausted back into the laboratory first passes through filters that are designed to remove biological and viral contaminants. The most popular type of biological filter is the high-energy particulate air (or HEPA) filter.

Biological fume hoods can have a moveable, protective glass partition at the front. Most hoods also have a gas source inside, so that sterile work, such as the flaming of inoculation loops, can be done. The fume hood should be positioned in an area of the laboratory where there is less traffic back and forth, which lessens the turbulence of air outside the fume hood.

The filtering system of biological fume hoods restricts its use to biological work. Work involving noxious chemicals and vapors needs to be conducted in another, specially designed chemical fume hood.

The construction of fume hoods is conducted according to strict protocols of safety and performance monitoring. In normal laboratory use, the continued performance of a fume hood is regularly monitored and test results recorded. Often such checks are a mandatory requirement of the ongoing certification of an analysis laboratory. Accordingly, laboratories must properly maintain and use fume hoods to continue to meet operating rules and regulations.

See also Bioterrorism, protective measures; Containment and release prevention protocol

FUNGAL GENETICS

Fungi possess strikingly different morphologies. They include large, fleshy, and often colorful mushrooms or toadstools, filamentous organisms only just visible to the naked eye, and single-celled organisms such as yeasts. Molds are important agents of decay. They also produce a large number of industrially important compounds like **antibiotics (penicillin**, griseofulvin, etc.), organic acids (citric acid, gluconic acid, etc.), **enzymes** (alpha-amylases, lipase, etc.), traditional foods (softening and flavoring of cheese, shoyu soy sauce, etc.), and a number of other miscellaneous products (gibberellins, ergot alkaloids, steroid bioconversions). As late as 1974 the only widely applicable techniques for strain improvement were mutation, screening, and **selection**. While these techniques proved dramatically successful in improving penicillin production, they deflected attempts to employ a more sophisti-

cated approach to genetic manipulation. The study of fungal genetics has recently changed beyond all recognition.

The natural genetic variation present in fungal species has been characterized using molecular methods such as electrophoretic karyotyping, restriction fragment length polymorphism, **DNA** finger printing, and DNA sequence comparisons. The causes for the variation include chromosomal polymorphism, changes in repetitive DNA, **transposons**, virus-like elements, and mitochondrial **plasmids**.

Genetic **recombination** occurs naturally in many fungi. Many industrially important fungi such as *Aspergilli* and *Penicillia* lack sexuality, so in these species parasexual systems (cycles) provide the basis for genetic study and breeding programs. The parasexual cycle is a series of events that can be induced when two genetically different strains are grown together in the laboratory. A heterokaryon, which is **mycelium** with two different nuclei derived from two different haploid strains, is produced by the fusion of **hyphae**. Increased penicillin titer in the haploid progeny of parasexual crosses has been achieved in *Penicillium chrysogenum*. A more direct approach has been developed using **protoplasts**. These are isolated from vegetative cells of fungi or yeasts by removing the cell wall by digestion using a cell wall degrading enzyme. Protoplasts from the two strains can be fused by treatment with polyethylene glycol. Protoplast fusion in fungi initiates the parasexual cycle, resulting in the formation of diploidy and mitotic recombination and segregation. A selection procedure to screen such fusants is done using genetic markers. A good example of applying this technique is the fusion of a fast growing but poor glucoamylase producer with a slow growing but excellent producer of glucoamylase. The desired result will be a strain that is both fast growing and an excellent producer of enzyme.

The realization that **transformation** of genetic material into fungi can occur came with the discovery that yeasts like *Saccharomyces cerevisiae* and filamentous fungi like *Podospora anserine* contain **plasmids**. Currently transformation technology is largely based on the use of *Neurospora crassa* and *Aspergillus nidulans,* though methods for use in filamentous organisms are being developed. The protocols used in transformation of filamentous fungi involve **cloning** the desired **gene** into the plasmid from *E. coli* or a plasmid constructed from genetic material from *E. coli* and *Saccharomyces cerevisiae*. Protoplasts from the recipient strains are then formed and mixed with the plasmid. After incubating for a short time to allow for the uptake of the plasmid DNA, the protoplasts are allowed to regenerate and the cells are screened for the presence of the specific marker.

The application of recombinant DNA to yeasts and filamentous fungi has opened up new possibilities in relation to the construction of highly productive strains. The filamentous fungi are now established as potent host organisms for the production of heterologous proteins. This is particularly useful as expression of specific proteins can reach relatively high levels. Using *Aspergillus* as a host for reproduction has led to the production of many recombinant products like human therapeutic proteins, including growth factors, **cytokines**, and hormones. While expression can be good in *E. coli,* lack of posttranslational modifications has limited their usage. The use of

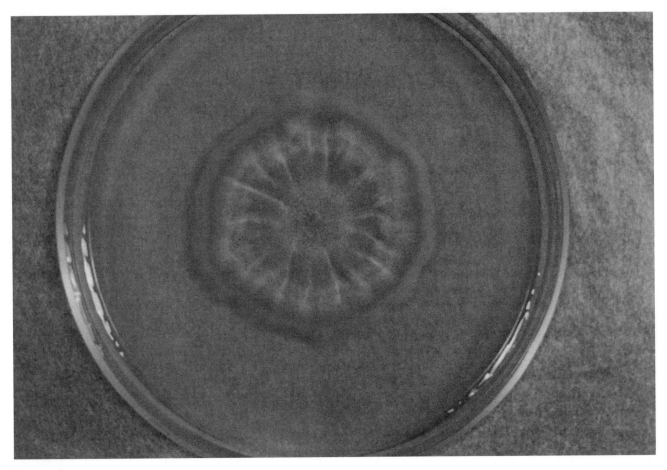

Fungus colony.

Saccharomyces species has not been highly successful for the production of extracellular proteins. Most of the initial advances for the production of heterologous proteins has been with filamentous fungi, namely *Aspergillus nidulans*. Although this organism is not of industrial importance it is nevertheless genetically well characterized; in addition, this organism has secretion signals that result in recombinant proteins being identical to mammalian cells. This allows the product from such systems to be used safely in human therapy. Other systems that have been used include Pichia and Trichoderma, which have been widely used in industry. Now that the complete genome of *S. cerevisiae* has been deciphered, and with more fungi genomes in the pipeline, an even better understanding of fungal genetics is certain.

See also Cell cycle (Eukaryotic), genetic regulation of; Microbial genetics

FUNGI

Fungi play an essential role in breaking down organic matter and thereby allowing nutrients to be recycled in nature. As such, they are important decomposers and without them living communities would become buried in their own waste. Some fungi, the saprobes, get their nutrients from nonliving organic matter, such as dead plants and animal wastes, clothing, paper, leather, and other materials. Others, the **parasites**, get nutrients from the tissues of living organisms. Both types of fungi obtain nutrients by secreting **enzymes** from their cells that break down large organic molecules into smaller components. The fungi cells can then absorb the nutrients.

Although the term fungus invokes unpleasant images for some people, fungi are a source of **antibiotics**, vitamins, and industrial chemicals. **Yeast**, a kind of fungi, is used to ferment bread and alcoholic beverages. Nevertheless, fungi also cause athlete's foot, yeast infections, food spoilage, wheat and corn diseases, and, perhaps most well known, the Irish potato famine of 1843–1847 (caused by the fungus *Phytophthora infestans*), which contributed to the deaths of 250,000 people in Ireland.

Fungi are not plants, and are unique and separate forms of life that are classified in their own kingdom. Approximately 75,000 species of fungi have been described, and scientists estimate that more than 90% of all fungi species on the planet have yet to be discovered. The fungi body, called **mycelium**, is composed of threadlike filaments called **hyphae**. All fungi can reproduce asexually by cell division, budding, fragmentation, or spores, although some reproduce sexually.

The main groups of fungi are chytrids, water molds, zygosporangium-forming fungi, sac fungi, and club fungi. Chyrids live in muddy or aquatic habitats and feed on decaying plants, though some live as parasites on living plants, animals, and other fungi. Water molds, distantly related to other fungi, play an important role as decomposers in aquatic habitats. Some, however, live as parasites on aquatic animals and terrestrial plants, including potato plants that can be destroyed by certain types of water molds. Zygosporangium-forming fungi also can be either saprobes, such as the well-known black bread **mold**, or parasites on insects, such as houseflies. Sac fungi, of which more than 30,000 species are known, include the yeast used to leaven bread and alcoholic beverages. However, many of these fungi also cause diseases in plants. Club fungi, numbering more than 25,000 species, include mushrooms, stinkhorns, and puffballs. While some fingi are edible, others produce deadly poisons.

See also Candidiasis; Chitin; Fermentation; Fungal genetics; History of the development of antibiotics; Lichens; Winemaking

FUNGICIDES

Fungicides are chemicals that inhibit the growth of **fungi**. Fungi can attack agricultural crops, garden plants, wood and wood products (dry rot in particular is a major problem), and many other items of use to humans. Fungicides usually kill the fungus that is causing the damage. Sulfur, sulfur-containing compounds, organic salts of iron, and heavy metals are all used as fungicides. Other fungicide types include carbamates or thiocarbamates such as benomyl and ziram, thiozoles such as etridiazole, triazines such as anilazine, and substituted organics such as chlorothalonil. Many non-drug fungicides have low mammalian tolerance for toxicity, and have been shown to cause cancer or reproductive toxicity in experimental animal studies.

Fungicides operate in different ways depending upon the species that they are designed to combat. Many are poisons and their application must be undertaken carefully or over-application may kill other plants in the area. Some fungicides disrupt some of the metabolic pathways of fungi by inhibiting energy production or biosynthesis, and others disrupt the fungal cell wall, which is made of **chitin**, as opposed to the cellulose of plant cell walls. Chitin is a structural polysaccharide and is composed of chains of N-acetyl-D-glucosamine units. Fungal pathogens come from two main groups of fungi, the ascomycetes (rusts and smuts) and the basidiomycetes (the higher fungi—mushrooms, toadstools, and bracket fungi).

Human fungal infections, such as athlete's foot, can be treated by fungicides normally referred to as antifungal agents or antimycotics. Compounds such as fluconazole, clotrimazole, and nystatin are used to treat human fungal infections.

See also Candidiasis; Mycology

G

GALLO, ROBERT C. (1937-   )
American virologist

Robert C. Gallo, one of the best-known biomedical researchers in the United States, is considered the co-discoverer, along with **Luc Montagnier** at the Pasteur Institute, of the **Human Immunodeficiency Virus** (**HIV**). Gallo established that the virus causes acquired **immunodeficiency** syndrome (**AIDS**), something that Montagnier had not been able to do, and he developed the blood test for HIV, which remains a central tool in efforts to control the disease. Gallo also discovered the **human T-cell leukemia virus** (**HTLV**) and the human T-cell growth factor interleukin–2.

Gallo's initial work on the isolation and identification of the AIDS virus has been the subject of a number of allegations, resulting in a lengthy investigation and official charges of scientific misconduct which were overturned on appeal. Although he has now been exonerated, the ferocity of the controversy has tended to obscure the importance of his contributions both to AIDS research and biomedical research in general. As Malcolm Gladwell observed in 1990 in the *Washington Post*: "Gallo is easily one of the country's most famous scientists, frequently mentioned as a Nobel Prize contender, and a man whose research publications were cited by other researchers publishing their own work during the last decade more often than those of any other scientist in the world."

Gallo was born in Waterbury, Connecticut, on March 23, 1937, to Francis Anton and Louise Mary (Ciancuilli) Gallo. He grew up in the house that his Italian grandparents bought after they came to the United States. His father worked long hours at the welding company which he owned. The dominant memory of Gallo's youth was of the illness and death of his only sibling, Judy, from childhood leukemia. The disease brought Gallo into contact with the nonfamily member who most influenced his life, Dr. Marcus Cox, the pathologist who diagnosed her disease in 1948. During his senior year in high school, an injury kept Gallo off the high school basketball team and forced him to think about his future. He began

to spend time with Cox, visiting him at the hospital, even assisting in postmortem examinations. When Gallo entered college, he knew he wanted a career in biomedical research.

Gallo attended Providence College, where he majored in biology, graduating with a bachelor's degree in 1959. He continued at Jefferson Medical College in Philadelphia, where he got an introduction to medical research. In 1961, he worked as a summer research fellow in Alan Erslev's laboratory at Jefferson. His work studying the pathology of oxygen deprivation in coal miners led to his first scientific publication in 1962, while he was still a medical student.

In 1961, Gallo married Mary Jane Hayes, whom he met while in Providence College. Together they had two children. Gallo graduated from medical school in 1963; on the advice of Erslev, he went to the University of Chicago because it had a reputation as a major center for blood-cell biology, Gallo's research interest. From 1963 to 1965, he did research on the biosynthesis of hemoglobin, the protein that carries oxygen in the blood.

In 1965, Gallo was appointed to the position of clinical associate at the National Institutes of Health (NIH) in Bethesda, Maryland. He spent much of his first year at NIH caring for cancer patients. Despite the challenges, he observed some early successes at treating cancer patients with **chemotherapy**. Children were being cured of the very form of childhood leukemia that killed his sister almost twenty years before. In 1966, Gallo was appointed to his first full-time research position, as an associate of Seymour Perry, who was head of the medicine department. Perry was studying how white blood cells grow in various forms of leukemia. In his laboratory, Gallo studied the **enzymes** involved in the synthesis of the components of **DNA** (**deoxyribonucleic acid**), the carrier of genetic information.

The expansion of the NIH and the passage of the National Cancer Act in 1971 led to the creation of the Laboratory of Tumor Cell Biology at the National Cancer Institute (NCI), a part of the NIH. Gallo was appointed head of the new laboratory. He had become intrigued with the possibility that certain kinds of cancer had viral origins, and he set up his new laboratory to study human **retroviruses**. Retroviruses are types of viruses that possess the ability to penetrate other cells and splice their own genetic material into the genes of their hosts, eventually taking over all of their reproductive functions. At the time Gallo began his work, retroviruses had been found in animals; the question was whether they existed in humans. His research involved efforts to isolate a virus from victims of certain kinds of leukemia, and he and his colleagues were able to view a retrovirus through electron microscopes. In 1975, Gallo and Robert E. Gallagher announced that they had discovered a human leukemia virus, but other laboratories were unable to replicate their results. Scientists to whom they had sent samples for independent confirmation had found two different retroviruses not from humans, but from animals. The samples had been contaminated by **viruses** from a monkey or a chimp.

Despite the setback, Gallo continued his efforts to isolate a human retrovirus. He turned his attention to T-cells, white blood cells which are an important part of the body's **immune system**, and developed a substance called T-cell growth factor (later called interleukin–2), which would sustain them outside the human body. The importance of this growth factor was that it enabled Gallo and his team to sustain cancerous T-cells long enough to discover whether a retrovirus existed within them. These techniques allowed Gallo and his team to isolate a previously unknown virus from a leukemia patient. He named the virus human T-cell leukemia virus, or HTLV, and he published this finding in *Science* in 1981. This time his findings were confirmed.

It was Gallo's experience with viral research that made him important in the effort to identify the cause of AIDS, after that disease had first been characterized by doctors in the United States. In further studies of HTLV, Gallo had established that it could be transmitted by breast-feeding, sexual intercourse, and blood transfusions. He also observed that the incidence of cancers caused by this virus was concentrated in Africa and the Caribbean. HTLV had these and other characteristics in common with what was then known about AIDS, and Gallo was one of the first scientists to hypothesize that the disease was caused by a virus. In 1982, the National Cancer Institute formed an AIDS task force with Gallo as its head. In this capacity he made available to the scientific community the research methods he had developed for HTLV, and among those whom he provided with some early technical assistance was Luc Montagnier at the Pasteur Institute in Paris.

Gallo tried throughout 1983 to get the AIDS virus to grow in **culture**, using the same growth factor that had worked in growing HTLV, but he was not successful. Finally, a member of Gallo's group named Mikulas Popovic developed a method to grow the virus in a line of T-cells. The method consisted, in effect, of mixing samples from various patients into a kind of a cocktail, using perhaps ten different strains of the virus at a time, so there was a higher chance that one would survive. This innovation allowed the virus to be studied, and observing the similarities to the retroviruses he had previously discovered, Gallo called it HTLV–3. In 1984, he and his colleagues published their findings in *Science*. Gallo and the

other scientists in his laboratory were able to establish that this virus caused AIDS, and they developed a blood test for the virus.

Almost a year before Gallo announced his findings, Montagnier at the Pasteur Institute had identified a virus he called LAV, though he was not able to prove that it caused AIDS. The two laboratories were cooperating with each other in the race to find the cause of AIDS and several samples of this virus had been sent to Gallo at the National Cancer Institute. The controversy which would embroil the American scientist's career for almost the next decade began when the United States government denied the French scientists a patent for the AIDS test and awarded one to his team instead. The Pasteur Institute believed their contribution was not recognized in this decision, and they challenged it in court. Gallo did not deny that they had preceded him in isolating the virus, but he argued that it was proof of the causal relationship and the development of the blood test which were most important, and he maintained that these advances had been accomplished using a virus which had been independently isolated in his laboratory.

This first stage of the controversy ended in a legal settlement that was highly unusual for the scientific community: Gallo and Montagnier agreed out of court to share equal credit for their discovery. This settlement followed a review of records from Gallo's laboratory and rested on the assumption that the virus Gallo had discovered was different from the one Montagnier had sent him. An international committee renamed the virus HIV, and in what Specter calls "the first such negotiated history of a scientific enterprise ever published," the American and French groups published an agreement about their contributions in *Nature* in 1987. In 1988, Gallo and Montagnier jointly related the story of the discoveries in *Scientific American*.

Questions about the isolation of the AIDS virus were revived in 1989 by a long article in the *Chicago Tribune*. The journalist, a Pulitzer Prize winner named John Crewdson, had spent three years investigating Gallo's laboratory, making over one hundred requests under the Freedom of Information Act. He directly questioned Gallo's integrity and implied he had stolen Montagnier's virus. The controversy intensified when it was established that the LAV virus which the French had isolated and the HTLV–3 virus were virtually identical. The genetic sequencing in the two were in fact so close that some believed they actually came from the same AIDS patient, and Gallo was accused of simply renaming the virus Montagnier had sent him. Gallo's claim to have independently isolated the virus was further damaged when it was discovered that in the 1984 *Science* article announcing his discovery of HTLV–3 he had accidently published a photograph of Montagnier's virus.

In 1990, pressure from a congressional committee forced the NIH to undertake an investigation. The NIH investigation found Popovic guilty of scientific misconduct but Gallo guilty only of misjudgment. A committee of scientists that oversaw the investigation was strongly critical of these conclusions, and the group expressed concern that Popovic had been assigned more than a fair share of the blame. In June 1992, the NIH investigation was superseded by the Office of Research Integrity (ORI) at the Department of Health and

Human Services, and in December of that year, ORI found both Gallo and Popovic guilty of scientific misconduct. Based largely on a single sentence in the 1984 *Science* article that described the isolation of the virus, the ORI report found Gallo guilty of misconduct for "falsely reporting that LAV had not been transmitted to a permanently growing cell line." This decision renewed the legal threat from the Pasteur Institute, whose lawyers moved to claim all the back royalties from the AIDS blood test, which then amounted to approximately $20 million.

Gallo strongly objected to the findings of the ORI, pointing to the fact that the finding of misconduct turned on a single sentence in a single paper. Other scientists objected to the panel's priorities, arguing that the charge of misconduct concerned a misrepresentation of a relatively minor issue which did not negate the scientific validity of Gallo's conclusions. Lawyers representing both Gallo and Popovic brought their cases before an appeals board at the Department of Health and Human Services. Popovic's case was heard first, and in December 1993, the board announced that he had been cleared of all charges. As quoted in *Time,* the panel declared: "One might anticipate... after all the sound and fury, there would be at least a residue of palpable wrongdoing. This is not the case." The ORI immediately withdrew all charges against Gallo for lack of proof.

According to *Time,* in December 1993, Gallo considered himself "completely vindicated" of all the allegations that had been made against him. He has established that before 1984 his laboratory had succeeded in isolating other strains of the virus that were not similar to LAV. Many scientists now argue that the problem was simply one of **contamination**, a mistake which may have been a consequence of the intense pressure for results in many laboratories during the early years of the AIDS epidemic. It has been hypothesized that the LAV sample from the Pasteur Institute contaminated the mixture of AIDS viruses that Popovic concocted to find one strain that would survive in culture; it is believed that this strain was strong enough to survive and be identified by Gallo and Popovic for a second time.

In 1990, when the controversy was still at its height, Gallo published a book about his career called *Virus Hunting,* which seemed intended to refute the charges against him, particularly the *Tribune* article by Crewdson. Gallo made many of the claims that were later supported by the appeals board, and in the *New York Times Book Review,* Natalie Angier called him "a formidable gladiator who firmly believes in the importance of his scientific contributions." Angier wrote of the book: "His description of the key experiments in 1983 and 1984 that led to the final isolation of the AIDS virus are intelligent and persuasive, particularly to a reader who was heard the other side of the story."

The many allegations and the long series of investigations have distracted many people from the accomplishments of a man whose name appears on hundreds of scientific papers and who has won most major awards in biomedical research except the Nobel Prize. Gallo received the coveted Albert Lasker Award twice, once in 1982 for his work on the viral origins of cancer, and again in 1986 for his research on AIDS. He

has also been awarded the American Cancer Society Medal of Honor in 1983, the Lucy Wortham Prize from the Society for Surgical Oncology in 1984, the Armand Hammer Cancer Research Award in 1985, and the Gairdner Foundation International Award for Biomedical Research in 1987. He has received eleven honorary degrees.

See also AIDS, recent advances in research and treatment; Antibody and antigen; Antibody formation and kinetics; Antibody-antigen, biochemical and molecular reactions; Viruses and responses to viral infection

GAS VACUOLES AND GAS VESICLES

Gas vacuoles are aggregates of hollow cylindrical structures called gas vesicles. They are located inside some **bacteria**. A membrane that is permeable to gas bound each gas vesicle. The inflation and deflation of the vesicles provides buoyancy, allowing the bacterium to float at a desired depth in the water.

Bacteria that are known as cyanobacteria contain gas vacuoles. Cyanobacteria, which used to be called **blue-green algae**, live in water and manufacture their own food from the photosynthetic energy of sunlight. Studies have demonstrated that the inflation and deflation of the gas vesicles is coordinated with the light. The buoyancy provided by the gas vacuoles enables the bacteria to float near the surface during the day to take advantage of the presence of sunlight for the manufacture of food, and to sink deeper at night to harvest nutrients that have sunk down into the water.

Gas vesicles are also found in some archae, bacteria that are thought to have branched off from a common ancestor of **eukaryotes** and prokaryotes at a very early stage in **evolution**. For example, the gas vesicles in the bacterium *Halobacterium NRC-1* allow the bacteria to float in their extremely salt water environments (the bacteria are described as halophilic, or "salt loving." The detailed genetic analysis that has been done with this bacterium indicates that at least 13 to 14 genes are involved in production of the two gas vesicle structural proteins and other, perhaps regulatory, proteins. For example, some proteins may sense the environment and act to trigger synthesis of the vesicles. Vesicle synthesis is known to be triggered by low oxygen concentrations.

The gas vesicles tend to be approximately 75 nanometers in diameter. Their length is variable, ranging from 200 to 1000 nanometers, depending on the species of bacteria. The vesicles are constructed of a single small protein. In at least some vesicles these proteins are linked together by another protein. The interior of the protein shell is very **hydrophobic** (water-hating), so that water is excluded from the inside of the vesicles. Yet it is still unclear how the regular arrangement of proteins produces a shell that is permeable to gas. Presumably there must be enough space in between the protein subunits to permit the passage of air.

See also Blue-green algae; Photosynthetic microorganisms

GASTROENTERITIS

Gastroenteritis is an **inflammation** of the stomach and the intestines. More commonly, gastroenteritis is called the stomach flu.

The symptoms of gastroenteritis always include diarrhea. Fever, and vomiting can also be present. Typically the symptoms associated with a bout of gastroenteritis typically last only several days and are self-limiting. But sometimes the malady can be more extended.

The diarrhea in gastroenteritis is very loose, even watery. Also, bowel movements are frequent, occurring even several times an hour as the body attempts to expel the offending microorganism. This large loss of fluid creates the potential for dehydration. Usually dehydration is not an issue in an adult, unless the person is incapable of caring for themselves and has no other caregiver. Dehydration is an important issue in children. If a child is hospitalized because of diarrhea, it is usually because of complications arising from dehydration, rather than from the actual stomach and intestinal infection.

The other symptoms of gastroenteritis are especially complicating in children. Vomiting makes it difficult to administer drugs to combat a **bacterial infection**. Also, the loss of stomach contents can exacerbate dehydration.

Gastroenteritis-induced diarrhea is one of the major causes of death in infants around the world. In Asia, Africa, and Latin America millions of deaths in the newborn to four years age group occurs every year.

Gastroenteritis can be caused by **viruses** and **bacteria**. Viruses are the more common cause. Many There **types of viruses** can cause gastroenteritis. These include rotaviruses, enteroviruses, **adenoviruses**, caliciviruses, astroviruses, Norwalk virus and a group of Norwalk-like viruses. Of these, rotavirus infections are the most common.

Viral gastroenteritis tends to appear quickly, within three days of ingestion of the virus, and diminishes within a week. Those whose **immune system** is compromised may experience symptoms for a longer period of time.

Rotavirus is a virus that contains **ribonucleic acid** as the genetic material. The genetic material is enclosed within a double shell of protein. The virus is a member of the Reoviridae family of viruses. There are three main groups of rotavirus with respect to the antibodies that are produced against them. These types are called groups A, B, and C. Group A rotavirus is the cause of more than three million cases of gastroenteritis in the United States every year. The group B rotavirus causes diarrhea in adults, and has been the cause a several major outbreaks of severe diarrhea in China. Finally, the group C rotavirus can cause diarrhea in both children and adults, but is encountered much less frequently than groups A and B.

Rotavirus gastroenteritis is very contagious, spreading from person to person in a fecal to oral route. Not surprisingly, the virus is frequently encountered in day care facilities, where the care of the soiled diapers of infants occurs regularly. Improper **hygiene**, especially hand washing, contributes directly to the spread of the virus. Infected individuals can shed large numbers of virus in their diarrhea. Infection can

also be spread by the **contamination** of eating utensils. Food can become contaminated if the food handler has not properly washed their hands after using the bathroom. Shellfish can also be a source of the virus. Because shellfish feed by filtering water through a special filter feeding apparatus, virus in the water can become trapped and concentrated inside the shellfish. Eating the shellfish, especially raw, spreads the virus.

Gastroenteritis due to the Norwalk virus tends to be more common in adults. However, more advanced immunological methods of detection have detected **antibody** to the virus in many children. Thus, children may be infected by the virus but show no symptoms. Infection in the adult years produces gastroenteritis, for reasons that are as yet unknown. Discovering the nature of the asymptomatic response of children could led to a therapeutic strategy for the adult infection.

Bacteria also cause gastroenteritis. The bacteria of concern include certain strains of **Escherichia coli, Salmonella, Shigella**, and *Vibrio cholerae*. In developed countries, where sanitary conditions and water treatment are established, bacterial gastroenteritis is infrequent. But the bacterial form remains problematic in the under-developed world, where water is more vulnerable to contamination. Bacterial gastroenteritis can also be caused by the ingestion of contaminated food. For example the presence of *Salmonella* in potato salad that has been improperly stored or of *E.coli O157:H7* in undercooked meat can cause the malady.

The protozoan *Cryptosporidium parvum* also causes gastroenteritis following the ingestion of contaminated water.

The bacterial and protozoan cases of gastroenteritis account for well below half of the reported cases. The majority of cases are of viral origin.

In the treatment of gastroenteritis it is important to establish whether the source of the condition is bacterial, viral, protozoan or another and non-biological factor. Intolerance to the digestion of the lactose constituent of milk can also cause gastroenteritis, for example. The need to establish the origin of the malady is important, since bacterial infections will respond to the administration of **antibiotics** while viral infections will not. Furthermore, the use of antibiotics in a viral infection can actually exacerbate the diarrhea.

In August 1998, a **vaccine** for rotavirus gastroenteritis was licensed for sale in the United States. From September 1998 until July 1999, 15 cases of intussusception (a condition where a segment of bowel folds inside an adjacent segment, causing an obstruction) were reported among infants who received the vaccine. Subsequently, the vaccine was withdrawn from the market. No other vaccine has as yet been licensed for use.

See also Enterobacterial infections; Transmission of pathogens

GENE

A gene is the fundamental physical and functional unit of heredity. Whether in a microorganism or in a human cell, a gene is an individual element of an organism's genome and determines a trait or characteristic by regulating biochemical structure or metabolic process.

Genes are segments of nucleic acid, consisting of a specific sequence and number of the chemical units of nucleic acids, the nucleotides. In most organisms, the nucleic acid is **DNA** (**deoxyribonucleic acid**), although in **retroviruses**, the genetic material is composed of **ribonucleic acid** (**RNA**). Some genes in a cell are active more or less all the time, which means they are continuously transcribed and provide a constant supply of their protein product. These "housekeeping" genes are always needed for basic cellular reactions. Others may be rendered active or inactive depending on the needs and functions of the organism under particular conditions. The signal that masks or unmasks a gene can come from outside the cell, for example, from a steroid hormone or a nutrient, or it can come from within the cell itself because of the activity of other genes. In both cases, regulatory substances can bind to the specific DNA sequences of the target genes to control the synthesis of transcripts.

In a paper published in 1865, Gregor Mendel (1823–1884), advanced a theory of inheritance dependent on material elements that segregate independently from each other in sex cells. Before Mendel's findings, inherited traits were thought to be passed on through a blending of the mother and father's characteristics, much like a blending of two liquids. The term "gene" was coined later by the Danish botanist Wilhelm Johannsen (1857–1927), to replace the variety of terms used up until then to describe hereditary factors. His definition of the gene led him to distinguish between **genotype** (an organism's genetic makeup) and **phenotype** (an organism's appearance). Before the chemical and physical nature of genes were discovered they were defined on the basis of phenotypic expression and algebraic symbols were used to record their distribution and segregation. Because sexually reproducing, eukaryotic organisms possess two copies of an inherited factor (or gene), one acquired from each parent, the genotype of an individual for a particular trait is expressed by a pair of letters or symbols. Each of the alternative forms of a gene is also known as alleles. Dominant and recessive alleles are denoted by the use of higher and lower case letters. It can be predicted mathematically, for example, that a single allele pair will always segregate to give a genotype ratio 1AA:2Aa:1aa, and the phenotype ratio 2A:1aa (where A represents both AA and Aa since these cannot be distinguished phenotypically if dominance is complete).

The molecular structure and activity of genes can be modified by **mutations** and the smallest mutational unit is now known to be a single pair of nucleotides, also known as a muton. To indicate that a gene is functionally normal it is assigned a plus (+) sign, whereas a damaged or mutated gene is indicated by a minus (–) sign. A wild-type *Escherichia coli* able to synthesize its own arginine would thus, be symbolized as *arg+* and strains that have lost this ability by mutation of one of the genes for arginine utilization would be *arg–* Such strains, known as arginine auxotrophs, would not be able to grow without a supplement of arginine. At this level of definition, the plus or minus actually refer to an **operon** rather than

a single gene, and finer genetic analysis can be used to reveal the exact location of the mutated gene.

The use of mutations in studying genes is well illustrated in a traditional genetic test called the "*cis–trans* test" which also gave the gene the alternative name, cistron. This is a complementation test that can be used to determine whether two different mutations (m^1 and m^2) occur in the same functional unit, i.e., within the same gene or cistron. It demonstrates well how genes can be defined phenomenologically and has been performed successfully in **microorganisms** such as yeasts. It works on the principle that pairs of homologous **chromosomes** containing similar genes can **complement** their action. Two types of heterozygotes of the test organism are prepared. Heterozygotes are organisms having different alleles in the two homologous chromosomes each of which was inherited from one parent. One heterozygote contains the mutations under investigation within the same chromosome, that is in the *cis*— configuration, which is symbolically designated ++/m^{1}m^2 (m^1 and m^2 are the two mutations under investigation and the symbol "+" indicates the same position on the homologous chromosome in the unmutated, wild type state). The second mutant is constructed to contain the mutations in such a way that one appears on each of the homologous chromosomes. This is called the *trans*— configuration and is designated, for example, by ^{2}+/+m^1. If two recessive mutations are present in the same cistron, the heterozygous *trans*— configuration displays the mutant phenotype, whereas the *cis*— configuration displays the normal, wild type, phenotype. This is because in the *cis*— configuration, there is one completely functional, unmutated, cistron (++) within the system which masks the two mutations on the other chromosome and allows for the expression of the wild type phenotype. If one or both mutations are dominant, and the *cis*– and *trans*– heterozygotes are phenotypically different, then both mutations must be present in the same cistron. Conversely, if the *cis*– and *trans*– heterozygotes are phenotypically identical, this is taken as evidence that the mutations are present in different cistrons.

In 1910, the American geneticist Thomas Hunt Morgan (1866–1945) began to uncover the relationship between genes and chromosomes. He discovered that genes were located on chromosomes and that they were arranged linearly and associated in linkage groups, all the genes on one chromosome being linked. For example the genes on the X and Y chromosomes are said to be sex-linked because the X and Y chromosomes determine the sex of the organisms, in humans X determining femaleness and Y determining maleness. Nonhomologous chromosomes possess different linkage groups, whereas homologous chromosomes have identical linkage groups in identical sequences. The distance between two genes of the same linkage group is the sum of the distances between all the intervening genes and a schematic representation of the linear arrangement of linked genes, with their relative distances of separation, is known as a genetic map. In the construction of such maps the frequency of **recombination** during crossing over is used as an index of the distance between two linked genes.

Advances in **molecular genetics** have allowed analysis of the structure and **biochemistry** of genes in detail. They are no longer the nebulous units described by Mendel purely in terms of their visible expression (phenotypic expression). It is now possible to understand their molecular structure and function in considerable detail. The biological role of genes is to carry, encode, or control information on the composition of proteins. The proteins, together with their timing of expression and amount of production are possibly the most important determinants of the structure and physiology of organisms. Each structural gene is responsible for one specific protein or part of a protein and codes for a single polypeptide chain via messenger RNA (mRNA). Some genes code specifically for transfer RNA (tRNA) or ribosomal RNA (rRNA) and some are merely sequences, which are recognized by regulatory proteins. The latter are termed regulator genes. In higher organisms, or **eukaryotes**, genes are organized in such a way that at one end, there is a region to which various regulatory proteins can bind, for example RNA polymerase during **transcription**, and at the opposite end, there are sequences encoding the termination of transcription. In between lies the protein encoding sequence. In the genes of many eukaryotes this sequence may be interrupted by intervening non-coding sequence segments called introns, which can range in number from one to many. Transcription of eukaryotic DNA produces pre–mRNA containing complementary sequences of both introns and the information carrying sections of the gene called exons. The pre–mRNA then undergoes post–transcriptional modification or processing in which the introns are excised and exons are spliced together, leaving the complete coding transcript of connected exons ready to code directly for the protein. When the central dogma of genetics was first established, a "one gene–one enzyme" hypothesis was proposed, but today it is more accurate to restate this as a one to one correspondence between a gene and the polypeptide for which it codes. This is because a number of proteins are now known to be constituted of multiple polypeptide subunits coded for by different genes.

See also Bacterial artificial chromosome (BAC); Chromosomes, eukaryotic; Chromosomes, prokaryotic; DNA (Deoxyribonucleic acid); Evolution and evolutionary mechanisms; Gene amplification; Genetic code; Genetic mapping; Genotype and phenotype; Immunogenetics; Microbial genetics; Molecular biology, central dogma of; Molecular biology and molecular genetics

GENE CHIPS · *see* DNA CHIPS AND MICROARRAYS

GENETIC CAUSES OF IMMUNODEFICIENCY

· *see* IMMUNODEFICIENCY DISEASE SYNDROMES

GENETIC CODE

The genetic code is the set of correspondences between the nucleotide sequences of nucleic acids such as **DNA (deoxyribonucleic acid)**, and the amino acid sequences of polypeptides. These correspondences enable the information encoded

in the chemical components of the DNA to be transferred to the **ribonucleic acid** messenger (mRNA), and then to be used to establish the correct sequence of amino acids in the polypeptide. The elements of the encoding system, the nucleotides, differ by only four different bases. These are known as adenine (A), guanine, (G), thymine (T) and cytosine (C), in DNA or uracil (U) in **RNA**. Thus, RNA contains U in the place of C and the nucleotide sequence of DNA acts as a template for the synthesis of a complementary sequence of RNA, a process known as **transcription**. For historical reasons, the term genetic code in fact refers specifically to the sequence of nucleotides in mRNA, although today it is sometimes used interchangeably with the coded information in DNA.

Proteins found in nature consist of 20 naturally occurring amino acids. One important question is, how can four nucleotides code for 20 amino acids? This question was raised by scientists in the 1950s soon after the discovery that the DNA comprised the hereditary material of living organisms. It was reasoned that if a single nucleotide coded for one amino acid, then only four amino acids could be provided for. Alternatively, if two nucleotides specified one amino acid, then there could be a maximum number of 16 (4^2) possible arrangements. If, however, three nucleotides coded for one amino acid, then there would be 64 (4^3) possible permutations, more than enough to account for all the 20 naturally occurring amino acids. The latter suggestion was proposed by the Russian born physicist, George Gamow (1904–1968) and was later proved correct. It is now well known that every amino acid is coded by at least one nucleotide triplet or codon, and that some triplet combinations function as instructions for the termination or initiation of **translation**. Three combinations in tRNA, UAA, UGA and UAG, are termination codons, while AUG is a translation start codon.

The genetic code was solved between 1961 and 1963. The American scientist Marshall Nirenberg (1927–), working with his colleague Heinrich Matthaei, made the first breakthrough when they discovered how to make synthetic mRNA. They found that if the nucleotides of RNA carrying the four bases A, G, C and U, were mixed in the presence of the enzyme polynucleotide phosphorylase, a single stranded RNA was formed in the reaction, with the nucleotides being incorporated at random. This offered the possibility of creating specific mRNA sequences and then seeing which amino acids they would specify. The first synthetic mRNA polymer obtained contained only uracil (U) and when mixed *in vitro* with the protein synthesizing machinery of *Escherichia coli* it produced a polyphenylalanine—a string of phenylalanine. From this it was concluded that the triplet UUU coded for phenylalanine. Similarly, a pure cytosine (C) RNA polymer produced only the amino acid proline so the corresponding codon for cytosine had to be CCC. This type of analysis was refined when nucleotides were mixed in different proportions in the synthetic mRNA and a statistical analysis was used to determine the amino acids produced. It was quickly found that a particular amino acid could be specified by more than one codon. Thus, the amino acid serine could be produced from any one of the combinations UCU, UCC, UCA, or UCG. In this way the genetic code is said to be degenerate, meaning that each of the 64 possible

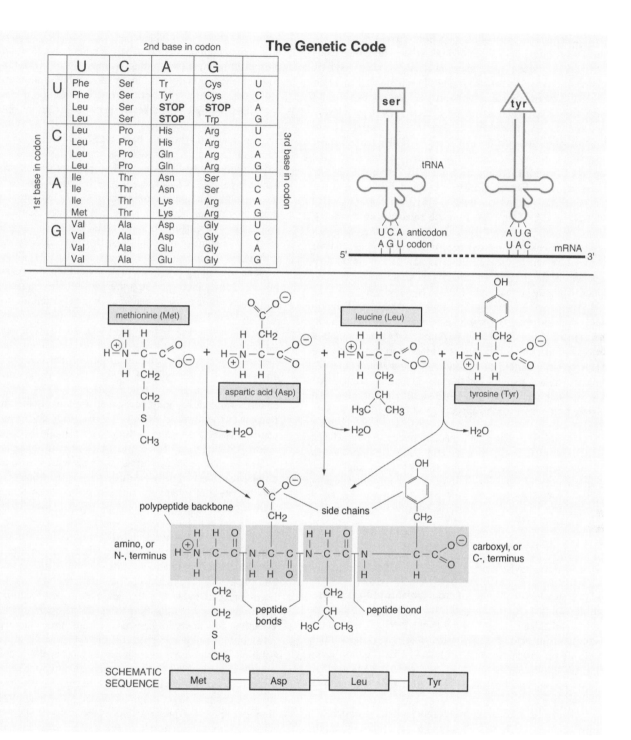

Genetic code related to models of amino acids inserting into a protein.

triplets have some meaning within the code and that several codons may encode a single amino acid.

This work confirmed the ideas of the British scientists **Francis Crick** (1916–) and **Sidney Brenner** (1927–). Brenner and Crick were working with **mutations** in the bacterial virus bactriophage T4 and found that the deletion of a single nucleotide could abolish the function of a specific **gene**. However, a second mutation in which a nucleotide was inserted at a different, but nearby position restored the function of that gene. These two mutations are said to be suppressors of each other, meaning that they cancel each other's mutant properties. It was concluded from this that the genetic code was read in a sequential manner starting from a fixed point in the gene. The insertion or deletion of a nucleotide shifted the reading frame in which succeeding nucleotides were read as codons, and was thus termed a frameshift mutation. It was also found that whereas two closely spaced deletions, or two closely spaced insertions, could not suppress each other, three closely spaced deletions or insertions could do so. Consequently, these observations established the triplet nature of the genetic code. The reading frame of a sequence is the way in which the sequence is divided into the triplets and is determined by the precise point at which translation is initiated. For example, the sequence CATCATCAT can be read CAT CAT CAT or C ATC ATC AT or CA TCA TCA T in the three possible reading frames. Sometimes, as in particular bacterial **viruses**, genes have been found that are contained within other genes. These are translated in different reading frames so the amino acid sequences of the proteins encoded by them are different. Such economy of genetic material is, however, quite rare

The same genetic code appears to operate in all living things, but exceptions to this universality are known. In human mitochondrial mRNA, AGA and AGG are termination or stop codons. Other differences also exist in the correspondences between certain codon sequences and amino acids. In ciliates, there are also unusual features in that UAA and UAG code for glutamine (CAA and CAG in other **eukaryotes**) and the only termination codon appears to be UGA.

See also Bacteriophage and bacteriophage typing; Gene amplification; Genetic identification of microorganisms; Genetic mapping; Genetic regulation of eukaryotic cells; Genetic regulation of prokaryotic cells; Genotype and phenotype; Immunogenetics

GENETIC IDENTIFICATION OF MICROORGANISMS

The genetic identification of **microorganisms** utilizes molecular technologies to evaluate specific regions of the genome and uniquely determine to which genus, species, or strain a microorganism belongs. This work grew out of the similar, highly successful applications in human identification using the same basic techniques. Thus, the genetic identification of microorganisms has also been referred to a microbial fingerprinting.

Genetic identification of microorganisms is basically a comparison study. To identify an unknown organism, appropriate sequences from the unknown are compared to documented sequences from known organisms. Homology between the sequences results in a positive test. An exact match will occur when the two organisms are the same. Related individuals have genetic material that is identical for some regions and dissimilar for others. Unrelated individuals will have significant differences in the sequences being evaluated. Developing a database of key sequences that are unique to and characteristic of a series of known organisms facilitates this type of analysis. The sequences utilized fall into two dif-

ferent categories, 1) fragments derived from the transcriptionally active, coding regions of the genome, and, 2) fragments present in inactive, noncoding regions. Of the two, the noncoding genomic material is more susceptible to mutation and will therefore show a higher degree of variability.

Depending on the level of specificity required, an assay can provide information on the genus, species, and/or strain of a microorganism. The most basic type of identification is classification to a genus. Although this general identification does not discriminate between the related species that comprise the genus, it can be useful in a variety of situations. For example, if a person is thought to have **tuberculosis**, a test to determine if *Mycobacterium* cells (the genus that includes the tuberculosis causing organism) are present in a sputum sample will most likely confirm the diagnosis. However, if there are several species within a genus that cause similar diseases but that respond to entirely different drugs, it would then be critical to know exactly which species is present for proper treatment. A more specific test using genomic sequences unique to each species would be needed for this type of discrimination. In some instances, it is important to take the analysis one step further to detect genetically distinct subspecies or strains. Variant strains usually arise as a result of physical separation and **evolution** of the genome. If one homogeneous sample of cells is split and sent to two different locations, over time, changes (**mutations**) may occur that will distinguish the two populations as unique entities. The importance of this issue can be appreciated when considering tuberculosis. Since the late 1980s, there has been a resurgence of this disease accompanied by the appearance of several new strains with antimicrobial resistance. The use of genetic identification for rapid determination of which strain is present has been essential to protect health care workers and provide appropriate therapy for affected individuals.

The tools used for genetic studies include standard molecular technologies. Total sequencing of an organism's genome is one approach, but this method is time consuming and expensive. Southern blot analysis can be used, but has been replaced by newer technologies in most laboratories. Solution-phase hybridization using **DNA** probes has proven effective for many organisms. In this procedure, probes labeled with a reporter molecule are combined with cells in solution and upon hybridization with target cells, a chemiluminescent signal that can be quantitated by a luminometer is emitted. A variation of this scheme is to capture the target cells by hybridization to a probe followed by a second hybridization that results in precipitation of the cells for quantitation. These assays are rapid, relatively inexpensive and highly sensitive. However, they require the presence of a relatively large number of organisms to be effective. Amplification technologies such as **PCR (polymerase chain reaction)** and LCR (ligase change reaction) allow detection of very low concentrations of organisms from cultures or patient specimens such as blood or body tissues. Primers are designed to selectively amplify genomic sequences unique to each species, and, by screening unknowns for the presence or absence these regions, the unknown is identified. Multiplex PCR has made it possible to discriminate between a number of different species in a

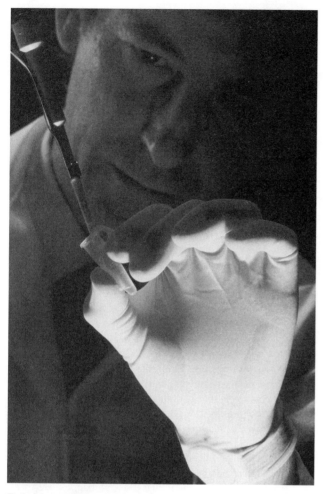

Technician making a genetic marker.

single amplification reaction. For **viruses** with a **RNA** genome, RT-PCR (reverse transcriptase PCR) is widely utilized for identification and quantitation.

The **anthrax** outbreak in the Unites States in the fall of 2001 illustrated the significance of these technologies. Because an anthrax infection can mimic **cold** or flu symptoms, the earliest victims did not realize they were harboring a deadly bacterium. After confirmation that anthrax was the causative agent in the first death, genetic technologies were utilized to confirm the presence of anthrax in other locations and for other potential victims. Results were available more rapidly than would have been possible using standard microbiological methodology and appropriate treatment regimens could be established immediately. Furthermore, unaffected individuals are quickly informed of their status, alleviating unnecessary anxiety.

The second stage of the investigation was to locate the origin of the anthrax cells. The evidence indicated that this event was not a random, natural phenomenon, and that an individual or individuals had most likely dispersed the cells as an act of **bioterrorism**. In response to this threat, government agencies collected samples from all sites for analysis. A key element in the search was the genetic identification of the cells found in patients and mail from Florida, New York, and Washington, D.C. The PCR studies clearly showed that all samples were derived from the same strain of anthrax, known as the "Ames strain" since the cell line was established in Iowa. Although this strain has been distributed to many different research laboratories around the world, careful analysis revealed minor changes in the genome that allowed investigators to narrow the search to about fifteen United States laboratories. Total genome sequencing of these fifteen strains and a one-to-one base comparison with the lethal anthrax genome may detect further variation that will allow a unique identification to be made.

The advent of molecular technologies and the application of genetic identification in clinical and forensic microbiology have greatly improved the capability of laboratories to detect and specifically identify an organism quickly and accurately.

See also Anthrax, terrorist use of as a biological weapon; Culture; Microbial genetics

GENETIC MAPPING

The aim of genetic mapping is to determine the linear sequence of genes in genetic material. The mapping can be performed at several levels of detail (resolution) that fall into two broad types: traditional genetic or linkage mapping and, more detailed, physical mapping.

Linkage mapping shows the relative rather than absolute positions of genes along a chromosome and is a technique that has been used since the early 1900s. Early geneticists determined that genes were found on **chromosomes**. They also reasoned that because the various forms of genes, or alleles, could be precisely exchanged during meiosis through crossovers between homologous chromosomes, the genes for specific characteristics must lie at precise points along each chromosome. It followed that the mapping of chromosomes could, therefore, be made from the observation of crossovers. Between 1912 and 1915, the American scientist Thomas Hunt Morgan (1866–1945) hypothesized that if genes were arranged linearly along chromosomes, then those genes lying closer together would be separated by crossovers less often than those lying further apart. Genes lying closer together would thus have a greater probability of being passed along as a unit. It follows that the percentage of crossovers would be proportional to the distance between two genes on a chromosome. The percentage crossover can be expressed as the number of crossovers between two genes in meiosis. One genetic map unit (m.u.) is defined as the distance between **gene** pairs for which one product out of 100 is recombinant (a product of crossover). The recombinant frequency (R.F.) of 0.01 (1%) is defined as 1 m.u. and a map unit is sometimes referred to as a centimorgan (cM) in honor of Thomas Hunt Morgan.

As an example of how linkage mapping might work, suppose two characteristics, A and B, show 26% crossover. Assign 26 crossover units to the distance between these two

•

genes. If a characteristic C turns out in breeding experiments to have 9% crossover with B and 17% crossover with A, it would then be located between A and B at a point 9 units from B and 17 units from A. Compiling the information from many such breeding experiments creates a chromosome map that indicates the relative positions of the genes that code for certain characteristics. Accordingly, the further apart any two genes are on the same chromosome, the greater the incidence of crossing over between them.

A linkage map is limited because **recombination** frequencies can be distorted relative to the physical distance between sites. As a result, the linkage map is not always the best possible representation of genetic material.

While linkage maps only indicate relative positions of genes, physical maps are more accurate and aim to show the actual number of nucleotides between each gene. Restriction maps are constructed by cleaving **DNA** into fragments with **restriction enzymes**. These **enzymes** recognize specific short DNA sequences and cut the duplex. The distances between the sites of cleavage are then measured. The positions of the target restriction sites for these enzymes along the chromosome can be used as DNA markers. Restriction sites generally exist in the same positions on homologous chromosomes so the positions of these target sites can be used rather like milestones along a road and can act as reference points for locating significant features in the chromosome.

A map of the positions of restriction sites can be made for a localized region of a chromosome. It is made by comparing the sizes of single enzyme breakages (digests) of the region of interest with double digests of the same region. This means that two different restriction enzymes are applied, one to each of two separate chromosome extracts of the region of interest, and subsequently the two enzymes are used together in a third digestion with the chromosome extract. The chromosome fragments resulting from the three digestions are then subjected to a biochemical procedure known as gel **electrophoresis**, which separates them and gives an estimation of their size. Comparison of the sizes of the chromosome fragments resulting from single and double restriction enzyme digestions allows for an approximate location of the target restriction sites. Thus, such maps represent linear sequences of restriction sites. As this procedure determines the sizes of digested chromosome fragments, the distances between sites in terms of the length of DNA can be calculated, because the size of a fragment estimated from an electrophoresis experiment is proportional to the number of base pairs in that fragment.

A restriction map does not intrinsically identify sites if genetic interest. For it to be of practical use, **mutations** have to be characterized in terms of their effects upon the restriction sites. In the 1980s, it was shown how restriction fragment length polymorphisms (RFLPs) could be used to map human disease genes. RFLPs are inherited by Mendelian segregation and are distributed in populations as classical examples of common genetic polymorphisms. If such a DNA variant is located close to a defective gene (which can not be tested directly), the DNA variant can be used as a marker to detect the presence of the disease-causing gene. The prenatal exami-

nation of DNA for particular enzyme sites associated with certain hereditary diseases has proved to be an important method of diagnosis. Clinically useful polymorphic restriction enzyme sites have been detected within the Beta-like globin gene cluster. For example, the absence of a recognition site for the restriction enzyme HpaI is frequently associated with the allele for sickle-cell anemia, and this association has been useful in prenatal diagnosis of this disease.

The ultimate genetic map is the complete nucleotide sequence of the DNA in the whole chromosome **complement**, or genome, of an organism. Today, several completed genome maps already exist. Simple prokaryotic organisms, e.g., **bacteria**, with their relatively small (one to two million base pairs) chromosomes of one to two million base pairs were the first to be mapped. Later, eukaryotic organisms such as the **yeast**, *Saccharomyces cerevisiae*, and the nematode worm, *Caenorhabditis elegans*, were mapped. In 2000, the Human Genome Project produced the first draft of the human genome. The project adopted two methods for mapping the 3 billion nucleotides. The earlier approach was a "clone by clone" method. In this, the entire genome was cut into fragments up to several thousand base pairs long, and inserted into synthetic chromosomes known as **bacterial artificial chromosomes (BACs)**. The subsequent mapping step involved positioning the BACs on the genome's chromosomes by looking for distinctive marker sequences called sequence tagged sites (STSs), whose location had already been pinpointed. Clones of the BACs are then broken into smaller fragments in a process known as **shotgun cloning**. Each small fragment was then sequenced and computer algorithms, that recognize matching sequence information from overlapping fragments, were used to reconstruct the complete sequence inserted into each BAC. It was later argued that the first mapping step was unnecessary and that the algorithms used to reassemble the shotgunned DNA fragments could be applied to cloned random fragments taken directly from the whole genome. In this whole genome shotgun strategy, fragments were first assembled by algorithms into larger scaffolds and the correct position of these scaffolds on the genome was worked out by STSs. The latter method speeded up the whole procedure considerably and is currently being used to sequence genomes from other organisms.

See also Cloning, application of cloning to biological problems; Fungal genetics; Gene amplification; Gene; Genetic code; Genetic identification of microorganisms; Genetic regulation of eukaryotic cells; Genetic regulation of prokaryotic cells; Genotype and phenotype; Microbial genetics

GENETIC REGULATION OF EUKARYOTIC CELLS

Although prokaryotes (i.e., non-nucleated unicellular organisms) divide through binary fission, **eukaryotes** undergo a more complex process of cell division because **DNA** is packed in several **chromosomes** located inside a cell **nucleus**. In eukaryotes, cell division may take two different paths, in accordance with the cell type involved. Mitosis is a cellular division resulting in two identical nuclei is performed by somatic cells. The process of meiosis results in four nuclei, each containing half of the original number of chromosomes. Sex cells or gametes (ovum and spermatozoids) divide by meiosis. Both prokaryotes and eukaryotes undergo a final process, known as cytoplasmatic division, which divides the parental cell into new daughter cells.

The series of stages that a cell undergoes while progressing to division is known as **cell cycle**. Cells undergoing division are also termed competent cells. When a cell is not progressing to mitosis, it remains in phase G0 (G zero). Therefore, the cell cycle is divided into two major phases: interphase and mitosis. Interphase includes the phases (or stages) G1, S and G2, whereas mitosis is subdivided into prophase, metaphase, anaphase and telophase.

The cell cycle starts in G1, with the active synthesis of **RNA** and proteins, which are necessary for young cells to grow and mature. The time G1 lasts, varies greatly among eukaryotic cells of different species and from one tissue to another in the same organism. Tissues that require fast cellular renovation, such as mucosa and endometrial epithelia, have shorter G1 periods than those tissues that do not require frequent renovation or repair, such as muscles or connective tissues.

The cell cycle is highly regulated by several **enzymes**, proteins, and **cytokines** in each of its phases, in order to ensure that the resulting daughter cells receive the appropriate amount of genetic information originally present in the parental cell. In the case of somatic cells, each of the two daughter cells must contain an exact copy of the original genome present in the parental cell. Cell cycle controls also regulate when and to what extent the cells of a given tissue must proliferate, in order to avoid abnormal cell proliferation that could lead to dysplasia or tumor development. Therefore, when one or more of such controls are lost or inhibited, abnormal overgrowth will occur and may lead to impairment of function and disease.

Cells are mainly induced into proliferation by growth factors or hormones that occupy specific receptors on the surface of the cell membrane, and are also known as extra-cellular ligands. Examples of growth factors are as such: epidermal growth factor (EGF), fibroblastic growth factor (FGF), platelet-derived growth factor (PDGF), insulin-like growth factor (IGF), or hormones. PDGF and FGF act by regulating the phase G2 of the cell cycle and during mitosis. After mitosis, they act again stimulating the daughter cells to grow, thus leading them from G0 to G1. Therefore, FGF and PDGF are also termed competence factors, whereas EGF and IGF are termed progression factors, because they keep the process of cellular progression to mitosis going on. Growth factors are also classified (along with other molecules that promote the cell cycle) as pro-mitotic signals. Hormones are also pro-mitotic signals. For example, thyrotrophic hormone, one of the hormones produced by the pituitary gland, induces the proliferation of thyroid gland's cells. Another pituitary hormone, known as growth hormone or somatotrophic hormone (STH), is responsible by body growth during childhood and early ado-

lescence, inducing the lengthening of the long bones and **protein synthesis**. Estrogens are hormones that do not occupy a membrane receptor, but instead, penetrate the cell and the nucleus, binding directly to specific sites in the DNA, thus inducing the cell cycle.

Anti-mitotic signals may have several different origins, such as cell-to-cell adhesion, factors of adhesion to the extra-cellular matrix, or soluble factor such as TGF beta (tumor growth factor beta), which inhibits abnormal cell proliferation, proteins p53, p16, p21, APC, pRb, etc. These molecules are the products of a class of genes called tumor suppressor genes. **Oncogenes**, until recently also known as proto-oncogenes, synthesize proteins that enhance the stimuli started by growth factors, amplifying the mitotic signal to the nucleus, and/or promoting the accomplishment of a necessary step of the cell cycle. When each phase of the cell cycle is completed, the proteins involved in that phase are degraded, so that once the next phase starts, the cell is unable to go back to the previous one. Next to the end of phase G1, the cycle is paused by tumor suppressor **gene** products, to allow verification and repair of DNA damage. When DNA damage is not repairable, these genes stimulate other intra-cellular pathways that induce the cell into suicide or apoptosis (also known as programmed cell death). To the end of phase G2, before the transition to mitosis, the cycle is paused again for a new verification and decision, either mitosis or apoptosis.

Along each pro-mitotic and anti-mitotic intra-cellular signaling pathway, as well as along the apoptotic pathways, several gene products (**proteins and enzymes**) are involved in an orderly sequence of activation and inactivation, forming complex webs of signal transmission and signal amplification to the nucleus. The general goal of such cascades of signals is to achieve the orderly progression of each phase of the cell cycle.

Interphase is a phase of cell growth and metabolic activity, without cell nuclear division, comprised of several stages or phases. During Gap 1 or G1, the cell resumes protein and RNA synthesis, which was interrupted during mitosis, thus allowing the growth and maturation of young cells to accomplish their physiologic function. Immediately following is a variable length pause for DNA checking and repair before cell cycle transition to phase S during which there is synthesis or semi-conservative replication or synthesis of DNA. During Gap 2 or G2, there is increased RNA and protein synthesis, followed by a second pause for proofreading and eventual repairs in the newly synthesized DNA sequences before transition to mitosis.

At the start of mitosis, the chromosomes are already duplicated, with the sister-chromatids (identical chromosomes) clearly visible under a light **microscope**. Mitosis is subdivided into prophase, metaphase, anaphase, and telophase.

During prophase there is a high condensation of chromatids, with the beginning of nucleolus disorganization and nuclear membrane disintegration, followed by the start of centrioles' migration to opposite cell poles. During metaphase the chromosomes organize at the equator of a spindle apparatus (microtubules), forming a structure termed metaphase plate.

The sister-chromatids are separated and joined to different centromeres, while the microtubules forming the spindle are attached to a region of the centromere termed kinetochore. During anaphase there are spindles, running from each opposite kinetochore, that pull each set of chromosomes to their respective cell poles, thus ensuring that in the following phase each new cell will ultimately receive an equal division of chromosomes. During telophase, kinetochores and spindles disintegrate, the reorganization of nucleus begins, chromatin becomes less condensed, and the nucleus membrane start forming again around each set of chromosomes. The cytoskeleton is reorganized and the somatic cell has now doubled its volume and presents two organized nucleus.

Cytokinesis usually begins during telophase, and is the process of cytoplasmatic division. This process of division varies among species but in somatic cells, it occurs through the equal division of the cytoplasmatic content, with the plasma membrane forming inwardly a deep cleft that ultimately divides the parental cell in two new daughter cells.

The identification and detailed understanding of the many molecules involved in the cell cycle controls and intracellular signal **transduction** is presently under investigation by several research groups around the world. This knowledge is crucial to the development of new anti-cancer drugs as well as to new treatments for other genetic diseases, in which a gene over expression or deregulation may be causing either a chronic or an acute disease, or the impairment of a vital organ function. Scientists predict that the next two decades will be dedicated to the identification of gene products and their respective function in the cellular microenvironment. This new field of research is termed **proteomics**.

See also Cell cycle (eukaryotic), genetic regulation of; Genetic code; Genetic identification of microorganisms; Genetic mapping

GENETIC REGULATION OF PROKARYOTIC CELLS

The ability of a bacterium to regulate the expression of the myriad of genes contained in the chromosome and **plasmids** is essential to the growth and survival of the microorganism. While a bacterium has many genes that code for a variety of proteins, these genes are not all expressed at the same time. Some genes are active all the time, while others are active only at specific times in the growth cycle of the bacterium or in response to a certain environmental condition. The amounts of proteins that are produced are not all the same. Moreover, the triggers that stimulate the expression of one **gene** can be quite different from the triggers for another gene. The ability of a prokaryotic cells (bacterial are the prototypical system) to orchestrate the expression of the repertoire of genes constitutes genetic regulation.

The activity of genes in the manufacture of compounds by the bacterium, such as in the biosynthetic pathways of the microbe, is often under a type of control known as feedback inhibition. In this type of genetic regulation, the object of the regulation is the first enzyme that is unique to the pathway (not to the gene that coeds for the enzyme). In biosynthetic pathways, there are typically a number of compounds that can be formed in the various enzymatic reactions within the pathway. Feedback inhibition occurs when the final product inhibits the first biosynthetic enzyme. Blocking the first enzymatic step prevent the remainder of the **enzymes** from having any material on which to act.

Feedback inhibition is possible because the biosynthetic enzymes have two binding regions. If both sites are occupied by the end product, the three-dimensional structure of the enzyme is changed such that it cannot bind any more of the protein it is supposed to enzymatically alter. But, when the amount of the end product decreases, one of the enzyme's binding sites is no longer occupied, and the enzyme can resume its function. The function of the enzyme can also be affected by modifying the structure of side groups that protrude from the enzyme molecule. This alteration is also reversible, when the concentration of the blocking end product is lowered.

Feedback inhibition is a genetic regulatory mechanism that allows a bacterium to rapidly respond to changes in concentration of a particular compound. The bacterium does not have to manufacture protein, as the molecules already exist and are primed to resume activity once conditions are favorable.

Regulation also operates directly at the level of the genes. This type of genetic regulation is called induction (when the gene is stimulated into action) or repression (when the gene's activity is reversible silenced). Regulating the activity of genes, rather than the activity of the proteins made by the genes can save a bacterium the energy of manufacturing the protein.

Induction and repression depend on the binding of a molecule known as **RNA** polymerase to regions that signal the beginning of a stretch of **DNA** that code for proteins. The three-dimensional shape of the polymerase-binding region influences the binding of the RNA polymerase. The binding of molecules called effectors can in turn influence the shape of this region. If an effector alters the shape of the polymerase-binding region so that the polymerase is able to bind, the effect is called induction. If the effector binding prevents the polymerase from binding, then the effect is known as repression.

Induction and repression tend to cycle back and forth, in response to the level of effector, and so in response to whatever environmental or other condition the particular effector is sensitive to. A visual analogy would the turning on and off of room light under the control of a very sensitive light meter, as clouds obscured the sunlight from one moment to the next.

Another genetic regulatory mechanism that operates only in procaryotes is termed attenuation. Attenuation requires a close coupling between the synthesis of **ribonucleic acid** from a DNA template (**transcription**) and the use of the RNA as another template to manufacture protein (**translation**). These processes are very closely coupled in procaryotes, particularly in the activity of enzymes that participate in the making of amino acids.

In the process of attenuation, a gene that codes for an enzyme required for the synthesis of an amino acid is not active until the level of that amino acid lowers to some threshold level. At this level, the molecules called **ribosomes** physically stall as they move down the beginning of the RNA template that encodes protein. The stalling prevents the formation of a signal that otherwise stops the onward movement of the ribosomes. After the pause, because the stop signal has not formed, the ribosomes resume their movement and the protein is produced. When the level of the critical amino acid is higher, the ribosomes do not stall, encounter a stop signal, and the synthesis of the protein does not occur.

These processes operate simultaneously for many genes in a bacterium. For some of these genes, the controlling factors are independent of one another. But for other proteins, a common factor, such as a sensory protein that can sense changes in the environment and provide a signal to the various regulatory processes, also operates. This genetic regulation pattern is referred to as global regulation. An example of global regulation is a phenomenon called diauxic growth, which is exemplified by the lactose **operon** (also called the lac operon). Diauxic growth allows a bacterium to preferentially utilize one nutrient (such as glucose) when two nutrients (such as glucose and lactose) are present. When the preferred source is exhausted, **metabolism** can switch so as to utilize the second source (lactose). This nutrient preference involves genetic regulation of protein production.

Other genetic regulatory mechanisms operate in response to fluctuations in temperature, **pH**, oxygen level, the attraction or repulsion of a bacterium from a compound (chemotaxis), and the production of a spore.

See also Cell cycle (prokaryotic), genetic regulation of; Microbial genetics

GENETICALLY ENGINEERED VACCINES •

see VACCINE

GENOTYPE AND PHENOTYPE

The term genotype describes the actual set (**complement**) of genes carried by an organism. In contrast, **phenotype** refers to the observable expression of characters and traits coded for by those genes. Although phenotypes are based upon the content of the underlying genes comprising the genotype, the expression of those genes in observable traits (phenotypic expression) is also, to varying degrees, influenced by environmental factors.

The term genotype was first used by Danish geneticist Wilhelm Johannsen (1857–1927) to describe the entire genetic or hereditary constitution of an organism, In contrast, Johannsen described displayed characters or traits (e.g., anatomical traits, biochemical traits, physiological traits, etc.) as an organism's phenotype.

Genotype and phenotype represent very real differences between genetic composition and expressed form. The geno-type is a group of genetic markers that describes the particular forms or variations of genes (alleles) carried by an individual. Accordingly, an individual's genotype includes all the alleles carried by that individual. An individual's genotype, because it includes all of the various alleles carried, determines the range of traits possible (e.g., a individual's potential to be afflicted with a particular disease). In contrast to the possibilities contained within the genotype, the phenotype reflects the manifest expression of those possibilities (potentialities). Phenotypic traits include obvious observable traits as height, weight, eye color, hair color, etc. The presence or absence of a disease, or symptoms related to a particular disease state, is also a phenotypic trait.

A clear example of the relationship between genotype and phenotype exists in cases where there are dominant and recessive alleles for a particular trait. Using an simplified monogenetic (one **gene**, one trait) example, a capital "T" might be used to represent a dominant allele at a particular locus coding for tallness in a particular plant, and the lowercase "t" used to represent the recessive allele coding for shorter plants. Using this notation, a diploid plant will possess one of three genotypes: TT, Tt, or tt (the variation tT is identical to Tt). Although there are three different genotypes, because of the laws governing dominance, the plants will be either tall or short (two phenotypes). Those plants with a TT or Tt genotype are observed to be tall (phenotypically tall). Only those plants that carry the tt genotype will be observed to be short (phenotypically short).

In humans, there is genotypic sex determination. The genotypic variation in sex **chromosomes**, XX or XY decisively determines whether an individual is female (XX) or male (XY) and this genotypic differentiation results in considerable phenotypic differentiation.

Although the relationships between genetic and environmental influences vary (i.e., the degree to which genes specify phenotype differs from trait to trait), in general, the more complex the biological process or trait, the greater the influence of environmental factors. The genotype almost completely directs certain biological processes. Genotype, for example, strongly determines when a particular tooth develops. How long an individual retains a particular tooth, is to a much greater extent, determined by environmental factors such diet, dental **hygiene**, etc.

Because it is easier to determine observable phenotypic traits that it is to make an accurate determination of the relevant genotype associated with those traits, scientists and physicians place increasing emphasis on relating (correlating) phenotype with certain genetic markers or genotypes.

There are, of course, variable ranges in the nature of the genotype-environment association. In many cases, genotype-environment interactions do not result in easily predictable phenotypes. In rare cases, the situation can be complicated by a process termed phenocopy where environmental factors produce a particular phenotype that resembles a set of traits coded for by a known genotype not actually carried by the individual. Genotypic frequencies reflect the percentage of various genotypes found within a given group (population) and phenotypic frequencies reflect the percentage of observed expression. Mathematical measures of phenotypic variance reflect the variability of expression of a trait within a population.

The exact relationship between genotype and disease is an area of intense interest to geneticists and physicians and many scientific and clinical studies focus on the relationship between the effects of a genetic changes (e.g., changes caused by **mutations**) and disease processes. These attempts at genotype/phenotype correlations often require extensive and refined use of statistical analysis.

See also Genetic code; Genetic identification of microorganisms; Genetic mapping; Genetic regulation of eukaryotic cells; Genetic regulation of prokaryotic cells; Immunogenetics; Microbial genetics

GENTAMICIN · *see* ANTIBIOTICS

GERM THEORY OF DISEASE

The germ theory is a fundamental tenet of medicine that states that **microorganisms**, which are too small to be seen without the aid of a **microscope**, can invade the body and cause certain diseases.

Until the acceptance of the germ theory, diseases were often perceived as punishment for a person's evil behavior. When entire populations fell ill, the disease was often blamed on swamp vapors or foul odors from sewage. Even many educated individuals, such as the prominent seventeenth century English physician William Harvey, assumed that **epidemics** were caused by miasmas, poisonous vapors created by planetary movements affecting the Earth, or by disturbances within the Earth itself.

The development of the germ theory was made possible by certain laboratory tools and techniques that permitted the study of **bacteria** during the seventeenth and eighteenth centuries. The invention of primitive microscopes by the English scientist **Robert Hooke** and the Dutch merchant and amateur scientist **Anton van Leeuwenhoek** in the seventeenth century, gave scientists the means to observe microorganisms. During this period, a debate raged among biologists regarding the concept of spontaneous generation.

Until the second part of the nineteenth century, many scientists held that some lower life forms could arise spontaneously from nonliving matter, for example, flies from manure and maggots from decaying corpses. In 1668, however, the Italian physician Francisco Redi demonstrated that decaying meat in a container covered with a fine net did not produce maggots. Redi asserted this was proof that merely keeping egg-laying flies from the meat by covering it with a net while permitting the passage of air into the containers was enough to prevent the appearance of maggots. However, the belief in spontaneous generation remained widespread even in the scientific community.

In the 1700s, more evidence that microorganisms can cause certain diseases was passed over by physicians, who did not make the connection between **vaccination** and microorganisms. During the early part of the eighteenth century, Lady Montague **(Mary Wortley Montague)**, wife of the British ambassador to that country, noticed that the women of Constantinople routinely practiced a form of **smallpox** prevention that included "treating" healthy people with pus from individuals suffering from smallpox. Lady Montague noticed that the Turkish women removed pus from the lesions of smallpox victims and inserted a small amount of it into an area of broken skin of the recipients.

While the practice generally caused a mild form of the illness, many of these same people remained healthy while others succumbed to smallpox epidemics. The reasons for the success of this preventive treatment, called variolation, were not understood at the time, and depended on the coincidental use of a less virulent smallpox virus and the fact that the virus was introduced through the skin, rather than through its usually route of entry, the respiratory tract.

Lady Montague introduced the practice of variolation to England, where physician **Edward Jenner** later modified and improved the technique. Jenner noticed that milkmaids who contracted **cowpox** on their hands from touching the lesions on the udders of cows with the disease rarely got smallpox. He showed that inoculating people with cowpox prevented smallpox. The success of this technique, which demonstrated that the identical substances need not be used to stimulate the body's protective mechanisms, still did not convince many scientists of the existence of disease-causing microorganisms.

Thus, the debate continued well into the 1800s. In 1848, **Ignaz P. Semmelweis**, a Hungarian physician working in German hospitals, discovered that a sometimes-fatal infection commonly found in maternity hospitals in Europe could be prevented by simple **hygiene**. Semmelweis demonstrated that medical students doing autopsies on the bodies of women who died from puerperal fever often spread that disease to maternity patients they subsequently examined. He ordered these students to wash their hands in chlorinated lime water before examining pregnant women. Although the rate of puerperal fever in his hospital plummeted dramatically, many other physicians continued to criticize this practice as time-consuming and useless.

In 1854, modern **epidemiology** was born when the English physician John Snow determined that the source of cholera epidemic in London was the contaminated water of the Broad Street pump. After he ordered the pump closed, the epidemic ebbed. Nevertheless, many physicians refused to accept that invisible organisms could spread disease. The argument took an important turn in 1857, however, when the French chemist **Louis Pasteur** discovered "diseases" of wine and beer. French brewers asked Pasteur to determine why wine and beer sometimes spoiled. Pasteur showed that, while yeasts produce alcohol from the sugar in the brew, bacteria could change the alcohol to vinegar. His suggestion that brewers heat their product enough to kill bacteria but not **yeast**, was a boon to the brewing industry, a process called **pasteurization**. In addition, the connection Pasteur made between food spoilage and microorganisms was a key step in demonstrating the link between microorganisms and disease. Pasteur observed that, "There are similarities between the diseases of animals or man and the diseases of beer and wine." The notion of spontaneous generation received another blow in 1858, when the German scientist Rudolf Virchow introduced the concept of biogenesis. This concept holds that living cells can arise only from preexisting living cells. This was followed in 1861 by Pasteur's demonstration that microorganisms present in the air can contaminate solutions that seemed sterile. For example, boiled nutrient media left uncovered will become contaminated with microorganisms, thus disproving the notion that air itself can create microbes.

In his classic experiments, Pasteur first filled short-necked flasks with beef broth and boiled them. He left some opened to the air to cool and sealed others. The sealed flasks remained free of microorganisms, while the open flasks were contaminated within a few days. Pasteur next placed broth in flasks that had open-ended, long necks. After bending the necks of the flasks into S-shaped curves that bent downward, then swept sharply upward, he boiled the contents. Even months after cooling, the uncapped flasks remained uncontaminated. Pasteur explained that the S-shaped curve allowed air to pass into the flask; however, the curved neck trapped airborne microorganisms before they could contaminate the broth.

Pasteur's work followed earlier demonstrations by both himself and Agostino Bassi, an amateur microscopist, showing that silkworm diseases can be caused by microorganisms. While these observations in the 1830s linked the activity of microorganisms to disease, it was not until 1876 that German physician **Robert Koch** proved that bacteria could cause diseases. Koch showed that the bacterium *Bacillus anthracis* was the cause of **anthrax** in cattle and sheep, and he discovered the organism that causes **tuberculosis**.

Koch's systematic methodology in proving the cause of anthrax was generalized into a specific set of guidelines for determining the cause of infectious diseases, now known as **Koch's postulates**. Thus, the following steps are generally used to obtain proof that a particular organism causes a particular disease:

1. The organism must be present in every case of the disease.
2. The organism must be isolated from a host with the corresponding disease and grown in pure **culture**.
3. Samples of the organism removed from the pure culture must cause the corresponding disease when inoculated into a healthy, susceptible laboratory animal.
4. The organism must be isolated from the inoculated animal and identified as being identical to the original organisms isolated from the initial, diseased host.

By showing how specific organisms can be identified as the cause of specific diseases, Koch helped to destroy the notion of spontaneous generation, and laid the foundation for modern medical microbiology. Koch's postulates introduced what has been called the "Golden Era" of medical bacteriology. Between 1879 and 1889, German microbiologists isolated the organisms that cause cholera, **typhoid fever**, **diphtheria**, **pneumonia**, **tetanus**, **meningitis**, **gonorrhea**, as well the *Staphylococcus* and *Streptococcus* organisms.

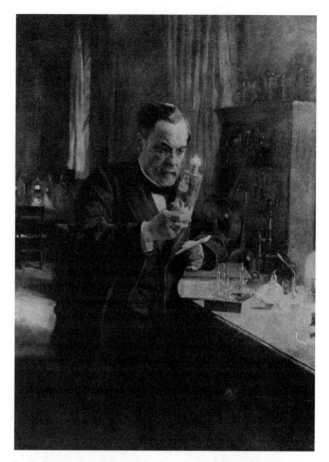

Louis Pasteur, one of the "fathers" of microbiology. Among his accomplishments was the demonstration of the involvement of microorganisms in disease.

Even as Koch's work was influencing the development of germ theory, the influence of the English physician **Joseph Lister** was being felt in operating rooms. Building on the work of both Semmelweis and Pasteur, Lister began soaking surgical dressings in carbolic acid (phenol) to prevent postoperative infection. Other surgeons adopted this practice, which was one of the earliest attempts to control infectious microorganisms.

Thus, following the invention of microscopes, early scientists struggled to show that microbes can cause disease in humans, and that **public health** measures, such as closing down sources of **contamination** and giving healthy people vaccines, can prevent the spread of disease. This led to reduction of disease transmission in hospitals and the community, and the development of techniques to identify the organisms that for many years were considered to exist only in the imaginations of those researchers and physicians struggling to establish the germ theory.

See also Bacteria and bacterial infection; Bacterial growth and division; Centers for Disease Control (CDC); Colony and colony formation; Contamination, bacterial and viral; Epidemics and pandemics; Epidemics, bacterial; Epidemics, viral; Epidemiology, tracking diseases with technology;

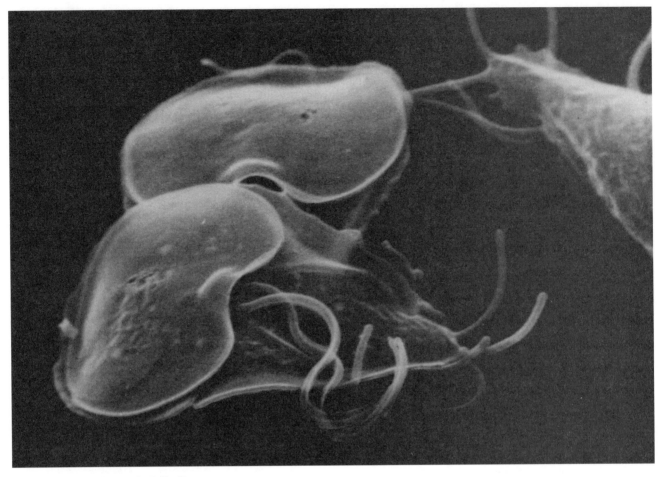

Scanning electron micrograph of *Giardia*.

History of microbiology; History of public health; History of the development of antibiotics; Infection and resistance; Laboratory techniques in microbiology

GIARDIA AND GIARDIASIS

Giardia is a protozoan parasite that can be transmitted to humans via drinking water that is contaminated with feces. The prototypical species is *Giardia lamblia*. The protozoan causes an intestinal malady, typified by diarrhea that is called giardiasis. The intestinal upset has also been dubbed "beaver fever."

The natural habitat of *Giardia* is the intestinal tract of warm-blooded animals. In the wild, warm-blooded creatures such as beavers and bears are natural reservoirs of the protozoan. Also, domestic dogs and cats can harbor the microbe. Typically, *Giardia* is passed onto humans by the fecal **contamination** of drinking water by these animals. The ingestion of only a few cysts is sufficient to establish an infection

Giardia has two distinct morphologies. In the environment, such as in water, *Giardia* is in the form of what is termed a cyst. An individual cyst is egg-shaped and contains four eye-like appearing nuclear bodies. This form is function-

ally analogous to a bacterial spore. It is a dormant form of the organism that is designed to allow preservation of the genetic material in a hostile environment. Cysts can remain capable of growth for months in water.

In the more hospitable intestinal tract, *Giardia* reverts to an actively growing and dividing form that is termed a trophozoite. A trophozoite has a distinctive "tear-drop" shape and flagella protruding from five regions on the surface. Two nuclei present the appearance of eyes and a darker central body looks somewhat like a mouth. The effect is to produce an image in the light **microscope** that is reminiscent of a face.

When excreted from an animal into water, the cyst form is particularly insidious because of the small size, which can allow the cyst to elude filtering steps in a drinking water treatment plant. Also, the cyst is resistant to chlorine, which is the most common means of disinfecting drinking water. Other documented routes of fecal to oral transmission are the sharing of toys in day care facilities (where hands are soiled) and via oral/anal sexual acts. Food borne transmission can occur, but is rare.

While in some people an infection with *Giardia* does not produce symptoms, many people experience prolonged diarrhea. Indeed, giardiasis is a major cause of intestinal upset in the world. In North America, giardiasis is the leading cause of non-bacterial diarrhea. The diarrhea typically persists for a few weeks to a few months, although in extreme cases the infection can persist for years. Infection produces a general malaise and considerable weight loss. The diarrhea tends to be mushy but, in contrast to the diarrhea produced in bacterial and amoebic **dysentery**, it is not bloody. Other symptoms of giardiasis include flatulence, sore abdomen, foul-smelling breath and, particularly in infants, the disruption of normal body growth. Research on animal models has also demonstrated that the infection disrupts the ability of the intestinal epithelial cells to absorb nutrients from the intestinal contents. The decreased absorption of compounds such as vitamin B_{12} and lactose can have deleterious effects on overall health.

The molecular basis of the infection is still not fully resolved. However, the trophozoite form of the protozoan is required, as is associated with the surface of the intestinal epithelial cells. In contrast to another intestinal disease causing microbe, *Entamoeba histolytica*, *Giardia lamblia* does not invade the host tissue. Studies with animal models have indicated that the symptoms of giardiasis may be due to a physical barrier to the absorption of nutrients, the disruption of intestinal structures called microvilli by the adherent **protozoa**, and production of a toxin that damages the epithelial cells.

During an active infection, trophozoites undergo division to new daughter trophozoites. Also, formation of cysts occurs and the cysts are excreted with the feces in huge numbers. These can be passed onto someone else to establish a new infection.

Treatment for giardiasis can include the use of **antibiotics**. Often, however, the malady is self-limiting without intervention. Prevention of giardiasis is a more realistic option, and involves proper treatment of drinking water and good hygienic practices, especially handwashing.

Currently, the detection of *Giardia* is based on the microscopic detection of either form of the protozoan, although animal models of the infection are being researched. The infection has been produced in gerbils. The lack of a routine detection method is problematic for water treatment. The need for rapid testing of drinking water for *Giardia* is pressing as the incidence of infection is increasing, with the encroachment of human habitation on previously pristine areas.

See also Amebic dysentery; Parasites; Water quality

GLIDING BACTERIA

Gliding **bacteria** is a term that refers to any bacteria that exhibit a gliding or creeping type of movement (also known as motility) when in contact with a solid surface.

There are hundred of types of gliding bacteria. Most are beneficial or benign to humans and animals. Some strains, such as the myxobacteria, produce **antibiotics** and compounds that act on tumors. In addition, some strains of gliding bacteria can degrade compounds, and so have potential in the biodegradation of pollutants. However, some strains are a major health concern. For example, gliding bacteria that live

in human saliva can cause gum disease, and can be life-threatening if they enter the bloodstream. Other types of gliding bacteria cause disease in animals and fish.

The gliding motility of myxobacteria is only one of several forms the organism can adopt. Another form consists of a stalk with fruiting bodies positioned at one end. When exhibiting gliding motility, a single cell can be in motion or a population of cells can move in concert with one another. The latter type of gliding seems to require the group of cells. If a cell moves out in front of the others, the lead cell will soon stop. The nature of the communal movement is unknown.

The gliding motility of bacteria such as those in the myxobacteria, the green nonsulfur group of bacteria (such as *Chloroflexus auranticus*) and the nonphotosynthetic gliding bacteria (such as *Herpetosiphon*) has long been a fascination to bacteriologists. The bacteria glide smoothly with no evidence of cellular involvement in the movement. In fact, the gliding motion may be the result of what have been termed "slime fibrils," a complex of proteins, which are attached to the bacterium at one end and to the solid surface at the other end. The exact mechanism of action of the slime fibrils is still unresolved. If the fibrils have to move to propel a bacterium along, the nature of this movement and how the movement is powered remain unknown.

Some gliding bacteria are known to exhibit a chemotactic response, that is, a concerted movement either in the direction of an attractant or concerted movement away from a repellent. The chemical sensing system must be coordinated with the gliding mechanism. Again, the nature of this coordination is unresolved.

See also Bacterial movement

GLOBULINS

Globulins are immune molecules that are produced by the **immune system** in response to invasion of the body of agents that are perceived by the system as being foreign. Some immune globulins are also known as antibodies. Examples of **microorganisms** that stimulate globulin production are **bacteria**, **viruses**, molds, and **parasites**.

The production of globulins is triggered by the presence of the foreign material (antigen). Through an intricately coordinated series of events, the immune system responds to the presence of an antigen by the production of a corresponding globulin. There are three divisions of globulins, based on the movement of the molecules through a gel under the influence of an electric current (in other words, based on their size and their charge character). The three types are alpha, beta, and gamma globulins.

Alpha globulins are manufactured mainly in the liver. There are a number of so-called alpha-1 and alpha-2 globulins. The functions of these globulins includes the inhibition of an enzyme that digests protein, an inhibitor of two compounds vital in the clumping (coagulation) of blood, and a protein that can transport the element copper.

Alpha and beta globulins function as **enzymes** and proteins that transport compounds in the body. Gamma globulins act as the **antibody** defense against antigen invasion.

Beta globulins are also manufactured predominantly in the liver. Akin to the alpha type globulins, there are beta-1 and beta-2 globulins. Examples of beta globulins include a protein that binds iron in the body, factors involved with the immune targeting of foreign material for immune destruction, and a species of immunoglobulin antibody termed IgM.

Gamma globulins are manufactured in cells of the immune system known as lymphocytes and plasma cells. These globulins, which are known as IgM, IgA, and IgG, represent antibodies. Depending on the nature of the invading antigen, a specific immun globulin will be produced in great numbers by a specific lymphocyte or plasma cell. Infection with a different antigen will stimulate the production of a different immune globulin. As the infection eases, the production of the immun globulin will decrease.

The quantities of the various globulins in the blood can be diagnostic of malfunctions in the body or specific diseases. Examples of maladies that affect the globulin levels are chronic microbial infections, liver disease, **autoimmune disorders**, leukemias, and rheumatoid arthritis.

See also Immunity: active, passive, and delayed; Immunity, cell mediated; Immunity, humoral regulation; Immunochemistry; Immunogenetics; Immunoglobulins and immunoglobulin deficiency syndromes; Immunologic therapies; Immunological analysis techniques; Laboratory techniques in immunology

GLYCOCALYX

The glycocalyx is a carbohydrate-enriched coating that covers the outside of many eukaryotic cells and prokaryotic cells, particularly **bacteria**. When on eukaryotic cells the glycocalyx can be a factor used for the recognition of the cell. On bacterial cells, the glycocalyx provides a protective coat from host factors. The possession of a glycocalyx on bacteria is associated with the ability of the bacteria to establish an infection.

The glycocalyx of bacteria can assume several forms. If in a condensed form that is relatively tightly associated with the underlying cell wall, the glycocalyx is referred to as a capsule. A more loosely attached glycocalyx that can be removed from the cell more easily is referred to as a slime layer.

The bacterial glycocalyx can vary in structure from bacteria to bacteria. Even particular bacteria can be capable of producing a glycocalyx of varying structure, depending upon the growth conditions and nutrients available. Generally, the glycocalyx is constructed of one or more sugars that are called saccharides. If more than one saccharide is present, the glycocalyx is described as being made of polysaccharide. In some glycocalyces, protein can also be present.

There are two prominent functions of the glycocalyx. The first function is to enable bacteria to become harder for the immune cells called phagocytes so surround and engulf. This is because the presence of a glycocalyx increases the effective diameter of a bacterium and also covers up components of the bacterium that the **immune system** would detect and be stimulated by. Thus, in a sense, a bacterium with a glycocalyx becomes more invisible to the immune system of a host.

Infectious strains of bacteria such as *Staphylococcus, Streptococcus,* and *Pseudomonas* tend to elaborate more glycocalyx than their corresponding non-infectious counterparts.

The second function of a bacterial glycocalyx is to promote the adhesion of the bacteria to living and inert surfaces and the subsequent formation of adherent, glycocalyx-enclosed populations that are called **biofilms**. Biofilm bacteria can become very hard to kill, party due to the presence of the glycocalyx material. Many persistent infections in the body are caused by bacterial biofilms. One example is the dental **plaque** formed by glycocalyx-producing *Streptococcus mutans*, which can become a focus for tooth enamel-digesting acid formed by the bacteria. Another example is the chronic lung infections formed in those afflicted with certain forms of cystic fibrosis by glycocalyx-producing *Pseudomonas aeruginosa*. The latter infections can cause sufficient lung damage to prove lethal.

See also Anti-adhesion methods; Bacterial surface layers

GOLGI, CAMILLO (1843-1926)
Italian histologist

Among other achievements in neurobiology, Camillo Golgi devised a method of staining nerve tissue using silver nitrate. Golgi-stained nerve tissue revealed unique structures with fine projections, which were later recognized as individual cells, or neurons.

Golgi was born in Corteno, Italy, on July 7, 1843. His hometown was later re-named Corteno-Golgi in his honor. Golgi studied medicine at the University of Pavia, where he received his M.D. in 1865. After graduation, he worked briefly in a psychiatric clinic, but eventually decided to pursue a career in histological research.

Financial difficulties forced him in 1872 to accept a position as chief medical officer at the Hospital for the Chronically Ill in Abbiategrasso, Italy. No research facilities were available there, however, and he was able to continue his studies only by converting an unused kitchen into a laboratory. By 1875, Golgi had earned sufficient fame to receive an appointment as lecturer in histology at the University of Pavia. Four years later, he was appointed Professor of Anatomy at the University of Siena, but he stayed only a year there before returning to Pavia as Professor of Histology.

Golgi's earliest research involved the study of neurons, or nerve cells. Neurons present a number of problems for researchers that other cells do not. While most cells are compact and have a relatively fixed shape, neurons are commonly very long and thin with structures that are difficult to see clearly. In the 1860s, techniques used to stain and study non-nerve cells were well developed, but they were largely useless with neurons. As a result, a great deal of uncertainty surrounded the structure and function of neurons and neuron networks.

In 1873, Golgi found that silver salts could be used to dye neurons. The neurons turned black and stood out clearly from surrounding tissue. Golgi perfected his technique so that the addition of just the right amount of dye for just the right period of time would highlight one or another part of the neuron, a single complete neuron, or a group of neurons.

Golgi's new technique resolved some questions about the nervous system, but not all. He was able, for example, to confirm the view of Wilhelm von Waldeyer-Hartz that neurons are separated by narrow gaps, synapses, and are not physically connected to each other. He was not able to completely explain, however, the complex, overlapping network of dendrites.

While studying the brain of a barn owl in 1896, Golgi made a second important discovery. He found previously undetected bodies near the nuclear membrane. The function of those bodies, now known as Golgi apparatus, or **Golgi bodies**, is still not understood. For his research on the nervous system, Golgi was awarded a share of the 1906 Nobel Prize for physiology or medicine.

Between 1885 and 1893, Golgi was also involved in research on **malaria**. He made one especially interesting discovery in this field, namely that all the malarial **parasites** in an organism reproduce at the same time, a time that corresponds to the recurrence of fever.

In addition to his scientific work, Golgi was active in Italian politics. He was elected a Senator in 1900 and served in a number of administrative posts at Pavia. Golgi died in Pavia on January 21, 1926.

See also Cell cycle and cell division; Cell membrane transport; Golgi body; Malaria and the physiology of parasitic inflections

GOLGI BODY

The Golgi body, or Golgi apparatus is a collection of flattened membrane sacks called cisternae that carry out the processing, packaging, and sorting of a variety of cellular products in higher plants and animals. This important cellular organelle was named in honor of **Camillo Golgi**, the Italian neuroanatomist who first described it in brain cells late in the nineteenth century. An individual Golgi apparatus is usually composed of four to eight cisternae, each a micron or less in diameter stacked on top of each other like pancakes. Many cisternal stacks interconnected by tubules and mobile transport vesicles make up a Golgi complex, which often is located near the **nucleus** in the center of the cell. In some animal cells, this complex can be huge, filling much of the cytoplasmic space. In some plant cells, on the other hand, many small, apparently independent Golgi apparatuses are distributed throughout the cell interior.

Each Golgi stack has a distinct orientation. The *cis* or entry face is the site at which transport vesicles bringing newly synthesized products from the endoplasmic reticulum dock with and add their contents to the Golgi cisternae. A complex network of anastomosing (connecting) membrane tubules attach to and cover the fenestrated cisternae on the *cis* face and serves as a docking site for transport vesicles. From the *cis*

face a flow of vesicles carry transport and chaperone proteins back to the endoplasmic reticulum, while secretory products move on into the medial cisternae where further processing takes place. Finally, the products move to the *trans* or exit face where they undergo final processing, sorting, and packaging into vesicles that will carry them to the cell surface for secretion or to other cellular organelles for storage or use. Complex oligosaccharides are synthesized in the Golgi apparatus, and glycoproteins are assembled as materials move through the compartments of this organelle. A unique set of **enzymes** and chaperone proteins occur in each of the Golgi compartments to direct and carry out this complex set of reactions.

See also Cell cycle and cell division; Cell membrane transport

GONORRHEA

Gonorrhea is among the most common **sexually transmitted diseases** (STD) and is also among the most common bacterial infections in adults. In the United States, between 2.5 and 3 million cases are reported each year, most occurring in people under age 30. In its early stages, gonorrhea may cause no symptoms and therefore, can be spread by unsuspecting victims. In females, gonorrhea often remains asymptomatic but can lead to vaginal itching, discharge, or uterine bleeding and other serious complications. An infected woman who gives birth can transmit the disease to her infant, often resulting in childhood blindness. As a precaution, silver nitrate is routinely administered to the eyes of newborns to prevent this condition. In males, gonorrhea causes infection of the urethra and painful urination. Though not deadly, the disease if untreated can infect other genital organs. If the infection spreads throughout the blood stream, it can cause an arthritis-dermatitis syndrome.

Gonorrhea was described in early writings from Egypt, China, and Japan. Warnings against "unclean discharge from the body" appear in the Bible. A diagnostic description of the disease was written in the Middle Ages. In the late fifteenth century, a **syphilis** epidemic raged throughout Europe, though at that time, syphilis was often confused with gonorrhea and some physicians assumed that gonorrhea was the first stage of syphilis. The gram-negative bacterium that causes gonorrhea was discovered in 1879 by Albert Neisser (1855–1916), a German physician who went on to identify the bacterial cause for **leprosy**. German immunologist **Paul Ehrlich** named the bacterium *Gonococcus*. Since then, five types of the *Gonococcus* organism have been identified.

A test for the presence of *Gonococcus* bacterium serves as the diagnostic tool. The first effective treatments for gonorrhea were the sulfonamides, which became available in 1937. During World War II, **penicillin** became widely available for the treatment of gonorrhea and other bacterial disease. However, while penicillin and related **antibiotics** are effective in about 90% of cases, some strains of the *Gonococcus* are becoming resistant to penicillin.

See also History of the development of antibiotics; History of public health

GOODPASTURE, ERNEST WILLIAM (1886-1960)

American pathologist

Ernest William Goodpasture created a means of culturing **viruses** in the laboratory without **contamination** from foreign **bacteria**. This research was instrumental in the development of most of the vaccines and inoculations used in medicine today. Additionally, Goodpasture developed an alternate way of staining specimens for examination under the **microscope**. He also pursued research interests in varying other fields of medicine, and identified a progressive and rare **immune system** illness that became known as Goodpasture's Syndrome.

Goodpasture was born in Montgomery County, Tennessee. He left home to study medicine in 1909, and received his doctorate from Johns Hopkins University. He then served as the Rockefeller Fellow in Pathology until 1914. Goodpasture returned to practicing medicine and served his residency at Peter Bent Brigham Hospital in Boston from 1915 to 1917. In 1917, he was offered a professorship at Harvard University, but only remained there for three years. Shortly thereafter, Goodpasture was appointed chair of pathology at Vanderbilt University. The position at Vanderbilt afforded Goodpasture the opportunity to return home, he accepted and remained with the university for the entirety of his career.

In 1931, Goodpasture, working with Alice Woodruff, devised a method for cultivating viruses that revolutionized **virology**. Because rickettsiae and other viruses will only grow on living tissue, scientists had to study viruses on living hosts or on tissue cells cultures in the lab. Before the advent of **antibiotics**, lab cultures were often tainted by bacteria. Thus, viruses remained illusive to scientific study. Little was known about their structure and behavior. Goodpasture used fertilized chicken eggs to **culture** his viruses, a method that proved not only successful, but also cost effective. The team first successfully cultured fowl pox virus, but quickly proved that a multitude of viruses could be studied using the technique. Within a span of a few years, other scientists used Goodpasture's technique to create vaccines for **yellow fever**, **smallpox**, and **influenza**.

Goodpasture himself worked to create a **vaccination** against the **mumps**. In 1934, Goodpasture and his colleague, C.D. Johnsen, proved that the mumps virus vas filterable. This prompted to team to devise a method by which the virus could be manipulated to produce a **vaccine**.

Throughout the course of his career, Goodpasture was chiefly concerned with infectious diseases, but he also conducted research in the formation of various types of cancers and genetic diseases. His name was given to a condition that he discovered working in tandem with doctors at Vanderbilt University Hospital. Goodpasture's Syndrome is a rare and often fatal autoimmune disorder that affects the kidneys.

See also Laboratory techniques in immunology; Laboratory techniques in microbiology

GOTSCHLICH, EMIL CLAUS (1935-)

German-American physician and bacteriologist

Emil Gotschlich's basic research on *Meningococcus, Gonococcus, Streptococcus, Haemophilus, Escherichia coli,* protein antigens, and polysaccharides has contributed much to the knowledge of **immunology**, vaccines, and the bacterial pathogenesis of **meningitis**, **gonorrhea**, and other diseases.

Gotschlich was born on January 17, 1935, in Bangkok, Thailand, to Emil Clemens Gotschlich, and his wife Magdalene, née Holst, both expatriate Germans. He immigrated to the United States in 1950 and became a naturalized American citizen in 1955, the same year that he received his A.B. from the New York University College of Arts and Sciences. After receiving his M.D. from the New York University School of Medicine in 1959, he interned at Bellevue Hospital in New York City until 1960, then joined the staff of Rockefeller University, where he built the rest of his career, except for serving as a captain in the Department of Bacteriology of the U.S. Army Medical Corps at the Walter Reed Institute for Research in Washington, D.C., from 1966 to 1968. At Rockefeller in 2002, he is simultaneously professor of bacteriology, head of the Bacterial Pathogenesis and Immunology Laboratory, vice president for medical sciences, and principal investigator of the General Clinical Research Center.

Gotschlich's team at Rockefeller continues to achieve important results in bacteriology and immunology and has published hundreds of scientific papers. As of 2000, Gotschlich was the author, lead author, or co-author of 135 of these papers. The main focus of his research is the *Neisseria* genus of **bacteria**, especially two pathogenic varieties: the meningococcus *Neisseria meningitidis* and the gonococci *Neisseria gonorrhoeae*. In the 1970s, he engaged in a fruitful scientific correspondence with **Harry A. Feldman** (1914–1985) about meningococcal diseases and won the 1978 Albert Lasker Award for his part in developing a polysaccharide **vaccine** against these diseases. In 1984, he outlined protocols for the development of a gonorrhea vaccine. In 2001, the United States **Centers for Disease Control** appointed him to its national review committee on **anthrax** vaccine safety and efficacy.

Medicine and medical research are a tradition in Gotschlich's family. His grandfather, Emil Carl Anton Constantin Gotschlich, a student of Carl Flügge and a colleague of Max Josef von Pettenkofer (1818–1901) and **Robert Koch** (1843–1910), was a prominent German academic physician, hygienist, and epidemiologist who specialized in cholera and tropical diseases. His great uncle, Felix Gotschlich (b. 1874), also studied cholera and in 1906 isolated *El Tor vibrio cholerae,* an epidemic strain of the cholera bacillus. His father was a physician in private practice in Thailand. His second wife, Kathleen Ann Haines (b. 1949), a pediatric allergist and immunologist in New York City; his son, Emil Christopher Gotschlich (b. 1961), an obstetrician/gynecologist in Portland, Maine; and his daughter, Hilda Christina Gartley (b. 1965), a pediatrician in Boston, Massachusetts, all continue this tradition.

See also Antibiotics; Antibody and antigen; Bacteria and

bacterial infection; Haemophilus; Infection control; Lipopolysaccharide and its constituents; Meningitis, bacterial and viral; Microbiology, clinical; Serology; Streptococci and streptococcal infections; Vaccine

GRAM, HANS CHRISTIAN JOACHIM
(1853-1938)
Danish pharmacologist

Hans Christian Joachim Gram was a Danish physician and bacteriologist who developed the most widely used method of staining bacterial cells for microscopic study.

Gram was born in Copenhagen, Denmark, on September 13, 1853. He received a B.A. in the natural sciences from the Copenhagen Metropolitan School in 1871 and served as an assistant to the zoologist Japetus Steenstrup from 1873 to 1874. He subsequently became interested in medicine and earned a medical degree from the University of Copenhagen in 1878. Gram, who worked in several areas of science and medicine, earned a gold medal in 1882 for a study on human erythrocytes. The following year he received a doctoral degree for his work in this field.

After obtaining his degree, Gram pursued post-doctoral studies in Berlin, focusing on bacteriology and pharmacology. It was in Berlin in 1884 that he published his work on the technique of staining cells, a procedure that became widely known as **Gram staining**.

At that time, the method of staining cells was not entirely new to scientific research and several methods were already being used. Gram borrowed from a procedure initially devised by **Paul Ehrlich**, who used alkaline aniline solutions to stain **bacteria** cells. Experimenting with pneumococci bacteria, Gram first applied Gentian violet, which stained the cells purple, and then washed the cells with Lugol's solution (iodine), which served as a mordant to fix the dye. He followed those steps by applying alcohol, which washed away any dye that was not permanently fixed. Gram found that some cells remained purple (Gram positive), while others stayed essentially unstained (Gram negative). Gram's method aided microscopic study of bacteria, as well as provided a means of differentiating and classifying bacteria cells. Several years later, the pathologist Carl Weigart improved upon Gram's method by adding another staining step, which consisted in dyeing the Gram-negative cells with saffranine.

Gram remained in Berlin working as an assistant in a hospital until 1891, when he was appointed as a professor of pharmacology at the University of Copenhagen. In 1889, Gram married Louise I. C. Lohse, and in 1892, advanced to the position of chief of internal medicine at the Royal Frederiks Hospital. Extremely active in the field of medical education, Gram also maintained a large internal medicine practice. From 1901 to 1921, Gram served as chairman of the Pharmacopoeia Commission, during which time he abolished the use of many useless and obsolete therapeutic treatments. In addition, he published a four-volume book on the importance of rational pharmacology in clinical science. After his retire-

ment in 1923, he returned to an earlier interest: the history of medicine. During his career, Gram received several honors including the Danneborg Commander's Cross, the Golden Medal of Merit, and an honorary M.D. Gram died in Copenhagen, on November 14, 1938.

See also Laboratory techniques in microbiology

GRAM STAINING

In the second half of nineteenth century, scientists proved that specific bacterial organisms caused specific diseases, and the field of microbiology was on its way to becoming a distinct science. The **microscope** was also further developed during that time, and scientists were concerned with identifying and classifying **bacteria**. Most bacteria are difficult to see with a compound microscope, but can be seen when there is obvious contrast between the bacteria cells and their surrounding medium. Various dyes are used to stain cells so that they are more easily seen. As early as the late eighteenth century, scientists had developed some basic methods of staining cells to aid in their study and used natural substances such as saffron, which stained some parts of a cell. The discovery of synthetic dyes in the mid-1800s enabled scientists to utilize more colors to stain cells.

In 1884, the Danish physician **Hans Christian Joachim Gram** further developed a method of staining bacteria originally developed by the German biologist **Paul Ehrlich**. Ehrlich used aniline water and gentian violet (a cationic dye) to stain cells, and the cell walls would appear purple after staining. Gram added a potassium triiodide solution, which acted as a mordant for the gentian violet dye, and then poured ethanol over the cells to wash away the unfixed dye. Gram found that some of the cells remained purple, while others did not. Bacteria that remained purple were termed positive and those that did not remain purple were called negative. A few years later, Carl Weigert, director of the Senckberg Foundation in Frankfurt, Germany, added another step to the staining method. Weigert followed Gram's procedure with a final staining using saffranine (an anionic dye), which subsequently stained the negative bacteria red. The Gram stain is still considered the definitive, differential test to determine the chemical make-up of a bacterium cell wall. On the basis of a cell's reaction to the Gram stain, bacteria are divided into two groups, Gram positive and Gram negative.

The distinguishing feature between Gram positive and negative bacteria is the difference in the structure of the cell walls. The cell wall of a Gram positive is a thick, single layer of a cross-linked polysaccharide that is easily stained by gentian violet, while the cell wall of a Gram negative bacterium consists of a thin layer of polysaccharide and is covered by a lipid layer that resists the gentian violet, but can be stained by saffranine. Many dyes, which are organic compounds, are positively charged and easily combine with the negatively charged, acidic polysaccharide wall. Other dyes are negatively charged and combine with protein-based cell constituents.

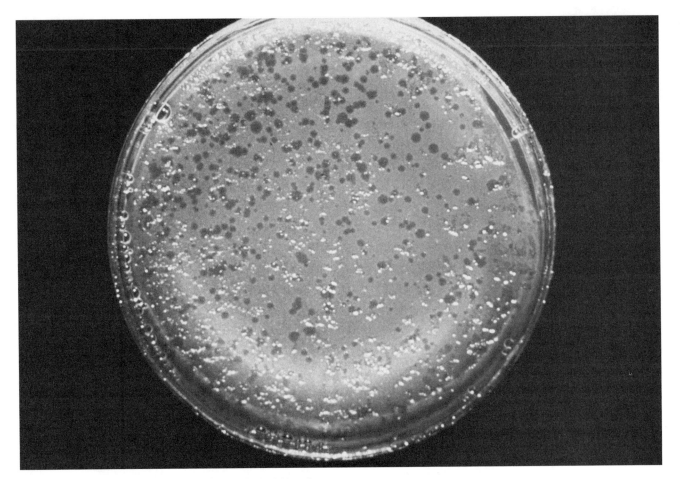

Growth of virus creates clearing in lawn of growing *Escherichia coli*.

The chemical make-up of the cell wall also determines the penetrability of the wall by various drugs. Knowing if a bacterium is Gram positive or negative determines what type of antibiotic is suitable for treatment, as some **antibiotics** act against Gram positive bacteria (i.e., **penicillin**), while others act against Gram negative bacteria (i.e., tetracycline or streptomycin). Another important consideration is the fact that some Gram negative bacteria release endotoxins, which can be fatal. When pharmaceutical companies develop new antibacterial drugs, the Gram stain is the method by which scientists determine the effectiveness of the drug.

See also Laboratory techniques in microbiology

GRAMICIDIN • *see* ANTIBIOTICS

GREEN FLUORESCENT PROTEIN • *see*

LABORATORY TECHNIQUES IN IMMUNOLOGY

GROWTH AND GROWTH MEDIA

The ability of all organisms, including **microorganisms**, to grow and divide is the fundamental underpinning of their continued existence. In the laboratory, the nutrients needed for growth are supplied in the form of growth media.

Microorganisms such as **bacteria, yeast**, and algae grow by increasing in size, replicating their genetic material and other internal factors such as proteins, manufacturing the required additional cell wall material to enclose the new cell, and finally dividing to form two so-called daughter cells. Vital materials are required by most microbes, including carbon, hydrogen, nitrogen, phosphorus, calcium, cobalt, magnesium, and manganese. Often these elements must be supplied in the growth media, because the microbes cannot manufacture them. Once supplied, however, such elements form the building blocks upon which the microorganism can construct some (but not all) amino aids, proteins, and even the **DNA (deoxyribonucleic acid)** and **ribonucleic acid (RNA)** genetic materials.

Provision of the necessary elements is not sufficient to permit growth, however. The level of oxygen, moisture content, and temperature are examples of other factors that must be adjusted to permit the growth of the target microbe. For example, *Escherichia coli* requires a temperature of around

37° C [98.6° F], to match the temperature of its normal intestinal habitat. Refrigeration temperature, which does support the growth of some bacteria, does not support the growth of *Escherichia coli*.

The nature of the growth requirements of bacteria has been used as a means of grouping bacteria together. Photoautotrophic bacteria are those that use sunlight as a source of energy. **Heterotrophic bacteria** utilize organic carbon as a type of fuel for growth, while lithotrophic bacteria use inorganic carbon sources. As a final example, **autotrophic bacteria** are those bacteria that use carbon dioxide as the only source of carbon. Similarly, bacteria can be grouped according to their growth requirements with respect to temperature, salinity, the hydrogen ion concentration (also known as the **pH**), and oxygen.

In the laboratory, growth media often requires the presence of a few growth factors that the bacteria or other microbe cannot make themselves. For example, depending on the particular bacteria being grown, certain amino acids may need to be supplied. Likewise, the inclusion of compounds known as purines and pyrimidines may be necessary for the manufacture of DNA or RNA. Lastly, some vitamins may need to be added, which allow some **enzymes** to function. Sometimes bacteria can become altered so that the daughter cell has specific nutritional requirements that the parent cell does not. The mutant strain is referred to as an auxotroph. For example, a strain of *Escherichia coli* that requires the amino acid tryptophane for growth is a tryptophan auxotroph and is designated as *Escherichia coli trp*. Auxotrophs can be very useful as markers, or indicators of the success of an experimental procedure.

Growth of microorganisms can occur in a liquid growth medium, which is termed a broth, or on a solid medium. **Agar and agarose** are two examples of solid growth media. Often a broth can be supplemented with the solidifying agent to form **agar**. Growth media can be very nonspecific with respect to nutrients. For example, Brain-Hear Infusion (BHI) broth or agar is a blended mixture of animal brain and heart. A medium such as BHI is also referred to as a complex medium. Other media contains defined amounts of specific components. This type of medium is also called a minimal medium.

Growth media can also be tailored to favor the growth of one or a few types of bacteria over the many other types of bacteria that would develop on a nonselective medium, or to provide an enriched environment for those bacteria that would other wise grow poorly or very slowly. An example of a medium that is both selective and enriched is that used to grow bacteria in the genus *Halococcus*. These bacteria require very high concentrations of salt. The high sodium chloride concentration of the medium is lethal for all other types of bacteria.

In conventional broth and agar cultures, the growth of microorganisms is uncontrolled. The cells grow as fast as possible for as long as possible. However, growth of bacteria is possible such that the rate of growth and division can be controlled. Devices that accomplish this are the chemostat and the turbidostat. Comparison of the chemical make-up of the same type of microbe under relatively fast growing or slow growing conditions can be very useful, particularly because in infec-

tions, **bacterial growth** can be slower than in the laboratory environment.

See also Agar and agarose; Blood agar, hemolysis, and hemolytic reactions; Colony and colony formation; Synchronous growth

VON GRUBER, MAX (1853-1927)
Austrian physician and bacteriologist

Max von Gruber's discovery of specific bacterial agglutination in 1896 laid the groundwork for significant advances in **serology** and **immunology**.

Gruber was born in Vienna, the son of a prominent physician, Ignaz Gruber (1803–1872), and his wife, née Gabrielle Edle von Menninger. His brother, Franz von Gruber (1837–1918), became famous as an architect, military engineer, and teacher. After preparing for college at the Schottengymnasium in Vienna, Gruber studied chemistry and physiology at the University of Vienna, earned his M.D. there in 1876, then took postgraduate instruction in the biosciences under Max Josef von Pettenkoffer (1818–1901) in Vienna, Carl von Voit (1831–1908) and Carl Wilhelm von Nägeli (1817–1891) in Munich, Germany, and Carl Friedrich Wilhelm Ludwig (1816–1895) in Leipzig, Germany. Among his fellow graduate students under Pettenkoffer was Hans Buchner (1850–1902), who urged Gruber toward bacteriology.

Gruber began lecturing on **hygiene** at the University of Vienna in 1882, became professor of hygiene at the University of Graz, Austria, in 1884, and assumed the same position in 1887 at the University of Vienna, where he remained until 1902. He was promoted in 1891 to full professor. He was unhappy in Vienna because he considered the facilities ill kept and substandard. Nevertheless, he was able to attract to Vienna such stellar graduate students as future Nobel laureate **Karl Landsteiner** (1868–1943), Alois Lode (b. 1866), and Herbert Edward Durham (1866–1945). From 1902 until he retired in 1923, Gruber was director of the Institute for Hygiene, Munich.

In March, 1896, Gruber and Durham published a landmark article in a prestigious journal, *Münchener medizinische Wochenschrift* [Munich Medical Weekly], which described how **bacteria** of similar size clump together in sera, in ways specific to or determined by each serum. Their research concerned the typhoid bacillus *Salmonella typhi*, the cholera bacillus *Vibrio cholerae*, and the respective sera of typhoid and cholera patients. This clumping process, agglutination, soon had wider implications for serology, immunology, bacteriology, and clinical medicine. The first important practical consequence of Gruber's work on bacterial agglutination occurred in June 1896, when the French physician Georges Fernand Isidor Widal (1862–1929) developed a diagnostic agglutination test for typhoid, thereafter known as the Gruber-Widal test or the Gruber-Widal reaction.

In the first decade of the twentieth century, Gruber's main interest shifted toward right-wing social theory, political eugenics, and so-called "racial hygiene." His *Hygiene des Geschlechtslebens* [Sexual Hygiene] first appeared in 1903, was reprinted or revised fifty-two times by 1925, and was translated into many languages, including English. With psychiatrist Ernst Rüdin (1874–1952), later a Nazi, Gruber co-edited *Fortpflanzung, Vererbung, und Rassenhygiene* [Propagation, Inheritance, and Racial Hygiene] in 1911. Thereafter, much of his work was political propaganda. Gruber attended Adolph Hitler's first big rally in 1921 and was impressed by Hitler's control of the crowd and command of issues. Gruber died in Berchtesgaden, Germany, on September 16, 1927.

See also Antibody-antigen, biochemical and molecular reactions; Bacteria and bacterial infection; History of immunology; Typhoid fever

H

HAEMOPHILUS

Haemophilus is a bacterial genus. The **bacteria** in this genus all share the characteristic of preferring to grow on solid laboratory media that contains blood cells. The blood supplies two factors that *Haemophilus* species require for growth. These are X factor and V factor. The utilization of these factors and of the blood cells causes the destruction of the cells and various characteristic reactions in the **blood agar**. Indeed, the name of the genus arise from these reactions.

Haemophilus are Gram negative in their **Gram staining** behavior and are very tiny rods in shape. The bacteria can display different shapes, and so is one of the types of bacteria known as pleomorphic bacteria. A hallmark of *Haemophilus* species is the formation of small colonies that are described as "satellites" around colonies of *Staphylococcus*.

In humans, *Haemophilus* is a normal resident of the throat and nose. However, spread of the bacteria beyond these sites can cause infections.

Haemophilus influenzae commonly infects children, causing a respiratory infection. This infection typically strikes those who already have the flu. The bacteria that cause these relatively severe reactions possess a **glycocalyx** that surrounds the each bacterium. The glycocalyx help thwart the host's immune response. Types of *Haemophilus influenzae* that cause less severe infections of the ears and the sinuses typically do not possess the glycocalyx.

Haemophilus influenzae infections can spread beyond the lungs. Spread to the central nervous system can result in an infection and **inflammation** of the sheath that surrounds nerve cells (**meningitis**). *Haemophilus influenzae* type b (which is also known as Hib) is particularly noteworthy in regard to meningitis. Hib can cause of fatal brain infection in young children.

Hib infections were once more common and dangerous. Now, however, the availability of a **vaccine** and the widespread requirement for a series of vaccinations early in life has greatly reduced the incidence of Hib meningitis.

Haemophilus can also spread to the airway. In that location, an infection known as epiglottits can be produced. The resulting obstruction of the airway in children less than 5 years of age can be fatal.

Other species of note include *Haemophilus aegyptius*, the cause of conjunctivitis (or pinkeye), a very contagious disease in children, and *Haemophilus ducreyi*, a sexually transmitted disease that causes genital ulceration.

See also Bacteria and bacterial infection; Blood agar, hemolysis, and hemolytic reactions

HALOPHILIC BACTERIA · *see* EXTREMOPHILES

HANCOCK, ROBERT ERNEST WILLIAM (1949-)
English bacteriologist

Robert (Bob) Hancock is a bacteriologist and professor of microbiology in the department of microbiology and **immunology** at the University of British Columbia (U.B.C.) in Vancouver, British Columbia, Canada. He is internationally renowned for his fundamental contributions to the study of **antibiotic resistance** of Gram-negative **bacteria**, particularly the antibiotic resistance of *Pseudomonas aeruginosa*.

Hancock was born in Merton, Surrey, England. Following his undergraduate education he obtained his Ph.D. at the University of Adelaide in Australia in 1974. Postdoctoral training followed at the University of Tübingen (1975–1977) and at the University of California at Berkeley (1977–1978). In 1978, Hancock became an assistant professor in the department of microbiology and immunology at U.B.C. In 1983, he became an associate professor with tenure, and became an associate member of the department of Pediatrics at U.B.C. (which has continued to the present day). In 1986, he became a professor at U.B.C.

From 1989 until 1996, he was the first Scientific Director of the newly established Canadian Bacterial Diseases Network. Under his direction, the network of academic and applied microbiologists and molecular biologists made fundamental discoveries of the mechanisms of **bacterial infection**. Presently, he is a board member of the network. From 1990 until 1993, Hancock was the Chair of the Medical/Scientific Advisory Committee of the Canadian Cystic Fibrosis Foundation. Finally, beginning in 1997, Hancock has been the Director of the Centre for Microbial Diseases and Host Defense Research at UBC.

Hancock has served on the editorial boards of ten international peer-reviewed journals and his expertise in bacterial pathogenesis and antibiotic resistance is utilized in a consultative and directorial role in a myriad of government and industrial settings.

Through his research, Hancock has revealed some of the molecular aspects of the mechanisms by which *Pseudomonas aeruginosa* is able to cause disease or death, particularly in those afflicted with cystic fibrosis. His research has determined the structure of some outer membrane proteins that functions as transport pores. Additionally, he is among the group that has completed the sequencing of the genome of the bacterium. The latter work will lead to further discoveries of genes that are vital in disease processes.

Hancock's best-known research has been the unraveling of what is termed the "self-promoted uptake" of aminoglycoside, polymyxin and cationic **antibiotics** and antimicrobial peptides. This uptake is a major reason for the acquisition of antibiotic resistance by the bacterium, and so will be the target of treatment strategies.

In recognition of his fundamental contributions to bacteriology, Hancock has been the recipient of numerous awards and honors, including the Canadian Society of Microbiologists Award in 1987, the 125th Anniversary of Canada Silver Medal in 1993, inclusion in the *American Men and Women in Science,* 1989–2000, and the MRC Distinguished Scientist Award, 1995–2000.

See also Bacterial adaptation; Infection and resistance

HAND-FOOT-MOUTH DISEASE

Hand-foot-mouth disease is a contagious illness that strikes predominantly infants and children that is characterized by fever, mouth sores, and a rash with blistering. Two types of **viruses** cause the disease. The majority of cases are due to several members of the Coxsackie virus group (subtypes A16, A5, and A10). A type of enterovirus designated as enterovirus 71 also causes the disease, but is of minor importance.

The name of the disease has caused confusion with the well-known hoof and mouth disease. However, hand-foot-mouth disease is entirely different from hoof and mouth disease that strikes cattle, sheep, and swine, causes entirely different symptoms, and which is caused by a different virus.

The disease was initially described and the viral agents determined in 1957.

Hand-foot-mouth disease begins with a general feeling of being unwell. A mild fever, poor appetite, and sore throat leads within a few days to the appearance of sores in the mouth. The blister-like rash develops soon thereafter on the palms of the hands, soles of the feet, on the inside of the mouth, and sometimes on the buttocks. The hands tend to be involved more than the other regions of the body. These symptoms are more inconvenient than threatening to health. Recovery is typically complete within a week or two. Rarely, a stiff neck and back pain reminiscent of **meningitis** can lead to hospitalization. This precaution is prudent, since one of the enteroviruses that causes hand-foot-mouth disease, enterovirus 71, can also cause viral meningitis. During outbreaks of hand-foot-mouth disease, cases of viral meningitis can concurrently appear.

Children fewer than ten years of age are most susceptible. However, the disease can occur in adults as well. In children the fever, which can peak in the range of 103 to 104° F (39.4 to 39.9° C), is a concern. Also, the sores in the mouth can discourage children from eating and drinking. Thus, an important aspect of managing the disease is the maintenance of a sufficient diet.

The disease is contagious and can be spread from person to person by direct contact with nose or throat fluids. There is no geographic restriction on the occurrence of the disease. There is some seasonal distribution, with the majority of cases being reported during the summer and early fall.

Treatment of hand-foot-mouth disease is confined to the relief of the symptoms, and observance of good hygienic practices to minimize the spread of the virus. **Antibiotics** are useless, given the viral nature of the disease. An actual cure, such as a **vaccine**, does not yet exist. Even if specific **immunity** to one episode of the disease has been produced, a subsequent infection with a different subtype of Coxsackie virus can cause another bout of the disease. In this sense, hand-foot-mouth disease is similar to the immune variation that is the hallmark of influenzae viruses.

HAND WASHING · *see* HYGIENE

HANTAVIRUS AND HANTA DISEASE

Hantavirus (family Bunyaviridae, genus Hantavirus) infection is caused by **viruses** that can infect humans with two serious illnesses: hemorrhagic fever with renal syndrome (HFRS), and Hantavirus pulmonary syndrome (HPS).

Hantaviruses are found without causing symptoms within various species of rodents and are passed to humans by exposure to the urine, feces, or saliva of those infected rodents. Infection is commonly associated with disturbing the droppings or nests of rodents within confined spaces. The disturbed particles are inhaled to cause infection. Ten different hantaviruses have been identified as important in humans.

Each is found in specific geographic regions, and therefore is spread by different rodent carriers. Further, each type of virus causes a slightly different form of illness in its human hosts. Hantaan virus is carried by the striped field mouse, and exists in Korea, China, Eastern Russia, and the Balkans. Hantaan virus often causes a severe form of hemorrhagic fever with renal syndrome (HFRS).

Puumula virus is carried by bank voles, and exists in Scandinavia, western Russia, and Europe. Puumula virus causes a milder form of HFRS, usually termed nephropathia epidemica.

Seoul virus is carried by a type of rat called the Norway rat, and exists worldwide, but causes disease almost exclusively in Asia. Seoul virus causes a form of HFRS which is slightly milder than that caused by Hantaan virus, but results in liver complications.

Prospect Hill virus is carried by meadow voles and exists in the United States, but has not been found to cause human disease. Sin Nombre virus, the most predominant strain in the United States, is carried by the deer mouse. This virus was responsible for severe cases of HPS that occurred in the Southwestern United States in 1993. A similar, but genetically distinct strain was responsible for an outbreak of HPS in Argentina in 1996, and was later termed the Andes virus. During the outbreak in Argentina, five of the victims were physicians, three of which were directly responsible for the care of an HPS patient. This, along with additional epidemiologic evidence (such as the low rodent population density in the area affected) suggest that person-to-person transmission was possible during this outbreak, a feature unique to any known hantavirus.

Black Creek Canal virus has been found in Florida. It is predominantly carried by cotton rats. New York virus strain has been documented in New York State. The vectors for this virus appear to be deer mice and white-footed mice. Bayou virus has been reported in Louisiana and Texas and is carried by the marsh rice rat.

Blue River virus has been found in Indiana and Oklahoma and seems to be associated with the white-footed mouse. Monongahela virus, discovered in 2000, has been found in Pennsylvania and is transmitted by the white-footed mouse.

Hantaviruses that produce forms of hemorrhagic fever with renal syndrome (HFRS) cause a classic group of symptoms, including fever, malfunction of the kidneys, and low platelet count. Because platelets are blood cells important in proper clotting, low numbers of circulating platelets can result in spontaneous bleeding, or hemorrhage.

Patients with HFRS have pain in the head, abdomen, and lower back, and may report bloodshot eyes and blurry vision. Tiny pinpoint hemorrhages, called petechiae, may appear on the upper body and the soft palate in the mouth. The patient's face, chest, abdomen, and back often appear flushed and red, as if sunburned. Around day eight of HFRS, kidney involvement results in multiple derangements of the body chemistry. Simultaneously, the hemorrhagic features of the illness begin to cause spontaneous bleeding, as demonstrated by bloody urine, bloody vomit, and in very serious cases, brain hemorrhages with resulting changes in consciousness and shock.

Hantavirus pulmonary syndrome (HPS) develops in four stages. They are: The incubation period. This lasts from one to five weeks from exposure. Here, the patient may exhibit no symptoms.

The prodrome, or warning signs, stage. The patient begins with a fever, muscle aches, backache, and abdominal pain and upset. Sometimes there is vomiting and diarrhea.

The cardiopulmonary stage. The patient slips into this stage rapidly, sometimes within a day or two of initial symptoms; sometimes as long as 10 days later. There is a drop in blood pressure, shock, and leaking of the blood vessels of the lungs, which results in fluid accumulation in the lungs, and subsequent shortness of breath. The fluid accumulation can be so rapid and so severe as to put the patient in respiratory failure within only a few hours. Some patients experience severe abdominal tenderness.

The convalescent stage. If the patient survives the respiratory complications of the previous stage, there is a rapid recovery, usually within a day or two. However, abnormal liver and lung functioning may persist for six months.

The diagnosis of infection by a hantavirus uses serologic techniques. The **ELISA (enzyme-linked immunosorbant assay)** is done in a laboratory to identify the presence of specific immune substances (antibodies), which an individual's body would only produce in response to the hantavirus. It is difficult to demonstrate the actual virus in human tissue or to grow cultures of the virus within the laboratory, so the majority of diagnostic tests use indirect means to demonstrate the presence of the virus.

Treatment of hantavirus infections is primarily supportive, because there are no agents available to kill the viruses and interrupt the infection. The diseases caused by hantaviruses are lethal. About 6–15% of people who contract HFRS have died. Almost half of all people who contract HPS will die. It is essential that people living in areas where the hantaviruses exist seek quick medical treatment, should they begin to develop an illness that might be due to a hantavirus. Preventative measures focus on vector control (elimination of rodents), and avoiding rodent infested areas.

See also Epidemics, viral; Epidemiology, tracking diseases with technology; Epidemiology; Hemorrhagic fevers and diseases; Virology

HAZARD ANALYSIS AND CRITICAL CONTROL POINTS PROGRAM (HACCP)

Hazard Analysis and Critical Control Points (HACCP) refers to a system that is established and instituted to monitor all stages of a processing or manufacturing operation to ensure that the final product is not compromised because of microbial **contamination**. Originally, HACCP was devised for the food processing industry. Now, HACCP has expanded to include the manufacture of pharmaceuticals and other products that could be affected by unwanted growth of **microorganisms**.

The global scope of the HACCP program reflects the susceptibility of, for example, a food to contamination from different microorganisms at different stages of the processing pathway. The altered storage conditions, physical state and chemistry of the food, and shipping conditions can select for the growth of different microbes. The absence of microbes as a food enters a plant is no guarantee that the food will remain uncontaminated. The monitoring of points along the production pathway that are deemed critical and susceptible to contamination can reveal problems and spur remediation of the problems.

The concept of HACCP arose in 1959 at the Pillsbury Company. At that time, the company was contracted to provide food products for the United States manned space program. A system of stringent quality control was needed, because astronauts would not have access to medical attention in the event of the development of a food poisoning or intoxication event in space. The concept of a controlled series of checks was born. In 1971, at the United States Conference on Food Protection, the principles of HACCP were formally described. The principles and procedures of a HACCP program have since been formalized by the National Advisory Committee on Microbiological Criteria for Foods.

Then, as now, there are three principles to the program. First is the identification of hazards found all the way from the field to the marketplace, and the determination of the urgency of each hazard in terms of remedy. Second is the formulation of steps to control or prevent the occurrence of those hazards that warrant remediation. Last is the establishment of a system to monitor the points in the manufacturing process that have been deemed either critical to product quality or a point at which contamination could occur.

A critical part of a HACCP program is the writing of what are known as standard operating procedures (or SOPs). A SOP documents exactly how a test or monitoring will be conducted, how often it will be conducted, and both how—and to whom—the results of the test or monitoring will be reported. This ensures that the food or other material that is being guarded from contamination will be treated the same way. In this way, if a problem occurs, there is a standard in place, which allows for a frame of reference in which to properly evaluate the problem.

A properly operating HACCP program is not, of course, a guarantee that no problems will occur. However, the chances of microbial contamination will be reduced, because problems will be noted as they develop (for example, the need to clean a piece of equipment or the accumulation of stagnant water in a pipeline), rather than being confronted by a contamination problem with no warning. Knowledge of the types of contamination problems that can arise can help pinpoint the source of a contamination, and so can minimize the time that a production line is shut down.

An important aspect of a HACCP program is that all remediative procedures that are contemplated must be capable of being routinely performed. If a solution is not easily done, the control step is meaningless. An adjunct to a successful HACCP is the industrial concept of Good Manufacturing Practices (abbreviated GMP). Essentially GMP is a series of

quality control measures designed to ensure that a process proceeds as planned.

Another important aspect of a HACCP program is the verification that the program is operating properly. This can involve the use of known strains of **bacteria** to verify that the examination techniques being used to monitor a process do indeed detect the bacteria. Such tests should be performed regularly (daily, weekly, monthly) and the results should be documented.

HACCP programs involving microorganisms typically are revised as more becomes known about the microbe of interest. As further information is learned of, for example, the microbe's habitat, growth conditions, and environmental niches, more monitoring or the use of additional examination techniques may need to be incorporated into the HACCP program.

See also Disinfection and disinfectants; Food safety

HAZEN, ELIZABETH (1885-1975)

American microbiologist

Elizabeth Hazen, through a long-distance collaboration with her colleague Rachel Brown, developed the first non-toxic drug treatment for fungal infections in humans.

Hazen was born in Rich, Mississippi, on August 24, 1885, and raised by relatives in Lula, Mississippi, after the death of her parents. Hazen attended the public schools of Coahoma County, Mississippi, and earned a B.S. from the State College for Women, now Mississippi University for Women. She began teaching high school science and continued her own education during summers at the University of Tennessee and University of Virginia.

In 1916, Hazen began studying bacteriology at Columbia University, where she earned an M.A. the following year. World War I provided some opportunities for women scientists, and Hazen served in the Army diagnostic laboratories and subsequently in the facilities of a West Virginia hospital. Following the war, she returned to Columbia University to pursue a doctorate in microbiology, which she earned in 1927 at age 42.

After a four-year stint at Columbia University as an instructor, Hazen joined the Division of Laboratories and Research of the New York State Department of Health. She was assigned to special problems of bacterial diagnosis and spent the next few years researching bacterial diseases. She investigated an outbreak of **anthrax**, tracing it to a brush factory in Westchester County. Hazen discovered unknown sources of **tularemia** in New York and was the first to identify imported canned seafood that had spoiled as the cause of type E toxin deaths.

Her discoveries led Hazen to try to better understand mycotic (fungal) diseases. In 1944, she was given the responsibility of investigating such diseases, and she acquired cultures of **fungi** from local laboratories and specialized collections. Although Hazen was learning more about mycotic diseases, fungal infections continued to spread in epidemic proportions among school children in New York City. In addition to **pneumonia**, many other fungal diseases caused widespread ailments, such as moniliasis (**thrush**), a mouth condition that makes swallowing painful. Despite personal health problems and stressful working conditions, Hazen persevered.

In the mid-1940s, she teamed up with Rachel Brown (1898–1980), a chemist at the Albany laboratory who prepared extracts from the cultures sent by Hazen. In the fall of 1950, Hazen and Brown announced at a National Academy of Sciences meeting that they had successfully produced two antifungal agents from an antibiotic. This led to their development of Nystatin, the first fungicide safe for treating humans. Nystatin was immediately used nationwide, earning $135,000 in its first year.

Nystatin, which is still sold as a medication today under various trade names, turned out to be an extremely versatile substance. In addition to curing serious fungal infections of the skin and digestive system, it can also combat Dutch Elm disease in trees and even restore artwork damaged by water and **mold**. Remarkably, Hazen and Brown chose not to accept any royalties from the patent rights for Nystatin. Instead, they established a foundation to support advances in science. The donated royalties totaled more than $13 million by the time the patent expired. Hazen died on June 24, 1975.

See also Candidiasis; Fungicide; Yeast, infectious

HEAT SHOCK RESPONSE

The heat shock response occurs in virtually all organisms, including **bacteria**. The response occurs when an environmental stress is imposed on the organism. The name of the response comes from its discovery following the application of a mild heat stress, only 5 to 10° C higher than the usual preferred growth temperature. However, the response, which can be more correctly thought of as an adaptive response, consisting of a temporary alteration in the **metabolism** of the organism, occurs in response to more than just excessive heat.

Hallmarks of the heat shock response are its rapid onset and short-term nature. The response is an emergency coping type of reaction to a conditions that is perceived by the organism as being threatening. The response is not a long-term commitment, such as the formation of a spore by a bacterium (although some proteins that are stimulated in the heat shock response of *Bacillus subtilis* also function in the formation of spores by the bacteria). Rather, a heat shock response allows the organism to cope and then to quickly resume normal function.

The alteration in the chromosome of the fruit fly *Drosophila* flowing an elevation in the temperature was reported in 1962. At the time and for some years thereafter, the observation was regarded as an interesting curiosity that was relevant only to the fruit fly. However, it is unequivocally clear that the genes encoding the responsive proteins and the structure of the proteins themselves are highly conserved in many species. For example, three heat shock proteins that were discovered in bacteria, which have been dubbed Hsp70, Hsp10, and Hsp60 are highly conserved in a large number of bacteria and in eukaryotic organisms.

Heat shock proteins are induced in large quantities in response to factors including nutrient depletion, addition of alcohols such as ethanol, change in the sodium concentration, presence of heavy metals, fever, interaction with cells of a host, and the presence of virus. The proteins are produced in non-stress conditions. But typically their quantities are much less. In non-stress conditions they function in the normal metabolic events within the cell.

The heat shock response in bacteria involves the elevated production of more than 20 proteins whose functions are varied. For example, some of the proteins degrade other proteins (proteases), while other proteins help transport molecules from one place to another while preserving their structure (these are known as **chaperones**). These induced proteins act to overcome the changes that would prove destructive to other proteins in the bacterium. By preventing protein alteration and destruction, the heat shock response ensure that the bacterium will be capable of normal function once the stress is removed.

Some bacteria also utilize the heat shock response to promote infection of host cells or tissue, or to survive within host cells. Examples of bacteria include *Escherichia coli*, *Legionella pneumophila*, and *Listeria monocytogenes*. Furthermore, the alteration in structure of bacteria can involve heat shock proteins. Examples include *Bacillus subtilis* spore formation and the formation of the so-called fruiting bodies by myxobacteria.

The principle trigger for the heat shock response in bacteria is at the level of **transcription**, where the genetic material, **DNA** (**deoxyribonucleic acid**), is used to manufacture **ribonucleic acid**. In *Escherichia coli* the response is controlled by what has been called a sigma factor. The sigma factor is capable of binding to various regions of the DNA that stimulate the transcription of the particular **gene** under their control. In other words, the single sigma factor is capable of stimulating the expression of multiple genes. The sigma factor is under a tight and complex control, which normally restricts its activity but leaves the factor primed for action. This is the reason for the rapid nature of the heat shock response.

Two other heat shock response controls in bacteria operate after the proteins are produced. These controls aid in maintaining the proteins for a bit longer than if they were produced under non-heat shock conditions. By preserving the structure and functions of the heat shock proteins, their activity is allowed to persist. But, once again, the protein activity does not last indefinitely, which allows the heat shock response to be rapidly "turned off."

The observations that bacterial heat shock proteins can be vital for the establishment of infections has made the heat shock response the subject of much study, with the aim of circumventing the response or devising vaccines that protect host cells.

See also Bacterial adaptation; Microbial genetics

HELICOBACTERIOSIS

Helicobacteriosis is an infection of the gastrointestinal tract that is caused by the Gram-negative, spiral-shaped bacterium called *Helicobacter pylori*. Ulcers on the lining of the stomach and upper intestinal tract characterize the malady. The ulceration may be a prelude to the development of cancer of the stomach.

Helicobacteriosis is established following the colonization of the stomach by *Helicobacter pylori*. How the **bacteria** are transmitted to a person is still unclear. The prevalence of the infection in overcrowded environments, especially where children are present, indicate that person-to-person transmission is most likely, and that personal **hygiene** plays a role in transmission. Following transmission, the bacterium is able to persist in the extremely acidic environment of the stomach by burrowing under the mucous overlay of the stomach epithelial cells, and because the bacteria produce an enzyme called urease. The enzyme is able to degrade the gastric acid in the stomach.

Helicobacteriosis invariably becomes chronic. Then, the infection can also be referred to as chronic gastritis. The infection can become chronic because initially the infection produces little or no symptoms. Thus, the **immune system** is not alerted to response to the infection, which provides an opportunity for the bacterial population to become more tenaciously established.

In about 15% of those who become infected, ulcers develop in the stomach or in a region of the upper intestine called the duodenum. The resulting burning feeling caused by increased secretion of acid is relieved by over-the-counter antacids, which can further dissuade people from seeking a physician's care for the malady. If the infection is diagnosed and the bacteria eliminated by antibiotic therapy, the elevated production of acid stops. But, in the absence of treatment, the painful ulcers will recur. Why only fifteen per cent of those who have infections develop ulcers while the other 85% of infected individuals do not is not clear.

Moreover, the molecular basis for the establishment of the ulcers is also still not clear. There has been some indication of toxin involvement. *Helicobacter pylori* produces a toxin called VacA and a protein called CagA.

More ominously, epidemiologic evidence strongly indicates that *Helicobacter pylori* stomach infections are associated with the development of various types of stomach cancers. For examples, the bacterial infection is nine times more common in those patients who are diagnosed with cancer of the stomach, and seven times more common in those people who have a tumor of the lymphatic tissue. Studies have demonstrated that even in these advanced cases, the elimination of *Helicobacter pylori* can produce a shrinking of the tumors.

Helicobacteriosis can be detected in three ways. The first way is by obtaining a sample of stomach tissue. Culturing of the stomach contents on growth media that selects for the growth of *Helicobacter pylori* over other bacteria is used to isolate the organism. If the region of the stomach where tissue is obtained is free from bacteria, then an infection can be missed.

A second way of detecting the presence of the bacteria is by a breath test. Breathing on a specially prepared support can detect the presence of the urease enzyme that is produced by *Helicobacter pylori*. Since this enzyme is not commonly produced, the detection of the enzyme is a strong indication of the presence of living bacteria. However, in the absence of the actual isolation of the bacteria, the breath test cannot be absolutely diagnostic.

Finally, antibodies produced in response to a *Helicobacter pylori* infection can be detected by a blood test.

Once detected, the bacterial infection does respond to antibiotic therapy. Elimination of the infection relieves the symptoms of helicobacteriosis in 80% of those people who are infected.

The discovery that helicobacteriosis has a bacterial origin and the relief of the symptoms upon bacterial eradication has reinforced the validity of a theory that proposes that many chronic and autoimmune diseases, such as certain types of heart disease and rheumatoid arthritis, are caused by an infection by bacteria or other microbe.

See also Bacteria and bacterial infection; Microbial flora of the stomach and gastrointestinal tract

HEMAGGLUTININ (HA) AND NEURAMINIDASE (NA)

Hemagglutinin (designated as HA) and neuraminidase (designated as NA) are glycoproteins. Hemagglutinin and neuraminidase protrude from the outer surface of the **influenza** virus and neuraminidase is a constituent of the enveloping membrane that surrounds the viral contents. A glycoprotein is a protein that contains a short chain of sugar as part of its structure. The hemagglutinin and neuraminidase glycoproteins are important in the ability of the virus to cause influenza.

A typical influenza virus particle contains some 500 molecules of hemagglutinin and 100 molecules of neuraminidase. These are studded over the surface of the virus.

The illness caused by the influenza virus can be devastating. For example, in 1918 a new genetic variant of the virus swept around the world and in just over a year over 20 million people succumbed to the influenza. The variation was due to alterations in both the hemagglutinin and neuraminidase components of the virus. Further antigenic variations of these molecules produced a virus that, at least for some time, was not recognized by the **immune system**. The result was localized outbreaks or worldwide outbreaks in 1957, 1962, 1964, 1976, and 1978.

Hemagglutinin derives its name from its activity. The glycoprotein confers upon the virus the ability to agglutinate, or clump together, red blood cells. The aggregation compromises the function of the red blood cells. The hemagglutinin glycoprotein also functions in the binding of the virus to cells, via the recognition of a chemical structure on the cells surface called sialic acid. The binding of hemagglutinin to sialic acid compounds on the surface of cells is the initial event in the association of the virus with human epithelial cells. These two activities associated with hemagglutinin are important activities in the infectious ability of the virus. Indeed, hemagglutinin is the major virulence (disease-causing) factor of the influenza virus.

There are three distinct haemagglutinins important in human infections that are encoded by genes in the virus. These are designated as H1, H2, and H3. Animal influenza **viruses** contain nine additional types of hemagglutinin.

Neuraminidase is the common name for acetyl-neuraminyl hydrolase. The glycoprotein compound is an enzyme. The enzyme removes residues called N-Acetyl-neuraminic acid from chains of sugars and from other glycoproteins. The disruption of the neuraminic acid residues allows the virus to both pass out of the human epithelial cells in which it is replicating, and enter new cells to initiate a new round of viral replication. The activity of neuraminidase disrupts the mucous fluid that is present in the respiratory tract. Also, possession of neuraminidase keeps the viruses from aggregating with other virus particles. The result of these activities is to ease the spread of the virus through the respiratory tract.

Two different species of neuraminidase, designated N1 and N2, are important in human infections, while seven additional species are important in animal influenza viruses.

Inhibitors of neuraminidase have been developed in an effort to thwart the viral infection. The inhibitors are structurally similar to the silica acid on the surface of human epithelial cells. The rational is that the virus will bind to the inhibitor rather than to the human cells, and the inhibitor-viral complex can be removed from the body.

Hemagglutinin and neuraminidase are used in the designation of the different antigenic types of the influenza virus that have and continue to appear. For example, Influenza A/Taiwan/86/H1N1 is an influenza A strain of the H1 hemagglutinin type and N1 neuraminidase type that was first isolated in Taiwan in 1986.

Both hemagglutinin and neuraminidase tend to undergo what is termed antigenic drift, which is a slight but frequent change in the antigenic character. The slight change is still usually enough to thwart the recognition capabilities of the immune system. Hence, annual vaccinations are necessary to minimize the chance of acquiring an influenza infection. A major antigenic change in one or both of the glycoproteins, as happened in the 1918 virus, is termed antigenic shift.

See also Flu, the great flu epidemic of 1918; Mutations and mutagenesis

HEMOLYSIS AND HEMOLYTIC REACTIONS

• *see* BLOOD AGAR, HEMOLYSIS, AND HEMOLYTIC REACTIONS

HEMOLYTIC REACTIONS · *see* BLOOD AGAR,

HEMOLYSIS, AND HEMOLYTIC REACTIONS

HEMORRHAGIC FEVERS AND DISEASES

Hemorrhagic diseases are caused by infection with **viruses** or **bacteria**. As the name implies, a hallmark of a hemorrhagic disease is copious bleeding. The onset of a hemorrhagic fever or disease can lead to relatively mild symptoms that clear up within a short time. However, hemorrhagic diseases are most recognized because of the ferocity and lethality of their symptoms as well as the speed at which they render a person extremely ill.

Virtually all the hemorrhagic diseases of microbiological origin that arise with any frequency are caused by viruses. The various viral diseases are also known as viral hemorrhagic fevers. Bacterial infections that lead to hemorrhagic fever are rare. One example is a bacterium known as scrub **typhus**.

The viruses that cause hemorrhagic diseases are members of four groups. These are the arenaviruses, filoviruses, bunyaviruses, and the flaviviruses. Arenaviruses are the cause of Argentine hemorrhagic fever, Bolivian hemorrhagic fever, Sabia-associated hemorrhagic fever, Lassa fever, Lymphocytic choriomeningitis, and Venezuelan hemorrhagic fever. The Bunyavirus group causes Crimean-Congo hemorrhagic fever, Rift Valley fever, and Hantavirus pulmonary syndrome. Filoviruses are the cause of Ebola hemorrhagic fever and Marburg hemorrhagic fever. Lastly, the Flaviviruses cause tick-borne encephalitis, **yellow fever**, Dengue hemorrhagic fever, Kyasanur Forest disease, and Omsk hemorrhagic fever.

While the viruses in the groups display differences in structure and severity of the symptoms they can cause, there are some features that are shared by all the viruses. For instance, all the hemorrhagic viruses contain **ribonucleic acid** as their genetic material. The nucleic acid is contained within a so-called envelope that is typically made of lipid. Additionally, all the viruses require a host in which to live. The animal or insect that serves as the host is also called the natural reservoir of the particular virus. This natural reservoir does not include humans. Infection of humans occurs only incidentally upon contact with the natural reservoir.

Hemorrhagic diseases can be devastating for the victim. The symptoms can progress from mild to catastrophic in only hours. As a result, an outbreak of hemorrhagic disease tends to be self-limiting in a short time. In some cases, this is because the high death rate of those who are infected literally leaves the virus with no host to infect. Often the outbreak fades away as quickly as it appeared.

Hemorrhagic fever related illnesses appear in a geographical area where the natural reservoir and human are both present. If the contact between the two species is close enough, then the disease causing microorganism may be able to pass from the species that is the natural reservoir to the human.

Although little is still clear about the state of the microbes in their natural hosts, it is reasonably clear now that the viruses do not damage these hosts as much as they do a human who acquires the **microorganisms**. Clarifying the reasons for the resistance of the natural host to the infections would be helpful in finding an effective treatment for human hemorrhagic diseases.

The speed at which hemorrhagic fevers appear and end in human populations, combined with their frequent occurrence in relatively isolated areas of the globe has made detailed study difficult. Even though some of the diseases, such as Argentine hemorrhagic fever, have been known for almost 50 years, knowledge of the molecular basis of the disease is lacking. For example, while it is apparent that some hemorrhagic viruses can be transmitted through the air as aerosols, the pathway of infection once the microorganism has been inhaled is still largely unknown.

The transmission of hemorrhagic viruses from the animal reservoir to humans makes the viruses the quintessential zoonotic disease. For some of the viruses the host has been determined. Hosts include the cotton rat, deer mouse, house mouse, arthropod ticks, and mosquitoes. However, for other viruses, such as the Ebola and Marburg viruses, the natural host still remains undetermined. Outbreaks with the Ebola and Marburg viruses have involved transfer of the virus to human via primates. But, whether the primate is the natural host, or acquired the virus as the result of contact with the true natural host is not clear.

Another fairly common feature of hemorrhagic diseases is that once humans are infected with the agent of the disease, human-to-human transmission can occur. Often this transmission can be via body fluids that accidently contact a person who is offering care to the afflicted person.

Hemorrhagic diseases typically begin with a fever, a feeling of tiredness, aching of muscles. These symptoms may not progress further, and recovery may occur within a short time. However, damage that is more serious can occur, which is characterized by copious bleeding, often from orifices such as the mouth, eyes, and ears. More seriously, internal bleeding also occurs, as organs are attacked by the infection. Death can result, usually not from loss of blood, but from nervous system failure, coma, or seizures.

Hemorrhagic diseases are difficult to treat. Vaccines are available to only yellow fever and Argentine hemorrhagic fever. For the remaining diseases, the best policy is to curb the potential for human interaction with the natural reservoir of the microbe. For example, in the case of hantavirus pulmonary syndrome, control of the rodent population, especially after a rainy season when numbers naturally increase, is a wise course. Insect vectors are controlled by a concerted campaign of spraying and observance of precautionary measures (e.g., use of insect repellent, proper clothing, insect netting over sleeping areas, etc.).

See also Public health, current issues; Viruses and response to viral infection

HEPADNAVIRUSES

Hepadnaviridae is a family of hepadnaviruses comprised by two genera, *Avihepadnavirus* and the *Orthohepadnavirus*. Hepadnaviruses have partially double strands **DNA** (partial dsDNA virion) and they replicate their genome in the host cells using reverse transcriptase and are therefore, termed

retroviruses. Their virion DNA, invades the hepatocytes (i.e., liver cells) of vertebrates, which are their natural hosts. When hepadna retroviruses invade a cell, a complete viral dsDNA is made before its random integration in one of the host's **chromosomes**, and is then transcribed into an intermediate messenger **RNA** (mRNA) into the hosts' **nucleus**. The viral mRNA then leaves the nucleus and undergoes reverse transcriptase, mediated by a viral reverse transcriptase enzyme that transcribes complementary strands of complementary dsDNA in the cell cytosol, thus forming new partial dsDNA virions.

Orthohepadnavirus is the pathogenic agent that causes chronic **hepatitis** (Hepatitis type B) in mammals, which may eventually lead to either cirrhosis or liver cancer if not detected and treated. Hepatitis B Virus or HBV, the prototype member of the family Hepadnaviridae, is transmitted by both infected blood (blood transfusions, grafts) and body fluids (usually through sexual relations with infected partners). HBV comprises several viral species that also infect the liver cells of orangutans, dogs, and other mammalians besides man. Vaccines for both human Hepatitis B and several forms of animal Hepatitis B (lions, cats, dogs) are available as a form of disease prevention. All Hepadnaviridae **viruses** have a high affinity with liver cells (hepatotropy) and the viruses of the genus *Avihepadnavirus,* also known as avian hepadnaviruses, have as targets the liver of birds, such as storks, ducks, herons, etc.

See also Animal models of infections; Antiviral drugs; Hepatitis, hepatitis viruses and tests; Interferons; Virology

HEPATITIS AND HEPATITIS VIRUSES

Hepatitis is **inflammation** of the liver, a potentially life-threatening disease most frequently caused by viral infections but which may also result from liver damage caused by toxic substances such as alcohol and certain drugs. Hepatitis **viruses** identified to date occur in six major types: hepatitis A HAV), hepatitis B (HBV), hepatitis C (HCV), hepatitis D (HDV), and hepatitis E (HEV) and hepatitis G (HGV). All types are potentially serious and, because clinical symptoms are similar, positive identification of the infecting strain is possible only through serologic testing (analyzing the clear, fluid portion of the blood). Symptoms may include a generalized feeling of listlessness and fatigue, perhaps including mental depression, nausea, vomiting, lack of appetite, dark urine and pale feces, jaundice (yellowing of the skin), pain in the upper right portion of the abdomen (where the liver is located), and enlargement of both the liver and the spleen. Severe cases of some types of hepatitis can lead to scarring and fibrosis of the liver (cirrhosis), and even to cancer of the liver.

Epidemics of liver disease were recorded as long ago as Hippocrates' time and, despite major advances in diagnosis and prevention methods over the past two decades, viral hepatitis remains one of the most serious global health problems facing humans today.

The incidence and spread of HAV is directly related to poor personal and social **hygiene** and is a serious problem not only in developing countries where sanitation and water purification standards are poor, but also in developed, industrialized nations, including the United States, where it accounts for 30% of all incidences of clinical hepatitis. Except in one to four percent of cases where sudden liver failure may result in death, chronic liver disease and serious liver damage very rarely develop, and "chronic carrier state," in which infected people with no visible symptoms harbor the virus and transfer the disease to non-infected individuals, never occurs. Also, reinfection seldom develops in recovered HAV patients because the body eventually develops antibodies, cells which provide a natural **immunity** to the specific virus attacking the host. Although HAV is self-limiting (after time, ends as a result of its own progress), there is as yet no effective treatment once it is contracted.

Apart from the symptoms described above, HAV commonly produces a medium-grade fever, diarrhea, headaches, and muscle pain. The primary route of HAV transmission is fecal-oral through ingestion of water contaminated with raw sewage, raw or undercooked shell-fish grown in contaminated water, food contaminated by infected food handlers, and close physical contact with an infected person. Heterosexual and homosexual activities with multiple partners, travel from countries with low incidences to countries with high rates of infected population, and, less frequently, blood transfusions and intravenous drug use also spread infection.

During the infectious stage, large numbers of viruses are eliminated with the stool. Although HAV infection occurs in all age groups, high rates of disease transmission occur in day-care centers and nursery schools where children are not yet toilet trained or able to wash their hands thoroughly after defecating. The disease may then be transmitted to day-care workers and carried home to parents and siblings. In areas of the world where living quarters are extremely crowded and many people live in unhygienic conditions, large outbreaks of HAV threaten people of all ages. Because during the viruses' incubation period—from 14 to 49 days—no symptoms are observable, and because symptoms seldom develop in young children, particularly those under the age of two, the disease is often unknowingly but readily transmitted before infected people can be isolated.

A **vaccine** against HAV is available. It appears to provide good protection, if the first **immunization** has been received at least four weeks prior to exposure. For adults, two immunizations about 6 months apart are recommended; for children, three immunizations are necessary (two a month apart, and the third six months later). High-risk groups who should receive HAV vaccine include child care workers, military personnel, Alaskan natives, frequent travelers to HAV endemic areas, laboratory technicians where HAV is handled, people who work with primates. The immunization lasts for 20 years.

If someone who is unimmunized is exposed to HAV, or if a traveler cannot wait four weeks prior to departure for an HAV endemic area, then immune globulin may be utilized to avoid infection. Immune globulin is a naturally occurring substance harvested from the plasma in human blood, then injected into an individual exposed to the HAV. Immune globulin prevents disease development in 80–90% of cases in clinical trials. It also seems to be effective in reducing the number of cases normally expected after outbreaks in schools and

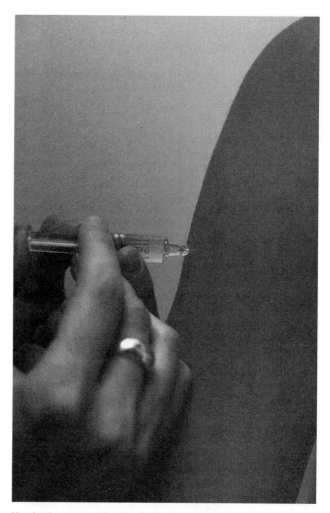

Vaccination against Hepatitis B virus.

other institutions. As yet, the most effective control mechanisms are public education regarding the importance of improved personal hygiene, which in many instances is as simple as washing hands thoroughly after using the toilet and before handing food, and concerted worldwide efforts to purify water supplies (including rivers and oceans) and improve sanitation methods.

Acute HBV is currently the greatest cause of viral hepatitis throughout the world. **World Health Organization** figures released in 1992 indicate that as many as 350 million people worldwide carry the highly infectious HBV. Because of its severity and often lengthy duration, 40% of those carriers—possibly as many as two million per year—will eventually die from resultant liver cancer or cirrhosis. HBV-related liver cancer deaths are second only to tobacco-related deaths worldwide. Infected children who survive into adulthood may suffer for years from the damage caused to the liver. In the United States alone, as many as 300,000 people become infected with HBV every year, medical costs amount to more than $1 million per day, and the death rate over the last 15 or so years has more than doubled in the United States and Canada.

If **serology** (blood) tests detect the presence of HBV six months or more from time of initial diagnosis, the virus is then termed "chronic." Chronic persistent hepatitis may develop following a severe episode of acute HBV. Within a year or two, however, this type usually runs its course and the patient recovers without serious liver damage. Chronic active hepatitis also may follow a severe attack of acute HBV infection, or it may simply develop almost unnoticed. Unlike persistent hepatitis, the chronic active type usually continues until fatal liver damage occurs. In long-term studies of 17 patients with chronic active hepatitis, 70% developed cirrhosis of the liver within two to five years.

Symptoms are similar to those manifested by HAV and may include weight loss, muscle aches, headaches, flu-like symptoms, mild temperature elevation, and constipation or diarrhea. By the time jaundice appears, the patient may feel somewhat better overall but the urine becomes dark, stools light or yellowish, the liver and possibly the spleen enlarged and painful, and fluid may accumulate around the abdominal area. Early in the disease's life, however, symptoms may be very slight or even virtually nonexistent, particularly in children, facilitating infection of others before isolation is implemented.

The incubation period for HBV varies widely—anywhere from four weeks to six months. Primary routes of transmission are blood or blood product transfusion; body fluids such as semen, blood, and saliva (including a bite by an infected human) organ and/or tissue transplants; contaminated needles and syringes in hospitals or clinical settings; contaminated needles or syringes in illegal intravenous drug use; and vertical transmission—from mother to baby during pregnancy, birth, or after birth through breast milk. Even though they may not develop symptoms of the disease during childhood, and will remain healthy, almost all infected newborns become chronic carriers, capable of spreading the disease. Many of these infected yet apparently healthy children, particularly the males, will develop cirrhosis and liver cancer in adulthood. Where the incidence of the disease is relatively low, the primary mode of transmission appears to be sexual and strongly related to multiple sex partners, particularly in homosexual men. In locations where disease prevalence is high, the most common form of transmission is from mother to infant.

Controlling HBV infection is an overwhelming task. In spite of the development of safe and effective vaccines capable of preventing HBV in uninfected individuals, and regardless of programs designed to vaccinate adults in high-risk categories such as male homosexuals, prostitutes, intravenous drug users, health-care workers, and families of people known to be carriers, the disease still remains relatively unchecked, particularly in developing countries.

Although effective vaccines have been available since the mid-1980s, the cost of mass immunization world-wide, and particularly in developing countries, was initially prohibitive, while immunizing high-risk adult populations did little to halt the spread of infection. Authorities now believe the most effective disease control method will be immunization of all babies within the first weeks following birth. Concerted efforts of researchers and health authorities worldwide, including the foundation in 1986 of an International Task Force for Hepatitis B Immunization are investigating various avenues for providing cost-effective, mass **vaccination** programs. These include incorporating HBV vaccination into the existing Expanded Program of Immunization controlled by the World Health Organization. Methods of cost containment, storing the vaccine, and distribution to midwives in remote villages (60% of the world's births occur at home), have been designed and are continually being refined to ultimately attain the goal of universal infant immunization. This will not only drastically decrease the number of babies infected through vertical transmission (which constitutes 40% of all HBV transmission in Asia), preventing them from becoming adult carriers, it also provides immunity throughout adulthood.

Finding an effective treatment for those infected with HBV presents a major challenge to researchers—a challenge equal to that posed by any other disease which still remains unconquered. And HBV may present yet another challenge: mutant forms of the virus seem to be developing in resistance to the current vaccines, thus finding a way to survive, replicate and continue its devastating course. Necessary measures in disease control include: education programs aimed at health care workers to prevent accidental HBV transfer—from an infected patient to an uninfected patient, or to themselves; strict controls over testing of blood, blood products, organs, and tissue prior to transfusion or transplantation; and the "passive" immunization with immunoglobulin containing HBV antibodies as soon as possible after exposure to the active virus. Treatment with Interferon and new drug, Lamivudine, have shown positive results in managing HBV.

Relatively recently discovered hepatitis viruses, often called non-A, non-B hepatitis, exist in more than 100 million carriers worldwide, with 175,000 new cases developing each year in the U.S. and Europe.

Not until 1990 were serology tests available to identify the hepatitis C virus (HCV). Research since then has determined that HCV is distributed globally and, like HBV, is implicated in both acute and chronic hepatitis, as well as liver cancer and cirrhosis. Eighty-five percent of all transfusion-related hepatitis is caused by HCV, and mother-baby and sexual transmission are also thought to spread the disease. Symptoms are similar but usually less severe than HBV; however, it results in higher rates of chronic infection and liver disease.

Control and prevention of HCV is a serious problem. First, infected people may show no overt symptoms and the likelihood that infection will become chronic means that many unsuspecting carriers will transmit the disease. Second, HCV infection does not appear to stimulate the development of antibodies, which not only means infected people often become reinfected, it creates a major challenge in the development of an effective vaccine. Third, HCV exists in the same general high-risk populations as does HBV. Combined, these factors make reducing the spread of infection extremely difficult. On a positive note, the development of accurate blood screening for HCV has almost completely eliminated transfusion-related spread of hepatitis in developed countries. Immunoglobulin injections do not protect people who have been exposed to HCV; the search is on for an adequate immunization, although this effort is hampered by characteristics of HCV, which include rapid mutation of the virus. Treatment with interferon remains the most effective measure in managing the long term effects of HCV.

Undiscovered until 1980, Hepatitis E virus (HEV) is thought to transmit in a similar fashion to HAV. HEV is most prevalent in India, Asia, Africa, and Central America. Contaminated water supplies, conditions that predispose to poor hygiene (as in developing countries), and travel to developing countries all contribute to the spread of HEV. Symptoms are similar to other hepatitis viruses and, like HAV, it is usually self-limiting, does not develop into the chronic stage, and seldom causes fatal liver damage. It does seem, however, that a higher percentage of pregnant women (from 10–20%) die from HEV than from HAV.

Research into the virus was slow because of the limited amounts which could be isolated and collected from both naturally infected humans and experimentally infected primates. Recently, successful genetic **cloning** (artificial duplication of genes) is greatly enhancing research efforts. Surprisingly, research found that antibodies exist in between one to five percent of people who have never been infected with hepatitis. Until an effective vaccine is developed, sanitation remains the most important factor in preventing the spread of HEV.

Because it is a "defective" virus requiring "coinfection" with HBV in order to live and reproduce, HDV alone poses no threat in the spread of viral hepatitis. It also poses no threat to people vaccinated against HBV. However, when this extremely infectious and potent virus is contracted by unsuspecting carriers of HBV, rapidly developing chronic and even fatal hepatitis often follows. The coexistent requirements of HDV as yet remain unclear. Research into development of an effective vaccine is ongoing, and genetic cloning may aid in this effort.

Little is currently known about a relatively recently discovered hepatitis virus, G. HGV appears to be passed through contaminated blood, as is HCV. In fact, many infections with HVG occur in people already infected with HCV. HGV, however, does not seem to change the disease course in people infected with both HCV and HGV. In cases of isolated HGV infection, little liver injury is noted, and there does not appear to be a risk of chronic liver injury. Much more information must be sought about this particular hepatitis virus, and its risks.

See also Epidemics, viral; Interferon actions; Public health, current issues; Viruses and responses to viral infection

HEPATITIS, AUTOIMMUNE · *see* AUTOIMMUNITY AND AUTOIMMUNE DISORDERS

HERPES AND HERPES VIRUS

Herpes is a name given to a common viral infection. The infection can occur in the mouth and in the genitals.

The two forms of herpes are caused by two forms of a herpes virus. Both forms are called herpes simplex virus. Oral

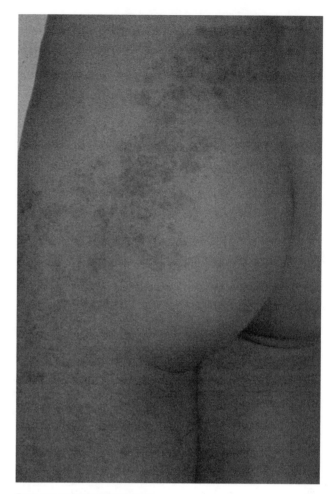

Rash due to Herpes zoster virus.

herpes is generally caused by herpes simplex type 1 (that is typically shortened to HSV–1). It is also known as human herpes virus 1 (HHV1). Genital herpes is generally caused by herpes simplex type 2 (shortened to HSV–2, which has also been called human herpes virus 2, or HHV2). However, HSV–1 can cause genital herpes and HSV–2 can cause oral herpes.

There are eight herpes virus types known in humans. HSV–1 (HHV1) and HSV-2 (HHV2) are the forms associated with oral and genital herpes. Human herpes virus 3 is also known as **varicella zoster virus**, and is the cause of chickenpox. HHV4 is the official name of **Epstein-Barr virus**, the major cause of infectious **mononucleosis**. HHV5 is also known as cytomegalovirus. It can cause mononucleosis, **hepatitis** in newborns, and complications in **AIDS** patients. HHV6 causes roseola in children and fever-associated seizures in infants. HHV7 has not yet been associated with any disease, and appears to be present in almost all people. Infection with HHV7 likely occurs early in life. Finally, HHV8 contributes to Kaposi's sarcoma, a relatively rare cancer that predominantly afflicts AIDS patients whose immune systems are failing.

Herpes simplex virus types 1 and 2 appear identical when examined using the high magnification power of the **electron microscope**. Both types are icosahedral in shape; that is, their surface consists of twenty equal-sized and equilateral triangles.

The oral form of herpes is manifest as cold sores or so-called fever blisters, and is common in young children. The virus can be passed from person to person very easily. Only a brief contact is needed for transmission. Cold sores are innocuous in children and adults. However, they can be a very serious health threat in newborns.

The genital form can be apparent as genital sores. These appear as clustered blistery-appearing sores on the vagina, vulva, cervix, penis, buttocks, or the anus. Pain, itching, and a burning feeling during urination can accompany the sores. In more severe cases, the lymph glands can be swollen, with a number of flu-like symptoms evident. These symptoms of what is referred to as primary herpes persist for several weeks then disappear. They can return, usually to a lesser extent, in anywhere from a few weeks to years later. Others who are infected may not display any symptoms whatsoever. Diagnosis of infection in asymptomatic people can still be made, based on the detection of viral antibodies in the blood.

Herpes affects some 80 million people in the United States alone, with one in six of these people having genital herpes. Herpes is spread by human contact. Typically this involves kissing, touching, or sexual contact. Typically, a person is contagious when he or she has open sores. Because of this, contact with others can be minimized when sores are present, thus minimizing the chance of spread. However, it has been proven that genital herpes can be spread even when no symptoms or sores are evident. The chance of this happening is about 10 percent. The spread of herpes via wet toilet seats and the like is now considered to be unlikely.

Studies have shown that the chances of pregnant women passing either herpes simplex virus to the developing fetus are rare. Transfer can occur during childbirth. If open sores are evident at this time, a caesarean section may be considered to avoid the chance of infection.

Herpes simplex virus replicates insides cells of the host. An association between a virus particle and the surface of the host cell starts this process. The host cell is typically that in nerves. This association is specific, involving the recognition of a host surface molecule. Another viral protein then associates with several of the host cell molecules that are collectively termed the herpes virus entry mediators. This second association leads to the fusion of the host and the viral membranes. The contents of the virus can then be emptied into the host cell.

Once in the host cell, the viral deoxyribonucleic acid genetic material somehow enters the **nucleus**. The viral **DNA** is then replicated using the **transcription** machinery of the host. The viral transcription process occurs immediately with certain stretches of the viral DNA and a bit later with other stretches of the DNA. The early **gene** products participate in the replication of the later regions of the viral DNA.

New virus particles can be produced very soon after infection. Or, alternatively, the infection may become what is described as latent. In a latent infection, no viral particles are produced. Viral DNA continues to be replicated along with host DNA until such time as a signal stimulates the transcription of viral genes that are involved in the assembly of new virus particles. Stress, surgery, menstruation, and **skin infections** such as sunburn are known to be signals, although the molecular nature of these stimuli is unclear.

Recurrence of symptoms can be more frequent with people whose immune systems are compromised, such as those with leukemia or acquired **immunodeficiency** syndrome (AIDS). Currently there is no cure for herpes. Physicians can prescribe one of three medications to treat genital herpes. These are acyclovir, famciclovir, and valacyclovir. With or without medication, in general the recurrences become fewer with the passage of time, often ending after five to six years.

Despite this fading of symptoms, the herpes simplex **viruses** can be debilitating aside from their direct affects. They can deplete the body's immune resources, leaving someone more vulnerable to infection by another microbial agent.

See also Latent viruses and diseases; Virus replication

HERSHEY, ALFRED DAY (1908-1997)
American microbiologist

By seeking to understand the reproduction of **viruses**, Alfred Day Hershey made important discoveries about the nature of **deoxyribonucleic acid** (**DNA**) and laid the groundwork for modern **molecular genetics**. Highly regarded as an experimental scientist, Hershey is perhaps best known for the 1952 "blender experiment" that he and Martha Chase conducted to demonstrate that DNA, not protein, was the genetic material of life. This discovery stimulated further research into DNA, including the discovery by **James Watson** and **Francis Crick** of the double-helix structure of DNA the following year. Hershey's work with bacteriophages, the viruses that prey on **bacteria**, was often carried out in loose collaboration with other scientists working with bacteriophages. Hershey shared the Nobel Prize in Physiology or Medicine in 1969 with Max Delbrück and Salvador Edward Luria. The Nobel Committee praised the three scientists for their contributions to **molecular biology**. Their basic research into viruses also helped others develop vaccines against viral diseases such as polio.

Hershey was born in Owosso, Michigan, to Robert Day Hershey and Alma Wilbur Hershey. Hershey's father worked for an auto manufacturer. Alfred attended public schools in Owosso and nearby Lansing. He received his B.S. in bacteriology from Michigan State College (now Michigan State University) in 1930 and his Ph.D. in chemistry from the same school in 1934. Hershey's interest in bacteriology and the **biochemistry** of life was already evident when he was a graduate student. His doctoral dissertation was on the chemistry of *Brucella,* the bacteria responsible for **brucellosis**, also known as undulant fever. After receiving his Ph.D., Hershey took a position as a research assistant in the Department of Bacteriology at the Washington University School of Medicine in St. Louis. There, he worked with Jacques Jacob

Bronfenbrenner, one of the pioneers in **bacteriophage** research in the United States. During the sixteen years he spent teaching and conducting research at Washington University, from 1934 to 1950, Hershey was promoted to instructor (1936), assistant professor (1938), and associate professor (1942).

Bacteriophages—known simply as phages—had been discovered in 1915, only nineteen years before Hershey began his career. Phages are viruses that reproduce by preying on bacteria, first attacking and then dissolving them. For scientists who study bacteria, phages are a source of irritation because they can destroy bacterial cultures. But other scientists are fascinated by this tiny organism. Perhaps the smallest living thing, phages consist of little more than the protein and DNA (the molecule of heredity) found in a cellular **nucleus.**

By studying viral replication, scientists hoped to learn more about the viral diseases that attack humans, like **mumps,** the common **cold,** German **measles,** and polio. But the study of bacteriophages also promised findings with implications that reached far beyond disease cures into the realm of understanding life itself. If Hershey and other researchers could determine how phages replicated, they stood to learn how higher organisms—including humans—passed genetic information from generation to generation.

Hershey's study of phages soon yielded several discoveries that furthered an understanding of genetic inheritance and change. In 1945, he showed that phages were capable of spontaneous mutation. Faced with a bacterial **culture** known to be resistant to phage attack, most, but not all, phages would die. By mutating, some phages survived to attack the bacteria and replicate. This finding was significant because it showed that **mutations** did not occur gradually, as one school of scientific thought believed, but immediately and spontaneously in viruses. It also helped explain why a viral attack is so difficult to prevent. In 1946, Hershey made another discovery that changed what scientists thought about viruses. He showed that if different strains of phages infected the same bacterial cell, they could combine or exchange genetic material. This is similar to what occurs when higher forms of life sexually reproduce, of course. But it was the first time viruses were shown to combine genetic material. Hershey called this phenomenon genetic **recombination.**

Hershey was not the only scientist who saw the potential in working with bacteriophages. Two other influential scientists were also pursuing the same line of investigation. Max Delbrück, a physicist, had been studying phages in the United States since he fled Nazi Germany in 1937. Studying genetic recombination independently of Hershey, he reached the same results that Hershey did in the same year. Similarly, Salvador Edward Luria, a biologist and physician who immigrated to the United States from Italy in 1940, had independently confirmed Hershey's work on spontaneous mutation in 1945. Although the three men never worked side by side in the same laboratory, they were collaborators nonetheless. Through conversation and correspondence, they shared results and encouraged each other in their phage research. Indeed, these three scientists formed the core of the self-declared "phage group," a loose-knit clique of scientists who encouraged research on

particular strains of bacteriophage. By avoiding competition and duplication, the group hoped to advance phage research that much faster.

In 1950, Hershey accepted a position as a staff scientist in the department of genetics (now the Genetics Research Unit) of the Carnegie Institute at Cold Spring Harbor, New York. It was at Cold Spring Harbor that Hershey conducted his most influential experiment. Hershey wished to prove conclusively that the genetic material in phages was DNA. Analysis with an **electron microscope** had showed that phages consist only of DNA surrounded by a protein shell. Other scientists' experiments had revealed that during replication some part of the parental phages was being transferred to their offspring. The task before Hershey was to show that it was the phage DNA that was passed on to succeeding generations and that gave the signal for replication and growth.

With Martha Chase, Hershey found a way to determine what role each of the phage components played in replication. In experiments done in 1951 and 1952, Hershey used radioactive phosphorus to tag the DNA and radioactive sulfur to tag the protein. (The DNA contains no sulfur and the protein contains no phosphorus.) Hershey and Chase then allowed the marked phage particles to infect a bacterial culture and to begin the process of replication. This process was interrupted when the scientists spun the culture at a high speed in a blender.

In this manner, Hershey and Chase learned that the shearing action of the blender separated the phage protein from the bacterial cells. Apparently while the phage DNA entered the bacterium and forced it to start replicating phage particles, the phage protein remained outside, attached to the cell wall. The researchers surmised that the phage particle attached itself to the outside of a bacterium by its protein "tail" and literally injected its nucleic acid into the cell. DNA, and not protein, was responsible for communicating the genetic information needed to produce the next generation of phage.

In 1953, a year after Hershey's blender experiment, the structure of DNA was determined in Cambridge, England, by James Dewey Watson and Francis Harry Compton Crick. Watson, who was only twenty-five years old when the structure was announced, had worked with Luria at the University of Indiana. For their discovery of DNA's double-helix structure, Watson and Crick received the Nobel Prize in 1962.

Hershey, Delbrück, and Luria also received a Nobel Prize for their contributions to molecular biology, but not until 1969. This seeming delay in recognition for their accomplishments prompted the *New York Times* to ask in an October 20, 1969, editorial: "Delbrück, Hershey and Luria richly deserve their awards, but why did they have to wait so long for this recognition? Every person associated with molecular biology knows that these are the grand pioneers of the field, the giants on whom others—some of whom received the Nobel Prize years ago—depended for their own great achievements." Yet other scientists observed that the blender experiment merely offered experimental proof of a theoretical belief that was already widely held. After the blender experiment, Hershey continued investigating the structure of phage DNA. Although human DNA winds double-stranded like a spiral staircase, Hershey found that some phage DNA is single-stranded and some is circular. In 1962, Hershey was named director of the Genetics Research Unit at Cold Spring Harbor. He retired in 1974.

Hershey was "known to his colleagues as a quiet man who avoids crowds and noise and most hectic social activities," according to the report of the 1969 Nobel Prize in the 17 October 1969 *New York Times*. His hobbies were woodworking, reading, gardening, and sailing. He married Harriet Davidson, a former research assistant, in 1945. She later became an editor of the *Cold Spring Harbor Symposia on Quantitative Biology*. Hershey and his wife had one son. Hershey died at his home in Syosset, New York, at age 89.

See also Bacteriophage and bacteriophage typing; Molecular biology and molecular genetics; Viral genetics

HETEROTROPHIC BACTERIA

Heterotrophic cells must ingest biomass to obtain their energy and nutrition. In direct contrast, autotrophs are capable of assimilating diffuse, inorganic energy and materials, and using these to synthesize biochemicals. Green plants, for example, use sunlight and simple inorganic molecules to photosynthesize organic matter. All heterotrophs have an absolute dependence on the biological products of autotrophs for their sustenance—they have no other source of nourishment.

All animals are heterotrophs, as are most **microorganisms** (the major exceptions being microscopic algae and blue-green **bacteria**). Heterotrophs can be classified according to the sorts of biomass that they eat. Animals that eat living plants are known as herbivores, while those that eat other animals are known as carnivores. Many animals eat both plants and animals, and these are known as omnivores. Animal **parasites** are a special type of carnivore that are usually much smaller than their prey, and do not usually kill the animals that they feed upon.

Heterotrophic microorganisms mostly feed upon dead plants and animals, and are known as decomposers. Some animals also specialize on feeding on dead organic matter, and are known as scavengers or detritivores. Even a few vascular plants are heterotrophic, parasitizing the roots of other plants and thereby obtaining their own nourishment. These plants, which often lack **chlorophyll**, are known as saprophytes.

Heterotrophic bacteria, therefore, are largely responsible for the process of organic matter decomposition. Many pathogenic (disease-causing) bacteria are heterotrophs. However, many species of heterotrophic bacteria are also abundant in the environment and are considered normal flora for human skin. The recycling of minerals in aquatic ecosystems, especially in estuaries, is also made possible by heterotrophic bacteria. Although monitored by health officials, the presence of heterotrophic bacteria in public water supplies is seldom considered a **public health** threat.

See also Autotrophic bacteria

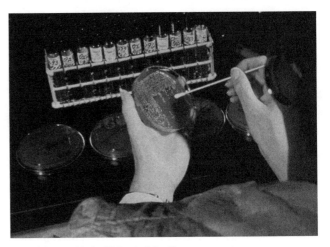

Technician working with bacterial cultures.

HETEROTROPHIC PLATE COUNT · *see*

LABORATORY TECHNIQUES IN MICROBIOLOGY

HIGH EFFICIENCY PARTICULATE AIR (HEPA) FILTER · *see* FUME HOOD

HISTAMINE

Histamine is a hormone that is chemically similar to the hormones serotonine, epinephrine, and norepinephrine. A hormone is generally defined as a chemical produced by a certain cell or tissue that causes a specific biological change or activity to occur in another cell or tissue located elsewhere in the body. Specifically, histamine plays a role in localized immune responses and in allergic reactions.

A select population of cells located in the brain manufactures histamine. After being made, the hormone is stored in a number of cells (e.g., mast cells, basophils, enterochromaffin cells).

Normally, there is a low level of histamine circulating in the body. However, the release of histamine can be triggered by an event such as a mosquito bite. Histamine causes the inconvenient redness, swelling and itching associated with the bite. For those with severe **allergies**, the sudden and more generalized release of histamine can be fatal (e.g., anaphylactic shock).

Mast cell histamine has an important role in the reaction of the **immune system** to the presence of a compound to which the body has developed an allergy. When released from mast cells in a reaction to a material to which the immune system is allergic, the hormone causes blood vessels to increase in diameter (e.g., vasodilation) and to become more permeable to the passage of fluid across the vessel wall. These effects are apparent as a runny nose, sneezing, and watery eyes. Other symptoms can include itching, burning and swelling in the skin, headaches, plugged sinuses, stomach cramps, and diarrhea. Histamine can also be released into the lungs, where it causes the air passages to become constricted rather than dilated. This response occurs in an attempt to keep the offending allergenic particles from being inhaled. Unfortunately, this also makes breathing difficult. An example of such an effect of histamine occurs in asthma.

Histamine has also been shown to function as a neurotransmitter (a chemical that facilitates the transmission of impulses from one neural cell to an adjacent neural cell).

In cases of an extreme allergic reaction, adrenaline is administered to eliminate histamine from the body. For minor allergic reactions, symptoms can sometimes be lessened by the use of antihistamines that block the binding of histamine to a receptor molecule.

See also Immune system

HISTOCOMPATIBILITY

Histocompatibility refers to the means by which a eukaryotic cell can be identified. The phenomenon is the result of the presence of proteins on the surface of cells. These proteins are referred to as histocompatibility molecules. The histocompatibility molecules on the cells of one individual of a species are unique. Thus, if the cell is transplanted into another person, the cell will be recognized by the **immune system** as being foreign. The histocompatibility molecules act as an antigen in the recipient, and so can also be called a histocompatibility antigen or transplantation antigen. This is the basis of the rejection of transplanted material.

Identical twins have the same histocompatibility molecules on their cells. Thus, tissue can be successfully transplanted from one individual to the other, because the tissue will essentially not be foreign. However, for unrelated individuals, cells will have their own signature chemistry with respect to the histocompatibility molecules. Tissue from one individual will be recognized as foreign in another individual.

The suite of histocompatibility molecules present on the surface of a cell is also referred to as the histocompatibility complex. There are two classes of these molecules. The first class is called class I molecules. These molecules are made up of a portion that is embedded in the cell membrane and a portion that protrudes out from the membrane's outer surface. The protruding portion is composed of both protein and sugar (carbohydrate). Some of the human leukocyte antigens are examples of class I molecules.

The class I molecules function to chemically tag a cell so that the cell will be recognized and categorized by the T lymphocyte cells of the immune system. The T cell will recognize a region of the histocompatibility complex as "self." Because of this recognition, there will not be an immune response initiated against the cell. But, in another host, where the same region is chemically different from class I groups on the host cells, the introduced cells would be recognized as foreign by the T lymphocytes.

Another class of histocompatibility molecules called class II are anchored into the cell membrane by have two segments of the molecule. At the outer surface of the cell the mol-

ecule contains an antigen that has been acquired from the surrounding environment when particles were taken in and degraded by host processes. This is called antigen presentation.

Class II molecules are on the surface of macrophages and B-lymphocytes. These immune cells function to process cells and present the antigens from these cells to T lymphocytes. This is done to increase the repertoire of antibodies that an organism possesses. Antigen presentation of histocompatibility molecules "primes" the immune system. When an invading organism is detected, the immune response can occur much more swiftly than if no exposure to the antigen had ever occurred.

The role of the histocompatibility complexes in immune recognition of "self " and "non-self" is the reason why transplants are typically accompanied by the administration of drugs that dampen down the immune response of the host. Only by nullifying the host recognition of the class I and class II histocompatibility complexes can the transplant be maintained.

The genes that encode the histocompatibility determinants are clustered together on the chromosome. These clusters are referred to as the major and minor histocompatibility complexes. The major compatibility genes are clustered together on one chromosome. The minor compatibility genes are located in several clusters throughout the genome.

Studies on mice, which also possess the histocompatibility complexes, have demonstrated that these complexes not only play a role in transplant rejection, but also function in the immune response to a variety of diseases. Mice that are genetically different for a given histocompatibility complex will respond differently to the same antigen. If a "non-self" histocompatibility complex is poorly recognized by the host immune system, then an inadequate immune response will ensue. The result can be the establishment of an infection.

See also Antibody and antigen; Immune system; Immunodeficiency diseases; Major histocompatibility complex (MHC)

HISTORY OF IMMUNOLOGY

In Western society, it was not until the late eighteenth century that a rational approach to the origin of disease developed. Prior to the discovery that disease was the result of pathogenic organisms, it was commonly accepted that disease was a punishment from God (or the Gods), or even a witches curse. Eastern cultures perceived disease as an imbalance in the energy channels within the body. Later, the great plagues of Europe were assumed the result of virulent or noxious vapors. Nevertheless, there were intimations as early as 430 B.C. that if one survived a disease, the person thereafter became "immune" to any subsequent exposures. However, this was never recognized as evidence of some type of internal defense system until the later part of the seventeenth century.

Although most historical accounts credit **Edward Jenner** for the development of the first **immunization** process, a previous similar procedure had become established in China by 1700. The technique was called variolation. This was derived from the name of the infective agent—the **variola virus**. The basic principal of variolation was to deliberately cause a mild infection with unmodified pathogen. The risk of death from variolation was around two to three percent. Although still a risk, variolation was a considerable improvement on the death rate for uncontrolled infection. **Immunity** to **smallpox** was conferred by inserting the dried exudate of smallpox pustules into the nose. This technique for the transfer of smallpox, as a form of limited infection, traveled to the west from China along the traditional trade routes to Constantinople where it spread throughout Europe. Hearing of this practice, the Royal family of England had their children inoculated against the disease in 1721, but the practice aroused severe opposition as physicians felt it was far too risky.

In 1798, Edward Jenner, noticed that milkmaids were protected from smallpox if they had been first infected with **cowpox**. It was not his intention to make medical history, as his interests were mostly scholarly and involved the transfer of infections from one species to another, especially from animals to humans. However, Jenner's work led him to the conclusion, that inoculation with cowpox (a bovine analogue of smallpox) could confer immunity to smallpox. Thus, the concept of **vaccination** was initiated. (Incidentally, the Latin word for cow is *vacca*). Jenner's ideas first made him a medical as well as a social pariah, as they were in opposition to both the church and popular beliefs. Because his method was much safer then variolation, however, the use of vaccinations gradually became widely accepted and most European countries had some form of compulsory program within fifty years of Jenner's discovery.

The idea that a pathogenic organism caused disease was not fully realized until certain technological advances had occurred. Initially, **Antoni van Leeuwenhoek**'s development of the **microscope** and the subsequent realization that entities existed that were not visible to the human eye, allowed the concept of germs to be appreciated. That these organisms were the causative agent of disease was not recognized until **Louis Pasteur** developed his **germ theory of disease**. His original interests were in **fermentation** in wine and beer, and he was the first to isolate the organisms that caused the fermentation process. Pasteur's work eventually led him to the development of **pasteurization** (heating) as a means of halting fermentation. While working with silk worms and **anthrax**, he was able to demonstrate that the same method for transferring the fermentation process also worked in transmitting disease from infected animals to unaffected animals. Finally, in 1878, Pasteur accidentally used an attenuated (weakened) chicken cholera **culture** and realized, when he repeated the experiment using a fresh culture, that the weakened form protected the chickens from the virulent form of the disease. Pasteur went on to develop an attenuated **vaccine** against **rabies** and swine erysipelas.

Pasteur was not the only proponent of the germ theory of disease. His chief competitor was **Robert Koch**. Koch was the first to isolate the anthrax microbe and, unaware of Pasteur's work, he was able to show that it caused the disease. Then in 1882, Koch was able to demonstrate that the germ theory of disease applied to human ailments as well as animals, when he isolated the microbe that caused **tuberculosis**. His "Koch's postulates" are still used to identify infective organisms.

Much of the basis for modern medicine, as well as the field of **immunology**, can be traced back to these two scientists, but the two major questions still to be answered were how did infection cause the degradation of tissue, and how did vaccines work? The first question was addressed in 1881 by **Emile Roux** and Alexander Yersin when they isolated a soluble toxin from **diphtheria** cultures. Later, **Emil von Behring** and **Shibasaburo Kitasato** were able to demonstrate passive immunity when they took serum from animals infected with diphtheria and injected into healthy animals. These same animals were found to be resistant to the disease. Eventually these serum factors were recognized in 1930 as antibodies. However, thirty years before antibodies were finally isolated and identified, **Paul Ehrlich** and others, recognized that a specific antigen elicited the production of a specific **antibody**. Ehrlich hypothesized that these antibodies were specialized molecular structures with specific receptor sites that fit each pathogen like a lock and key. Thus, the first realization that the body had a specific defense system was introduced. In addition, sometime later, he realized that this powerful effector mechanism, used in host defense would, if turned against the host, cause severe tissue damage. Ehrlich termed this *horror autotoxicus*. Although extremely valuable, his work still left a large gap in understanding how the **immune system** fights a pathogenic challenge. The idea that specific cells could be directly involved with defending the body was first suggested in 1884 by **Élie Metchnikoff**. His field was zoology and he studied **phagocytosis** in single cell organisms. Metchnikoff postulated that vertebrates could operate in a similar manner to remove pathogens. However, it was not until the 1940s that his theories were accepted and the cell mediated, as opposed to the humoral, immune response was recognized.

The clarification of the immune response and the science of immunology did not progress in a systematic or chronological order. Nonetheless, once scientists had a basic understanding of the cellular and humoral branches of the immune system, what remained was the identification of the various components of this intricate system, and the mechanisms of their interactions. This could not have been accomplished without the concomitant development of **molecular biology** and genetics.

Milestones in the history of immunology include:

1798 Edward Jenner initiates smallpox vaccination.

1877 Paul Erlich recognizes mast cells.

1879 Louis Pasteur develops an attenuated chicken cholera vaccine.

1883 Elie Metchnikoff develops cellular theory of vaccination.

1885 Louis Pasteur develops rabies vaccine.

1891 Robert Koch explored delayed type hypersensitivity.

1900 Paul Erlich theorizes specific antibody formation.

1906 Clemens von Pirquet coined the word allergy.

1938 John Marrack formulates antigen-antibody binding hypothesis.

1942 Jules Freund and Katherine McDermott research

adjuvants.

1949 Macfarlane Burnet & Frank Fenner formulate immunological tolerance hypothesis.

1959 Niels Jerne, David Talmage, Macfarlane Burnet develop clonal **selection** theory.

1957 Alick Isaacs & Jean Lindemann discover interferon (cytokine).

1962 Rodney Porter and team discovery the structure of antibodies.

1962 Jaques Miller and team discover thymus involvement in cellular immunity.

1962 Noel Warner and team distinguish between cellular and humoral immune responses.

1968 Anthony Davis and team discover T cell and B cell cooperation in immune response.

1974 Rolf Zinkernagel and Peter Doherty explore **major histocompatibility complex** restriction.

1985 Susumu Tonegawa, Leroy Hood, and team identify immunoglobulin genes.

1987 Leroy Hood and team identify genes for the T cell receptor.

1985 Scientists begin the rapid identification of genes for immune cells that continues to the present.

See also Antibody and antigen; B cells or B lymphocytes; Germ theory of disease; History of the development of antibiotics; History of public health; Immunity, active, passive and delayed; Immunity, cell mediated; Immunity, humoral regulation; Infection and resistance; T cells or T-lymphocytes

HISTORY OF MICROBIOLOGY

Microbiology was born in 1674 when **Antoni van Leeuwenhoek** (1632–1723), a Dutch drapery merchant, peered at a drop of lake water through a carefully ground glass lens. Through this he beheld the first glimpse of the microbial world. Perhaps more than any other science, the development of microbiology depended on the invention and improvement of a tool, the **microscope**. Since **bacteria** cannot be seen individually with the unaided eye, their existence as individuals can only be known through microscopic observations. Indeed, it is interesting to speculate on how microbiology might have developed if the limits of resolution of the microscope were poorer.

The practical and scientific aspects of microbiology have been closely woven from the very beginning. Perhaps it is for this reason that microbiology as a field of study did not really develop until the twentieth century. Nineteenth century "microbiologists" were chemists and physicians and a few were botanists. At that stage, the science of microbes was developing to solve very practical problems in two clear scientific fields, the science of **fermentation** and in medicine.

Although medicine and fermentation presented the practical problems that stimulated the development of microbiology, the first studies that put the subject on a scientific basis arose from a problem of pure science. This was the con-

troversy over spontaneous generation. Although the crude ideas of spontaneous generation (e.g., maggots from meat) were dispelled by Francesco Redi (1626?–1698?) in the seventeenth century, more subtle ideas such as that **protozoa** and bacteria can arise from vegetable and animal infusions, were still accepted in the nineteenth century. The controversy also involved fermentations, since it was considered that the **yeast** fermentation was of spontaneous origin.

Many workers became involved in the study of fermentation and spontaneous generation, but **Louis Pasteur** (1822–1895) stands out as a giant. He came into biology from the field of chemistry and was apparently able to remove all the philosophical hurdles that blocked the thinking of others. Within a period of four years after he began his studies, he had clarified the problems of spontaneous generation so well that the controversy died a natural death.

Pasteur was also able to go easily from fermentation into the field of medical microbiology, which occupied the later part of his life. His contributions in that field were numerous, and his work in fields such as microbial attenuation and **vaccination** has been the basis of many modern medical practices. It should be emphasized that the development of **sterilization** methods by researchers such as Pasteur and John Tyndall (1820–1893), so necessary to the solution of the spontaneous generation controversy, were essential to put the science of microbiology on a firm foundation. The workers did not set out to develop these methods, but they evolved as a bonus that was received for solving the spontaneous generation question.

Other important developments were in medicine. The microbiological aspects of medicine arose out of considerations of the nature of contagious disease. Although the phenomenon of contagion, especially with respect to diseases such as **smallpox**, was recognized far back in antiquity, its nature and relationship to **microorganisms** was not understood. It was probably the introduction of **syphilis** into Europe, which served to crystallize thinking as here was a disease that could only be transmitted by contact and helped to formulate the question, what is being transmitted? Gerolamo Fracastoro (1478–1553) gave syphilis its name in the sixteenth century and came close to devising a **germ theory of disease**, an idea that later attracted a number of workers all the way down to the nineteenth century. By the late 1830s, Schwann and Cagniard-Latour had shown that alcoholic fermentation and putrefaction were due to living, organized beings. If one accepted the fact that the decomposition of organic materials was due to living organisms, it was only a step further to reason that disease, which in many ways appears as the decomposition of body tissues, was due to living agents. Jacob Henle, in 1840, further commented on this similarity and with the newfound knowledge on the nature of fermentation, he proceeded to draw rather clear conclusions also saying that experimental proof would be required to clinch this hypothesis. That evidence came later from **Robert Koch** provided, in 1867, the final evidence proving the germ theory. He established the etiologic role of bacteria in **anthrax** and as a result proposed a set of rules to be followed in the establishment of etiology. The key to Koch's observation was the isolation of

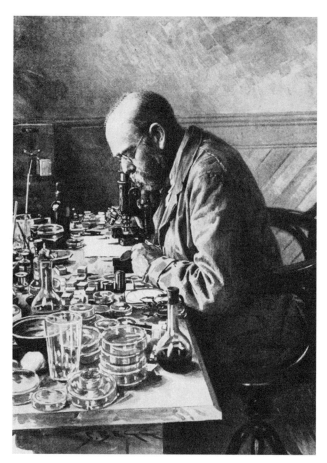

Robert Koch in his laboratory in the late nineteenth century.

the organism in pure **culture**. While limiting dilutions could have been used (as described previously by **Joseph Lister**, 1827–1912), Koch promoted the use of solid media, giving rise to separate colonies and the use of stains. In 1882, Koch identified the tubercle bacillus and so formalized the criteria of Henle for distinguishing causative pathogenic microbes. This set of criteria is known as **Koch's postulates**.

One of the most important applied developments in microbiology was in understanding the nature of specific acquired **immunity** to disease. That such immunity was possible was known for a long time, and the knowledge finally crystallized with the prophylactic treatment for smallpox introduced by **Edward Jenner** (1749–1823). Using **cowpox**, Jenner introduced the first vaccination procedures in 1796. This occurred long before the germ theory of disease had been established. Later workers developed additional methods of increasing the immunity of an individual to disease, but the most dramatic triumph was the discovery of the **diphtheria** and **tetanus** antitoxins by von Behring and Kitisato in the 1890s. This work later developed into a practical tool by **Paul Ehrlich** (1854–1915) and it was now possible to cure a person suffering from these diseases by injecting some antitoxic serum prepared by earlier **immunization** of a horse or other large animal. This led for the first time to rational cures for infectious dis-

eases, and was responsible for Ehrlich's later conception of **chemotherapy**. The **antibiotics** era, which followed the groundbreaking work of **Alexander Fleming** (1881–1955) with **penicillin**, was another important step in the understanding of microbiology.

Most of the most recent work in the development of microbiology has been in the field of **microbial genetics** and how it evolved into a separate discipline known as **molecular biology**. This work really began in the 1940s, when **Oswald Avery, Colin MacLeod** and **Maclyn McCarty** demonstrated that the transforming principle in bacteria, previously observed by Frederick Griffiths in 1928, was **DNA**. **Joshua Lederberg** and **Edward Tatum** demonstrated that DNA could be transferred from one bacterium to another in 1944. With the determination of the structure of DNA in 1953, a new and practical aspect of microbiology suddenly became realised, and the foundations of genetic engineering were laid. It is perhaps important to realize that if it were not for bacteria and their characteristics, genetic engineering would not be possible. The concept of DNA transfer was essentially born in the 1940s. Later on, in the late 1960s bacterial **restriction enzymes** were discovered and the possibilities of splicing and rearranging DNA emerged. The advances in molecular biology following these major breakthroughs have been immense but it is important to realize that the field of microbiology lies at their root.

See also Antibiotics; Fermentation; Microscope and microscopy; Vaccine

HISTORY OF PUBLIC HEALTH

Infections caused by **microorganisms** are often spread more easily in an unsanitary environment. Even today, for example, *Escherichia coli* infections of food and between people are still commonly caused by poor hygienic practices, such as the failure to properly wash hands after toileting.

Because of the association between microbial infection and sanitary conditions, many **public health** initiatives and regulations have been instituted around the world. Before the recognition that microbes caused infections, and even before the realization that microbes existed, public health was a foreign concept. The history of public health parallels advances in the understanding of microorganisms and disease.

Prior to the fourteenth century, public health was nonexistent. The sanitary environment in urban centers was appalling by today's standards. However, at that time there was no knowledge that, for example, the flow of raw sewage alongside streets was connected to illness. The occurrence of **bubonic plague** in Europe in 1348 began to change this view. Between 1348 and 1350, the infection caused by *Yersinia pestis* killed almost two-thirds of the population in the major urban centers of Europe. In the aftermath of this devastation came an increased awareness of the influence of health conditions and disease. In the 1350s, Italian government initiatives sought to improve sanitary and living conditions. These initiatives occurred even though the existence of microorganisms was not

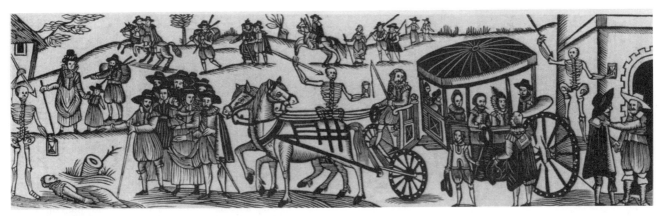

The scourge of epidemics.

yet known. By the sixteenth century, the idea of a microbial cause of disease (e.g., "contagion") was being debated.

In the United States, the organized public health initiative that is today's Public Health Service began in the late eighteenth century. Legislation passed by the United States Congress in 1798 provided care and relief for afflicted mariners. Hospitals to serve seamen were established on the eastern seaboard and later in cities on the Great Lakes, Gulf coast and Pacific coast. In 1870, the control of these hospitals became the responsibility of the newly formed Marine Hospital Service, headquartered in Washington, DC.

Because mariners were often the carriers of infectious diseases acquired in other countries, the Marine Hospital Service soon became concerned with infectious diseases. In 1887, a small bacteriology laboratory (the Hygienic Laboratory) was created at a marine hospital on Staten Island in the New York harbor. The laboratory was later relocated to Washington, DC, where it became the National Institutes of Health.

The increasing responsibility for infectious disease treatment and research prompted a name change of the organization to the Public Health and Marine Service (1902) and the Public Health Service (1912). In the twentieth century, the services' role in controlling infectious microbial diseases and funding infectious disease research expanded. For example, among the agencies that comprise the Public Health Service are the **Centers for Disease Control**, the National Institutes of Health, and the Food and Drug Administration. Approximately 60,000 people are employees of the Public Health Service, whose annual budget now exceeds 15 billion dollars.

As the public health infrastructure was growing in the nineteenth century, public health nursing was also growing in the United States. In 1898, Los Angeles became the first city to employ a nurse to care for sick people in their homes. Thereafter, more governments recognized that caring for the populace in the homes and workplaces had a positive effect on the society as a whole, in terms of reducing the spread of infectious diseases.

During the nineteenth century, microbiologists such as **Louis Pasteur** and **Robert Koch** demonstrated the involvement of **bacteria** in disease. The importance of maintaining a hygienic atmosphere in hospitals was recognized. Indeed,

Joseph Lister's implementation of the use of a disinfectant spray and fresh changes of operating smocks for surgeons greatly decreased the mortality rate associated with operations. Because of these public health efforts, operations moved from a position of last resort to a procedure that could improve the health and alleviate suffering in people.

The increasing disparity between the developed and underdeveloped countries of the world spawned major international public health efforts in the twenty-first century. The most prominent example is the **World Health Organization (WHO)**, created in 1948. Other agencies are noteworthy as well, such as the United Nations International Children's Emergency Fund (UNICEF), which was created in 1946 to aid children victimized by World War II.

At the time of the creation of UNICEF and the WHO, the average life expectancy in the world was 46 years. As of the late 1990s, this average life expectancy had risen to 65 years of age. Much of this increase is attributable to organized public health initiatives such as **vaccination**, medical care and hydration programs.

The recognition of the involvement of microorganisms and disease has continued to the present day. Since the 1970s, a series of microbiologically related diseases (i.e., Acquired **Immunodeficiency** Syndrome) has prompted renewed emphasis on public health. Other diseases that were thought to be due to a genetic or physiological abnormality (e.g., stomach ulcers, heart disease) have been demonstrated to be at least partially due to chronic bacterial infections. Lessening the chances of exposure to such infectious agents has become another public health concern.

Another watershed in the history of public health has occurred in the latter decades of the twenty-first century. Then, the importance of the adherent bacterial populations known as biofilms to the establishment and maintenance of long-lasting infections that are extremely resistant to treatments became known. **Biofilms** are important in environments ranging from the operating room to the drinking water treatment plant. This importance has focused public health efforts on the prevention of biofilm build-up and on the creation of strategies that eliminate the biofilm bacteria.

See also AIDS; Bacteria and bacterial infection; Epidemics and pandemics; Infection control; Public health, current issues

HISTORY OF THE DEVELOPMENT OF ANTIBIOTICS

The great modern advances in **chemotherapy** have come from the chance discovery that many **microorganisms** synthesize and excrete compounds that are selectively toxic to other microorganisms. These compounds are called **antibiotics** and have revolutionized medicine. The period since World War II has seen the establishment and extremely rapid growth of a major industry, using microorganisms for the synthesis of, amongst other compounds, chemotherapeutic agents. The development of this industry has had a dramatic and far-reaching impact. Nearly all bacterial infectious diseases that were, prior to the antibiotic era, major causes of human death have been brought under control by the use of chemotherapeutic drugs, including antibiotics. In the United States, bacterial infection is now a less frequent cause of death than suicide or traffic accidents.

The first chemotherapeutically effective antibiotic was discovered in 1929 by **Alexander Fleming** (1881–1955), a British bacteriologist, who had long been interested in the treatment of wound infections. On returning from a vacation in the countryside, he noticed among a pile of petri dishes on his bench one that had been streaked with a **culture** of *Saphyloccocus aureus* which was also contaminated by a single **colony** of **mold**. As Fleming observed the plate, he noted that the colonies immediately surrounding the mold were transparent and appeared to by undergoing lysis. He reasoned that the mould was excreting into the medium a chemical that caused the surrounding colonies to lyse. Sensing the possible chemotherapeutic significance of his observation, Fleming isolated the mold, which proved to be a species of *Penicillium,* and established that culture filtrates contained an antibacterial substance, which he called **penicillin.**

Although it has often been suggested that many bacteriologists must have observed petri dishes that were similarly contaminated and therefore similar in appearance to Fleming's dish, such speculation is undoubtedly false. As subsequent experiments have shown, a highly unusual series of events must have occurred in order to produce the results seen on Fleming's plate: **contamination** must have occurred at the time the plate was streaked with **bacteria** (prior growth of either would have prevented growth of the other in the immediate vicinity); the inoculated petri dish must not have been incubated (if it had been the bacterium would have outgrown the mold); the room temperature of the laboratory must have been below 68°F [20° C] (a temperature that probably did occur during a brief cold storm in London in the summer of 1928).

Penicillin proved to be chemically unstable and Fleming was unable to purify it. Working with impure preparations, he demonstrated its remarkable effectiveness in inhibiting the growth of many Gram-positive bacteria, and he even used it with success for the local treatment of human **eye infections**.

In the meantime, the chemotherapeutic effectiveness of other, non-antibiotic compounds such as sulfonamides had been discovered, and Fleming, discouraged by the difficulties in purifying penicillin, abandoned further work on the problem.

Ten years later a group of British scientists headed by **H.W. Florey** (1898–1968) and **E. Chain** (1906–1979) resumed the study of penicillin. Clinical trials with partly purified material were dramatically successful. By this time, however, Britain was at war; and the industrial development of penicillin was undertaken in the United States, where an intensive program of research and development was begun in many laboratories. Within three years, penicillin was being produced on an industrial scale. Today it remains one of the most effective chemotherapeutic agents for the treatment of many bacterial infections.

Rather than being a single substance, penicillin turned out to be a class of compounds. The various penicillins vary with respect to the chemical composition of their side chain. The penicillin that was first isolated in Peoria, Illinois, designated penicillin G, carried a benzyl side chain. The penicillin isolated soon after in England, designated penicillin F, carried an isopentanyl side chain. By varying the composition of the fungal growth media, a variety of penicillins collectively termed biosynthetic penicillins, have been synthesized. Penicillin G proved the most successful and later it became possible to remove the side chain and replace it by a variety of chemical substituents, thereby producing semisynthetic penicillins. For example, penicillin V is resistant to acid and therefore can be administered orally because it is not inactivated in the stomach; ampicillin is also acid resistant and also effective against enteric bacteria; oxacillin is resistant to the action of B-lactamase, the enzyme produced by certain "penicillin-resistant" strains of bacteria.

The remarkable chemotherapeutic efficacy of penicillin for certain bacterial infections, primarily those caused by Gram-positive bacteria, prompted intensive research into new antibiotics. In the 1940s, a second clinically important antibiotic, streptomycin, effective against both Gram-negative bacteria and *Mycobacterium tuberculosis,* was discovered by A. Schatz and **S. Waksman**. This was the first example of a broad-spectrum antibiotic. Other antibiotics with even broader spectra of activity, such as the tetracyclines, were subsequently discovered. The search for new antibiotics remains an empirical enterprise. So far, they have proved very effective as antibacterial agents, although some bacteria do acquire resistance to antibiotics, so there is a continuous search for new and effective antibacterial agents. Antibiotics have proved less effective in the treatment of fungal infections. Antifungal antibiotics, such as nystatin and amphoterecin B are considerably less successful therapeutically than their bacterial counterparts, at least in part because their toxicity is far less selective. There are no known antiviral antibiotics.

Since 1945, thousands of different antibiotics produced by **fungi**, actinomycetes or unicellular bacteria have been isolated and characterized. A small fraction of these are of therapeutic value. Their nomenclature is complicated as one antibiotic may be sold under several different names. For example in the United States the compound, which in Europe

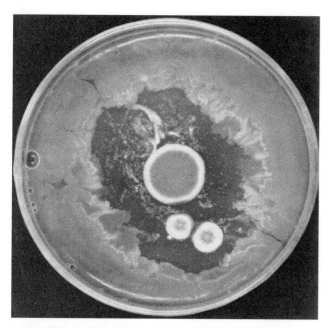

Photograph of the original culture plate of the fungus *Penicillum notatum* made by the Scottish bacteriologist Alexander Fleming in 1928.

has the generic name rifampicin, is called rifampin. Its proper chemical class name is rifamycin and it is also sold under the trade names Rifactin and Rifadin, among others.

See also Bacteria and bacterial infection; Fungicide; History of microbiology; History of public health; Streptococci and streptococcal infections; Sulfa drugs

HIV · *see* Human immunodeficiency virus (HIV)

Hobby, Gladys Lounsbury (1910-1993)
American microbiologist

Gladys Lounsbury Hobby was one of the few women who were part of the extensive network that brought **penicillin** from the laboratory to the clinic. Discovered by Sir **Alexander Fleming** in 1928, penicillin was one of the first **antibiotics**. In her book, *Penicillin: Meeting the Challenge,* Hobby detailed the efforts in the early 1940s to discover a way to manufacture large amounts of penicillin, which would greatly aid in the treating of war wounded. In addition to her work as a microbiologist, Hobby wrote many articles and was a teacher.

Hobby was born November 19, 1910, in New York City. She received her Bachelor of Arts degree from Vassar College in 1931; she then attended Columbia University, receiving her master's degree in 1932 and her doctorate in bacteriology three years later. From 1934 to 1943, she worked on perfecting penicillin specifically for several infectious diseases as

part of a research team at the Columbia Medical School, while also being professionally involved at Presbyterian Hospital in New York City. In 1944, Hobby went to work for Pfizer Pharmaceuticals in New York, where she researched streptomycin and other antibiotics, discovering how antimicrobial drugs worked. In 1959, Hobby became chief of research at the Veteran's Administration Hospital in East Orange, New Jersey, where she worked on chronic infectious diseases. Before retiring in 1977, she was assistant research clinical professor in **public health** at Cornell Medical College.

Retirement for Hobby meant continuing her work. Hobby became a freelance science writer and a consultant. It was during this time that she penned her book, *Penicillin: Meeting the Challenge,* about the drug's odyssey from the laboratory to the hands of the clinician. Hobby, having taken meticulous notes, detailed each researcher's contribution to producing a safe penicillin on a large scale basis. She also authored more than two hundred articles and was the founder and editor of the journal *Antimicrobial Agents and Chemotherapy.*

Hobby was a member of several professional organizations, including the American Association for the Advancement of Science, the American Academy of Microbiology, and the American Society of Microbiology. Hobby died suddenly of a heart attack on July 4, 1993, at her home in Pennsylvania.

See also History of the development of antibiotics

HOLDFAST · *see* Caulobacter

Hooke, Robert (1635-1703)
English physicist

One of the preeminent scientists of the seventeenth century, Robert Hooke is perhaps best remembered for the wide variety of fields to which he contributed, including physics, astronomy, microscopy, biology, and architecture, among others. Although Hooke introduced many concepts previously unimagined or unexamined, his ability to formulate these ideas usually did not match his intuition, and the credit for many scientific breakthroughs inspired by Hooke's ideas is often given to such scientists as Isaac Newton and Christiaan Huygens, who brought the work to its fruition. Still, Hooke remains an important pioneer of science.

Born on Britain's Isle of Wight, Hooke was a sickly child. As a youth, his perpetual ill health made it impossible for him to attend classes regularly, and he was unable to enter the ministry as his father, a minister, had wished. Instead, Hooke was allowed to pursue his interest in mechanics, which he first demonstrated as a small child by constructing elaborate toys. He attended Westminster School and later Oxford, where he became the laboratory assistant to Robert Boyle. It was in Boyle's lab that Hooke's talent for designing scientific instruments was noticed, as he constructed the improved air pump used to establish Boyle's gas laws. In fact, it has been speculated that Hooke himself may have been the author of Boyle's law, since, customarily, any findings from research done in the lab would have been credited to the professor.

Along with some of his colleagues from Oxford and the surrounding area, Hooke helped to establish what would soon become the Royal Society, to which he was appointed Curator of Experiments. During his time as Curator he had many other successes attributed to him such as the compound **microscope**, an improved barometer, the reflecting telescope, and the universal joint.

Although Hooke was not the first to experiment using a microscope, he was the first to dedicate a major intensive volume to microscopy. His 1665 publication *Micrographia* describes the structures of insects, fossils, and plants in unprecedented detail. While studying the porous structure of cork, Hooke noted the presence of tiny rectangular holes that he called cells, a word that has been adopted as the cornerstone of microbiology. *Micrographia* also contains illustrations in Hooke's own hand that remain among the best renderings of microscopic views.

In the years following the great London fire of 1666, Hooke became a surveyor and, eventually, an architect, constructing numerous famous buildings. Because his architectural interests took much time away from his scientific work, he was ultimately forced to retire as Curator of Experiments for the Royal Society in favor of his new vocation.

See also History of microbiology; Microscope and microscopy

HTLV · *see* HUMAN T-CELL LEUKEMIA VIRUS (HTLV)

HUANG, ALICE SHIH-HOU (1939-   )

Chinese-born American microbiologist

Alice Shih-hou Huang's discovery of reverse transcriptase, an enzyme that allows **viruses** to convert their genetic material into **DNA** (**deoxyribonucleic acid**)—the molecular basis of heredity—led to a major breakthrough in understanding how viruses function. Searching for clues on how to prevent viruses from replicating, Huang also isolated a rabies-like virus that produced mutant strains that interfered with viral growth.

The youngest of four children, Huang was born in Kiangsi, China, on March 22, 1939. Her father, the Right Reverend Quentin K. Y. Huang, was the second Chinese bishop ordained by the Anglican Episcopal Ministry in China. Her mother, Grace Betty Soong Huang, undertook a career of her own by entering nursing school at the age of forty-five. In 1949, when communism pervaded China, the Huangs sent their children to the United States, hoping for a more stable life and greater opportunities.

Huang was ten years old when she arrived in the United States. She studied at an Episcopalian boarding school for girls in Burlington, New Jersey, and at the National Cathedral

School in Washington, D.C., and became a United States citizen her senior year in high school. While in China, Huang had seen many people suffering from illness and decided to become a physician. She attended Wellesley College in Massachusetts from 1957 to 1959, and subsequently enrolled in a special program at the Johns Hopkins University School of Medicine, where she earned her B.A. in 1961 and her M.A. in 1963. While at Johns Hopkins, she chose to pursue medicine not as a physician, but as a microbiologist. She published several papers on viruses, including the **herpes** simplex viruses, and earned her Ph.D. from Johns Hopkins in 1966. That same year Huang served as a visiting assistant professor at the National Taiwan University. In 1967, Huang worked as a postdoctoral fellow with **David Baltimore** at the Salk Institute for Biological Studies in San Diego, California. Huang and Baltimore married in 1968; they have one daughter.

Huang and Baltimore took their work to the Massachusetts Institute of Technology in 1968. At the time, scientists understood that the genetic material DNA in cells was converted into **ribonucleic acid** (**RNA**, nucleic acids associated with the control of chemical activities within cells), and then into proteins. But one of the viruses Huang studied had an enzyme that did something different—it made RNA from RNA. The work led to Baltimore's research on **tumor viruses** and his discovery of the enzyme called reverse transcriptase, which threw the usual process in reverse by converting RNA to DNA. Baltimore and American oncologist Howard Temin, who had independently discovered reverse transcriptase, were awarded the Nobel Prize in medicine in 1975 for their work on tumor viruses.

Huang became assistant professor of microbiology and **molecular genetics** at Harvard Medical School in 1971, was promoted to associate professor in 1973, and to full professor in 1979. She also served as an associate at the Boston City Hospital from 1971 to 1973 and director of the infectious diseases laboratory at the Children's Hospital in Boston from 1979 to 1989. Huang studied a rabies-like virus that produced mutant strains, which interfered with further growth of the viral infection. She sought to understand where the **mutants** originated and how they affected the viral population, knowledge she hoped could be applied to halt the spread of viral infections in humans. For this research, Huang was awarded the Eli Lilly Award in Microbiology and **Immunology** in 1977. In 1987, she was appointed trustee of the University of Massachusetts. The following year Huang became president of the American Society for Microbiology, the first Asian American to head a national scientific society in the United States. She is also a member of the American Association for the Advancement of Science, the American Society for **Biochemistry** and **Molecular Biology**, and the Academia Sinica in Taiwan. Huang remained at Harvard until 1991, when she was appointed Dean for Science at New York University.

Though Huang sees her role in administration at New York University as important and necessary, her first love remains basic research. Huang has numerous research publications to her credit, and has served on the editorial boards of *Intervirology, Journal of Virology, Reviews of Infectious Diseases, Microbial Pathogenesis,* and *Journal of Women's*

Health. She became a trustee of Johns Hopkins University in 1992, and joined the council of the Johns Hopkins-Nanjing University Center for Chinese and American Studies in 1993. In addition to her duties as university administrator, scientist, and mother, Huang is an avid reader of mystery novels, and enjoys sailing.

See also Viral genetics; Virology; Virus replication; Viruses and responses to viral infection

HUMAN IMMUNODEFICIENCY VIRUS (HIV)

The Human **Immunodeficiency** Virus (HIV) belongs to a class of **viruses** known as the **retroviruses**. These viruses are known as **RNA** viruses because they have RNA as their basic genetic material instead of **DNA**. The retroviruses are unable to replicate outside of living host cells, because they contain only RNA. However, they have the enzyme reverse transcriptase that can make DNA from the RNA and allow them to integrate into the host cell genome. The retroviruses are composed of three subgroups, two of which are pathogenic to humans. They are the oncarnovirus subgroup and the lentivirus (meaning, slow virus) subgroup. The Human Immunodeficiency Virus, which belongs to the lentivirus subgroup, is further divided into two types based on the diseases they produce. The HIV-1 produces the acquired immunodeficiency syndrome (**AIDS**), while the HIV-2 produces a similar disease that is at present, largely restricted to West Africa.

The genetic material of the HIV virus consists of two short strands of RNA about 9,200 nucleotides long, enclosed in an outer lipid envelope. A viral glycoprotein (gp120) is displayed on the surface of the envelope. This protein recognizes and binds to the CD4 receptor on T-helper cells. The HIV genome contains a long terminal repeat (LTR) and the gag, pol, env, and tax/rex genes. The LTR helps in the integration of the virus into the host cell DNA. The gag **gene** codes for the proteins that make up the outer core or capsid while the env gene codes for the envelope glycoprotein including the outer envelope glycoprotein (gp 120) and the transmembrane glycoprotein (gp141). The major proteins coded by the pol gene are the reverse transcriptase, protease, and the integrase. The tax/rex gene codes for certain factors that have a regulatory role.

The HIV infects cells that have the CD4 receptor molecule on their surface. In macrophages and cells lacking this molecule, an alternate receptor molecule (such as the Fc receptor, or the **complement** receptor site) may be used for entry of HIV. The immune cells such as the blood monocytes, macrophages, **T cells**, **B cells**, natural killer (NK) cells, dendritic cells, hematopoietic stem cells, etc are the primary targets of HIV infection.

After entering the body, the virus attaches itself by fusion to a cell with the appropriate CD4 receptor molecule. On gaining entry into the cell, the viral particle uncoats from its envelope and releases the RNA. The reverse transcriptase encoded by the pol gene, reverse transcribes the viral RNA

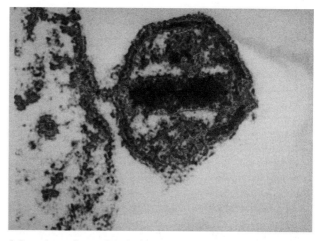

Color enhanced scanning electron microscope image of the Human Immunodeficiency Virus (HIV) on a hemocyte.

into DNA, and the integrase enzyme (also coded by the pol gene) inserts the HIV proviral DNA into the genomic DNA of the host cell. The HIV provirus is replicated by the host cell and transcribed to produce new progeny RNA molecules. The infected host cells either release the new HIV virions by lysis, or the viruses can escape by surface budding. These go on to infect additional host cells.

The primary target of the HIV is the **immune system** itself, with a special affinity for CD4 (T-helper) cells. Following infection, there is a latent phase during which the viral replication continues actively, accompanied with a progressive destruction of the CD4 cells. During latency, there are enough immune cells remaining to provide an immune response and fight infections. Eventually, when a significant number of T cells are destroyed, and the rate of production of the cells cannot match the rate of destruction, there is a loss of both cell-mediated and humoral **immunity**. This failure of the immune system leads to the appearance of clinical AIDS. The patients generally die of secondary causes such as Kaposi's sarcoma (a rare form of cancer that occurs in HIV-infected individuals) or bacterial and fungal infections.

Primary HIV infection may go undetected in more than half the cases, because the symptoms produced are mild and they subside quickly. This is followed by a clinical latent period, which could last on an average 8–11 years. The latency period varies from person to person and depends on a variety of factors including the person's health status and life style. In cases of acute HIV infection, the most common symptoms are fever, swelling of the lymph glands, a red, diffuse rash all over the body, sore throat or upper respiratory infection, muscle ache, diarrhea, and headache. These symptoms subside in a couple of months. Within three months of infection, the body mounts an additional immune response to the virus, and detectable levels of antibodies are seen. Both humoral and cell-mediated immune responses play a role. There is a decline in the viral counts and the levels of CD4 T-helper cells increase. In rare cases, it may take as long as six months for the immune response to develop. Therefore, the **Centers for Disease Control** (CDC) recommends testing for HIV at six months after the last possible exposure to the virus (through unprotected sex or sharing needles).

HIV is primarily spread as a **sexually transmitted disease**. However, one can also acquire the virus through either intravenous drug use or transfusions. The virus can be present in a variety of body fluids and secretions, but the presence of HIV in blood, and genital secretions, and to a lesser extent breast milk, is significant for the spread of HIV. In addition, HIV infection can be acquired as a congenital infection during birth or in infancy. Mothers with HIV infection can pass the virus either transplacentally at the time of delivery through the birth canal or through breast milk. The diagnosis of clinical AIDS often occurs because of the presence of rare diseases such as Kaposi's sarcoma, **pneumonia**, or other serious recurrent infections. The patient's lifestyle, and medical history could also provide clues. Laboratory diagnosis of the infection is based on **serology**, measuring the antibodies to HIV using **ELISA**. Positive results are further confirmed with another test known as a Western Blot. Together, the two tests are more than 99.9% accurate.

No vaccines are currently available to prevent infection by HIV. However, scientists and researchers the world over are working on making a **vaccine** to HIV and have some interesting leads. The drugs used to treat HIV fall into three categories: the nucleosides, non-nucleosides, and the protease inhibitors. The nucleoside and non-nucleoside inhibit the reverse transcriptase enzyme, while the third category of drugs inhibits the enzyme protease. These drugs are given in combinations of two or three to attack the HIV in different ways.

See also AIDS, recent advances in research and treatment; Antibody and antigen; Antiviral drugs; Immunity, active, passive and delayed; Immunity, cell mediated; Immunity, humoral regulation; Infection and resistance; Public health, current issues; T cells or T lymphocytes; Virology; Virus replication; Viruses and responses to viral infection

HUMAN LEUKOCYTE ANTIGEN (HLA)

The human leukocyte **antigen** (HLA) is not a single antigen, but is rather a group of proteins that are located on the surface of white blood cells. These proteins have a pivotal role in the body's immune response to foreign material. Because the HLA is a chemical tag that distinguishes "self" from "non-self," the antigen is important in the rejection of transplanted tissue and in the development of certain diseases (e.g., insulin-dependent diabetes).

The HLA is the human version of a complex that is known as the **major histocompatibility complex**. Similar complexes exist in other species. Indeed much of the early knowledge of the antigen complex came from work on mice in the early decades of the twentieth century. Research on human blood cells in the 1950s identified three genes associated with the HLA (HLA-A, HLA-B, HLA-C). In the 1970s, another **gene** was identified (HLA-D). With the advent of molecular

technology beginning in the 1980s, more genes that code for proteins that function in the antigen complex have continued to be identified.

The HLA evolved to serve two functions. The first is to chemically label a cell in a manner that is unique to that cell. White blood cells from all but an identical twin will have differently structured HLAs on their surface. Thus, if white blood cells from one person are injected into someone else, the injected cells will be recognized as foreign. This recognition occurs because the HLA groups are "read" by an immune cell called the T cell. Essentially the different HLA arrangement on cells allows the **immune system** to develop an inventory of "self" antigens in the body. Knowing the "self" antigen allows the immune system to rapidly distinguish foreign antigens.

HLAs are a class of what is referred to as the major **histocompatibility** complex. These molecules are made up of a portion that is embedded in the cell membrane and a portion that protrudes out from the membrane's outer surface. The molecules function to identify a cell to the T lymphocyte cells of the immune system. The T cell will recognize a region of the histocompatibility complex as a host structure, and no immune reaction will be initiated towards the cell. In another host, the same region could be recognized as foreign by the T lymphocytes.

HLA-D is a so-called class II major histocompatibility molecule. Class II molecules have two segments that are embedded in the membrane. At the outer surface of the cell the molecule contains an antigen that has been acquired from the surrounding environment. Particles are engulfed, broken down into their constituent parts, and some of the components end up incorporated into the class II histocompatibility complex. Thus phenomenon is referred to as antigen presentation.

Class II molecules are not present on all cells the way class I molecules are. Rather, class II molecules are on the surface of immune cells such as macrophages and B-lymphocytes that are designed to process cells and present the antigens from these cells to T lymphocytes. This is done to increase the repertoire of antibodies that an organism possesses.

The two classes of histocompatibility molecules allow an organism to in essence establish an inventory of what cells are "self" and to expose foreign antigens to the immune system so that antibodies to these antigens can be made. In the future, an invading organism that possesses one or some of these "non-self" antigens will be swiftly recognized as an invader and will be dealt with.

Defects in the structure of the HLAs is the cause of some diseases where the body's immune system perceives a host antigen as foreign and begins to attack the body's own tissue. An example is insulin-dependent diabetes, where a host immune response causes the destruction of insulin producing cells.

See also Histocompatibility; Immune system; Immunodeficiency diseases

HUMAN T-CELL LEUKEMIA VIRUS (HTLV)

Two types of human T-cell Leukemia Virus (HTLV) are known. They are also known as human T-cell lymphotrophic **viruses**. HTLV-1 often is carried by a person with no overt symptoms being apparent. However, HTLV-I is capable of causing a number of maladies. These include abnormalities of the **T cells** and **B cells**, a chronic infection of the myelin covering of nerves that causes a degeneration of the nervous system, sores on the skin, and an **inflammation** of the inside of the eye. HTLV-II infection usually does not produce any symptoms. However, in some people a cancer of the blood known as hairy cell leukemia can develop.

At one time there was a third HTLV virus. However, what once called HTLV-III is now referred to as the **Human Immunodeficiency Virus** (**HIV**). HIV is generally accepted to be the causative agent of acquired **immunodeficiency** syndrome.

HTLV is a type of virus called a retrovirus. These viruses are unique in that they possess an enzyme that enables them to manufacture **deoxyribonucleic acid** from their constituent **ribonucleic acid**.

HTLV-I is most commonly associated with a disease called adult T-cell leukemia, which is a rapidly spreading cancerous growth that affects the T cells of the **immune system**. Indeed, the virus was first isolated in 1980 from a patient with T-cell lymphoma. Once the symptoms of the disease appear, deterioration of the individual occurs quickly. However, the symptoms may not appear for decades after the virus has infected someone. The reason for this extended period of latency is not known. HTLV-I has also been isolated from people who have maladies that include arthritis, Kaposi's sarcoma, and non-Hodgkin's lymphoma. Whether the virus is a contributor to such maladies, or is coincidentally expressed, is not yet clear.

The HTLV-I form of the virus is found all over the world. However, it is more prevalent in some countries, such as Japan, than in other countries, such as the United States.

HTLV-II was isolated in 1982 from a patient with hairy cell leukemia. Even so, the virus still has not been definitively established as the cause of that malady. However, the frequent isolation of HTLV-II from patients with this form of leukemia, as well as other types of leukemia's and lymphomas, lends credence to the theory that the virus is vital for the development of the malignancies.

HTLV-II is found in many intravenous drug users. Transmission of the virus from person to person via the contaminated blood in the needles used for drug injection has been documented. HTLV-II can also be spread by exchange of other body fluids, such as occurs in sexual contact.

In spite of the above conditions associated with HTLV-II, the majority of those infected with the virus do not display any symptoms.

The virus can be passed from person to person by the transfer of contaminated blood or via the intimate association of sexual contact. Also, the virus is capable of being passed from mother to infant via breast milk. Blood donor programs in many countries now rigorously test for the presence of HTLV in donated blood and plasma.

HTLV infections are incurable. However, the progressive physical deterioration associated with the infections can be lessened somewhat if the infections are diagnosed early. Screening for the virus relies on the detection of antibodies. Typically, antigen-antibody agglutination tests or the **enzyme-linked immunosorbent assay** (**ELISA**) is used. Confirmation of infections is provided by demonstrating the presence of viral protein in electrophoretic gels following the application of an **antibody** (the technique is dubbed the Western Blot).

See also AIDS; Immunodeficiency

HUMORAL IMMUNE RESPONSE · *see*
IMMUNITY, HUMORAL REGULATION

HYDROPHOBIC AND HYDROPHILIC

Hydrophobic and hydrophilic forces are interactions that serve to keep chemical groups positioned close to one another. Such associations are vital for the structure of the components of **microorganisms**.

Hydrophobic ("water hating") interactions are created because of the uncharged nature of the involved chemical groups. An example of such a chemical group is CH_3. All the bonds around the carbon atom are occupied. The chemical group is described as being nonpolar. Thus, a water molecule—a polar molecule—is unable to establish an association with the non-polar chemical group. This tends to create instability in the network of water molecules, and so is undesirable. The repulsive force of the surrounding water molecules acts to force hydrophobic regions into an association with like regions. The effect tends to be the formation of a hydrophobic "pocket" or "envelope" in a protein or a carbohydrate molecule or matrix.

Hydrophilic ("water loving) interactions are possible with polar chemical group. Water is polar because oxygen is far more electronegative than hydrogen and thus the electrons involved in an oxygen-hydrogen bond spend more time in proximity to the oxygen atom. Because of this unequal electron sharing, the oxygen atom takes on a partial negative charge and the hydrogen atom a partial positive charge. In addition, the bonds in a water molecule (oriented at 105° in a "bent" molecular shape) cannot cancel each other out. Other polar groups can then form ionic type bonds with water. Regions of proteins and other biological materials that are exposed to the environment are typically hydrophilic.

Hydrophobic and hydrophilic interactions can affect protein shape. Because of the polar or nonpolar nature of the constituent amino acid building blocks, as well as in carbohydrate and lipid constituents of microorganisms, molecules and sometimes whole microorganisms can assume shapes and orientations that depend on the intracellular or extracellular environment.

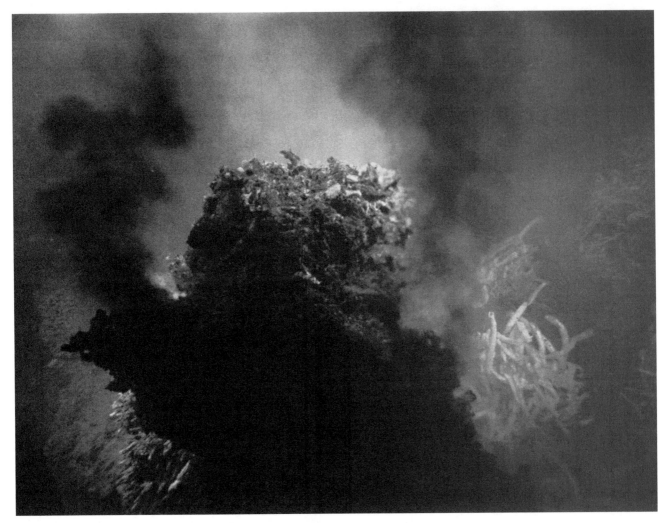

"Black smoker" hydrothermal vent, with tubes of worms growing to the right.

The tendency for hydrophobic regions of a protein of a lipid molecule to associate away from water is a main driving force in the folding of proteins into their dimensional configuration. Furthermore, the formation of biological membranes would be extremely difficult in the absence of hydrophobic and hydrophilic interactions. The biological molecules known as **phospholipids** have a hydrophilic "head" region and a nonpolar, hydrophobic "tail." These forces cause the phospholipid molecules to aggregate together so that the polar heads are oriented towards the water and the hydrophobic tails are buried inside. The effect is to spontaneously establish a membrane. Insertion of functionally specialized proteins into this so-called phospholipid bilayer acts to create a biological membrane of great complexity.

See also Bacterial membranes and cell wall; Biochemical analysis techniques; Biochemistry; Cell membrane transport; Membrane fluidity

HYDROTHERMAL VENTS

A hydrothermal vent is a geyser that is located on the floor of the sea. The first such vent was discovered in 1977 on the floor of the Pacific Ocean. Since then, vents have been discovered at a variety of locations in the Pacific and Atlantic Oceans.

The vents tend to be located deep in the ocean. For example, in the Atlantic ocean, some 7000 feet beneath the surface, hydrothermal vents are associated with underwater mountain chain called the Mid-Ocean Ridge. This ridge is geologically active with an upwelling of hot magma and volcanic activity. The tectonic plate movements cause faulting and seawater that then enters the cracks is superheated by the molten magma. The superheated water and steam and spews out through hydrothermal vents.

Some vents, known as "black smokers," spew out a black-colored mixture of iron and sulfide. "White smokers" spew out a whitish mix of barium, calcium, and silicon.

This eruption through the hydrothermal vents is continuous, in contrast with the sporadic eruptions of surface geysers. The material that emerges from hydrothermal vents is extremely hot (up to 750° F [398.89° C]) and is very rich in minerals such as sulfur. The minerals can precipitate out of solution to form chimneys. The construction of a chimney can occur quickly. Growth of 30 feet in 18 months is not unusual. The tallest of these chimneys that has been measured was the height of a 15 story building.

A vibrant community of **bacteria**, tubeworms that are unique to this environment, and other creatures exists around hydrothermal vents. The entire ecosystem is possible because of the activity of the bacteria. These bacteria have been shown, principally through the efforts of the **Holger Jannasch** (1927–1998) of Woods Hole Oceanographic Institution, to accomplish the conversion of sulfur to energy in a process that does not utilize sunlight called chemosynthesis. The energy is then available for use by the other life forms, which directly utilize the energy, consume the bacteria, or consume the organisms that rely directly on the bacteria for nourishment. For example, the tubeworms have no means with which to take in or process nutrients. Their existence relies entirely on the bacteria that live in their tissues.

See also Chemoautotrophic and chemolithotrophic bacteria; Extremophiles; Sulfur cycle in microorganisms

HYGIENE

Hygiene refers to the health practices that minimize the spread of infectious **microorganisms** between people or between other living things and people. Inanimate objects and surfaces, such as contaminated cutlery or a cutting board, may be a secondary part of this process.

One of the bedrock fundamentals of hygiene is handwashing. The recognition of the link between handwashing and reduction in microbial illness dates back to the mid-nineteenth century. Then, Florence Nightingale, based on her nursing experiences during the Crimean War, wrote about her perceived relationship between unsanitary conditions and disease. At about the same time, the Viennese physician **Ignaz Philipp Semmelweis** noted the connection between mortalities in hospital patients and the movement of physicians from patient to patient without an intervening washing of their hands. After Semmelweis introduced hand washing with a solution containing chloride, the incidence of mortality due to puerperal fever (infection after childbirth) diminished from 18% to less than 3%. Now, hand washing with similar antiseptic agents and even with plain soap and water is known to reduce illness and death from hospital acquired infections.

Proper hygienic practices in the hospital setting not only save lives, but save a great deal of money also. According to the **Centers for Disease Control**, the cost of dealing with the 2.4 million hospital acquired urinary tract infections, blood stream infections, respiratory infections and infections of incisions, which are caused each year by microbes transferred from hospital staff to the patient, and which could be prevented by proper hand washing, is over 4 billion dollars in the United States alone.

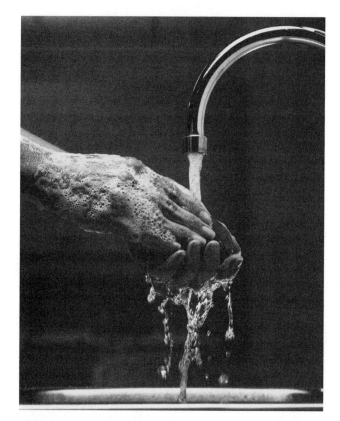

Hand washing is a means of preventing the spread of bacterial and viral infections.

Similarly, in the home and other social settings, hand washing can prevent the spread of infectious microorganisms. A common route of infection is from the bathroom to the kitchen. Improper hand washing fails to remove microorganisms, such as *Escherichia coli* and *Salmonella* acquired from fecal excretion. Handling of food transfers the organisms to the food.

Hygiene is not so concerned with the bacterial flora that normally resides on the skin. These **bacteria** include *Corynebacterium*, *Proprionibacterium*, and *Acinetobacter*. These organisms are tenaciously associated with the skin and so are not as easily removed by the mechanical scrubbing action of hand washing. Rather, hygienic efforts such as hand washing attempt to remove organisms, such as *Escherichia coli* that become transiently associated with the skin. The transient organisms tend be removed more easily and are more apt to be infectious.

In medical environments, hygiene is not only mandatory, but must be done according to established procedures. For example, both before and after seeing a patient, a physician must wash his/her hands with an alcohol-based preparation if hands are not visibly dirty, and with soap and water if dirt is apparent. This practice is also done if any contact with microorganisms has occurred or is even suspected of occurring (for example, handling a surgical instrument that is not wrapped in a sterile package) and after removing surgical gloves. The latter is important since the interior of a surgical glove can be an ideal breeding ground for bacteria. Furthermore, the act of handwashing is to be done for a specified period of time and with vigorous rubbing together of the hands and fingers. This is because the removal of microorganisms is accomplished not only by the presence of the soap but also by the friction of the opposing skin surfaces rubbing together.

Other hygienic practices in a laboratory include wiping the lab bench with a disinfectant compound before and after use and keeping the work area orderly and free of debris. Protective clothing can also be worn to minimize the spread of microorganisms. Such clothing includes hair nets, disposal boots and gloves, and lab coats. These items are worn in the vicinity of the work bench or other areas where microorganisms are expected, but are removed when exiting such locations.

Mechanical aids to hygiene exist. For example, many labs contain a **fume hood**, in which airflow is directed inward. Such laminar flow hoods do not allow the contaminated air inside the hood to move outward into the laboratory. Another standard feature of a microbiological laboratory is a small flame source. The flame is used to sterilize the lip of test tubes and vials before and after opening the containers, and to heat-sterilize the metal inoculating loops used to transfer microorganisms from one place to another.

While necessary for the protection of patients and to prevent **contamination** in the laboratory, the use of hygienic substances can have adverse effects. In the late 1980s the so-called "hygiene hypothesis" proposed that the increased use of disinfectants, particularly in the home, had decrease the exposure of people to substances that stimulated their **immune system**, and so had rendered the immune system less capable of dealing with environmental antigens. The result was proposed to be an increase in **allergies**. Time has strengthened this hypothesis to the point where the overuse of disinfectants has become a legitimate concern.

In addition to the development of allergic reactions, the inadequate or improper use of a hygienic compound can select for organisms that are more capable of causing disease. For example, certain disinfectants containing the compound triclosan have been shown to not only fail to kill the entire target *Escherichia coli* population, but to actually stimulate the development of resistance in those microbes that survive. In a setting such as a kitchen, the results could be problematic.

See also Acne, microbial basis of; Antiseptics; Disinfection and disinfectants; Transmission of pathogens

HYPHAE

One of the biological characteristics that distinguish multicellular **fungi** from other organisms is their constitutional cells, or hyphae (singular, hypha). Hyphae are nucleated cells in the shape of thin tubes, externally enveloped in a rigid chitin-rich cell wall and presenting an internal plasmatic membrane. They contain cellular organelles such as mitochondria, Golgi apparatus, **ribosomes**, endoplasmatic reticulum, which is also found in other **Eukaryotes** as well as cytoplasmatic vesicles bound to the plasmatic membrane. Hyphal cytoskeleton is organized by microtubules. Hyphae are separated by walls termed septae (singular, septum), usually bearing pores and regulatory structures that prevent cellular leaking due to cell disruption. For instance, the septum of Ascomycetes contains the Woronin body, an oily structure that blocks the pore if cell disruption occurs, whereas **Basidomycetes** have a dolipore septum, with the hyphae containing distinctly layered wall structures and endoplasmatic reticulum next to the pore. Hyphal growth and proliferation form structures similar to fine branches, which form the **mycelium** or vegetative hyphal network. However, Zygomycetes and Chytridiomycetes have non-septate vegetative mycelium, except for the reproductive structures.

As fungi grow, the older layers of hyphae gradually die because growth occurs through the proliferation and branching of the apical cell of the mycelium (i.e., cell at the mycelium tip). Growth takes place when two cytoplasmatic vesicles bound to the internal membrane fuse at the apical hypha, enlarging the hyphal tip because of the accumulation of biomass, leading to septum formation and branching. Branching is due to the growth of another apical cell inside the sub apical region of the mother cell. The growth process so far described is directed into new regions of the organic substrate, from which the fungus is feeding, and is termed the extension zone. The aerial part of the fungus, consisted of older hyphae forming aerial mycelia, may develop and differentiate to form structures bearing spores, and is termed the productive zone.

For most fungi, the haploid spore is the starting point from which the haploid hypha will develop and form the monokaryotic mycelium. The joining of two haploid mycelia leads to diploidization of the apical cells, resulting in two cells containing two separate nuclei, known as a dikaryotic mycelium. These cells are capable of producing spores and in Basidomycetes, are termed basidia (singular, basidium) whereas in Ascomycetes, they are termed ascus. Usually, a typical basidium produces four sexual spores and the ascus can produce eight spores, although the amount of spores can vary among the species of a given phylum. In the basidium, for instance, the two nuclei are duplicated and then merged when the cell is about to undergo meiosis twice, thus resulting in the formation of four haploid spores. Some Ascomycetes as well as a few Basidomycetes may also produce asexual spores; and asexual reproduction is the way Zygomycetes and Chytridiomycetes reproduce themselves.

See also Fungal genetics; Fungi; Mycology; Parasites; Yeast

I

IGA • *see* IMMUNOGLOBULINS AND IMMUNOGLOBULIN DEFI-
CIENCY SYNDROMES

IGA DEFICIENCY • *see* IMMUNODEFICIENCY DISEASE
SYNDROMES

IGD • *see* IMMUNOGLOBULINS AND IMMUNOGLOBULIN DEFI-
CIENCY SYNDROMES

IGE • *see* IMMUNOGLOBULINS AND IMMUNOGLOBULIN DEFI-
CIENCY SYNDROMES

IGG • *see* IMMUNOGLOBULINS AND IMMUNOGLOBULIN DEFI-
CIENCY SYNDROMES

**IGG SUBCLASS AND SPECIFIC ANTIBODY
DEFICIENCIES** • *see* IMMUNODEFICIENCY DISEASE SYN-
DROMES

IGM • *see* IMMUNOGLOBULINS AND IMMUNOGLOBULIN DEFI-
CIENCY SYNDROMES

IMMUNE COMPLEX TEST

The immune complex test is a test designed to evaluate the status or proper functioning of the **immune system**. The criterion used to evaluate the operation of the immune system is via the presence of so-called immune complexes.

An immune complex is an association formed between large numbers of antigens and the corresponding antibodies. The latter are produced in a specific response to the presence of the **antigen**, which has been perceived as being foreign by the body's immune system. The individual antigen-antibody complexes can associate together to form the interlocking network that represents an immune complex.

Normally, immune complexes are removed from the bloodstream by specialized cells of the spleen called macrophages and by other specialized cells located in the liver. However, if this clearance does not occur, the immune complexes will continue to circulate, and will become trapped in the kidneys, lung, skin, joints, or blood vessels. The specific location depends on the composition of the complex. Their presence will cause **inflammation** and can lead to tissue damage.

Immune complexes can develop as a result of what is termed a low-grade persistent infection. Examples include *Streptococcus viridans* infection of the blood, *Staphylococcus* heart infections, and viral **hepatitis**. Second, immune complexes can form in response to the continued exposure to an antigen, such as the repeated inhalation of **mold** in a farming or animal care facility. Finally, immune complexes are often a hallmark of autoimmune diseases. The continual response of the body's immune system overloads the ability of the body to remove the immune complexes that form. Examples of autoimmune diseases for which an immune test is beneficial in terms of diagnosis are systemic lupus erythematosus, rheumatoid arthritis, **Lyme disease** and **human immunodeficiency virus** infection.

Being able to test for the presence of abnormal levels of immune complexes can alert the physician to an abnormal function of the immune system, such as an autoimmune disorder.

Immune complexes can be detected by the application of special stains to tissue that has been obtained from a patient. The stains contain antibodies that bind to the complexes and this binding is highlighted by the presence of the staining agent. This test is useful because it directly detects the presence of the immune complexes. However, for routine clinical use, this method is cumbersome and invasive. This has stimulated the development of blood tests that indirectly detect the complexes in the blood serum.

There are several methods available. Often more than one will be used to test the same sample. This is because the

　　　　●　　　　

test methods are not yet uniformly standardized across the medical community. But, if the results from several tests are positive for immune complexes, the validity of the diagnosis is ensured.

Immune complex tests include the Raji cell, C1q binding, conglutinin, and anti-C3 assays. The Raji cell assay, for example, detects the immune complexes following the binding of the complexes with an immune molecule called **complement**. In addition, the complement has been labeled with a compound known as fluorescein isothiocyanate. The latter compound is able to fluoresce when light of a certain wavelength is shone on it. The detection occurs in a machine called a flow cytometer, in which fluid moves past a detector that is programmed to detect certain chemical aspects. In the Raji cell assay, detection of the fluorescent isothiocyanate indicates the presence of the immune complex.

A normal result in an immune complex test is a negative result. In other words, immune complexes are normally absent.

See also Antibody-antigen, biochemical and molecular reactions; Laboratory techniques in immunology

IMMUNE STIMULATION, AS A VACCINE

Immune stimulation refers to the stimulation of the **immune system** by an external source. The stimulation can confer a protective effect against **microorganisms**. As well, immune stimulation shows promise as a means of obtaining an immune response to conditions such as cancer.

Conventionally, the immune system is stimulated into producing antibodies or other infection-fighting constituents in response to an infection. Immune stimulation seeks to elicit the immune reaction before infection or other malady strikes, as a means of preventing the infection or malady. This approach is analogous to the administration of components of weakened or inactive **influenza** virus to protect people from the subsequent onset of influenza.

The roots of the use of immune stimulation as a **vaccine** date back to the late nineteenth century. Then, William Coley, a New York bone surgeon, began treatments in which he injected cancer sufferers with a preparation consisting of dissolved *Streptococcus pyogenes* **bacteria**. Anecdotal evidence claimed remission of tumor growth in 40% of the treated patients. Then, in the 1980s, it was discovered that the observed anti-tumor activity of a bacteria known as *Bacillus Calmette-Guerin* was a property of the construction of the bacterial genetic material. Indeed, the bacterial genetic material is able to stimulate the immune system such that the target sequence of the bacterial **gene** is distinguished from the host genetic material. The resulting immune stimulation boosts **antibody** levels as well as another aspect of the immune system known as cell-mediated **immunity**.

Synthetic peptides have also proved useful as agents of immune stimulation. These compounds are made up of chains of amino acids. They are called synthetic because they are not naturally occurring, but rather are constructed in the labora-

tory. The peptide can contain amino acids in which a chemical group is oriented in a mirror image of that which is normally found in nature.

The mirror image arrangement proves lethal to various bacteria. For example, synthetic peptides swiftly kill populations of *Staphylococcus aureus* and *Enterococcus faecium* that are resistant to an array of **antibiotics**. The peptide binds to the outer surface of the bacterium and is able to punch a hole through the cell wall. The punctured bacteria die. Furthermore, as the bacteria release their contents, the immune system is stimulated to produce antibodies to the bacterial constituents. The synthetic peptide both kills bacteria directly and stimulates an immune response that acts to kill more bacteria.

Thus far, immune stimulation as a vaccine has been developed towards so-called extracellular infections. These are infection caused by bacteria that adhere to host cells or that proliferate in fluids such as blood. For these types of infections, the immune stimulation aims to produce antibodies. Defense against intracellular infections, which are caused by bacteria invading host cells, requires the stimulation of other immune components, such as phagocytic cells. Furthermore, defense against viral infections requires stimulation of immune components called killer cells.

Synthetic peptides can also stimulate the immune system to recognize a surface constituent of a certain type of cancer cell called a melanoma cell. Melanoma is also commonly referred to as skin cancer. The synthetic peptide can mimic the peptide produced on a tumor that the immune system can recognize and respond to. By supplying the target externally, the immune system has more opportunity to mount a defense against the offending peptide. The resulting antibody molecules would target the peptide on the tumor cells.

While shrinkage of tumors was evident in laboratories studies, confirmation of the clinical power of the technique requires a clinical trial where many people are given the treatment and their progress monitored. Nonetheless, it has been demonstrated that synthetic peptides are capable of stimulating the ability of the immune system to distinguish between antigens that are an innate part of the body from those **antigen** that come from outside of the body. In the case of many cancers, such immune stimulation is required, as the disease can compromise the natural immune defenses.

See also Immunization; Immunologic therapies

IMMUNE SYNAPSE

Before they can help other immune cells respond to a foreign protein or pathogenic organism, helper **T cells** must first become activated. This process occurs when an antigen-presenting cell submits a fragment of a foreign protein, bound to a Class II **MHC** molecule (virus-derived fragments are bound to Class I MHC molecules) to the helper T cell. Antigen-presenting cells are derived from bone marrow, and include both dendritic cells and Langerhans cells, as well as other specialized cells. Because T cell responses depend upon direct contact with their target cells, their **antigen** receptors, unlike antibodies made by **B cells**, exist bound to the membrane only. In the intercellular gap between the T cell and the antigen-presenting cell, a special pattern of various receptors and complementary ligands forms that is several microns in size. This patterned collection of receptors is called the immune synapse.

The immune synapse can be compared to a molecular machine that controls T cell activation. Physically it consists of a group of T cell receptors surrounded by a ring of integrin-like adhesion molecules as well as other accessory proteins like the CD3 complex. Integrins are a family of cell-surface proteins that are involved in binding to extracellular matrix components. This specialized cell-cell junction was named the immunological synapse because it is thought to be involved in the transfer of information across the T cell-APC junction. Specifically, the immune synapse appears to play an essential role in organizing the immune response, the level of control, and the nature of that response. The formation of the synapse requires several minutes and it appears to be stable for several hours. The structural protein actin seems to have an important role in that stability as T-cell activation is blocked by disruption of actin filaments. There also appears to be a temporal spatial component in that signals that modulate T-cell maturity and functions are received in a serial manner as well as simultaneously. Further clarification of the structure of the immune synapse will help develop further insights into T cell recognition as well as the mechanism of T cell receptor signaling - how information transfer occurs across the synapse. The duration of signaling in immature T cells may control CD4 and CD8 lineage decisions. This would be useful in determining the degree to which different types and developmental stages rely on alternative signaling mechanisms.

See also Antibody and antigen; Antibody formation and kinetics; Antibody-antigen, biochemical and molecular reactions; T cells or T-lymphocytes

IMMUNE SYSTEM

The immune system is the body's biological defense mechanism that protects against foreign invaders. Only in the last century have the components of that system and the ways in which they work been discovered, and more remains to be clarified.

The true roots of the study of the immune system date from 1796 when an English physician, **Edward Jenner**, discovered a method of **smallpox vaccination**. He noted that dairy workers who contracted **cowpox** from milking infected cows were thereafter resistant to smallpox. In 1796, Jenner injected a young boy with material from a milkmaid who had an active case of cowpox. After the boy recovered from his own resulting cowpox, Jenner inoculated him with smallpox; the boy was immune. After Jenner published the results of this and other cases in 1798, the practice of Jennerian vaccination spread rapidly.

It was **Louis Pasteur** who established the cause of infectious diseases and the medical basis for **immunization**. First,

Pasteur formulated his **germ theory of disease**, the concept that disease is caused by communicable **microorganisms**. In 1880, Pasteur discovered that aged cultures of fowl cholera **bacteria** lost their power to induce disease in chickens but still conferred **immunity** to the disease when injected. He went on to use attenuated (weakened) cultures of **anthrax** and **rabies** to vaccinate against those diseases. The American scientists Theobald Smith (1859–1934) and Daniel Salmon (1850–1914) showed in 1886 that bacteria killed by heat could also confer immunity.

Why vaccination imparted immunity was not yet known. In 1888, Pierre-Paul-Emile Roux (1853–1933) and Alexandre Yersin (1863–1943) showed that **diphtheria** bacillus produced a toxin that the body responded to by producing an antitoxin. **Emil von Behring** and **Shibasaburo Kitasato** found a similar toxin-antitoxin reaction in **tetanus** in 1890. Von Behring discovered that small doses of tetanus or diphtheria toxin produced immunity, and that this immunity could be transferred from animal to animal via serum. Von Behring concluded that the immunity was conferred by substances in the blood, which he called antitoxins, or antibodies. In 1894, Richard Pfeiffer (1858–1945) found that antibodies killed cholera bacteria (bacterioloysis). Hans Buchner (1850–1902) in 1893 discovered another important blood substance called **complement** (Buchner's term was alexin), and **Jules Bordet** in 1898 found that it enabled the antibodies to combine with antigens (foreign substances) and destroy or eliminate them. It became clear that each **antibody** acted only against a specific **antigen**. **Karl Landsteiner** was able to use this specific antigen-antibody reaction to distinguish the different blood groups.

A new element was introduced into the growing body of immune system knowledge during the 1880s by the Russian microbiologist Elie Metchnikoff. He discovered cell-based immunity: white blood cells (leucocytes), which Metchnikoff called phagocytes, ingested and destroyed foreign particles. Considerable controversy flourished between the proponents of cell-based and blood-based immunity until 1903, when **Almroth Edward Wright** brought them together by showing that certain blood substances were necessary for phagocytes to function as bacteria destroyers. A unifying theory of immunity was posited by **Paul Ehrlich** in the 1890s; his "side-chain" theory explained that antigens and antibodies combine chemically in fixed ways, like a key fits into a lock. Until this time, immune responses were seen as purely beneficial. In 1902, however, Charles Richet and Paul Portier demonstrated extreme immune reactions in test animals that had become sensitive to antigens by previous exposure. This phenomenon of hypersensitivity, called **anaphylaxis**, showed that immune responses could cause the body to damage itself. Hypersensitivity to antigens also explained **allergies**, a term coined by Pirquet in 1906.

Much more was learned about antibodies in the mid-twentieth century, including the fact that they are proteins of the gamma globulin portion of plasma and are produced by plasma cells; their molecular structure was also worked out. An important advance in **immunochemistry** came in 1935 when Michael Heidelberger and Edward Kendall (1886–1972) developed a method to detect and measure amounts of different antigens and antibodies in serum. Immunobiology also advanced. **Frank Macfarlane Burnet** suggested that animals did not produce antibodies to substances they had encountered very early in life; Peter Medawar proved this idea in 1953 through experiments on mouse embryos.

In 1957, Burnet put forth his clonal **selection** theory to explain the biology of immune responses. On meeting an antigen, an immunologically responsive cell (shown by C. S. Gowans (1923–) in the 1960s to be a lymphocyte) responds by multiplying and producing an identical set of plasma cells, which in turn manufacture the specific antibody for that antigen. Further cellular research has shown that there are two types of lymphocytes (nondescript lymph cells): B-lymphocytes, which secrete antibody, and **T-lymphocytes**, which regulate the B-lymphocytes and also either kill foreign substances directly (killer **T cells**) or stimulate macrophages to do so (helper T cells). Lymphocytes recognize antigens by characteristics on the surface of the antigen-carrying molecules. Researchers in the 1980s uncovered many more intricate biological and chemical details of the immune system components and the ways in which they interact.

Knowledge about the immune system's role in rejection of transplanted tissue became extremely important as organ transplantation became surgically feasible. Peter Medawar's work in the 1940s showed that such rejection was an immune reaction to antigens on the foreign tissue. Donald Calne (1936–) showed in 1960 that immunosuppressive drugs, drugs that suppress immune responses, reduced transplant rejection, and these drugs were first used on human patients in 1962. In the 1940s, George Snell (1903–1996) discovered in mice a group of tissue-compatibility genes, the **MHC**, that played an important role in controlling acceptance or resistance to tissue grafts. Jean Dausset found human MHC, a set of antigens to human leucocytes (white blood cells), called **HLA**. Matching of HLA in donor and recipient tissue is an important technique to predict compatibility in transplants. Baruj Benacerraf in 1969 showed that an animal's ability to respond to an antigen was controlled by genes in the MHC complex.

Exciting new discoveries in the study of the immune system are on the horizon. Researchers are investigating the relation of HLA to disease; certain types of HLA molecules may predispose people to particular diseases. This promises to lead to more effective treatments and, in the long run, possible prevention. Autoimmune reaction, in which the body has an immune response to its own substances, may also be a cause of a number of diseases, like multiple sclerosis, and research proceeds on that front. Approaches to cancer treatment also involve the immune system. Some researchers, including Burnet, speculate that a failure of the immune system may be implicated in cancer. In the late 1960s, Ion Gresser (1928–) discovered that the protein interferon acts against cancerous tumors. After the development of genetically engineered interferon in the mid-1980s finally made the substance available in practical amounts, research into its use against cancer accelerated. The invention of monoclonal antibodies in the mid-1970s was a major breakthrough. Increasingly sophisticated knowledge about the workings of the immune system holds out the hope of finding an effective method to combat one of the most serious immune system disorders, **AIDS**.

Avenues of research to treat AIDS includes a focus on supporting and strengthening the immune system. (However, much research has to be done in this area to determine whether strengthening the immune system is beneficial or whether it may cause an increase in the number of infected cells.) One area of interest is **cytokines**, proteins produced by the body that help the immune system cells communicate with each other and activate them to fight infection. Some individuals infected with the AIDS virus **HIV** (**human immunodeficiency virus**) have higher levels of certain cytokines and lower levels of others. A possible approach to controlling infection would be to boost deficient levels of cytokines while depressing levels of cytokines that may be too abundant. Other research has found that HIV may also turn the immune system against itself by producing antibodies against its own cells.

Advances in immunological research indicate that the immune system may be made of more than 100 million highly specialized cells designed to combat specific antigens. While the task of identifying these cells and their functions may be daunting, headway is being made. By identifying these specific cells, researchers may be able to further advance another promising area of immunologic research, the use of recombinant **DNA** technology, in which specific proteins can be mass-produced. This approach has led to new cancer treatments that can stimulate the immune system by using synthetic versions of proteins released by **interferons**.

See also Antibody and antigen; Antibody formation and kinetics; Antibody, monoclonal; Antibody-antigen, biochemical and molecular reactions; B cells or B lymphocytes; Bacteria and bacterial infection; Germ theory of disease; Immunity, active, passive and delayed; Immunity, cell mediated; Immunity, humoral regulation; Immunochemistry; Immunodeficiency; Immunogenetics; Immunologic therapies; Immunological analysis techniques; Immunology, nutritional aspects; Immunology; Immunosuppressant drugs; Infection and resistance; Invasiveness and intracellular infection; Major histocompatibility complex (MHC); T cells or T-lymphocytes; Transmission of pathogens; Transplantation genetics and immunology; Viruses and responses to viral infection

IMMUNITY: ACTIVE, PASSIVE, AND DELAYED

Active, passive, and delayed immunity are all variations on the operation of the **immune system**, whereby antibodies are produced in response to the presence of an **antigen** considered to be foreign.

Active immunity occurs due to the production of an **antibody** as a result of the presence of the target antigen either as part of an intact infecting organism, or because of the introduction of the specific antigen in the form of a **vaccine**. The immunity is provided by an individual's own immune system.

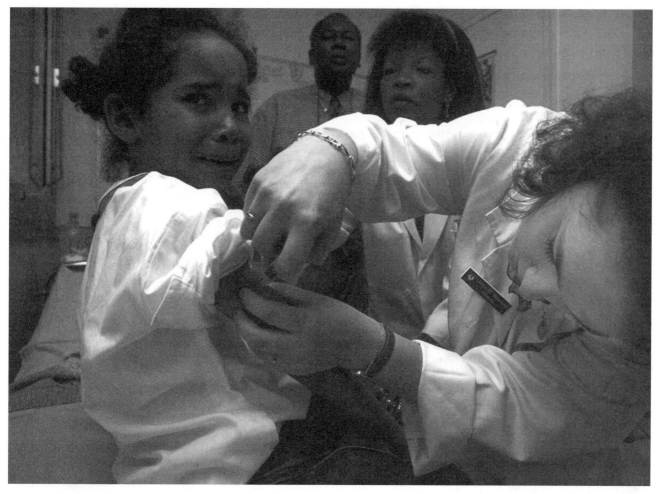

Vaccination against hepatitis.

The type of immunity invoked by the active response tends to be permanent. Once the antibody has been produced, an individual will be protected against the presence of the target antigen for a lifetime. The immune system has a capacity for memory of the antigen. If presented with the antigen challenge again, the immune machinery responsible for the formation of the corresponding antibody is rapidly triggered into action.

An example of active immunity is the injection into healthy individuals of the disabled toxins of **bacteria** such as *Corynebacterium diphtheriae*, the agent causing **diphtheria**, and *Clostridium tetani*, the agent that causes **tetanus**. This rational was first proposed by **Paul Ehrlich**. In 1927, Gaston Ramon attempted his suggestion. He separately injected inactivated version of the bacterial toxins and was able to demonstrate an immune response to both toxins. This rationale has carried forward to the present day. A combination vaccine containing both inactivated toxins is a routine inoculation in childhood.

Another historical development associated with active immunity involved **Louis Pasteur**. In 1884, Pasteur used weakened cultures of *Bacillus anthracis*, the causative agent of **anthrax**, and inactivated sample from the spinal cords of

rabbits infected with the **rabies** virus to produce immunity to anthrax and rabies. Pasteur's method spurred the development of other active immune protective vaccines. Just one example is the oral **poliomyelitis** vaccine developed by **Albert Sabin** in the 1950s.

Passive immunity also results in the presence of antibody. However, the particular individual does not produce the antibody. Rather, the antibody, which has been produced in someone else, is introduced to the recipient. An example is the transfer of antibodies from a mother to her unborn child in the womb. Such antibodies confer some immune protection to the child in the first six months following birth. Indeed, the transient nature of the protection is a hallmark of passive immunity. Protection fades over the course of weeks or a few months following the introduction of the particular antibody. For example, a newborn carries protective maternal antibodies to several diseases, including **measles**, **mumps** and rubella. But by the end of the individual's first year of life, **vaccination** with the MMR vaccine is necessary to maintain the protection.

Another example of passive **immunization** is the administration to humans of tetanus antitoxin that is produced in a horse in response to the inactivated tetanus toxin. This procedure is typically done if someone has been exposed to a situation where the possibility of contracting tetanus exists. Rather than rely on the individual's immune system to respond to the presence of the toxin, neutralizing antibodies are administered right away.

Active and passive immunity are versions of what is known as antibody-mediated immunity. That is, antibodies bind to the antigen and this binding further stimulates the immune system to respond to the antigen threat. Antibody-mediated immunity is also called humoral immunity.

A third type of immunity, which is known as delayed immunity or delayed-type hypersensitivity, is represents a different sort of immunity. Delayed immunity is a so-called cell-mediated immunity. Here, immune components called T-cells bind to the surface of other cells that contain the antigen on their surface. This binding triggers a further response by the immune system to the foreign antigen. The response can involve components such as white blood cells.

An example of delayed immunity is the tuberculin test (or the Mantoux test), which tests for the presence of *Mycobacterium tuberculosis*, the bacterium that causes **tuberculosis**. A small amount of bacterial protein is injected into the skin. If the individual is infected with the bacteria, or has ever been infected, the injection site becomes inflamed within 24 hours. The response is delayed in time, relative to the immediate response of antibody-based immunity. Hence, the name of the immunity.

See also Antibody formation and kinetics; Immunization

IMMUNITY, CELL MEDIATED

The **immune system** is a network of cells and organs that work together to protect the body from infectious organisms. Many different types of organisms such as **bacteria**, **viruses**, **fungi**, and **parasites** are capable of entering the human body and causing disease. It is the immune system's job to recognize these agents as foreign and destroy them.

The immune system can respond to the presence of a foreign agent in one of two ways. It can either produce soluble proteins called antibodies, which can bind to the foreign agent and mark them for destruction by other cells. This type of response is called a humoral response or an **antibody** response. Alternately, the immune system can mount a cell-mediated immune response. This involves the production of special cells that can react with the foreign agent. The reacting cell can either destroy the foreign agents, or it can secrete chemical signals that will activate other cells to destroy the foreign agent.

During the 1960s, it was discovered that different types of cells mediate the two major classes of immune responses. The T lymphocytes, which are the main effectors of the cell-mediated response, mature in the thymus, thus the name T cell. The **B cells**, which develop in the adult bone marrow, are responsible for producing antibodies. There are several different types of **T cells** performing different functions. These

diverse responses of the different T cells are collectively called the "cell-mediated immune responses."

There are several steps involved in the cell-mediated response. The pathogen (bacteria, virus, fungi, or a parasite), or foreign agent, enters the body through the blood stream, different tissues, or the respiratory tract. Once inside the body, the foreign agents are carried to the spleen, lymph nodes, or the mucus-associated lymphoid tissue (MALT) where they will come in contact with specialized cells known as antigen-presenting cells (APC). When the foreign agent encounters the antigen-presenting cells, an immune response is triggered. These **antigen** presenting cells digest the engulfed material, and display it on their surface complexed with certain other proteins known as the Major **Histocompatibility** Class (**MHC**) of proteins.

Next, the T cells must recognize the antigen. Specialized receptors found on some T cells are capable of recognizing the MHC-antigen complexes as foreign and binding to them. Each T cell has a different receptor in the cell membrane that is capable of binding a specific antigen. Once the T cell receptor binds to the antigen, it is stimulated to divide and produce large amounts of identical cells that are specific for that particular foreign antigen. The T lymphocytes also secrete various chemicals (**cytokines**) that can stimulate this proliferation. The cytokines are also capable of amplifying the immune defense functions that can eventually destroy and remove the antigen.

In cell-mediated immunity, a subclass of the T cells mature into cytotoxic T cells that can kill cells having the foreign antigen on their surface, such as virus-infected cells, bacterial-infected cells, and tumor cells. Another subclass of T cells called helper T cells activates the B cells to produce antibodies that can react with the original antigen. A third group of T cells called the suppressor T cells is responsible for regulating the immune response by turning it on only in response to an antigen and turning it off once the antigen has been removed.

Some of the B and T lymphocytes become "memory cells," that are capable of remembering the original antigen. If that same antigen enters the body again while the memory cells are present, the response against it will be rapid and heightened. This is the reason the body develops permanent immunity to an infectious disease after being exposed to it. This is also the principle behind **immunization**.

See also Antibody and antigen; Antibody-antigen, biochemical and molecular reactions; Antibody formation and kinetics; Antibody, monoclonal; Antigenic mimicry; Immune stimulation, as a vaccine; Immune synapse; Immune system; Immunity, active, passive and delayed; Immunity, humoral regulation; Immunization; Immunochemistry

IMMUNITY, HUMORAL REGULATION

One way in which the **immune system** responds to pathogens is by producing soluble proteins called antibodies. This is known as the humoral response and involves the activation of a special set of cells known as the **B lymphocytes**, because they originate in the bone marrow. The humoral immune response helps in the control and removal of pathogens such as **bacteria**, **viruses**, **fungi**, and **parasites** before they enter host cells. The antibodies produced by the **B cells** are the mediators of this response.

The antibodies form a family of plasma proteins referred to as **immunoglobulins**. They perform two major functions. One function of an **antibody** is to bind specifically to the molecules of the foreign agent that triggered the immune response. A second antibody function is to attract other cells and molecules to destroy the pathogen after the antibody molecule is bound to it.

When a foreign agent enters the body, it is engulfed by the antigen-presenting cells, or the B cells. The B cell that has a receptor (surface immunoglobulin) on its membrane that corresponds to the shape of the **antigen** binds to it and engulfs it. Within the B cell, the antigen-antibody pair is partially digested, bound to a special class of proteins called MHC-II, and then displayed on the surface of the B cell. The helper **T cells** recognize the pathogen bound to the MHC-II protein as foreign and becomes activated.

These stimulated T cells then release certain chemicals known as **cytokines** (or lymphokines) that act upon the primed B cells (B cells that have already seen the antigen). The B cells are induced to proliferate and produce several identical cells capable of producing the same antibody. The cytokines also signal the B cells to mature into antibody producing cells. The activated B cells first develop into lymphoblasts and then become plasma cells, which are essentially antibody producing factories. A subclass of B cells does not differentiate into plasma cells. Instead, they become memory cells that are capable of producing antibodies at a low rate. These cells remain in the immune system for a long time, so that the body can respond quickly if it encounters the same antigen again.

The antibody destroys the pathogen in three different ways. In neutralization, the antibodies bind to the bacteria or toxin and prevent it from binding and gaining entry to a host cell. Neutralization leads to a second process called **opsonization**. Once the antibody is bound to the pathogen, certain other cells called macrophages engulf these cells and destroy them. This process is called **phagocytosis**. Alternately, the immunoglobulin IgM or IgG can bind to the surface of the pathogen and activate a class of serum proteins called the **complement**, which can cause lysis of the cells bearing that particular antigen.

In the humoral immune response, each B cell produces a distinct antibody molecule. There are over a million different B lymphocytes in each individual, which are capable of recognizing a corresponding million different antigens. Since each antibody molecule is composed of two different proteins (the light chain and the heavy chain), it can bind two different antigens at the same time.

See also Antibody and antigen; Antibody-antigen, biochemical and molecular reactions; Antibody formation and kinetics; Immune system; Immunity, active, passive and delayed; Immunity, cell mediated

IMMUNIZATION

When a foreign disease-causing agent (pathogen) enters the body, a protective system known as the **immune system** comes into play. This system consists of a complex network of organs and cells that can recognize the pathogen and mount an immune response against it.

Any substance capable of generating an immune response is called an **antigen** or an immunogen. Antigens are not the foreign **bacteria** or **viruses** themselves; they are substances such as toxins or **enzymes** that are produced by the microorganism. In a typical immune response, certain cells known as the antigen-presenting cells trap the antigen and present it to the immune cells (lymphocytes). The lymphocytes that have receptors specific for that antigen binds to it. The process of binding to the antigen activates the lymphocytes and they secrete a variety of **cytokines** that promotes the growth and maturation of other immune cells such as cytotoxic T lymphocytes. The cytokines also act on **B cells** stimulating them to divide and transform into **antibody** secreting cells. The foreign agent is then either killed by the cytotoxic **T cells** or neutralized by the antibodies.

The process of inducing an immune response is called immunization. It may be either natural, i.e., acquired after infection by a pathogen, or, the **immunity** may be artificially acquired with serum or vaccines.

In order to make vaccines for immunization, the organism, or the poisonous toxins of the microorganism that can cause diseases, are weakened or killed. These vaccines are injected into the body or are taken orally. The body reacts to the presence of the **vaccine** (foreign agent) by making antibodies. This is known as active immunity. The antibodies accumulate and stay in the system for a very long time, sometimes for a lifetime. When antibodies from an actively immunized individual are transferred to a second non-immune subject, it is referred to as passive immunity. Active immunity is longer lasting than passive immunity because the memory cells remain in the body for an extended time period.

Immunizations are the most powerful and cost-effective way to prevent infectious disease in children. Because they have received antibodies from their mother's blood, babies are immune to many diseases when they are born. However, this immunity wanes during the first year of life. Immunization programs, therefore, are begun during the first year of life.

Each year in the United States, thousands of adults die needlessly from vaccine-preventable diseases or their complications. Eight childhood diseases (**measles, mumps**, rubella, **diphtheria, tetanus, pertussis**, *Hemophilus influenzae* type b, and polio) are preventable by immunization. With the exception of tetanus, all the other diseases are contagious and could spread rapidly, resulting in **epidemics** in an unvaccinated population. Hence, vaccinations are among the safest and most cost-efficient **public health** measures. Vaccinations against flu (**influenza**), **hepatitis** A, and pneumococcal disease are also recommended for some adolescents and adults. The vaccines indicated for adults will vary depending on lifestyle factors, occupation, chronic medical conditions and travel plans.

See also Antibody and antigen; Antibody formation and kinetics; Immunity, active, passive and delayed; Immunity, cell mediated; Immunity, humoral regulation

IMMUNOCHEMISTRY

Immunochemistry is the study of the chemistry of immune responses.

An immune response is a reaction caused by the invasion of the body by an **antigen**. An antigen is a foreign substance that enters the body and stimulates various defensive responses. The cells mainly involved in this response are macrophages and T and **B lymphocytes**. A macrophage is a large, modified white blood cell. Before an antigen can stimulate an immune response, it must first interact with a macrophage. The macrophage engulfs the antigen and transports it to the surface of the lymphocytes. The macrophage (or neutrophil) is attracted to the antigen by chemicals that the antigen releases. The macrophage recognizes these chemicals as alien to the host body. The local cells around the infection will also release chemicals to attract the macrophages; this is a process known as chemotaxis. These chemicals are a response to the infection. This process of engulfing the foreign body is called **phagocytosis**, and it leads directly to painful swelling and **inflammation** of the infected area.

Lymphocytes are also cells that have been derived from white blood cells (leucocytes). Lymphocytes are found in lymph nodes, the spleen, the thymus, bone marrow, and circulating in the blood plasma. Those lymphocytes that mature inside mammalian bone marrow are called **B cells**. Once B cells have come into contact with an antigen, they proliferate and differentiate into **antibody** secreting cells. An antibody is any protein that is released in the body in direct response to infection by an antigen. Those lymphocytes that are formed inside the thymus are called T lymphocytes or **T cells**. After contact with an antigen, T cells secrete lymphokines—a group of proteins that do not interact with the antigens themselves, instead they stimulate the activity of other cells. Lymphokines are able to gather uncommitted T cells to the site of infection. They are also responsible for keeping T cells and macrophages at the site of infection. Lymphokines also amplify the number of activated T cells, stimulate the production of more lymphokines, and kill infected cells. There are several types of T cells. These other types include T helper cells that help B cells mature into antibody-secreting cells, T suppresser cells that halt the action of B and T cells, T cytotoxic cells that attack infected or abnormal cells, and T delayed hypersensitivity cells that react to any problems caused by the initial infection once it has disappeared. This latter group of cells are long lived and will rapidly attack any remaining antigens that have not been destroyed in the major first stages of infection.

Once the antibodies are released by the B and T cells, they interact with the antigen to attempt to neutralize it. Some antibodies act by causing the antigens to stick together; this is a process known as agglutination. Antibodies may also cause the antigens to fall apart, a process known as cell lysis. Lysis is caused by **enzymes** known as lytic enzymes that are secreted by the antibodies. Once an antigen has been lysed, the remains of the antigen are removed by phagocytosis. Some antigens are still able to elicit a response even if only a small part of the antigen remains intact. Sometimes the same antibody will cause agglutination and then lysis. Some antibodies are antitoxins, which directly neutralize any toxins secreted by the antigens. There are several different forms of antibody that carry out this process depending upon the type of toxin that is produced.

Once antibodies have been produced for a particular antigen they tend to remain in the body. This provides **immunity**. Sometimes immunity is long term and once exposed to a disease we will never catch the disease again. At other times, immunity may only be short lived. The process of active immunity is when the body produces its own antibodies to confer immunity. Active immunity occurs after an initial exposure to the antigen. Passive immunity is where antibodies are passed form mother to child through the placenta. This form of immunity is short lived. Artificial immunity can be conferred by the action of **immunization**. With immunization, a **vaccine** is injected into the body. The vaccine may be a small quantity of antigen, it may be a related antigen that causes a less serious form of the disease, it may be a fragment of the antigen, or it may be the whole antigen after it has been inactivated. If a fragment of antigen is used as a vaccine, it must be sufficient to elicit an appropriate response from the body. Quite often viral coat proteins are used for this. The first vaccine was developed by **Edward Jenner** (1749–1823) in 1796 to inoculate against **smallpox**. Jenner used the mild disease **cowpox** to confer immunity for the potentially fatal but biochemically similar smallpox.

Within the blood there are a group of blood serum proteins called **complement**. These proteins become activated by antigen antibody reactions. Immunoglobulin is an antibody secreted by lymphoid cells called plasma cells. **Immunoglobulins** are made of two long polypeptide chains and two short polypeptide chains. These chains are bound together in a Y-shaped arrangement, with the short chains forming the inner parts of the Y. Each arm of the Y has specific antigen binding properties. There are five different classes of immunoglobulin that are based on their antigen-binding properties. Different classes of immunoglobulins come into play at different stages of infection. Immunoglobulins have specific binding sites with antigens.

One class of compounds in animals has antigens that can be problematical. This is the group called the **histocompatibility** complex. This is the group of usually surface proteins that are responsible for rejections and incompatibilities in organ transplants. These antigens are genetically encoded and they are present on the surface of cells. If the cells or tissues are transferred from one organism to another or the body does not recognize the antigens, it will elicit a response to try to rid the body of the foreign tissue. A body is not interested where foreign proteins come from. It is interested in the fact that they are there when they should not be. Even if an organ is human in origin, it must be genetically similar to the host body or it will be rejected. Because an organ is much larger than a small infection of an antigen when it elicits an immune response, it can be a greater problem. With an organ trans-

plant, there can be a massive cascade reaction of antibody production. This will include all of the immune responses of
which the body is capable. Such a massive response can over-
load the system and it can cause death. Thus, tissue matching
in organ transplants is vitally important. Often, a large range
of immunosuppressor drugs are employed until the body integrates a particular organ. In some cases, this may necessitate a
course of drugs for the rest of the individuals life.
Histocompatibility problems also exist with blood.
Fortunately, the proteins in blood are less specific and blood
transfusions are a lot easier to perform than organ transplants.
The blood-typing systems that are in use are indications of the
proteins that are present. If blood is mixed from the wrong
types, it can cause lethal clotting. The main blood types are A,
B, O, and AB. Group O individuals are universal donors, they
can give blood to anyone. Group AB are universal recipients
because they can accept blood from anyone. Type A blood has
A antigens on the blood cells and B antibodies in the plasma.
The combination of B antibodies and B antigens will cause
agglutination. There are also subsidiary blood proteins such as
the rhesus factor (rh) that can be positive (present) or negative
(absent). If only small amounts of blood are transfused, it is
not a problem due to the dilution factor.

Immunochemistry is the chemistry of the **immune system**. Most of the chemicals involved in immune responses are
proteins. Some chemicals inactivate invading proteins, others
facilitate this response. The histocompatibility complex is a
series of surface proteins on organs and tissues that elicit an
immune response when placed in a genetically different individual.

See also Biochemistry; History of immunology; Immune
stimulation, as a vaccine; Immunity, active, passive and
delayed; Immunity, cell mediated; Immunity, humoral regulation; Immunization; Immunological analysis techniques;
Laboratory techniques in immunology; Major histocompatibility complex (MHC)

IMMUNODEFICIENCY

The **immune system** is the body's main system to fight infections. Any defect in the immune system decreases a person's
ability to fight infections. A person with an immunodeficiency
disorder may get more frequent infections, heal more slowly,
and have a higher incidence of some cancers.

The normal immune system involves a complex interaction of certain types of cells that can recognize and attack
"foreign" invaders, such as **bacteria**, **viruses**, and **fungi**. It also
plays a role in fighting cancer. The immune system has both
innate and adaptive components. Innate **immunity** is made up
of immune protections present at birth. Adaptive immunity
develops the immune system to fight off specific invading
organisms throughout life. Adaptive immunity is divided into
two components: humoral immunity and cellular immunity.

The innate immune system is made up of the skin
(which acts as a barrier to prevent organisms from entering the
body), white blood cells called phagocytes, a system of pro-

teins called the **complement** system, and chemicals called
interferons. When phagocytes encounter an invading organism, they surround and engulf it to destroy it. The complement
system also attacks bacteria. The elements in the complement
system create a hole in the outer layer of the target cell, which
leads to the death of the cell.

The adaptive component of the immune system is
extremely complex, and is still not entirely understood.
Basically, it has the ability to recognize an organism or tumor
cell as not being a normal part of the body, and to develop a
response to attempt to eliminate it.

The humoral response of adaptive immunity involves a
type of cell called **B lymphocytes**. B lymphocytes manufacture
proteins called antibodies (which are also called **immunoglobulins**). Antibodies attach themselves to the invading foreign
substance. This allows the phagocytes to begin engulfing and
destroying the organism. The action of antibodies also activates the complement system. The humoral response is particularly useful for attacking bacteria.

The cellular response of adaptive immunity is useful for
attacking viruses, some **parasites**, and possibly cancer cells.
The main type of cell in the cellular response is T lymphocytes. There are helper T lymphocytes and killer T lymphocytes. The helper T lymphocytes play a role in recognizing
invading organisms, and they also help killer T lymphocytes to
multiply. As the name suggests, killer T lymphocytes act to
destroy the target organism.

Defects can occur in any component of the immune system or in more than one component (combined immunodeficiency). Different **immunodeficiency diseases** involve
different components of the immune system. The defects can
be inherited and/or present at birth (congenital), or acquired.

Congenital immunodeficiency is present at the time of
birth, and is the result of genetic defects. Even though more
than 70 different types of congenital immunodeficiency disorders have been identified, they rarely occur. Congenital
immunodeficiencies may occur as a result of defects in B lymphocytes, T lymphocytes, or both. They can also occur in the
innate immune system.

If there is an abnormality in either the development or
function of B lymphocytes, the ability to make antibodies will
be impaired. This allows the body to be susceptible to recurrent infections. Bruton's agammaglobulinemia, also known as
X-linked agammaglobulinemia, is one of the most common
congenital immunodeficiency disorders. The defect results in
a decrease or absence of B lymphocytes, and therefore a
decreased ability to make antibodies. People with this disorder
are particularly susceptible to infections of the throat, skin,
middle ear, and lungs. It is seen only in males because it is
caused by a genetic defect on the X chromosome. Since males
have only one X chromosome, they always have the defect if
the **gene** is present. Females can have the defective gene, but
since they have two X **chromosomes**, there will be a normal
gene on the other X chromosome to counter it. Women may
pass the defective gene on to their male children.

Another type of B lymphocyte deficiency involves a
group of disorders called selective immunoglobulin deficiency
syndromes. Immunoglobulin is another name for **antibody,**

and there are five different types of immunoglobulins (called IgA, IgG, IgM, IgD, and IgE). The most common type of immunoglobulin deficiency is selective IgA deficiency. The amounts of the other antibody types are normal. Some patients with selective IgA deficiency experience no symptoms, while others have occasional lung infections and diarrhea. In another immunoglobulin disorder, IgG and IgA antibodies are deficient and there is increased IgM. People with this disorder tend to get severe bacterial infections.

Common variable immunodeficiency is another type of B lymphocyte deficiency. In this disorder, the production of one or more of the immunoglobulin types is decreased and the antibody response to infections is impaired. It generally develops around the age of 10-20. The symptoms vary among affected people. Most people with this disorder have frequent infections, and some will also experience anemia and rheumatoid arthritis. Many people with common variable immunodeficiency develop cancer.

Severe defects in the ability of T lymphocytes to mature results in impaired immune responses to infections with viruses, fungi, and certain types of bacteria. These infections are usually severe and can be fatal.

DiGeorge syndrome is a T lymphocyte deficiency that starts during fetal development, but it isn't inherited. Children with DiGeorge syndrome either do not have a thymus or have an underdeveloped thymus. Since the thymus is a major organ that directs the production of **T-lymphocytes**, these patients have very low numbers of T-lymphocytes. They are susceptible to recurrent infections, and usually have physical abnormalities as well. For example, they may have low-set ears, a small receding jawbone, and wide-spaced eyes. In some cases, no treatment is required for DiGeorge syndrome because T lymphocyte production improves. Either an underdeveloped thymus begins to produce more T lymphocytes or organ sites other than the thymus compensate by producing more T lymphocytes.

Some types of immunodeficiency disorders affect both B lymphocytes and T lymphocytes. For example, **severe combined immunodeficiency** disease (**SCID**) is caused by the defective development or function of these two types of lymphocytes. It results in impaired humoral and cellular immune responses. SCID is usually recognized during the first year of life. It tends to cause a fungal infection of the mouth (**thrush**), diarrhea, failure to thrive, and serious infections. If not treated with a bone marrow transplant, a person with SCID will generally die from infections before age two.

Disorders of innate immunity affect phagocytes or the complement system. These disorders also result in recurrent infections.

Acquired immunodeficiency is more common than congenital immunodeficiency. It is the result of an infectious process or other disease. For example, the **Human Immunodeficiency Virus** (**HIV**) is the virus that causes acquired immunodeficiency syndrome (**AIDS**). However, this is not the most common cause of acquired immunodeficiency. Acquired immunodeficiency often occurs as a complication of other conditions and diseases. For example, the most common causes of acquired immunodeficiency are malnutrition, some types of cancer, and infections. People who weigh less than

70% of the average weight of persons of the same age and gender are considered to be malnourished. Examples of types of infections that can lead to immunodeficiency are chickenpox, cytomegalovirus, German **measles**, measles, **tuberculosis**, infectious **mononucleosis** (**Epstein-Barr virus**), chronic **hepatitis**, lupus, and bacterial and fungal infections.

Sometimes, acquired immunodeficiency is brought on by drugs used to treat another condition. For example, patients who have an organ transplant are given drugs to suppress the immune system so the body will not reject the organ. Also, some **chemotherapy** drugs, which are given to treat cancer, have the side effect of killing cells of the immune system. During the period of time that these drugs are being taken, the risk of infection increases. It usually returns to normal after the person stops taking the drugs.

Congenital immunodeficiency is caused by genetic defects, and they generally occur while the fetus is developing in the womb. These defects affect the development and/or function of one or more of the components of the immune system. Acquired immunodeficiency is the result of a disease process, and it occurs later in life. The causes, as described above, can be diseases, infections, or the side effects of drugs given to treat other conditions.

People with an immunodeficiency disorder tend to become infected by organisms that don't usually cause disease in healthy persons. The major symptoms of most immunodeficiency disorders are repeated infections that heal slowly. These chronic infections cause symptoms that persist for long periods of time.

Laboratory tests are used to determine the exact nature of the immunodeficiency. Most tests are performed on blood samples. Blood contains antibodies, lymphocytes, phagocytes, and complement components—all of the major immune components that might cause immunodeficiency. A blood cell count will determine if the number of phagocytic cells or lymphocytes is below normal. Lower than normal counts of either of these two cell types correlates with immunodeficiencies. The blood cells are also checked for their appearance. Sometimes a person may have normal cell counts, but the cells are structurally defective. If the lymphocyte cell count is low, further testing is usually done to determine whether any particular type of lymphocyte is lower than normal. A lymphocyte proliferation test is done to determine if the lymphocytes can respond to stimuli. The failure to respond to stimulants correlates with immunodeficiency. Antibody levels can be measured by a process called **electrophoresis**. Complement levels can be determined by immunodiagnostic tests.

There is no cure for immunodeficiency disorders. Therapy is aimed at controlling infections and, for some disorders, replacing defective or absent components.

In most cases, immunodeficiency caused by malnutrition is reversible. The health of the immune system is directly linked to the nutritional health of the patient. Among the essential nutrients required by the immune system are proteins, vitamins, iron, and zinc. For people being treated for cancer, periodic relief from chemotherapy drugs can restore the function of the immune system.

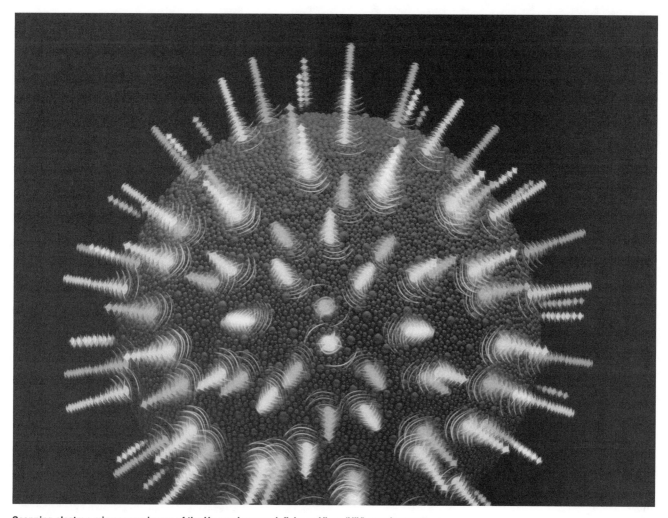

Scanning electron microscope image of the Human Immunodeficiency Virus (HIV) on a hemocyte.

In general, people with immunodeficiency disorders should maintain a healthy diet. This is because malnutrition can aggravate immunodeficiencies. They should also avoid being near people who have colds or are sick because they can easily acquire new infections. For the same reason, they should practice good personal **hygiene**, especially dental care. People with immunodeficiency disorders should also avoid eating undercooked food because it might contain bacteria that could cause infection. This food would not cause infection in normal persons, but in someone with an immunodeficiency, food is a potential source of infectious organisms. People with immunodeficiency should be given **antibiotics** at the first indication of an infection.

There is no way to prevent a congenital immunodeficiency disorder. However, someone with a congenital immunodeficiency disorder might want to consider getting genetic counseling before having children to find out if there is a chance they will pass the defect on to their children.

Some of the infections associated with acquired immunodeficiency can be prevented or treated before they cause problems. For example, there are effective treatments for tuberculosis and most bacterial and fungal infections. HIV infection can be prevented by practicing "safe sex" and not using illegal intravenous drugs. These are the primary routes of transmitting the virus. For people who don't know the HIV status of the person with whom they are having sex, safe sex involves using a condom.

See also AIDS, recent advances in research and treatment; Immunity, active, passive and delayed; Immunity, cell mediated; Immunity, humoral regulation; Immunodeficiency disease syndromes; Immunodeficiency diseases; Infection and resistance

IMMUNODEFICIENCY DISEASE SYNDROMES

An effective **immune system** requires that any antigens that are not native to the body be quickly recognized and destroyed, and that none of the antigens native to the body be identified as foreign. Excesses in the latter constitute the autoimmune diseases. Deficiencies in the body's ability to recognize antigens as foreign or a diminished capacity to respond to recognized antigens constitute the **immunodeficiency** syndromes.

There are many causes associated with immunodeficiencies. Primary immunodeficiencies are inherited conditions in which specific genes or **gene** families are corrupted by **mutations** or chromosome deletions. These syndromes are discussed elsewhere in this volume. Secondary immunodeficiencies are acquired conditions that may result from infections, cancers, aging, exposure to drugs, chemicals or radiation, or a variety of other disease processes.

Bacteria, viral, **fungi**, **protozoa**, and even parasitic infections can result in specific deficiencies of **B cells**, **T cells**, macrophages, and granulocytes. The best characterized of the infectious diseases is the acquired immunodeficiency syndrome (**AIDS**).

Infection by two **viruses**, HIV-1 and HIV-2, is associated with a wide range of responses in different people from essentially asymptomatic to a full-blown AIDS in which cell-mediated **immunity** is seriously compromised. HIV-1 and HIV-2 are **retroviruses** that attack humans and compromise cellular function. In contrast, the human T cell lymphotrophic viruses (**HTLV**) tend to provoke lymphoid neoplasms and neurologic disease. AIDS is most often associated with HIV-1 infection. The chance of developing AIDS following infection with HIV-1 is approximately one to two percent per year initially, and increases to around five percent per year after the fifth year of infection. Roughly, half of those infected with the virus will develop AIDS within ten years. In between those who are asymptomatic, and those with AIDS who are symptomatic with conditions associated with AIDS.

In AIDS, cellular immunity mechanisms are disrupted. Some immunologic cells are reduced in number and others, such as natural killer cells, have reduced activity despite their normal numbers. **HIV** infects primarily T helper lymphocyte cells and a variety of cells outside of the lymphoid system such as macrophages, endothelial, and epithelial cells. Because the T helper cells normally express a surface glycoprotein called CD4, counts of CD4 cells are helpful in predicting immunologic depression in HIV-infected individuals. The amount of viral **RNA** in circulation is also a helpful predictor of immunologic compromise. In addition to cell-mediated immunity, **antibody** responses (humoral immunity) are also muted in individuals with AIDS.

Initially, there is a period of several weeks to months where the host remains HIV antibody negative and viral replication occurs rapidly. Some subjects develop an acute response that appears like the flu or **mononucleosis**. Symptoms typically include fever, malaise, joint pain, and swollen lymph nodes. As the initial symptoms dissipate, patients enter an antibody positive phase without symptoms associated with AIDS. A variety of relatively mild symptoms like **thrush**, diarrhea, fever, or other viral infections may manifest along with a wide array of partial anemias. Nerve function can become compromised resulting in weakness, pain, or sensory loss. Eventually, life threatening opportunistic infections resulting from decreased immunologic function occur and may be accompanied by

wasting, dementia, **meningitis**, and encephalitis. Drug therapy in the form of antiretroviral agents is directed toward inhibition of proteases and reverse transcriptase **enzymes** which are critical for replication of the viruses.

Although not nearly as well known as AIDS, there are a variety of other acquired immunodeficiencies. Infections other than HIV can significantly alter the numbers and functions of other cells within the immune system. While individually these various infections may appear to be relatively uncommon, depression in the numbers of platelets, T cells, B cells, natural killer (NK) cells, and granulocytes can lead to immunologic dysfunction. The manifestations of these various conditions will depend on the specific cell population that is involved and its normal function within the immune system. B cell deficiencies tend to result in an increased susceptibility to bacterial infections. Decreased natural killer cell activity can result in the survival of tumor cells which would otherwise be destroyed by the immune system.

Chemical and physical agents (such as radiation) also can potentially depress various fractions of cells within the immune system, and like the immunodeficiencies caused by infectious agents, the manifestations of these agents will differ depending on the cells which are influenced. Cancer chemotherapeutic agents are often immunosuppressive. Likewise, immune function often declines with age. T cell populations (including the T helper cells) decline as the thymus gland activity decreases. Frequently, B cell populations proliferate at an accelerated rate in older people. Over production of cells within the immune system such as leukemias, lymphomas, and related disorders also may disturb immune function by radically altering the distribution of white cells. A number of other diverse disease processes can alter or compromise immune function. These include diabetes, liver disease, kidney disease, sickle cell anemia, Down syndrome, and many of the autoimmune diseases.

See also AIDS, recent advances in research and treatment; Autoimmunity and autoimmune diseases; Immunodeficiency diseases, genetic causes

IMMUNODEFICIENCY DISEASES, GENETIC CAUSES

The complex workings of the **immune system** requires the cooperation of various organs, tissues, cells and proteins and thus, it can be compromised in a number of different ways. People who have normal immune function at birth who later acquire some form of **immunodeficiency** are said to have secondary or acquired immunodeficiency diseases. Examples would include **AIDS**, age-related immune depression, and other immune deficiencies caused by infections, drug reactions, radiation sickness, or cancer. Individuals who are born with an intrinsically reduced capacity for immunologic activity usually have some genetic alteration present at birth. There are varieties of different genes involved, and they render people susceptible to infection by an assortment of different germs. Some of these diseases are relatively mild with onset in adolescence or adulthood. Others are severely debilitating and severely compromise daily activity. Clinically significant primary immunodeficiencies are relatively rare with 1 in 5,000 to 1 in 10,000 people in developed countries afflicted.

The most common form of primary immunodeficiency, selective IgA deficiency, is a very mild deficiency and may affect as many as 1 in every 300 persons, most of whom will never realize they have an immunodeficiency at all. B-cells are lymphocytes that produce antibodies and this component of the immune system is often called humoral **immunity**. Defects in humoral immunity predispose the body to viral infections. T-cells are lymphocytes that are processed in the thymus gland. Granulocytes are cells which consume an destroy **bacteria**.

There are now thought to be around 70 different primary immunodeficiency diseases. Of the more common forms, the vast majority of these conditions are recessive. This means that a single working copy of the **gene** is generally sufficient to permit normal immune functioning. Some of the genes are found on the X chromosome. Since males receive only a single X chromosome, recessive **mutations** of these genes will result in disease. Females have two copies of the X chromosome, and so rarely will express X-linked recessive diseases.

The most widely known of the primary immunodeficiencies is severe combined immune deficiency (**SCID**) and it conjures pictures of a child who must live his life encased in a plastic bubble to keep out germs. SCID is manifest in early childhood as a severe combined T cell and B cell deficiency, and can be caused by a number of different gene mutations. The most common form is X-linked, and so primarily affects boys. It can also be caused by an enzyme called adenosine deaminase. When ADA is deficient, toxic chemicals kill off the lymphocytes. Until recently, SCID was uniformly lethal. In recent years, the elucidation of the genes responsible has made possible interventions based on gene therapy. SCID often presents in early childhood as persistent diaper rash or **thrush**. **Pneumonia**, **meningitis**, blood poisoning, and many common viral infections are serious threats to children born with SCID. Diagnosis demands immediate medical attention and bone marrow transplants are a common form of treatment for SCID. Children with ADA deficiency may be treated with ADA infusions to correct the enzyme deficiency. Partial combined immune deficiencies are milder conditions in which cellular and humoral immunity are both compromised but not completely shut down. These are generally accompanied by other physical symptoms and so constitute syndromes. Wiskott-Aldrich syndrome, for example, is an X-linked partial combined syndrome in which the repeated infections are combined with eczema and a tendency toward bleeding. Another combined B and T cell deficiency is ataxia telangiectasia (AT). In AT, the combined B and T cell deficiency causes repeated respiratory infections, and is accompanied by a jerky movement disorder and dilated blood vessels in the eyes and skin. The thymus gland where T-cells are processed is underdeveloped.

Deficiency of the B cell population results in decreased **antibody** production and thus, an increased risk of viral or **bacterial infection**. X-linked agammaglobulinemia (XLA) is a condition in which boys (because it is X-linked) produce little to no antibodies due to an absence of **B cells** and plasma cells in circulation. As these children grow, they deplete the antibodies transmitted through the mother, and they become susceptible to repeated infections. Common variable immunodeficiency (CVID) is a group of disorders in which the number of B cells is normal, but the levels of antibody production are reduced.

DiGeorge anomaly is an example of a T cell deficiency produced by an underdeveloped thymus gland. Children with DiGeorge anomaly often have characteristic facial features, developmental delays, and certain kinds of heart defects usually stemming from small deletions on chromosome 22 (or more rarely, chromosome 10). In rare cases, there is an autosomal dominant gene mutation rather than a chromosome deletion.

Phagocytosis, the ability of the granulocytes to ingest and destroy bacteria, can also be the chief problem. One example of this is chronic granulomatous disease (CGD). There are four known genes that cause CGD; all are recessive. One is on the X chromosome, and the other three are on autosomes. These children do well until around age three when they begin to have problems with staphylococcal infections and infections with **fungi** which are generally benign in other people. Their granulosa cells may aggregate in tissues forming tumor like masses. Similarly, leukocyte adhesion defect (LAD) is a condition in which granulocytes fail to work because they are unable to migrate to the site of infections. In Chediak-Higashi syndrome (CHS), not only granulocytes, but also melanocytes and platelets are diminished. CHS is generally fatal in adolescence unless treated by bone marrow transplantation.

One other class of primary immunodeficiencies, the **complement** system defects, result from the body's inability to recognize and/or destroy germs that have been bound by antibodies. Complement fixation is a complex multi step process, and thus a number of different gene mutations can potentially corrupt the normal pathway. Complement system defects are rare and often not expressed until later in life.

The prospect of the development of effective and safe gene therapies holds hope for the primary immunodeficiency diseases. As these genes and their genetic pathways are more fully understood, interventions which replace the missing gene product will likely provide effective treatments.

See also Immunity, cell mediated; Immunity, humoral regulation; Microbial genetics; Microbiology, clinical

IMMUNOELECTRON MICROSCOPY, THEORY, TECHNIQUES AND USES · *see*

ELECTRON MICROSCOPIC EXAMINATION OF MICROORGANISMS

IMMUNOELECTROPHORESIS

Immunoelectrophoresis is a technique that separates proteins on the basis of both their net charge (and so their movement in an electric field) and on the response of the **immune system** to the proteins. The technique is widely used in both clinical and research laboratories as a diagnostic tool to probe the protein composition of serum.

Petr Nikolaevich Grabar, a French immunologist, devised the technique in the 1950s. In essence, immunoelectrophoresis separates the various proteins in a sample in an electric field and then probes the separated proteins using the desired **antiserum**.

The most widely used version of the technique employs an apparatus, which consists basically of a **microscope** slide-sized plate. The plate is the support for a gel that is poured over top and allowed to congeal. The construction of the gel can vary, depending on the separation to be performed. **Agar**, such as that used in microbiological growth media, and another material called agarose can be used. Another popular choice is a linked network of a chemical known as acrylamide. The linked up acrylamide chains form what is designated as polyacrylamide.

The different types of gel networks can be most productively envisioned as a three-dimensional overlay of the crossed linked chains. The effect is to produce snaking tunnels through the matrix of various diameters. These diameters, which are also referred to as pore sizes, can be changed to a certain extent by varying the concentrations of some of the ingredients of the gel suspension. Depending on the size and the shape of the protein, movement through this matrix will be relatively slow or fast. As well, depending on the net charge a protein molecule has, the protein will migrate towards the positively charged electrode or the negatively charged electrode when the electric current is passed through the gel matrix. Thus, the various species of protein will separate from each other along the length of the gel.

In some configurations of the immunoelectrophoretic set-up, the samples that contain the proteins to be analyzed are added to holes on either side of the gel plate. For example, one sample could contain serum from a health individual and another sample could contain serum from someone with an infection. The middle portion of the plate contains a trough, into which a single purified species of **antibody** or known mixture of antibodies is added. The antibody molecules diffuse outward from the trough solution into the gel. Where an antibody encounters a corresponding **antigen**, a reaction causes the formation of a visual precipitate. Typically, the precipitation occurs in arc around the antigen-containing sample. In the example, the pattern of precipitation can reveal antigenic differences between the normal serum and the serum from a infected person.

This type of immunoelectrophoresis provides a qualitative ("yes or no") answer with respect to the presence or absence of proteins, and can be semi-quantitative. The shape of the arc of precipitation is also important. An irregularly shaped arc can be indicative of an abnormal protein or the presence of more than one antigenically similar protein.

Immunoelectrophoresis can also be used to detect a particular antigenic site following the transfer of the proteins from a gel to a special support, such as nitrocellulose. Addition of the antibody followed by a chemical to which bound antibody reacts produces a darkening on the support wherever antibody has bound to antigen. One version of this technique is termed Western Blotting. An advantage of this technique is that, by running two gels and using just one gel for the transfer of proteins to the nitrocellulose, the immune detection of a protein can be performed without affecting the protein residing in the other gel.

Another application of immunoelectrophoresis is known as capillary immunoelectrophoresis. In this application, a sample can be simultaneously drawn up into many capillary tubes. The very small diameter of the tubes means that little sample is required to fill a tube. Thus, a sample can be subdivided into very many sub volumes. Each volume can be tested against a different antibody preparation. Often, the reaction between antigen and antibody can be followed by the use of compounds that fluoresces when exposed to laser light of a specific wavelength. Capillary immunoelectrophoresis is proving to be useful in the study of Bovine Spongiform Encephalopathy in cattle, where sample sizes can be very small.

In the clinical laboratory setting, immunoelectophoresis is used to examine alterations in the content of serum, especially changes concerned with **immunoglobulins**. Change in the immunoglobulin profile can be the result of immunodeficiencies, chronic bacterial or viral infections, and infections of a fetus. The immunoglobulin most commonly assayed for are IgM, IgG, and IgA. Some of the fluids that can be examined using immunoelectrophoresis include urine, cerebrospinal fluid and serum. When concerned with immunoglobulins, the technique can also be called gamma globulin **electrophoresis** or immunoglobulin electrophoresis.

See also Antibody-antigen, biochemical and molecular reactions; Immunological analysis techniques

IMMUNOFLUORESCENCE

Immunofluorescence refers to the combination of an **antibody** and a compound that will fluoresce when illuminated by light of a specific wavelength. The duo is also referred to as a fluorescently labeled antibody. Such an antibody can be used to visually determine the location of a target **antigen** in biological samples, typically by microscopic observation.

The fluorescent compound that is attached to an antibody is able to absorb light of a certain wavelength, the particular wavelength being dependent on the molecular construction of the compound. The absorption of the light confers additional energy to the compound. The energy must be relieved. This is accomplished by the emission of light, at a higher wavelength (and so a different color) than the absorbed radiation. It is this release of radiant energy that is the underpinning for immunofluorescence.

Immunofluorescence microscopy can revel much detail about the processes inside cells. In a light microscopic application of the technique, sections of sample are exposed to the fluorescently labeled antibody. The large wavelength of visible light, relative to other forms of illumination such as laser light, does not allow details to be revealed at the molecular level. Still, details of the trafficking of a protein from the site of its manufacture to the surface of a cell, for example, is possible, by the application of different antibodies. The antibodies can be labeled with the same fluorescent compound but are applied at different times. An example of the power of this type of approach is the information that has been obtained concerning the pathway that the **yeast** known as *Saccharomyces cervisiae* uses to shuttle proteins out of the cell.

Resolution of details to the molecular level has been made possible during the 1990s with the advent of the technique of confocal laser microscopy. This technique employs a laser to sequentially scan samples at selected depths through the sample. These so-called optical sections can be obtained using laser illumination at several different wavelengths simultaneously. Thus, the presence of different antibodies that are labeled with fluorescent compounds that fluoresce at the different wavelengths can produce an image of the location of two antigens in the same sample at the same time.

The use of immunofluorescent compounds in combination with confocal microscopy has allowed the fluorescent probing of samples which do not need to be chemically preserved (or "fixed") prior to examination. The thin sections of sample that are examined in light microscopy often require such chemical fixation. While the fixation regimens have been designed to avoid change of the sample's internal structure, especially the chemistry and three-dimensional structure of the site of the antigen to which the antibody will bind, the avoidance of any form of chemical modification is preferred.

There are a multitude of fluorescent compounds available. Collectively these compounds are referred to as fluorochromes. A well-known example in biological and microbiological studies is the green fluorescent protein. This molecule is ring-like in structure. It fluoresces green when exposed to light in the ultraviolet or blue wavelengths. Other compounds such as fluorescein, rhodamine, phycoerythrin, and Texas Red, fluoresce at different wavelength and can produce different colors.

Immunofluorescence can be accomplished in a one-step or two-step reaction. In the first option, the fluorescently labeled antibody directly binds to the target antigen molecule. In the second option the target antigen molecule binds a so-called secondary antibody. Then, other antigenic sites in the sample that might also bind the fluorescent antibody are "blocked" by the addition of a molecule that more globally binds to antigenic sites. The secondary antibody then can itself be the target to which the fluorescently labeled antibody binds.

The use of antibodies to antigen that are critical to disease processes in **microorganisms** allow immunofluorescence to act as a detection and screening tool in the monitoring of a variety of materials. Foe example, research to adapt immunofluorescence to food monitoring is an active field. In the present, immunofluorescence provides the means by which organisms can be sorted using the technique of flow cytometry. As individual **bacteria**, for example, pass by a detector, the presence of fluorescence will register and cause the bacterium to be shuttled to a special collection reservoir. Thus, bacteria with a certain surface factor can be separated from the other bacteria in the population that do not possess the factor

See also Fluorescent dyes; Microscopy

IMMUNOGENETICS

Immunogenetics is the study of the mechanisms of autoimmune diseases, tolerance in organ transplantation, and **immunity** to infectious diseases—with a special emphasis on the role of the genetic make-up of an organism in these processes. The **immune system** evolved essentially to protect vertebrates from a myriad species of potentially harmful infectious agents such as **bacteria**, virus, **fungi** and various eukaryotic **parasites**. However, the growing understanding of the immune system has influenced a variety of different biomedical disciplines, and is playing an increasingly important role in the study and treatment of many human diseases such as cancer and autoimmune conditions.

There are two broad types of immune systems. The innate immune system of defense depends on invariant receptors that recognize common features of pathogens, but are not varied enough to recognize all types of pathogens, or specific enough to act effectively against re-infection by the same pathogen. Although effective, this system lacks both specificity and the ability to acquire better receptors to deal with the same infectious challenge in the future, a phenomenon called immunological memory. These two properties, specificity and memory, are the main characteristics of the second type of immune system, known as the specific or adaptive immune system, which is based on **antigen** specific receptors. Besides these two families of different receptors that help in immune recognition of foreign infectious agents, both the innate and the adaptive immune systems rely on soluble mediators like the different **cytokines** and kemokines that allow the different cells involved in an immune response to communicate with each other. The major focus of immunogeneticists is the identification, characterization, and sequencing of genes coding for the multiple receptors and mediators of immune responses.

Historically, the launch of immunogenetics could be traced back to the demonstration of Mendelian inheritance of the human ABO blood groups in 1910. The importance of this group of molecules is still highlighted by their important in blood transfusion and organ transplantation protocols. Major developments that contributed to the emergence of immunogenetics as an independent discipline in **immunology** were the rediscovery of allograft reactions during the Second World War and the formulation of an immunological theory of allograft reaction as well as the formulation of the clonal **selection** hypothesis by Burnett in 1959. This theory proposed that clones of immunocompetent cells with unique receptors exist prior to exposure to antigens, and only cells with specific receptors are selected by antigen for subsequent activation.

The molecular understanding of how the diverse repertoire of these receptors is generated came with the discovery of somatic **recombination** of receptor genes, which is the paradigm for studying **gene** rearrangement during cell maturation.

The most important influence on the development of immunogenetics is, however, the studies of a gene family known as the MCH, or **major histocompatibility complex**. These highly polymorphic genes, first studied as white-cell antigens of the blood and therefore named human leukocyte antigens (**HLA**), influence both donor choice in organ transplantation and the susceptibility of an organism to chronic diseases. The **MHC** is also linked with most of all the important autoimmune diseases such as rheumatoid arthritis and diabetes.

The discovery in 1972 that these MHC molecules are intimately associated with the specific immune response to **viruses** led to an explosion in immunogenetic studies of these molecules. This has led to the construction of very detailed genetic and physical maps of this complex and ultimately to its complete sequence in an early stage of the human genome-sequencing project.

Other clusters of immune recognition molecules that are well established at the center of the immunogenetics discipline are the large arrays of rearranging gene segments that determine B-cell **immunoglobulins** and T-cell receptors. Immunoglobulins, which mediate the humoral immune response of the adaptive immune system, are the antibodies that circulate in the bloodstream and diffuse in other body fluids, where they bind specifically to the foreign antigen that induced them. This interaction with the antigen most often leads to its clearance. T cell receptors, which are involved in the cell-mediated immune response of the adaptive immune system, are the principle partners of the MHC molecules in mounting a specific immune response. An antigen that is taken up by specialized cells called antigen presenting cells is usually presented on the surface of this cell in complex with either MHC class I or class II to **T cells** that use specific receptors to recognize and react to the infectious agent. The reacting T cells can kill the host cells that bear the foreign antigen or secrete mediators (cytokines and lynphokines) that activate professional phagocytic cells of the immune system that eliminate the antigen. It is believed that during disease **epidemics**, some forms of class I and class II MHC molecules stimulate T-cell responses that better favor survival. Which MHC molecule is more favorable depends on the infectious agents encountered. Consequently, human populations that were geographically separated and have different disease histories differ in the sequences and frequencies of the HLA class I and class II alleles.

Other immune recognition molecules that were studied in great details in immunogenetics are two families of genes that encode receptors on the surface for natural killer (NK) cells. These large lymphocytes participate in the innate immune system and provide early defense from a pathogens attack, a response that distinguish them from B and T cells which become useful after days of infection. Some NK-cell receptors bind polymorphic determinants of MHC class I molecules and appear to be modulated by the effects that infectious agents have upon the conformation of these determinants.

One of the most important applications of immunogenetics in clinical medicine is HLA-typing in order to help match organ donors and recipients during transplantation surgery. Transplantation is a procedure in which an organ or tissue that is damaged and is no longer functioning is replaced with one obtained from another person. Because HLA antigens can be recognized as foreign by another person's immune system, surgeons and physicians try to match as many of the HLA antigens as possible, between the donated organ and the recipient. In order to do this, the HLA type of every potential organ recipient is determined. When a potential organ donor becomes available, the donor's HLA type is determined as well to make absolutely sure that the donor organ is suitable for the recipient.

See also Autoimmunity and autoimmune diseases; Immunity, active, passive and delayed; Immunity, cell mediated; Immunity, humoral regulation; Immunologic therapies; Immunosuppressant drugs; *In vitro* and *in vivo* research; Laboratory techniques in immunology; Major histocompatibility complex (MHC); Medical training and careers in immunology; Molecular biology and molecular genetics; Mutations and mutagenesis; Oncogenetic research; Transplantation genetics and immunology; Viral genetics

IMMUNOGLOBULIN DEFICIENCY • *see*

IMMUNODEFICIENCY DISEASE SYNDROMES

IMMUNOGLOBULINS AND IMMUNOGLOBU-LIN DEFICIENCY SYNDROMES

Immunoglobulins are proteins that are also called antibodies. The five different classes of immunoglobulins are formed in response to the presence of antigens. The specificity of an immunoglobulin for a particular **antibody** is exquisitely precise

The five classes of immunoglobulins are designated IgA, IgD, IgG, IgE, and IgM. These share a common structure. Two so-called heavy chains form a letter "Y" shape, with two light chains linked to each of the upper arms of the Y. The heavy chains are also known as *alpha, delta, gamma, epsilon,* or *mu.* The light chains are termed *lambda* or *kappa.*

The IgG class of immunoglobulin is the most common. IgG antibody is routinely produced in response to bacterial and viral infections and to the presence of toxins. IgG is found in many tissues and in the plasma that circulates throughout the body. IgM is the first antibody that is produced in an immune response. IgA is also produced early in a body's immune response, and is commonly found in saliva, tears, and other such secretions. The activity of IgD is still not clear. Finally, the IgE immunoglobulin is found in respiratory secretions.

The different classes of immunoglobulins additionally display differences in the sequence of amino acids comprising certain regions within the immunoglobulin molecule. For example, differences in the antigen-binding region, the variable region, accounts for the different **antigen** binding specificities of the various immunoglobulins. Differences in their structure outside of the antigen binding region, in an area known as the constant region, accounts for differences in the immunoglobulin in other functions. These other functions are termed effector functions, and include features such as the recognition and binding to regions on other cells, and the stimulation of activity of an immune molecule known as **complement**.

The vast diversity of immunoglobulin specificity is due to the tremendous number of variations that are possible in the variable region of an immunoglobulin. A certain immune cell known as a B cell produces each particular immunoglobulin. Thus, at any particular moment in time, there are a myriad of **B cells** actively producing a myriad of different immunoglobulins, in response to antigenic exposure.

Immunoglobulins can exist in two forms. They can be fixed to the surface of the B cells that have produced them. Or they can float freely in body fluids, essentially patrolling until a recognizable antigen is encountered. The protection of the body from invading antigens depends on the production of immunoglobulins of the required type and in sufficient quantity.

Conditions where an individual has a reduced number of immunoglobulins or none at all of a certain type is known as an immunoglobulin deficiency syndrome. Such syndromes are typically the result of damage to B cells.

People with immunoglobulin deficiencies are prone to more frequent illness than those people whose immune systems are fully functional. Often the illnesses are caused by **bacteria**, in particular bacteria that are able to form a capsule surrounding them. A capsule is not easily recognized by even an optimally performing **immune system**. As well, immunoglobulin deficiency can render a person more susceptible to some viral infections, in particular those caused by echovirus, enterovirus, and **hepatitis** B.

Immunoglobulin deficiencies can take the form of a primary disorder or a secondary disorder. A secondary deficiency results from some other ongoing malady or treatment. For example, **chemotherapy** for a cancerous illness can compromise the immune system, leading to an **immunodeficiency**. Once the treatment is stopped the immunodeficiency can be reversed. A primary immunodeficiency is not the result of an illness or medical treatment. Rather, it is the direct result of a genetic disorder or a defect to B cells or other immune cells.

X-linked agammaglobulinemia results in an inability of B cells to mature. This results in the production of fewer B cells and in a lack of "memory" of an infection. Normally, the immune system is able to rapidly respond to antigen that has been encountered before, because of the "memory" of the B cells. Without this ability, repeated infections caused by the same agent can result.

Another genetically based immunoglobulin deficiency is known as selective IgA deficiency. Here, B cells fail to switch from producing IgM to produce IgA. The limited amount of IgA makes someone more prone to infections of mucosal cells. Examples of such infections include those in the nose, throat, lungs, and intestine.

Genetic abnormalities cause several other immunodeficiency syndromes. A missing stretch of information in the **gene** that codes for the heavy chain of IgG results in the pro-

duction of an IgG that is structurally incomplete. The result is a loss of function of the IgG class of antibodies, as well as the IgA and IgE classes. On a subtler level, another genetic malfunction affects the four subclasses of antibodies within the IgG class. The function of some of the subclasses are affected more so than other subclasses. Finally, another genetic mutation destroys the ability of B cells to switch from making IgM to manufacture IgG. The lack of flexibility in the antibody capability of the immune system adversely affects the ability of the body to successfully fight infections.

Transient hypogammaglobulinemia is an immunodeficiency syndrome that is not based on a genetic aberration. Rather, the syndrome occurs in infants and is of short-term in duration. The **T cells** of the immune system do not function properly. Fewer than normal antibodies are produced, and those that are made are poor in their recognition of the antigenic target. However, as the immune system matures with age the proper function of the T cells is established. The cause of the hypogammaglobulinemia is not known.

Immunoglobulin deficiency syndromes are curable only by a bone marrow transplant, an option exercised in life-threatening situations. Normally, treatment rather than cure is the option. Prevention of infection, through the regular use of antimicrobial drugs and scrupulous oral health are important to maintain health in individuals with immunoglobulin deficiency syndromes.

See also Immunochemistry; Immunodeficiency disease syndromes; Immunodeficiency diseases; Immunodeficiency; Immunogenetics; Immunologic therapies; Immunological analysis techniques; Immunology; Immunosuppressant drugs

IMMUNOLOGIC THERAPIES

Immunologic therapy is defined as the use of medicines that act to enhance the body's immune response as a means of treating disease. The drugs can also aid in the recovery of the body from the harmful effects of immune-compromising treatments like **chemotherapy** and radiation.

Both microorganism-related infections and other maladies that are due to immune deficiency or cell growth defects are targets of immunologic therapy.

The emphasis in immunologic therapy is the application of synthetic compounds that mimic immune substances that are naturally produced in the body. For example, a compound called aldesleukin is an artificial form of interkeukin-2, a natural compound that assists white blood cells in recognizing and dealing with foreign material. Other examples are filgrastim and sargramostim, which are synthetic version of **colony** stimulating factors, which stimulate bone marrow to make the white blood cells, and epoetin, an artificial version of erythropoietin, which stimulates the marrow to produce red blood cells. Thrombopoietin encourages the manufacture of platelets, which are plate-shaped components of the blood that are vital in the clotting of blood. As a final example, synthetic forms of interferon are available and can be administered to aid the natural forms of interferon in battling infections and even cancer.

Research has provided evidence that the infusion of specific **enzymes** can produce positive results with respect to some neurological disorders. While not strictly an immunologic therapy, the supplementation of the body's natural components is consistent with the aim of the immune approach.

The use of immunologic therapy is not without risk. Paradoxically, given their longer-term enhancement of the immune defenses, some of the administered drugs reduce the body's ability to fight off infection because of a short-term damping-down of some aspects of the **immune system**. As well, certain therapies carry a risk of reduced clotting of the blood and of seizures.

As with other therapies, the use of immunologic therapies is assessed in terms of the risks of the therapy versus the health outcome if therapy is not used. Typically, the immediate health threat to a patient outweighs the possible side effects from therapy. Immunologic therapies are always administered under a physician's care, almost always in a hospital setting. As well, frequent monitoring of the patients is done, both for the abatement of the malady and the development of adverse effects.

Immunologic therapy can provide continued treatment following chemotherapy or the use of radiation. The latter two treatments cannot be carried on indefinitely, due to toxic reactions in the body. Immunologic therapy provides another avenue of treatment. For example, some tumors that are resistant to chemical therapy are susceptible to immune attack. By enhancing the immune response, such tumors may be productively treated. Moreover, despite their side effects, immunologic therapies usually are less toxic than either chemotherapy or the use of radiation.

See also Immune system; Laboratory techniques in immunology

IMMUNOLOGICAL ANALYSIS TECHNIQUES

Immunological techniques are the wide varieties of methods and specialized experimental protocols devised by immunologists for inducing, measuring, and characterizing immune responses. They allow the immunologists to alter the **immune system** through cellular, molecular and genetic manipulation. These techniques are not restricted to the field of **immunology**, but are widely applied by basic scientists in many other biological disciplines and by clinicians in human and veterinary medicine.

Most immunological techniques available are focused on the study of the adaptive immune system. They classically involve the experimental induction of an immune response using methods based on **vaccination** protocols. During a typical experiment called **immunization**, immunologists inject a test **antigen** to an animal or human subject and monitor for the appearance of immune responses in the form of specific antibodies and effector **T cells**. Monitoring the **antibody** response usually involves the analysis of crude preparations of serum from the immunized subject. The analysis of the immune

responses mediated by T cells are usually performed only on experimental animals and involves the preparation of these cells from blood or from the lymphoid organs, such as the spleen and the lymph nodes. Typically, any substance that has a distinctive structure or conformation that may be recognized by the immune system can serve as an antigen. A wide range of substances from simple chemicals like sugars, and small peptides to complex macromolecules and **viruses** can induce the immune system. Although the antigenic determinant of a test substance is usually a minor part of that substance called the epitope, a small antigen referred to as a hapten can rarely elicit an immune response on its own. It is not an immunogen and would therefore need to be covalently linked to a carrier in order to elicit an immune response. The induction of such a response to even large immunogenic antigen is not easy to achieve and the dose, the form and route of administration of that antigen can profoundly affect whether a response can occur. Especially the use of certain substances called adjuvants is necessary to alert the immune system and produce a strong immune response.

According to the clonal **selection** theory, antibodies produced in a typical immunization experiment are products of different clones of B-lymphocytes that are already committed to making antibodies to the corresponding antigen. These polyclonal antibodies are multi-subunit proteins that belong to the **immunoglobulins** family. They have a basic Y-shaped structure with two identical Fab domains, which form the arms and interact with the antigen, and one Fc domain that forms the stem and determines the isotype subclass of each antibody. There are five different isotype subclasses, IgM, Ig G, IgA, IgE, and IgD, which show different tissue distribution and half-life *in vivo*. They determine the biological function of the antibodies and appear during different stages of the immunization process. Knowledge about the biosynthesis and structure of these antibodies is important for their detection and use both as diagnostic and therapeutic tools.

Antibodies are highly specific for their corresponding antigen, and are able to detect one molecule of a protein antigen out of around a billion similar molecules. The amount and specificity of an antibody in a test serum can be measured by its direct binding to the antigen in assays usually referred to as primary interaction immunoassays. Commonly used direct assays are radioimmunoassay (RIA), enzyme-linked immunosorbent assay (**ELISA**), and immunoblotting techniques. In both ELISA and RIA, an enzyme or a radioisotope is covalently linked to the pure antigen or antibody. The unlabeled component, which most often is the antigen, is attached to the surface of a plastic well. The labeled antibody is allowed to bind to the unlabeled antigen. The plastic well is subsequently washed with plenty of **buffer** that will remove any excess non-bound antibody and prevent non-specific binding. Antibody binding is measured as the amount of radioactivity retained by the coated wells in radioimmunoassay or as fluorescence emitted by the product of an enzymatic reaction in the case of ELISA. Modifications of these assays known as competitive inhibition assays can be used that will allow quantifying the antigen (or antibody) in a mixture and determining the affinity of the antibody-antigen interaction by using mathematical models. Immunoblotting is usually performed in the form of Western blotting, which is reserved to the detection of proteins and involves an **electrophoresis** separation step followed by electroblotting of the separated proteins from the gel to a membrane and then probing with an antibody. Detection of the antigen protein antibody interaction is made in a similar way as in RIA or ELISA depending on whether a radiolabeled or enzyme-coupled antibody is used.

Antibodies can also be monitored through immunoassays that are based on the ability of antibodies to alter the physical state of their corresponding antigens and typically involve the creation of a precipitate in a solid or liquid medium. The hemmaglutination assay used to determine the ABO type of blood groups and match compatible donors and recipients for blood transfusion is based on this assay. Currently, the most common application of this immunoassay is in a procedure known as immunoprecipitation. This method allows antibodies to form complexes with their antigen in a complex mixture like the cytosol, the **nucleus** or membrane complexes of the cell. The antigen-antibody complex is precipitated either by inducing the formation of even larger complexes through the addition of excess amounts of anti-immunoglobulin antibodies or by the addition of agarose beads coupled to a special class of bacterial proteins that bind the Fc region of the antibody. The complex can also be precipitated by covalently linking the antibody to agarose beads forming a special affinity matrix. This procedure will also allow the purification of the antigen by immunoaffinity, a special form of affinity chromatography. Immunoprecipitation is a valuable technique that led to major discoveries in immunology an all disciplines of molecular and cellular biology. It allows the precipitation of the antigen in complex with other interacting proteins and reagents and therefore gives an idea on the function of the antigen.

The T cell immune response is detected by using monoclonal antibodies, a specific family of antibodies that recognize surface markers that are expressed by lymphocytes upon their activation. These monoclonal antibodies are highly specific, and are produced by special techniques from single clones of **B cells** and are therefore, homogenous groups of immunoglobulins with the same isotype and antigen binding affinity. These antibodies are used to identify characterize cells by flow cytometry (FACS), immunocytochemistry, **immunofluorescence** techniques. The difficulty to isolate antigen specific T cells is due to the fact that these T cells recognize the antigen in the context of a tri-molecular complex involving the T cell receptor and the **MHC** molecules on the surface of specialized cells called antigen-presenting cells. These interactions are subtle, have low affinity and are extremely complex to study. Novel and powerful techniques using tetramers of MHC molecules were developed in 1997 that are now used to identify and isolate antigen specific T cell clones. These tetramer-based assays are proving useful in separating very rare cells, and could be used in clinical medicine. In fact, virus and tumor specific T cells usually give a stronger response and are usually more effective in killing virus infected and tumor cells. Testing for the function of activated, antigen specific T cells known as effector T cells is routinely

done *in vitro* by testing for cytokine production, cytotoxicity to other cells and proliferation in response to antigen stimulation. Local reactions in the skin of animals and humans provide information about T cell responses to an antigen, a procedure that is very used in testing for allergic reactions and the efficacy of vaccination procedures. Experimental manipulations of the immune system in vivo are performed to reveal the functions of each component of the immune system *in vivo*. **Mutations** through irradiation, or mutations produced by **gene** targeting (e.g., knock-out and knock-in techniques), as well as animal models produced by transgenic breeding, are proving helpful to researchers in evaluating this highly complex system.

See also Immune complex test; Immune stimulation, as a vaccine; Immune synapse; Immunity, active, passive and delayed; Immunity, cell mediated; Immunity, humoral regulation; Immunization; Immunochemistry; Immunodeficiency; Immunoelectrophoresis; Immunofluorescence; Immunogenetics; Immunologic therapies; Immunology; Immunomodulation; Immunosuppressant drugs; *In vitro* and *in vivo* research; Laboratory techniques in immunology

IMMUNOLOGICAL ASPECTS OF REPRODUCTION • *see* REPRODUCTIVE IMMUNOLOGY

IMMUNOLOGY

Immunology is the study of how the body responds to foreign substances and fights off infection and other disease. Immunologists study the molecules, cells, and organs of the human body that participate in this response.

The beginnings of our understanding of **immunity** date to 1798, when the English physician **Edward Jenner** (1749–1823) published a report that people could be protected from deadly **smallpox** by sticking them with a needle dipped in the material from a **cowpox** boil. The French biologist and chemist **Louis Pasteur** (1822–1895) theorized that such **immunization** protects people against disease by exposing them to a version of a microbe that is harmless but is enough like the disease-causing organism, or pathogen, that the **immune system** learns to fight it. Modern vaccines against diseases such as **measles**, polio, and chicken pox are based on this principle.

In the late nineteenth century, a scientific debate was waged between the German physician **Paul Ehrlich** (1854–1915) and the Russian zoologist **Élie Metchnikoff** (1845–1916). Ehrlich and his followers believed that proteins in the blood, called antibodies, eliminated pathogens by sticking to them; this phenomenon became known as humoral immunity. Metchnikoff and his students, on the other hand, noted that certain white blood cells could engulf and digest foreign materials: this cellular immunity, they claimed, was the real way the body fought infection.

Modern immunologists have shown that both the humoral and cellular responses play a role in fighting disease.

They have also identified many of the actors and processes that form the immune response.

The immune response recognizes and responds to pathogens via a network of cells that communicate with each other about what they have "seen" and whether it "belongs." These cells patrol throughout the body for infection, carried by both the blood stream and the lymph ducts, a series of vessels carrying a clear fluid rich in immune cells.

The **antigen** presenting cells are the first line of the body's defense, the scouts of the immune army. They engulf foreign material or **microorganisms** and digest them, displaying bits and pieces of the invaders—called antigens—for other immune cells to identify. These other immune cells, called T lymphocytes, can then begin the immune response that attacks the pathogen.

The body's other cells can also present antigens, although in a slightly different way. Cells always display antigens from their everyday proteins on their surface. When a cell is infected with a virus, or when it becomes cancerous, it will often make unusual proteins whose antigens can then be identified by any of a variety of cytotoxic T lymphocytes. These "killer cells" then destroy the infected or cancerous cell to protect the rest of the body. Other T lymphocytes generate chemical or other signals that encourage multiplication of other infection-fighting cells. Various types of T lymphocytes are a central part of the cellular immune response; they are also involved in the humoral response, encouraging **B lymphocytes** to turn into antibody-producing plasma cells.

The body cannot know in advance what a pathogen will look like and how to fight it, so it creates millions and millions of different lymphocytes that recognize random antigens. When, by chance, a B or T lymphocyte recognizes an antigen being displayed by an antigen presenting cell, the lymphocyte divides and produces many offspring that can also identify and attack this antigen. The way the immune system expands cells that by chance can attack an invading microbe is called clonal **selection**.

Some researchers believe that while some B and T lymphocytes recognize a pathogen and begin to mature and fight an infection, others stick around in the bloodstream for months or even years in a primed condition. Such memory cells may be the basis for the immunity noted by the ancient Chinese and by Thucydides. Other immunologists believe instead that trace amounts of a pathogen persist in the body, and their continued presence keeps the immune response strong over time.

Substances foreign to the body, such as disease-causing **bacteria**, **viruses**, and other infectious agents (known as antigens), are recognized by the body's immune system as invaders. The body's natural defenses against these infectious agents are antibodies—proteins that seek out the antigens and help destroy them. Antibodies have two very useful characteristics. First, they are extremely specific; that is, each **antibody** binds to and attacks one particular antigen. Second, some antibodies, once activated by the occurrence of a disease, continue to confer resistance against that disease; classic examples are the antibodies to the childhood diseases chickenpox and measles.

The second characteristic of antibodies makes it possible to develop vaccines. A **vaccine** is a preparation of killed or weakened bacteria or viruses that, when introduced into the body, stimulates the production of antibodies against the antigens it contains.

It is the first trait of antibodies, their specificity, that makes monoclonal antibody technology so valuable. Not only can antibodies be used therapeutically, to protect against disease; they can also help to diagnose a wide variety of illnesses, and can detect the presence of drugs, viral and bacterial products, and other unusual or abnormal substances in the blood.

Given such a diversity of uses for these disease-fighting substances, their production in pure quantities has long been the focus of scientific investigation. The conventional method was to inject a laboratory animal with an antigen and then, after antibodies had been formed, collect those antibodies from the blood serum (antibody-containing blood serum is called **antiserum**). There are two problems with this method: It yields antiserum that contains undesired substances, and it provides a very small amount of usable antibody.

Monoclonal antibody technology allows the production of large amounts of pure antibodies in the following way. Cells that produce antibodies naturally are obtained along with a class of cells that can grow continually in cell **culture**. The hybrid resulting from combining cells with the characteristic of "immortality" and those with the ability to produce the desired substance, creates, in effect, a factory to produce antibodies that work around the clock.

A myeloma is a tumor of the bone marrow that can be adapted to grow permanently in cell culture. Fusing myeloma cells with antibody-producing mammalian spleen cells, results in hybrid cells, or hybridomas, producing large amounts of monoclonal antibodies. This product of cell fusion combined the desired qualities of the two different types of cells, the ability to grow continually, and the ability to produce large amounts of pure antibody. Because selected hybrid cells produce only one specific antibody, they are more pure than the polyclonal antibodies produced by conventional techniques. They are potentially more effective than conventional drugs in fighting disease, because drugs attack not only the foreign substance but also the body's own cells as well, sometimes producing undesirable side effects such as nausea and allergic reactions. Monoclonal antibodies attack the target molecule and only the target molecule, with no or greatly diminished side effects.

While researchers have made great gains in understanding immunity, many big questions remain. Future research will need to identify how the immune response is coordinated. Other researchers are studying the immune systems of non-mammals, trying to learn how our immune response evolved. Insects, for instance, lack antibodies, and are protected only by cellular immunity and chemical defenses not known to be present in higher organisms.

Immunologists do not yet know the details behind allergy, where antigens like those from pollen, poison ivy, or certain kinds of food make the body start an uncomfortable, unnecessary, and occasionally life-threatening immune response. Likewise, no one knows exactly why the immune system can suddenly attack the body's tissues—as in autoimmune diseases like rheumatoid arthritis, juvenile diabetes, systemic lupus erythematosus, or multiple sclerosis.

The hunt continues for new vaccines, especially against parasitic organisms like the **malaria** microbe that trick the immune system by changing their antigens. Some researchers are seeking ways to start an immune response that prevents or kills cancers. A big goal of immunologists is the search for a vaccine for **HIV**, the virus that causes **AIDS**. HIV knocks out the immune system—causing immunodeficiency—by infecting crucial T lymphocytes. Some immunologists have suggested that the chiefly humoral response raised by conventional vaccines may be unable to stop HIV from getting to lymphocytes, and that a new kind of vaccine that encourages a cellular response may be more effective.

Researchers have shown that transplant rejection is just another kind of immune response, with the immune system attacking antigens in the transplanted organ that are different from its own. Drugs that suppress the immune system are now used to prevent rejection, but they also make the patient vulnerable to infection. Immunologists are using their increased understanding of the immune system to develop more subtle ways of deceiving the immune system into accepting transplants.

See also AIDS, recent advances in research and treatment; Antibody, monoclonal; Biochemical analysis techniques; BSE, scrapie and CJD: recent advances in research; History of immunology; Immunochemistry; Immunodeficiency disease syndromes; Immunodeficiency diseases; Immunodeficiency; Immunogenetics; Immunological analysis techniques; Immunology, nutritional aspects; Immunosuppressant drugs; Infection and resistance; Laboratory techniques in immunology; Reproductive immunology; Transplantation genetics and immunology

IMMUNOLOGY, HISTORY OF · *see* HISTORY OF IMMUNOLOGY

IMMUNOLOGY, NUTRITIONAL ASPECTS

The role of nutrition is central to the development and modulation of the **immune system**. The importance of nutrition has been made clear by the burgeoning field of sports medicine. It appears the immune system is enhanced by moderate to severe exercise, although many components of the immune response exhibit adverse change for a period of from 3 to 72 hours after prolonged intense exertion. This "window of opportunity" for opportunistic bacterial and viral infections seems to be increased for "elite" athletes that are more prone to over-train. The elements of the immune response most affected by the strenuous activity that leads to the impairment of the immune system are lymphocyte concentrations, depressed natural killer activity, and elevated levels of IgA in the saliva.

The possible basis for this prolonged immunosuppression may include reduced plasma glutamine concentrations, altered plasma glucose levels, and proliferation of neutrophils and monocytes that increases prostaglandin concentrations. Exercise produces oxidative stress and so concomitantly, there are elevated free radical levels along with an attendant depletion of antioxidant levels. Therefore, antioxidants that help protect against oxidative stress are considered the most promising for further study, but those nutrients that heal the gut show potential also. These nutrients include Vitamin E, Vitamin C, zinc, and glutamine. Glutamine and nucleotides show a direct effect on lymphocyte proliferation. Free radicals and other reactive oxygen species that can damage cells as well as tissues are an integral part of the immune system, so the body has developed systems that protect from their damage. These products function by destroying invading organisms and damaged tissues, as well as enhance interleukin-I, Interleukin-8 and tumor necrosis factor concentrations as part of the inflammatory response. The purpose of supplementing the diet is to provide a balance to the immune system's pro-oxidant function. Carbohydrate supplementation has additionally shown impressive results. Increased plasma levels, a depressed cortisol and growth hormone response, fewer fluctuations in blood levels of immune competent cells, decreased granulocyte and monocyte **phagocytosis**, reduced oxidative stress and a diminished pro-inflammatory and anti-inflammatory cytokine response are all associated with an increase in complex carbohydrate consumption.

Besides exercise-associated immune suppression, malnutrition plays a pivotal role in modulating the immune response. Nowhere is this more important then during pregnancy and gestation. Besides genetics, no other factor is more important for the developing immune system then optimal nutrition. The immune response of low-birth-weight babies is compromised as well as those of children born to mothers without adequate nutrition. Especially important is the role of Vitamin E and selenium in preventing immune impairment. Animal studies showed that progeny of Vitamin E and selenium-deficient mothers never adequately developed immune competent cell lines.

Because nutrition plays such a vital role in the immune response, a special branch of **immunology** is developing called immunonutrition. These scientists are particularly interested in the interaction of genetics and nutrition. Preliminary work suggests that individual genotypes vary in their response to healing, infection, and dietary supplementation.

See also Immunogenetics; Infection and resistance; Metabolism

IMMUNOMODULATION

From a therapeutic point of view, immunomodulation refers to any process in which an immune response is altered to a desired level. **Microorganisms** are also capable of modulating the response of the **immune system** to their presence, in order to establish or consolidate an infection. Thus, immunomodulation can be beneficial or detrimental to a host.

Many providers of nutritional supplements claim that a product enhances certain aspects of the immune system so as to more vigorously shield the body from infection or the development of maladies such as cancer. However, rigorous testing of these claims is typically lacking and so the claims of nutritional links with immune system improvement are at present tenuous.

A firmer link exists between exercise and immunomodulation. Moderately active people are known to have macrophages that are more capable of killing tumors, due to the increased production of a compound called nitric oxide. This population also displays lower incidence rates for cancer and other chronic diseases. Even sporadic exercise increases the ability of an immune system component called natural killer cells to eradicate tumors.

Conversely, too much exercise is associated with increased susceptibility to respiratory tract infections, indicating that the immune system is impaired in the ability to thwart infections.

Immunomodulation by microorganisms is directed at several aspects of the immune system. One target are the small molecules known as **cytokines**, which function as messengers of the immune system. In other words, cytokines stimulate various immune responses such as **inflammation** of the manufacture of antibodies. Other cytokines are involved in downregulating the immune responses.

Some microorganisms are able to produce and excrete proteins that mimic the structure and function of cytokines. Often the result is a suppression of the host's inflammatory response. Examples of microbes that produce cytokine-like molecules are the **Epstein-Barr virus**, poxvirus, vaccinia virus.

Other microbes, such as the protozoan *Trypanosoma cruzi* blocks the activation of cytokines by an as yet unknown mechanism. The result is a severe suppression of the immune system. **Adenoviruses** also block cytokine expression, at the level of **transcription**.

The manipulation of cytokine expression and action may also be exploited to produce vaccines. For example, vaccines designed to nullify or enhance the activity of certain cytokines could cause greater activity of certain components of the immune system. While vaccines have yet to achieve this level of activity, specific experimental targeting of **deoxyribonucleic acid** has suppressed certain cytokines.

Another portion of the immune system capable of immunomodulation is **complement**. **Herpes** simplex virus types 1 and 2, the **viruses** responsible for cold sores and genital herpes in humans, resist the action of complement. The presence of specific viral proteins are required, and may act by disrupting a key enzyme necessary for complement manufacture.

Vaccinia virus can also evade complement action, via a protein that structurally resembles a host protein to which complement binds. Also, another viral protein, called the inflammation modulatory protein, acts to decrease the inflammatory response at the site of infection, thus preserving host tissue from damage and providing the virus particles with relatively undamaged cells in which to grow.

The protozoan *Trypanosoma cruzi* can regulate the activity of complement before infecting human cells. Once inside the cells of the host, the parasite can evade an immune response.

A variety of **bacteria**, viruses, and **parasites** are also able to modulate the immune system by affecting the way antigens are exposed on their surfaces. **Antigen** presentation is a complex series of steps. By controlling or modulating even one of these steps, the antigen presentation process can be disrupted. The formation of **antibody** is thus affected.

Aside from biological agents, physiological factors can cause immunomodulation. For example, stress is known to be capable of suppressing various aspects of the cellular immune response. The release of various hormones may disrupt in the normal expression of cytokines. Specifically, those cytokines that suppress inflammation are more evident, either because of their increased production or the decreased production of cytokines that activate inflammation.

See also Immunologic therapies

IMMUNOPRECIPITATION • *see* ANTIBODY-ANTIGEN, BIOCHEMICAL AND MOLECULAR REACTIONS

IMMUNOSUPPRESSANT DRUGS

Immunosuppressant drugs are medications that reduce the ability of the **immune system** to recognize and respond to the presence of foreign material. Such drugs were developed and still have an important use as a means of ensuring that transplanted organs and tissues are not rejected by the recipient.

Rejection of transplanted organs or tissue is a natural reaction of a person's immune system. In a very real sense, the transplanted material is foreign and is treated, as would be an infectious microorganism. The immune system attacks and tries to destroy the foreign matter. Suppressing the immune system allows the transplanted material to be retained.

Drugs to suppress the immune system are available only with a physician's authorization. Some commonly prescribed drugs are azathioprine, cyclosporine, prednisolone, and tacrolimus. These can be taken orally, both in solid and liquid forms, or can be injected.

The main target of such immunosuppressant drugs are the white blood cells (which are also called lymphocytes). The main function of lymphocytes is to patrol the body and root out foreign material. Then these cells, in combination with other immune system components, destroy the foreign material.

Transplantation of animal kidneys into humans was tried in the early 1900s, and human-to-human transplant attempts were first made in 1933. These attempts were unsuccessful. It was not until the years of World War II that the immunological basis for these failures was deciphered. Then, **Peter Medawar** observed that a skin graft survived about a week before being rejected, but a subsequent graft was rejected much more quickly. This led him to propose that an immunological response was at play in the rejection of transplanted material. This led to the first successful transplant in 1954, when the kidney of one identical twin was transplanted to the other twin. In the twins, the absence of genetic differences in their tissues would eliminate an immunological response.

As the role of the immune system in transplantation failure became more clear, the use of compounds to suppress the immune system began in the 1960s. In the 1960s and 1970s, the antigenic basis of immune recognition of foreign and nonforeign tissue became evident. With these discoveries came the recognition that the suppression of the immune system could aid in maintaining transplanted tissue. Successful transplantation of the liver was achieved in 1963, of the heart and small bowel in 1967.

In the 1980s, cyclosporin was discovered and shown to be effective in maintaining transplanted material. The clinical use of cyclosporin became standard. By the end of that decade, the use of immunosuppressant drugs just prior to and forever after a transplant had boosted the one-year transplant success rate to more than 80 per cent for all transplants except for the small intestine. In the present day, the survival rate of a kidney transplant is 86 percent even after five years.

Immunosuppressant drugs have other uses as well. Suppressing the immune system can lessen the disfigurement caused by severe forms of skin disorders such as psoriasis. Other examples include rheumatoid arthritis, Crohn's disease (which is an ongoing **inflammation** of the intestinal tract) and alopecia areata (nonuniform hair loss). In such cases the use of immunosuppressant therapy needs to be evaluated carefully, especially when the condition is not life threatening. This is because the deliberate suppression of the immune system can leave the individual vulnerable to other infections. Also, the clotting of blood can be inhibited, which could produce uncontrolled bleeding.

Another potential risk in the use of immunosuppressant drugs involves the administration of vaccines. The use of vaccines is not advisable when immunosuppressant drugs are being used, especially vaccines that utilize living but weakened **bacteria** or a virus as the agent designed to elicit protection. The deliberately immunocompromised individual could develop the disease for which the **vaccine** is intended to prevent.

The same risk analysis applies to the possible side effects of immunosuppressant drugs, which can include a higher than normal risk of developing some kinds of cancer later in life. The link between immunosuppressant drugs and cancer is not yet clear. The link was assumed to be a consequence of the interference with the ability of the body to detect and respond to cancerous cells. Conversely, cancer development has been viewed as being due partially to a failure of the immune system. Yet people with acquired **immunodeficiency** system, whose immune systems are also compromised, do not show increased rates of cancer. Instead, immunosuppressant drugs such as cyclosporine may themselves encourage the development of cancer by activating a cellular factor that makes cells more invasive.

It is now well known that the deliberate suppression of the immune system carries risks. However, the risks of a side effect or developing another illness, is usually less than the immediate health risk associated with not suppressing the immune system.

See also Autoimmunity and autoimmune diseases; Immunodeficiency

IN VITRO AND *IN VIVO* RESEARCH

In vitro research is generally referred to as the manipulation of organs, tissues, cells, and biomolecules in a controlled, artificial environment. The characterization and analysis of biomolecules and biological systems in the context of intact organisms is known as *in vivo* research.

The basic unit of living organisms is the cell, which in terms of scale and dimension is at the interface between the molecular and the microscopic level. The living cell is in turn divided into functional and structural domains such as the **nucleus**, the **cytoplasm**, and the secretory pathway, which are composed of a vast array of biomolecules. These molecules of life carry out the chemical reactions that enable a cell to interact with its environment, use and store energy, reproduce, and grow. The structure of each biomolecule and its subcellular localization determines in which chemical reactions it is able to participate and hence what role it plays in the cell's life process. Any manipulation that breaks down this unit of life, that is, the cell into its non-living components is, considered an *in vitro* approach. Thus, *in vitro,* which literally means "in glass," refers to the experimental manipulation conducted using cell-free extracts and purified or partially purified biomolecules in test tubes. Most of the biochemical and molecular biological approaches and techniques are considered genetic manipulation research. Molecular **cloning** of a **gene** with the aim of expressing its protein product includes some steps that are considered *in vitro* experiments such as the **PCR** amplification of the gene and the ligation of that gene to the expression vector. The expression of that gene in a host cell is considered an *in vivo* procedure. What characterizes an *in vitro* experiment is in principle the fact the conditions are artificial and are reconstructions of what might happen *in vivo.* Many *in vitro* assays are approximate reconstitutions of biological processes by mixing the necessary components and reagents under controlled conditions. Examples of biological processes that can be reconstituted *in vitro* are enzymatic reactions, folding and refolding of proteins and **DNA**, and the replication of DNA in the PCR reaction.

The definition of *in vitro* and *in vivo* research depends on the experimental model used. Microbiologists and **yeast** geneticists working with single cells or cell populations are conducting *in vivo* research while an immunologist who works with purified lymphocytes in tissue **culture** usually considers his experiments as an *in vitro* approach. The *in vivo* approach involves experiments performed in the context of the large system of the body of an experimental animal. In the case of *in vitro* fertilization, physicians and reproductive biologists are manipulating living systems, and many of the biological processes involved take place inside the living egg and sperm. This procedure is considered an *in vitro* process in order to distinguish it from the natural fertilization of the egg in the intact body of the female.

In vivo experimental research became widespread with the use **microorganisms** and animal models in genetic manipulation experiments as well as the use of animal models to study drug toxicity in pharmacology. Geneticists have used prokaryotic, unicellular **eukaryotes** like yeast, and whole organisms like *Drosophila*, frogs, and mice to study genetics, **molecular biology** and toxicology. The function of genes has been studied by observing the effects of spontaneous **mutations** in whole organisms or by introducing targeted mutations in cultured cells. The introduction of gene cloning and *in vitro* mutagenesis has made it possible to produce specific mutations in whole animals thus considerably facilitating *in vivo* research. Mice with extra copies or altered copies of a gene in their genome can be generated by transgenesis, which is now a well-established technique. In many cases, the function of a particular gene can be fully understood only if a mutant animal that does not express the gene can be obtained. This is now achieved by gene knock-out technology, which involves first isolating a gene of interest and then replacing it *in vivo* with a defective copy.

Both *in vitro* and *in vivo* approaches are usually combined to obtain detailed information about structure-function relationships in genes and their protein products, either in cultured cells and test tubes or in the whole organism.

See also Immunogenetics; Immunologic therapies; Immunological analysis techniques; Laboratory techniques in immunology; Laboratory techniques in microbiology; Molecular biology and molecular genetics

INDICATOR SPECIES

Indicator organisms are used to monitor water, food or other samples for the possibility of microbial **contamination**. The detection of the designated species is an indication that harmful microbes, which are found in the same environment as the indicator species, may be present in the sample.

Indicator organisms serve as a beacon of fecal contamination. The most common fecal microorganism that is used have in the past been designated as fecal coliforms. Now, with more specific growth media available, testing for *Escherichia coli* can be done directly. The detection of *Escherichia coli* indicates the presence of fecal material from warm-blooded animals, and so the possible presence of disease producing **bacteria**, such as *Salmonella, Shigella,* and *Vibrio.*

To be an indicator organism, the bacteria must fulfill several criteria. The species should always be present in the sample whenever the bacterial pathogens are present. The indicator should always be present in greater numbers than the pathogen. This increases the chances of detecting the indicator. Testing directly for the pathogen, which can be more expensive and time-consuming, might yield a negative result

if the numbers of the pathogen are low. Thirdly, the indicator bacterial species should be absent, or present in very low numbers, in clean water or other uncontaminated samples. Fourth, the indicator should not grow more abundantly than the pathogen in the same environment. Fifth, the indicator should respond to **disinfection** or **sterilization** treatments in the same manner as the pathogen does. For example, *Escherichia coli* responds to water disinfection treatments, such as **chlorination**, ozone, and ultra-violet irradiation, with the same sensitivity as does *Salmonella*. Thus, if the indicator organism is killed by the water treatment, the likelihood of *Salmonella* being killed also is high.

Another indicator bacterial species that is used are of the fecal *Streptococcus* group. These have been particularly useful in salt water monitoring, as they persist longer in the salt water than does *Escherichia coli*. In addition, the ratio of fecal coliform bacteria to fecal **streptococci** can provide an indication of whether the fecal contamination is from a human or another warm-blooded animal.

The use of indicator bacteria has long been of fundamental importance in the monitoring of drinking water. Similar indicator organisms will be needed to monitor water against the emerging protozoan threats of **giardia** and **cryptosporidium**.

See also Antibiotic resistance, tests for; Water quality

INDUSTRIAL MICROBIOLOGY · *see* ECONOMIC
USES AND BENEFITS OF MICROORGANISMS

INFECTION AND RESISTANCE

Infection describes the process whereby harmful **microorganisms** enter the body, multiply, and cause disease. Normally the defense mechanisms of the body's **immune system** keep infectious microorganisms from becoming established. Those organisms, however, that can evade or diffuse the immune system and therapeutic strategies (e.g., the application of **antibiotics**) are able to increase their population numbers faster than they can be killed. The population increase usually results in host illness.

There are a variety of ways by which harmful microorganisms can be acquired. Blood contaminated with microbes, such as the viral agents of **hepatitis** and acquired **immunodeficiency** syndrome, is one source. Infected food or water is another source that causes illness and death to millions of people around the world every year. A prominent example is the food and water-borne transmission of harmful strains of *Escherichia coli* **bacteria**. Harmful microbes can enter the body through close contact with infected creatures. Transmission of the **rabies** virus by an infected raccoon bite and of encephalitis virus via mosquitoes are but two examples. Finally, breathing contaminated air can cause illness. Bacterial spores of the causative bacterial agent of **anthrax** are readily aerosolized and inhaled into the lungs, where, if sufficient in

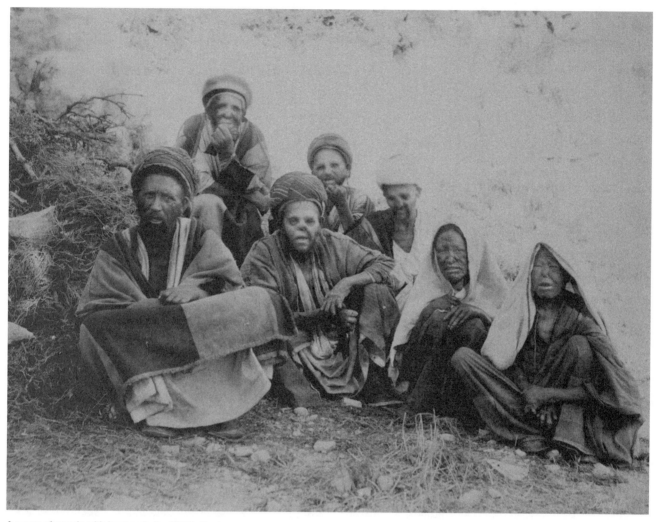

A group of people with leprosy in the Middle East.

large enough numbers, can germinate and cause severe illness and even death.

To establish an infection, microbes must defeat two lines of defense of the body. The first line of defense is at body surfaces that act as a barrier guard the boundaries between the body and the outside world. These barriers include the skin, mucous membranes in the nose and throat, and tiny hairs in the nose that act to physically block invading organisms. Organisms can be washed away from body surfaces by tears, bleeding, and sweating. These are non-specific mechanisms of resistance.

The body's second line of defense involves the specific mechanisms of the immune system, a coordinated response involving a variety of cells and protein antibodies, whereby an invading microorganism is recognized and destroyed. The immune system can be strengthened by **vaccination**, which supplies or stimulates the creation of antibodies to an organism that the body has not yet encountered.

An increasing cause of **bacterial infection** is the ability of the bacteria to resist the killing action of antibiotics. Within the past decade, the problem of antibiotic resistant bacteria has become a significant clinical issue. Part of the reason for the development of resistance has been the widespread and sometimes inappropriate use of antibiotics (e.g., use of antibiotics for viral illness because antibiotics are not effective against **viruses**).

Resistance can have molecular origins. The membrane(s) of the bacteria may become altered to make entry of the antibacterial compound more difficult. Also, **enzymes** can be made that will destroy or inactivate the antibacterial agent. These resistance mechanisms can be passed on to subsequent generations of bacteria that will then be able to survive in increasing numbers.

Bacteria can also acquire resistance to antibiotics and other antibacterial agents, even components of the immune system, by growing on body surfaces, passages, and tissues. In this mode of growth, termed a biofilm, the bacteria are enmeshed in a sticky polymer produced by the cells. The polymer and the slow, almost dormant, growth rate of the bacteria protect them from antibacterial compounds that would otherwise kill them, and can encourage the bacteria to become resistant to the compounds. Examples of such resistance includes the chronic *Pseudomonas aeruginosa* lung infections experienced by those with cystic fibrosis and infection of artificially implanted material, such as urinary catheters and heart pacemakers.

Bacteria and viruses can also evade immune destruction by entering host cells and tissues. Once inside the host structures they are shielded from immune recognition.

See also Antibody and antigen; Antibody formation and kinetics; Antibody-antigen, biochemical and molecular reactions; Bacteria and bacterial infection; Bacterial adaptation; Biofilm formation and dynamic behavior; Immune system; Immunity, active, passive and delayed; Immunity, cell mediated; Immunity, humoral regulation; Immunodeficiency; Microbiology, clinical; Viruses and responses to viral infection

INFECTION CONTROL

Microorganisms are easily transmitted from place to place via vectors such as insects or animals, by humans that can harbor the infectious organism and shed them to the environment, and via movement through the air (in the case of some **bacteria**, **yeast**, and **viruses**). Microorganisms can adapt to antimicrobial treatments (the best example being the acquisition of inheritable **antibiotic resistance** by bacteria). Thus, the potential for the spread of infection by disease-causing microbes is substantial unless steps are taken to limit the spread. Such strategies are collectively termed infection control.

For many microorganisms, particularly bacteria, contact transmission is a common means of spread of infection. This can involve the fecal-oral route, where hands soiled by exposure to feces are placed in the mouth. Day care workers and the infants under their charge are a significant focus of such *Escherichia coli* infections. As well, touching a contaminated inanimate surface is a means of transmitting an infectious microorganism.

The contact route of transmission is the most common route in the hospital setting. Various steps can be taken to control the spread of infection through contact with contaminated surfaces. Proper handwashing, in fact, is the single most effective means of preventing the spread of infection. Thorough handwashing prevents spread of bacteria to others and also prevents **contamination** of work or food preparation surfaces.

The operating theatre is an example of a place where the importance of infection control measures is apparent. In the nineteenth century, before the importance of hygienic procedures was recognized, operations were used as a last resort because of the extremely high mortality rate after surgery. Pioneering efforts by scientists such as **Joseph Lister** made operating rooms much cleaner, which resulted in a drop in the death rate attributable to surgically acquired infections. In the present day, operating rooms are places where personal **hygiene** is meticulous, instruments and clothing is sterile, and where post-operative clean up is scrupulous.

In hospitals and particularly in research settings, the control of infections involves the use of filters that can be placed in the ventilation systems. Such filters prevent the movement of particles even as small as viruses from a containment area to other parts of a building. Work surfaces are kept free of clutter and are exposed to disinfectant both before and after work with microbes, to kill any transient organisms that may be on the inanimate surface. Laboratories often contain containment structures called fume hoods, in which organisms can be worked with isolated from the airflow of the remainder of the lab. Even the nature of the work surface is designed to thwart infection. Surfaces are constructed so as to be very smooth and to be watertight. The presence of crevasses and cracks at the junction between surfaces are ideal spots for the collection and breeding of infectious microorganisms.

Some infectious microorganisms can be transferred by animal or insect vectors. One example is the viral agent of **Yellow Fever**, which is transmitted to humans via the mosquito. Control of such an infection can be challenging. Typically a concerted campaign to kill the breeding population of the vector is required, along with measures to protect people from those vectors that might escape the eradication campaign. To use the Yellow Fever example, spraying in mosquito breeding sites could be supplemented with the use of mosquito netting over the beds of people in particularly susceptible regions.

Another strategy of infection control is the use of antimicrobial or antiviral agents in an effort to either defeat an infection or, in the case of vaccines, to protect against the spread of an infection. **Antibiotics** are an antimicrobial agent. They have been in common use for less than 75 years, and already history is showing that antibiotics achieve success but that this success should not be assumed to be everlasting. Bacteria are proving to be adept at acquiring resistance to many antibiotics. Indeed, already strains of enterococci and *Staphylococcus aureus* are known to be resistant to virtually all antibiotics currently in use.

Immunization against infection is a widely practiced and successful infection control strategy. Depending upon the target microbe, the **vaccination** program may be undertaken to prevent the seasonal occurrence of a malady such as **influenza**, or to eradicate the illness on a worldwide scale. An example of the latter is the World Health Organization's effort to eradicate polio.

One breeding ground for the development of resistant microbial populations is the hospital. Antibiotics and disinfectants are an important part of the infection control strategy in place in most hospitals. Bacteria are constantly exposed to antibacterial agents. The pressure to adapt is constant.

The degree of infection control is tailored to the institution. For example, in a day care facility, the observance of proper hygiene and proper food preparation may be adequate to protect staff and children. However, in a hospital or nursing home, where people are frequently immunocompromised, additional measures need to be taken to ensure that microbes do not spread. Such measures can include regular **disinfection** of surfaces, one-time use of specific medical equipment such as disposable needles, and well-functioning ventilation systems.

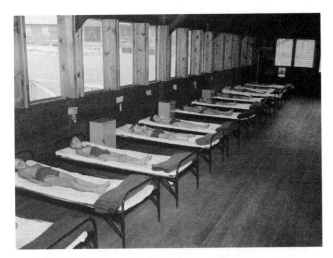
Young children lying on beds in a hospital ward.

The focus of infection control strategies has shifted with the emerging knowledge in the 1970s and 1980s of the existence and medical relevance of the adherent bacterial populations known as biofilms. These adherent growths can remain viable on surfaces after being treated with concentrations of chemicals that swiftly kill their free-floating counterparts. Infection control in areas such as physician and dentist offices, now focus on ensuring that equipment is free from biofilms, because the bacteria could be easily transferred from the equipment to a patient.

See also Bacteria and bacterial infection; Disinfection and disinfectants; Epidemics and pandemics; Hygiene

INFLAMMATION

Inflammation is a localized, defensive response of the body to injury, usually characterized by pain, redness, heat, swelling, and, depending on the extent of trauma, loss of function. The process of inflammation, called the inflammatory response, is a series of events, or stages, that the body performs to attain homeostasis (the body's effort to maintain stability). The body's inflammatory response mechanism serves to confine, weaken, destroy, and remove **bacteria**, toxins, and foreign material at the site of trauma or injury. As a result, the spread of invading substances is halted, and the injured area is prepared for regeneration or repair. Inflammation is a nonspecific defense mechanism; the body's physiological response to a superficial cut is much the same as with a burn or a **bacterial infection**. The inflammatory response protects the body against a variety of invading pathogens and foreign matter, and should not be confused with an immune response, which reacts to specific invading agents. Inflammation is described as acute or chronic, depending on how long it lasts.

Within minutes after the body's physical barriers, the skin and mucous membranes, are injured or traumatized (for example, by bacteria and other **microorganisms**, extreme heat or

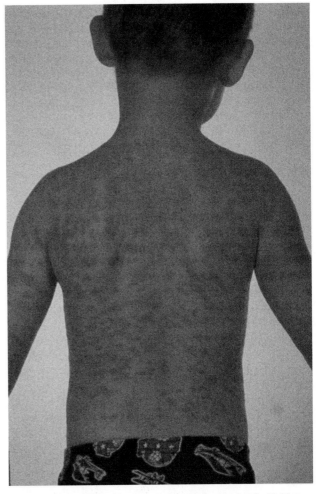
An example of inflammation, showing the rash associated with hives.

cold, and chemicals), the arterioles and capillaries dilate, allowing more blood to flow to the injured area. When the blood vessels dilate, they become more permeable, allowing plasma and circulating defensive substances such as antibodies, phagocytes (cells that ingest microbes and foreign substances), and fibrinogen (blood-clotting chemical) to pass through the vessel wall to the site of the injury. The blood flow to the area decreases and the circulating phagocytes attach to and digest the invading pathogens. Unless the body's defense system is compromised by a preexisting disease or a weakened condition, healing takes place. Treatment of inflammation depends on the cause. Anti-inflammatory drugs such as aspirin, acetaminophen, ibuprofen, or a group of drugs known as NSAIDs (non-steroidal anti-inflammatory drugs) are sometimes taken to counteract some of the symptoms of inflammation.

INFLUENZA

Influenza (commonly known as flu) is a highly contagious illness caused by a group of **viruses** called the orthomyx-

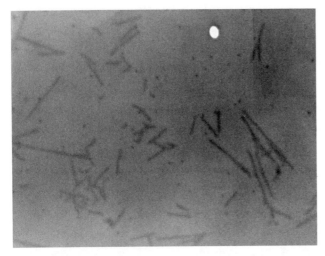

Microscopic view of Infuenza virus.

oviruses. Infection with these viruses leads to a self-limiting illness usually characterized by fever, muscle aches, fatigue, and upper respiratory infection and **inflammation**. Children and young adults usually recover from influenza within 3–7 days with no complications; however, in older adults, especially those over 65 with underlying conditions such as heart disease or lung illnesses, influenza can be deadly. Most of the hospitalizations and deaths from influenza occur in this age group. Although an influenza **vaccine** is available, it does not confer complete protection against all strains of influenza viruses.

Like all viruses, orthomyxoviruses cause illness by entering host cells and replicating within them. The new viruses then burst from the host cell and infect other cells. Orthomyxoviruses are sphere-shaped viruses that contain **ribonucleic acid (RNA)**. The viruses use this RNA as a blue-print for replication within host cells. The outer envelope of an orthomyxovirus is studded with protein spikes that help the virus invade host cells. Two different types of spikes are present on the virus's outer envelope. One type, composed of **hemagglutinin** protein (HA), fuses with the host cell membrane, allowing the virus particle to enter the cell. The other type of spike, composed of the protein neuraminidase (NA), helps the newly formed virus particles to bud out from the host cell membrane.

The only way a virus can be neutralized and stopped is through the body's immune response. At the present time, no cure or treatment is available that completely destroys viruses within the body. The HA spikes and proteins in the orthomyxovirus envelope stimulate the production of antibodies, immune proteins that mark infected cells for destruction by other immune cells. In a healthy person, it takes about three days for antibodies to be formed against an invading virus. People with impaired immune function (such as people with Acquired Immune Deficiency Syndrome, the elderly, or people with underlying conditions) may not be able to mount an effective immune response to the influenza virus. Therefore, these people may develop serious complications, such as **pneumonia**, that may lead to hospitalization or death.

Three types of orthomyxoviruses cause illness in humans and animals: types A, B, and C. Type A causes epidemic influenza, in which large numbers of people become infected during a short period of time. Flu **epidemics** caused by Type A orthomyxoviruses include the worldwide outbreaks of 1918, 1957, 1968, and 1977. Type A viruses infect both humans and animals and usually originate in the Far East, where a large population of ducks and swine incubate the virus and pass it to humans. The Far East also has a very large human population that provides a fertile ground for viral replication. In 1997, a new strain of influenza A jumped from the poultry population in Hong Kong to the human population. H5N1, as the strain was named, was contracted through contact with the feces of chicken. The illness it caused (dubbed avian flu) was severe, and sometimes fatal. Although it was strongly believed that humans could not get the disease from eating properly cooked chicken, the decision was ultimately made to destroy and bury all of the chickens in Hong Kong. This massive effort was carried out in December 1997.

Type B influenza viruses are not as common as type A viruses. Type B viruses cause outbreaks of influenza about every two to four years. Type C viruses are the least common type of influenza virus and cause sporadic and milder infections.

The hallmark of all three kinds of influenza viruses is that they frequently mutate. Due to the small amount of RNA genetic material within a virus, mutation of the genetic material is very common. The result of this frequent mutation is that each flu virus is different, and people who have become immune to one flu virus are not immune to other flu viruses. The ability to mutate frequently therefore allows these viruses to cause frequent outbreaks.

Influenza is characterized by a sudden onset of fever, cough, and malaise. The incubation period of influenza is short, only 1–3 days. The cells that the influenza virus target are the cells of the upper respiratory tract, including the sinuses, bronchi, and alveoli. The targeting of the upper respiratory tract by the viruses accounts for the prominence of respiratory symptoms of flu. In fact, flu viruses are rarely found outside the respiratory tract. Most of the generalized symptoms of flu, such as muscle aches, are probably due to toxin-like substances produced by the virus.

Symptoms last for about 3–6 days; however, lethargy and cough may persist for several days to weeks after a bout with the flu. Children may have more severe symptoms due to a lack of general **immunity** to influenza viruses. Children also have smaller airways, and thus may not be as able to compensate for respiratory impairment as well as adults.

The most common complication of influenza is pneumonia. Pneumonia may be viral or bacterial. The viral form of pneumonia that occurs with influenza can be very severe. This form of pneumonia has a high mortality rate. Another form of pneumonia that is seen with influenza is a bacterial pneumonia. If the respiratory system becomes severely obstructed during influenza, **bacteria** may accumulate in the lungs. This type of pneumonia occurs 5–10 days after onset of the flu. Because it is bacterial in origin, it can be treated with **antibiotics**.

Other complications of influenza include infections of the heart and heart lining, infections of the brain, and Guillain-Barre syndrome (GBS). GBS is a paralytic disease in which the body slowly becomes paralyzed. Paralysis starts in the facial muscles and moves downward. GBS is treated symptomatically and usually resolves by itself. Another complication of influenza is Reye's syndrome. Occurring typically in children, Reye's syndrome is associated with aspirin intake during an attack of influenza. Reye's syndrome is characterized by nausea, vomiting, and progressive neurological dysfunction. Because of the risk of Reye's syndrome, children should not be given aspirin if they have the flu. Non-aspirin pain relievers, such as acetaminophen, should be given instead of aspirin.

Flu is treated with rest and fluids. Maintaining a high fluid intake is important, because fluids increase the flow of respiratory secretions, which may prevent pneumonia. Antiviral medications (amantadine, rimantadine) may be prescribed for people who have initial symptoms of the flu and who are at high risk for complications. This medication does not prevent the illness, but reduces its duration and severity.

A flu vaccine is available that is formulated each year against the current type and strain of flu virus. The virus is grown in chicken eggs, extracted, and then rendered noninfective by chemicals. The vaccine is also updated to the current viral strain by the addition of proteins that match the current strain's composition. The vaccine would be most effective in reducing attack rates if it was effective in preventing influenza in schoolchildren; however, in vaccine trials the vaccine has not been shown to be effective in flu prevention in this age group. In certain populations, particularly the elderly, the vaccine is effective in preventing serious complications of influenza and thus lowers mortality.

Vaccine research is ongoing. One of the more exciting advances in flu vaccines involves research studies examining an influenza vaccine mist, which is sprayed into the nose. This is predicted to be an excellent route of administration, which will confer even stronger immunity against influenza. Because it uses a live virus, it encourages a strong immune response. Furthermore, it is thought to be a more acceptable **immunization** route for schoolchildren, an important reservoir of the influenza virus.

See also Flu: The great flu epidemic of 1918; Viruses and responses to viral infection

INSTITUTE FOR GENOMIC RESEARCH •

see THE INSTITUTE FOR GENOMIC RESEARCH (TIGR)

INTERFERON ACTIONS

Interferons are species-specific proteins, which induce antiviral and antiproliferative responses in animal cells. They are a major defense against viral infections and abnormal growths (neoplasms). Interferons are produced in response to penetration of animal cells by viral (or synthetic) nucleic acid and then leave the infected cell to confer resistance on other cells of the organism. In contrast to antibodies, interferons are not virus specific but host specific. Thus, viral infections of human cells are inhibited only by human interferon. The human genome contains 14 nonallelic and 9 allelic genes of α-interferon (macrophage interferon), as well as a single **gene** for β-interferon (fibroblast interferon). Genes for any two or more variants of interferon, which have originated from the same wild-type gene are called allelic genes and will occupy the same chromosomal location (locus). Variants originating from different standard genes are termed non allelic. α- and β-interferons are structurally related glycoproteins of 166 and 169 amino acid residues. In contrast, γ-interferon (also known as immune interferon) is not closely related to the other two and is not induced by virus infection. It is produced by T-cells after stimulation with the cytokine interleukin-2. It enhances the cytotoxic activity of T-cells, macrophages and natural killer cells and thus has antiproliferative effects. It also increases the production of antibodies in response to antigens administered simultaneously with α-interferon, possible by enhancing the antigen-presenting function of macrophages.

Interferons bind to specific receptors on the cell surface, and induce a signal in the cell interior. Two induction mechanisms have been elucidated. One mechanism involves the induction of protein kinase by interferon, which, in the presence of double-stranded **RNA**, phosphorylates one subunit of an initiation factor of **protein synthesis** (eIF-2B), causing the factor to be inactivated by sequestration in a complex. The second mechanism involves the induction of the enzyme 2',5'-oligoadenylate synthetase (2',5'-oligo A synthetase). In the presence of double-stranded RNA, this enzyme catalyses the polymerization of ATP into oligomers of 2 to 15 adenosine monophosphate residues which are linked by phosphodiester bonds between the position 2' of one ribose and 5' of the next. These 2',5'-oligoadenylates activate an interferon specific RNAase, a latent endonuclease known as RNAase L which is always present but not normally active. RNAase cleaves both viral and cellular single stranded mRNA. Interferons therefore do not directly protect cells against viral infection, but rather render cells less suitable as an environment for viral replication. This condition is known as the antiviral state.

See also Antibody and antigen; Immune system; Immunology; Viruses and responses to viral infection

INTERFERONS

Interferon is the name given to a group of proteins known primarily for their role in inhibiting viral infections and in stimulating the entire **immune system** to fight disease. Research has also shown that these proteins play numerous roles in regulating many kinds of cell functions. Interferons can promote or hinder the ability of some cells to differentiate, that is, to become specialized in their function. They can inhibit cell division, which is one reason why they hold promise for stopping cancer growth. Recent studies have also found that one interferon may play an important role in the early biological processes of pregnancy. Although once thought to be a potential cure-all for a number of viral diseases and cancers, subsequent research has shown that interferons are much more limited in their potential. Still, several interferon proteins have been approved as therapies for diseases like chronic **hepatitis**, genital warts, multiple sclerosis, and several cancers.

The first interferon was discovered in 1957 by Alick Isaacs and Jean Lindenmann. During their investigation, the two scientists found that virus-infected cells secrete a special protein that causes both infected and noninfected cells to produce other proteins that prevent **viruses** from replicating. They named the protein interferon because it interferes with infection. Initially, scientists thought there was only one interferon protein, but subsequent research showed that there are many different interferon proteins.

Interferons are members of a larger class of proteins called **cytokines** (proteins that carry signals between cells). Most interferons are classified as alpha, beta, or gamma interferons, depending on their molecular structure. Two other classes of interferons, omega and tau, have also been discovered. So far, more than 20 different kinds of interferon-alpha have been discovered but few beta and gamma interferons have been identified.

Interferons are differentiated primarily through their amino acid sequence. (Amino acids are molecular chains that make up proteins.) Interferon-alpha, -beta, -tau, and -omega, which all have relatively similar amino acid sequences, are classified as type I interferons. Type I interferons are known primarily for their ability to make cells resistant to viral infections. Interferon-gamma is the only type II interferon, classified as such because of its unique amino acid sequence. This interferon is known for its ability to regulate overall immune system functioning.

In addition to their structural makeup, type I and type II interferons have other differences. Type I interferons are produced by almost every cell in the body, while the type II interferon-gamma is produced only by specialized cells in the immune system known as T lymphocytes and natural killer cells. The two classes also bind to different kinds of receptors, which lie on the surface of cells, and attract and combine with specific molecules of various substances.

Interferons work to stop a disease when they are released into the blood stream and then bind to cell receptors. After binding, they are drawn inside the cell's **cytoplasm**, where they cause a series of reactions that produce other proteins that fight off disease. Scientists have identified over 30 disease-fighting proteins produced by interferons.

In addition to altering a cell's ability to fight off viruses, interferons also control the activities of a number of specialized cells within the immune system. For example, type I interferons can either inhibit or induce the production of **B lymphocytes** (white blood cells that make antibodies for fighting disease). Interferon-gamma can also stimulate the production of a class of T lymphocytes known as suppressor CD8 cells, which can inhibit **B cells** from making antibodies.

Another role of interferon-gamma is to increase immune system functioning by helping macrophages, still another kind of white blood cell, to function. These scavenger cells attack infected cells while also stimulating other cells within the immune system. Interferon-gamma is especially effective in switching on macrophages to kill tumor cells and cells that have been infected by viruses, **bacteria**, and **parasites**.

Interferon-tau, first discovered for its role in helping pregnancy to progress in cows, sheep, and goats, also has antiviral qualities. It has been shown to block tumor cell division, and may interfere with the replication of the acquired immune deficiency, or **AIDS**, virus. Because it has fewer unwanted side-effects (flu-like symptoms and decreased blood cell production) than the other interferons, interferon-tau is becoming a new focal point for research.

In 1986, interferon-alpha became the first interferon to be approved by the Food and Drug Administration (FDA) as a viable therapy, in this case, for hairy-cell leukemia. (Interferons are used therapeutically by injecting them into the blood stream.) In 1988, this class of interferons was also approved for the treatment of genital warts, proving effective in nearly 70% of patients who do not respond to standard therapies. In that same year, it was approved for treatment of Kaposi's Sarcoma, a form of cancer that appears frequently in patients suffering from AIDS. In 1991, interferon-alpha was approved for use in chronic hepatitis C, a contagious disease for which there was no reliable therapy. Interferon has been shown to eliminate the disease's symptoms and, perhaps, prevent relapse. Interferon-alpha is also used to treat Hodgkin's lymphoma and malignant melanoma.

In 1993, another class of interferon, interferon-gamma, received FDA approval for the treatment of a form of multiple sclerosis characterized by the intermittent appearance and disappearance of symptoms. It has also been used to treat chronic granulomatous diseases, inherited immune disorders in which white blood cells fail to kill bacterial infections, thus causing severe infections in the skin, liver, lungs, and bone. Interferon-gamma may also have therapeutic value in the treatment of leishmaniasis, a parasitic infection that is prevalent in parts of Africa, America, Europe, and Asia.

Although all of the disease fighting attributes of interferon demonstrated in the laboratory have not been attained in practice, continued research into interferons will continue to expand their medical applications. For example, all three major classes of interferons are under investigation for treating a variety of cancers. Also, biotechnological advances making genetic engineering easier and faster are making protein drugs like interferons more available for study and use. Using recombinant **DNA** technology, or **gene** splicing, genes that code for interferons are identified, cloned, and used for experimental studies and in making therapeutic quantities of protein. These modern DNA manipulation techniques have made possible the use of cell-signaling molecules like interferons as medicines. Earlier, available quantities of these molecules were too minute for practical use.

See also AIDS, recent advances in research and treatment; Interferon actions; Viral genetics; Viral vectors in gene therapy; Virology; Virus replication; Viruses and responses to viral infection

INVASIVENESS AND INTRACELLULAR INFECTION

Microorganisms that establish infections in humans do so by a number of means. For example, some **bacteria** remain associated with the surface of host cells, but elaborate a coating that provides protection from host immune defenses and external antimicrobial agents, such as **antibiotics**. Another strategy that is used by a number of disease-causing bacteria, virtually all **viruses**, single-celled eukaryotic **parasites**, and **protozoa** is the invasion of the host cells to which the microorganisms adhere. Once inside the host cell, the invading microbe is shielded from host defenses and therapeutic antimicrobial compounds.

Following the invasion of host cells, the microorganisms can establish an infection inside the host cells. This is referred to as intracellular infection. Once again, by remaining inside the host, the bacteria or protozoa are shielded from attack.

Intracellular infection presents a problem for the host, since the infection cannot be dealt with without damage to the host's own tissue. Many disease-causing microorganisms have adopted this mode of infection, including all viruses, some protozoa, and some bacteria. Indeed, some of these intracellular parasites depend absolutely on this mode of growth and cannot survive outside of the host cells. Two examples are the bacteria *Chlamydia* and *Rickettsia*. These bacteria are transmitted to another host only by direct contact of host cells, such as in sexual activity, or when they are sucked up by a biting insect and subsequently expelled into another host.

The molecular nature of invasiveness has been well studied in a number of Gram-negative bacteria. One example is designated as enteropathogenic *Escherichia coli*, or EPEC. This bacterium causes a severe, debilitating, and sometimes life-threatening diarrhea in infants, particularly in underdeveloped countries. EPEC associates with host epithelial cells in the intestinal tract by means of appendages known as fimbriae. Once adhesion is established, the bacterium produces a number of proteins that are then passed across the cell wall to the surface. Studies with **mutants** that do not manufacture one or more of these proteins have shown that the proteins are essential for invasion of the host cell. The exact function of these proteins in the invasive process is still unclear. But current data indicates that they have a role in altering the processes by which host cells transport compounds, and so may facilitate the movement of bacterial disease-causing compounds into the host cell. Finally, the bacteria form a protein that functions as an anchor, to irreversibly bind the bacterial cell to the host cell. Thus, while EPEC are not fully taken into the host cell, an intracellular invasion pathway is established.

A bona fide invasion of host cells is accomplished by the bacterium *Salmonella*. The bacteria have a number of genes, which are clustered together on the bacterial genome, which are activated following association of a bacterium with a host intestinal epithelial cell. The products of the genes operate in a similar fashion as those of EPEC. That is, they provide a conduit for the transport of bacterial compounds into the host cell. *Salmonella* additionally produces a protein that enters the host cell and modifies a scaffolding system in the cell that is called the actin cytoskeleton. The alteration is thought to cause the host cell membrane to become more pliable and capable of becoming much more wavy. This so-called ruffling can entrap a bacterium, enabling it to be taken into the host cell in a membrane-bound bag that is called a vacuole. Once inside the host, other proteins produced by the bacterium cause cell damage and allow the establishment of an infection. The bacteria remain inside the vacuole

Another Gram-negative species called *Shigella flexneri* also promotes the ruffling of the host membrane, which results in the uptake of the bacteria into the host cell. In contrast to *Salmonella*, *Shigella flexneri* break out of the vacuole and produce more copies of themselves in the cellular fluid of the host cell. In the host fluid a bacterium becomes coated with host molecules called actin. By propelling itself against the end of a host cell, a bacterium is able to use the stiff actin filament as a kind of battering ram, to punch a hole through to the neighbouring host cell. This enables the **bacterial infection** to spread from cell to cell without ever contact the surface of the host cells.

Other host cells can be invaded. For example, another Gram-negative bacterial species called *Legionella pneumophila* invades macrophages. Macrophages are white blood cells that are part of the **immune system**. By invading a macrophage, the bacteria can render the macrophage incapable of functioning in defending the body from infection. Thus, invasion serves not only to provide the bacteria with a safe haven for replication, but also compromises the immune system, facilitating the establishment of a bacterial infection.

Invasion of host cells and replication inside the cells can be a stage in the infectious cycle of microorganisms. For example, the single-celled eukaryotic parasites called *Entamoeba histolytica* and *Entamoeba dispar* can invade epithelial cells in the colon. Following the intracellular invasion the amoeba can become dispersed throughout the body via the bloodstream, leading to persistent infections, such as in the liver.

The protozoan called *Cryptosporidium parvum* causes a debilitating diarrhea, typically after being ingested in feces-contaminated drinking water. A key feature of the protozoan infection is the invasion of host epithelial cells in the ileum by a specialized form of the protozoan known as the sporozoite. Replication occurs inside the host cell with the progeny protozoa being released upon rupture of the host cell. The progeny can then go on to invade adjacent host tissue.

The wide spread distribution of host cell invasion and intracellular replication among microorganisms is indicative of the success of the strategy.

See also Bacteria and bacterial infection

ISOTYPES AND ALLOTYPES

Isotype and allotype are terms that relate to the structure of a component of the **immune system** that is called an immunoglobulin.

Immunoglobulins bind their corresponding **antigen**. An immunoglobulin can be static, as part of a membrane-bound receptor to which an antigen binds, or can be floating freely in the body as an **antibody**. The antigen-binding capacity of an immunoglobulin is related to the three-dimensional shape of the molecule. Immunoglobulin isotype and allotype determines the diversity in shape of immunoglobulins.

Immunoglobulins are structured with two Y-shaped "heavy" chains. To each of these a shorter "light" chain is linked. Within each chain there are regions whose amino acid sequence remains constant from immunoglobulin to immunoglobulin. There are also regions whose amino acid sequence is somewhat different and markedly different between the myriad of immunoglobulins that can be made.

The type of heavy chain an immunoglobulin has determines the isotype. Immunoglobulins of the same isotype have the same amino acid structure in two specific regions of the heavy chain. The similarity in amino acid sequence extends to the three-dimensional structure that the immunoglobulin adopts. Thus, immunoglobulins of the same isotype have similar shapes and so similar antigen binding characteristics. The different classes and subclasses of antibody protein arising from the amino acid variations represent the different isotypes.

In humans, there are five immunoglobulin isotypes: IgA, IgD, IgG, IgE, and IgM. All humans whose immune system is functioning correctly possess all these isotypes. Thus, no antigenic response would be elicited if an IgA from one person was injected into another.

Immunoglobulins can also be classified by their so-called allotypes. Allotypes are also determined by the amino acid sequences of the heavy and light chains. Allotypes focus on the variable regions of the chains. By their variable nature, differences in the amino acid sequence can exist even between members of the same species. Allotypes represent what is termed polymorphisms within certain heavy or light chains.

Not all members of a species such as man possess any particular allotype. In contrast to isotypes, the injection of a specific allotype from one person into another could elicit an antigenic reaction in the recipient.

See also Antibody-antigen, biochemical and molecular reactions

IVANOVSKY, DMITRI IOSIFOVICH (1864-1920)
Russian botanist

Dmitri Ivanovsky, in studying a disease that affects tobacco plants, paved the way for the discovery of the infectious particle known as a virus.

Ivanovsky, the son of a landowner, was born in Gdov, Russia. He attended the Gymnasium of Gdov and later graduated as a gold medalist from the Gymnasium of St. Petersburg in 1883. At the University of St. Petersburg, he enrolled in the natural science department and studied under several prominent Russian scientists. While a student, he became interested in diseases that destroy tobacco plants. He graduated in 1888 after presenting his thesis *On Two Diseases of Tobacco Plants*.

The following year, he was asked by the directors of the Department of Agriculture to study a new tobacco disease, called tobacco mosaic, that had afflicted plants in the Crimean region. He crushed the infected leaves, which were distinguished by their mosaic pattern, into sap and then forced the material through a Chamberland bacterial filter that was known to remove all **bacteria**. Despite following this procedure, the sap, when brushed on the leaves of healthy plants, was still toxic enough to cause disease. Ivanovsky's 1892 report on the tobacco mosaic disease detailed what he maintained must be an agent smaller than bacteria. It was the first study in which factual evidence was offered concerning the existence of this new kind of infectious pathogen.

Ivanovsky's work was ignored by the scientific community, and he eventually abandoned his study of this pathogen without understanding the implications of his research. The Dutch botanist, **Martinus Willem Beijerinck**, repeated Ivanovsky's experiments with this new pathogenic source, giving it the name filterable virus in 1898.

See also Tobacco mosaic virus (TMV); Virology

J

JACOB, FRANÇOIS (1920-   )
French molecular biologist

François Jacob made several major contributions to the field of genetics through successful collaborations with other scientists at the famous Pasteur Institute in France. His most noted work involved the formulation of the Jacob-Monod **operon** model, which helps explain how genes are regulated. Jacob also studied messenger **ribonucleic acid** (mRNA), which serves as an intermediary between the **deoxyribonucleic acid** (**DNA**), which carries the **genetic code**, and the **ribosomes**, where proteins are synthesized. He also demonstrated that **bacteria** follow the same general rules of natural **selection** and **evolution** as higher organisms. In recognition of their work in genetic control and **viruses**, Jacob and two other scientists at the Pasteur Institute, **Jacques Lucien Monod** and André Lwoff, shared the 1965 Nobel Prize for Physiology or Medicine.

Jacob was born in Nancy, France, to Simon Jacob, a merchant, and the former Thérèse Franck. Jacob attended school at the Lycée Carnot in Paris before beginning his college education. He began his studies toward a medical degree at the University of Paris (Sorbonne), but was forced to cut his education short when the German Army invaded France during World War II in 1940. He escaped on one of the last boats to England and joined the Free French forces in London, serving as an officer and fighting with the Allies in northern Africa. During the war, Jacob was seriously wounded. His injuries impaired his hands and put an abrupt end to his hopes of becoming a surgeon. For his service to his country, he received the Croix de Guerre and the Companion of the Liberation, two of France's highest military honors.

Despite this physical setback, Jacob continued his education at the University of Paris. In his autobiography, *The Statue Within,* Jacob said he got the idea for his thesis from his place of work, the National **Penicillin** Center, where a minor antibiotic called tyrothricin was manufactured and commercialized. For his thesis, Jacob manufactured and evaluated the drug. Nearing thirty years old, he earned his M.D. degree in

1947, the same year he married Lysiane "Lise" Bloch, a pianist. They would eventually have four children.

With his professional future unsure, Jacob continued to work for a while at the National Penicillin Center. The tide turned when he and his wife had dinner with her cousins, including Herbert Marcovich, a biologist working in a genetics lab. Jacob recalled, "As Herbert spoke, I felt an excitement rising like a storm. If a man of my generation could still go into research without making himself ridiculous, then why not I?" He decided to become a biologist the next day.

Jacob joined the Pasteur Institute in 1950 as an assistant to André Lwoff. Lwoff's laboratory location and its cramped quarters earned it the name of "the attic." The year 1950 was an exciting one in Lwoff's lab. Lwoff had been working with lysogenic bacteria, which are destroyed (lysed) when attacked by bacteria-infecting virus particles called bacteriophages. The bacteriophages invade the bacterial cell, then multiply within it, eventually bursting the cell and releasing new bacteriophages. According to Lwoff's research, the **bacteriophage** first exists in the bacterial cell in a non-infectious phase called the prophage. He could stimulate the prophage to begin producing infective virus by adding ultraviolet light. These new findings helped to give Jacob the background he would need for his future research.

Jacob continued his education at the University of Paris during his first years at the Pasteur Institute, earning his bachelor of science in 1951 and studying toward his doctor of science degree, which he received in 1954. For his doctoral dissertation, Jacob reviewed the ability of certain radiations or chemical compounds to inducethe prophage, and proposed possible mechanisms of **immunity**.

Once on staff in the lab, Jacob soon formed what would become a fruitful collaboration with Élie Wollman, also stationed in Lwoff's laboratory. In the summer of 1954 he and Wollman discovered what they termed erotic induction in the bacteria *Escherichia coli.* They later changed the name of the phenomenon to zygotic induction. In zygotic induction, the chromosome of a male bacterial cell carrying a prophage

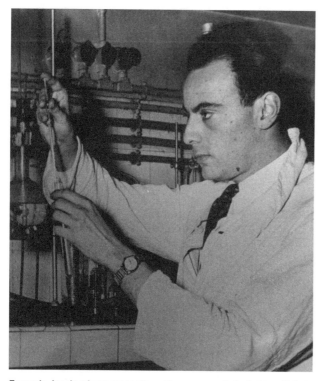

François Jacob, whose research on the operon culminated in a Nobel Prize.

could be transferred to a female cell which was not carrying the prophage, but not vice versa. Zygotic induction showed that both the expression of the prophage and immunity was blocked in the latter instance by a variable present in the **cytoplasm** that surrounds the cell's **nucleus**.

In another experiment, he and Wollman mated male and female bacterial cells, separating them before they could complete **conjugation**. This also clipped the chromosome as it was moving from the male to the female. They found that the female accepted the chromosome bit by bit, in a certain order and at a constant speed, rather similar to sucking up a piece of spaghetti. Their study became known as the "spaghetti experiment," much to Wollman's annoyance.

In the book *Phage and the Origins of Molecular Biology,* Wollman explained that by following different genetic markers in the male, they could determine each gene's time of entry into the zygote and correctly infer its position on the DNA. Jacob and Wollman also used an **electron microscope** to photograph the conjugating bacteria and time the transmission of the genes. "With Élie Wollman, we had developed a tool that made possible genetic analysis of any function, any "system," Jacob said in his autobiography. The two scientists also discovered and defined **episomes**, genetic strains which automatically replicate as part of the development of **chromosomes**.

Jacob and Wollman also demonstrated that bacteria could mutate and adapt in response to drugs or bacteriophages. Evolution and natural selection worked in bacteria as well as in higher life forms. Jacob and Wollman summarized their

research in the July, 1956, issue of *Scientific American:* "There is little doubt that the basic features of genetic **recombination** must be similar whether they occur in bacteria or in man. It would be rather surprising if the study of sexual reproduction in bacteria did not lead to deeper understanding of the process of genetic recombination, which is so vital to the survival and evolution of higher organisms."

In 1956 Jacob accepted the title of laboratory director at the Pasteur Institute. Within two years Jacob began to work with Jacques Monod, who had left Lwoff's lab several years earlier to direct the department of cellular **biochemistry** at the Pasteur Institute. Arthur Pardée also often joined in the research. Jacob and Monod studied how an intestinal enzyme called galactosidase is activated to digest lactose, or milk sugar. Galactosidase is an inducible enzyme, that is, it is not formed unless a certain substrate—in this case lactose—is present. Inducible **enzymes** differ from constitutive enzymes which are continuously produced, whether or not the inducer is present. By pairing a normal inducible male bacteria with a constitutive female, they showed that inducible enzyme processes take precedence over constitutive enzyme synthesis. In the experiments conducted by Jacob and Monod, the inducer, lactose, served to inhibit the **gene** that was regulating the synthesis of galactosidase.

Afterward, Jacob realized that his work with Monod and his earlier work with Wollman on zygotic induction were related. In *The Statue Within,* he said, "In both cases, a gene governs the formation of a cytoplasmic product, of a repressor blocking the expression of other genes and so preventing either the synthesis of the galactosidase or the multiplication of the virus." Their chore then was to determine the location of the repressor, which appeared to be on the DNA.

By the end of the decade, Jacob and Monod had discovered messenger **RNA**, one of the three types of ribonucleic acid. (The other two are ribosomal RNA and transfer RNA.) Each type of RNA has a specific function. MRNA is the mediator between the DNA and ribosomes, passing along information about the correct sequence of amino acids needed to make up proteins. While their work continued, Jacob accepted a position as head of the Department of Cell Genetics at the Pasteur Institute.

In 1961, they explained the results of their research involving the mRNA and the now-famous Jacob-Monod operon model in the paper, "Genetic Regulatory Mechanisms in the Synthesis of Proteins," which appeared in the *Journal of Molecular Biology* Molecular biologist Gunther S. Stent in *Science* described the paper "one of the monuments in the literature of molecular biology."

According to the Jacob-Monod operon model, a set of structural genes on the DNA carry the code that the messenger RNA delivers to the ribosomes, which make proteins. Each set of structural genes has its own operator gene lying next to it. This operator gene is the switch that turns on or turns off its set of structural genes, and thus oversees the synthesis of their proteins. Jacob and Monod called each grouping of an operator and its structural genes an operon. Besides the operator gene, a regulator gene is located on the same chromosome as the structural genes. In an inducible system, like the lactose operon (or lac operon as it is called), this regulator gene codes for a repressor protein. The repressor protein does one of two things. When no lactose is present, the repressor protein attaches to the operator and inactivates it, in turn, halting structural gene activity and **protein synthesis**. When lactose is present, however, the repressor protein binds to the regulator gene instead of the operator. By doing so, it frees up the operator and permits protein synthesis to occur. With a system such as this, a cell can adapt to changing environmental conditions, and produce the proteins it needs when it needs them.

A year after publication of this paper, Jacob won the Charles Leopold Mayer Prize of the French Academy of Sciences. In 1964, Collège de France also recognized his accomplishments by establishing a special chair in his honor. His greatest honor, however, came in 1965 when he, Lwoff, and Monod shared the Nobel Prize for Physiology or Medicine. The award recognized their contributions "to our knowledge of the fundamental processes in living matter which form the bases for such phenomena as adaptation, reproduction and evolution."

During his career, Jacob wrote numerous scientific publications, including the books *The Logic of Life: A History of Hereditary* and *The Possible and the Actual*. The latter, published in 1982, delves into the theory of evolution and the line that he believes must be drawn between the use of evolution as a scientific theory and as a myth.

See also Bacteriophage and bacteriophage typing; Evolution and evolutionary mechanisms; Evolutionary origin of bacteria and viruses; Genetic regulation of eukaryotic cells; Genetic regulation of prokaryotic cells; Immunogenetics; Molecular biology and molecular genetics; Molecular biology, central dogma of; Viral genetics

JANNASCH, HOLGER WINDEKILDE (1927-1998)
German marine microbiologist

Holger Jannasch was a marine microbiologist who made fundamental contributions to the study of microbial life in the extreme environment of the deep-sea. His discoveries helped reveal a hitherto unknown type of **bacterial growth** and broadened human knowledge about the diversity of life on Earth.

Jannasch was born in Holzminden, Germany. After a short stint as a lumberjack, he returned to school. His educational experiences and a job as a warden at a coastal bird sanctuary stimulated an interest in both biological life and the ocean. These interests were pursued during graduate studies at the University of Göttingen. He received his Ph.D. in biology in 1955. From 1956 to 1960 he was an assistant scientist at the Max Planck Society. At the same time he was also a post-doctoral fellow at the Scripps Institution of Oceanography in San Diego, California, and at the University of Wisconsin. From 1961 to 1963 he served as an assistant professor in the Department of Microbiology at the University of Göttingen.

He also held the position of Privatdozent at that University from 1963 until his death.

Visits to the Woods Hole Oceanographic Institution in the early 1960s lead to his joining the institution in 1963. He remained there for the remainder of his career and life.

While at Woods Hole, Jannasch proved to be a consummate mentor and educator. As well, he was a prolific researcher. His main interests were the growth of **microorganisms** in the sea, the existence of microbes at the low temperature and high pressure of the ocean depths, and the microbial processes taking place at **hydrothermal vents** on the ocean floor. Indeed, it was Jannasch who discovered hydrothermal vents.

Jannasch's research on the hydrothermal vents and their associated bacterial populations became classic papers that inspired other microbiologists to similar research. His discovery of sulfur-utilizing **bacteria** that support an entire hydrothermal ecosystem has had major implications for deep sea microbial ecology and may be of fundamental importance to providing insight into the **origin of life** on Earth.

Jannasch was also a seminal influence of the field of microbial ecology. He was a participating author on some 200 research publications. For these and other accomplishments in microbial ecology, a new microorganism was named for him in 1966: *Methanococcus jannaschii*. That same year Woods Hole established the Holger W. Jannasch Chair in recognition of his accomplishments.

Many other awards and honors were bestowed on Jannasch during his career. Foe example, in 1995 he was one of only a handful of non-United States citizens elected to the National Academy of Sciences.

See also Extremophiles

JENNER, EDWARD (1749-1823)
English physician

Edward Jenner discovered the process of **vaccination**, when he found that injection with **cowpox** protected against **smallpox**. His method of **immunization** via vaccination ushered in the new science of **immunology**.

Jenner was born in Berkeley, England, the third son and youngest of six children of Stephen Jenner, a clergyman of the Church of England. He was orphaned at age five and was raised by his older sister, who was married to a clergyman. When Jenner was thirteen years old, he was apprenticed to a surgeon. Then in 1770, he moved to London, England, to work with John Hunter (1728 – 1798), an eminent Scottish anatomist and surgeon who encouraged Jenner to be inquisitive and experimental in his approach to medicine. Jenner returned to Berkeley in 1773, and set up practice as a country doctor.

During and prior to Jenner's lifetime, smallpox was a common and often fatal disease worldwide. Many centuries before Jenner's time, the Chinese had begun the practice of blowing flakes from smallpox scabs up the nostrils of healthy persons to confer **immunity** to the disease. By the seventeenth century, the Turks and Greeks had discovered that, when injected into the skin of healthy individuals, the serum from the

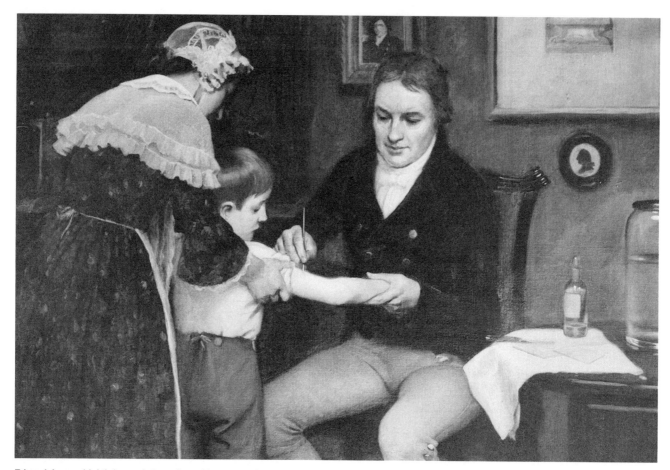

Edward Jenner (right), innoculating a boy with cowpox virus as a protection against smallpox.

smallpox pustule induced a mild case of the disease and subsequent immunity. This practice of inoculation, termed variolation, reached England by the eighteenth century. However, it was quite risky as those who were inoculated frequently suffered a severe or fatal case of smallpox. Despite the risk, people willingly agreed to inoculation because of the widespread incidence of smallpox and the fear of suffering from terribly disfiguring pockmarks that resulted from the disease.

As a young physician, Jenner noted that dairy workers who had been exposed to cowpox, a disease like smallpox only milder, seemed immune to the more severe infection. He continually put forth his theory that cowpox could be used to prevent smallpox, but his contemporaries shunned his ideas. They maintained that they had seen smallpox victims who claimed to have had earlier cases of cowpox.

It became Jenner's task to transform a country superstition into an accepted medical practice. For up until the mid – 1770s, the only documented cases of vaccinations using cowpox came from farmers such as Benjamin Jesty of Dorsetshire who vaccinated his family with cowpox using a darning needle.

After observing cases of cowpox and smallpox for a quarter century, Jenner took a step that could have branded him a criminal as easily as a hero. On May 14, 1796, he removed the fluid from a cowpox lesion from dairymaid Sarah Nelmes, and inoculated James Phipps, an eight-year-old boy, who soon came down with cowpox. Six weeks later, he inoculated the boy with smallpox. The boy remained healthy. Jenner had proved his theory. He called his method vaccination, using the Latin word *vacca*, meaning cow, and *vaccinia*, meaning cowpox. He also introduced the word virus.

The publication of Jenner's *An Inquiry into the Causes and Effects of the Variolae Vaccinae* set off an enthusiastic demand for vaccination throughout Europe. Within 18 months, the number of deaths from smallpox had dropped by two-thirds in England after 12,000 people were vaccinated. By 1800, over 100,000 people had been vaccinated worldwide. As the demand for the **vaccine** rapidly increased, Jenner discovered that he could take lymph from a smallpox pustule and dry it in a glass tube for use up to three months later. The vaccine could then be transported.

Jenner was honored and respected throughout Europe and the United States. At his request, Napoleon released several Englishmen who had been jailed in France in 1804, while France and Great Britain were at war. Across the Atlantic Ocean, Thomas Jefferson received the vaccine from Jenner and proceeded to vaccinate his family and neighbors at Monticello. However, in his native England, Jenner's medical colleagues refused to allow him entry into the College of

Physicians in London, insisting that he first pass a test on the theories of Hippocrates and Galen. Jenner refused to bow to their demands, saying his accomplishments in conquering smallpox should have qualified him for election. He was never elected to the college. Jenner continued his medical practice, as well as collecting fossils and propagating hybrid plants in his garden, until his death from a stroke at the age of 73.

Nearly two centuries after Jenner's experimental vaccination of young James, the **World Health Organization** declared endemic smallpox to be eradicated.

See also Antibody and antigen; Antibody formation and kinetics; Immunity, active, passive and delayed; Immunity, cell mediated; Immunity, humoral regulation

JERNE, NIELS K. (1911-1994)
Danish immunologist

Often considered the founder of modern cellular **immunology**, Niels K. Jerne shared the 1984 Nobel Prize for medicine or physiology with **César Milstein** and Georges J. F. Köhler for his body of work that explained the function of the **immune system**, the body's defense mechanism against disease and infection. He is best known for three theories showing how antibodies—the substances which protect the body from foreign substances such as **viruses** and poisons—are produced, formed, and regulated by the immune system. His theories were initially met with skepticism, but they later became the cornerstones of immunological knowledge. By 1984, when Jerne received the prize, colleagues agreed that he should have been recognized for his important contributions to the field much earlier than he was. Jerne's theories became the starting point from which other scientists, notably 1960 Nobel Prize winner Frank MacFarlane Burnett, furthered understanding of how the body protects itself against disease.

Niels Kaj (sometimes translated Kai) Jerne was born in London, England, to Danish parents Else Marie Lindberg and Hans Jessen Jerne. The family moved to the Netherlands at the beginning of World War I. Jerne earned his baccalaureate in Rotterdam in 1928, and studied physics for two years at the University of Leiden. Twelve years later, he entered the University of Copenhagen to study medicine, receiving his doctorate in 1951 at the age of forty. From 1943 until 1956 he worked at the Danish State Serum Institute, conducting research in immunology.

In 1955, Jerne traveled to the United States with noted molecular biologist Max Delbrück to become a research fellow at the California Institute of Technology at Pasadena. The two worked closely together, and it was not until his final two weeks at the institute that Jerne completed work on his first major theory—on selective **antibody formation**. At this time, scientists accepted that specific antibodies do not exist until an antigen—any substance originating outside the body (e.g., a virus, snake venom, transplanted organs, etc.)—is introduced, and acts as a template from which cells in the immune system create the appropriate **antibody** to eliminate it. Antigens and antibodies have surface patches, called combining sites, with

distinct patterns. When an **antibody and antigen** with complementary combining sites meet, they become attached, fitting together like a lock and key. Jerne's theory postulated instead that the immune system inherently contains all the specific antibodies it needs to fight specific antigens. The appropriate antibody, one of millions that are already present in the body, attaches to the **antigen**, thus neutralizing or destroying the antigen and its threat to the body.

Not until some months after developing his theory did Jerne shared it with Delbrück, who sent it to the *Proceedings of the National Academy of Sciences* for publication. Jerne later noted that his theory probably would have been forgotten, except that it caught the attention of Burnett, leading him to the development in 1959 of his clonal **selection** theory, which built on Jerne's hypothesis to show how specific antibody-producing cells multiply to produce necessary quantities of an antigen's antibody. The following year, Jerne left his research in immunology to become chief medical officer with the **World Health Organization** in Geneva, Switzerland, where he oversaw the departments of biological standards and immunology. From 1960 to 1962, he served on the faculty at the University of Geneva's biophysics department.

From 1962 to 1966, Jerne was professor of microbiology at the University of Pittsburgh in Pennsylvania. During this period, he developed a method, now known as the Jerne **plaque** assay, to count antibody-producing cells by first mixing them with other cells containing antigen material, causing the cells to produce an antibody that combines with red blood cells. Once combined, the blood cells are then destroyed, leaving a substance called plaque surrounding the original antibody-producing cells, which can then be counted. Jerne became director of the **Paul Ehrlich** Institute, in Frankfurt, Germany, in 1966, and, in 1969, established the Basel Institute for Immunology in Switzerland, where he remained until taking emeritus status in 1980.

In 1971, Jerne unveiled his second major theory, which deals with how the immune system identifies and differentiates between self molecules (belonging to its host) and nonself molecules (invaders). Noting that the immune system is specific to each individual, immunologists had concluded that the body's self-tolerance cannot be inherited, and is therefore learned. Jerne postulated that such immune system "learning" occurs in the thymus, an organ in the upper chest cavity where the cells that recognize and attack antigens multiply, while those that could attack the body's own cells are suppressed. Over time, **mutations** among cells that recognize antigens increase the number of different antibodies the body has at hand, thereby increasing the immune system's arsenal against disease.

Jerne introduced what is considered his most significant work in 1974—the network theory, wherein he proposed that the immune system is a dynamic self-regulating network that activates itself when necessary and shuts down when not needed. At that time, scientists knew that the immune system contains two types of immune system cells, or lymphocytes: **B cells**, which produce antibodies, and **T cells**, which function as "helpers" to the B cells by killing foreign cells, or by regulating the B cells either by suppressing or stimulating their antibody producing activity. Further, antibody molecules produced by the B cells also contain antigen-like components that can attract another antibody (anti-idiotype), allowing one antibody to recognize another antibody as well as an antigen. Jerne's theory expanded on this knowledge, speculating that a delicate balance of lymphocytes and antibodies and their idiotypes and anti-idiotypes exists in the immune system until an antigen is introduced. The antigen, he argued, replaces the anti-idiotype attached to the antibody. The immune system then senses the displacement and, in an attempt to find the anti-idiotype a "mate," produces more of the original antibody. This chain-reaction strengthens the body's **immunity** to the invading antigen. Experiments later demonstrated that **immunization** with an anti-idiotype would stimulate the production of the required antibody. It may well be that because of Jerne's network theory, vaccinations of the future will administer antibodies rather than antigens to bring about immunity to disease.

Jerne retired to southern France with his wife. A citizen of both Denmark and Great Britain, Jerne received honorary degrees from American and European universities, was a foreign honorary member of the American Academy of Arts and Sciences, a member of the Royal Danish Academy of Sciences, and won, among other honors, the Marcel Benorst Prize in 1979, and the Paul Ehrlich Prize in 1982.

See also B cells or B lymphocytes; Immunity, active, passive and delayed; Immunity, cell mediated; Immunity, humoral regulation; Immunochemistry; T cells or T lymphocytes

K

KELP AND KELP FORESTS

Brown algae, also known as kelps, are a group of seaweeds in the order Phaeophyta. They attach to rocks on the sea bottom by a tissue known as their holdfast, from which their flexible stems (known as a stipe) and leaf-like tissue (or fronds) grow into the water column. In some species, the fronds are kept buoyant by gas-filled bladders. Kelp tissues are extremely tough only the strongest storms are capable of tearing their fronds or ripping their holdfasts from the rocky bottom. When this happens, however, large masses of kelp biomass can float around as debris known as "paddies," or wash onto the shore as "wrack."

In some temperate marine habitats, large species of brown algae can be extremely abundant. These ecosystems are known as kelp forests. Because they are extremely productive ecosystems, and have a great deal of physical structure associated with their seaweed biomass, kelp forests provide habitat for a wide range of marine organisms. These include a diversity of species of smaller algae, invertebrates, fish, marine mammals, and birds. The kelp forests of the Pacific coast of North America are estimated to support more than 1,000 species of marine plants and animals.

Kelp forests occur in many parts of the world, including the Atlantic and Pacific coasts of North America. However, the tallest, best-developed kelp forests are in waters 20–210 ft (6–70 m) deep over rocky bottoms off the coast of California. This ecosystem is dominated by the giant kelp (*Macrocystis pyrifera*), which ranges from central California to Baja California (the genus also occurs on the west coast of South America, and off South Africa, southern Australia, and New Zealand). This enormous seaweed is also known as the giant bladder kelp because of the flotation structures attached to its fronds. The giant kelp begins its life as a microscopic spore, but can grow as immensely long as 200 ft (60 m) and live for 4–7 years. Most of its photosynthetic activity occurs in the upper part of its tall canopy, because the lower areas are intensely shaded and do not receive much sunlight.

Other, somewhat smaller species of *Macrocystis* occur more widely along the Pacific coast, as far north as southern Alaska. Other giant seaweeds of kelp forests of the Pacific coast include the bull kelp (*Nereocystis leutkeana*), the elk horn kelp (*Pelagophycus porra*), the feather boa kelp (*Egregia menziesii*), and the Fucalean alga (*Cystoseira osmundacea*).

Sea urchins are marine invertebrates that feed voraciously on kelp biomass (they are herbivores meaning that plants are their primary source of food). Periodically, sea urchins of the genus *Strongylocentrotus* can become extremely abundant and cause an intense disturbance to the kelp-forest ecosystem. They do this by feeding on the holdfasts and causing the kelp to detach from their rocky anchors, resulting in an ecosystem known as an "urchin barren" because it sustains so little biomass of seaweeds or other species. This sort of natural ecological damage has been observed numerous times, in various parts of the world.

Off the coast of western North America, however, sea otters (*Enhydra lutris*) feed on the urchins and can prevent them from becoming too abundant, thereby keeping the kelp forests intact. This ecological balance among sea urchins, sea otters, and kelps became upset during the nineteenth century, when the populations of the otters were virtually wiped out by excessive hunting for the fur trade. Because of the collapse of otter populations, the urchins became more abundant. Their excessive feeding on kelps greatly reduced the extent and luxuriance of the kelp forests. Fortunately, this balance has since been restored by the cessation of the hunting of sea otters, allowing them to again control the abundance of the urchins. In turn, the productive kelp forests have been able to redevelop.

Seaweed biomass contains a number of useful chemicals, such as alginates used as thickeners and gelling agents in a wide variety of manufactured products. A minor use is as a food supplement. In some regions, kelps are being harvested as an economic resource to supply these industrial chemicals. Off the coast of California, for example, kelp harvesting amounts to as much as 176,000 tons (160,000 metric tons) per year. If the harvesting method takes care to not damage the holdfasts and other deeper tissues of the kelps, then the forest can regenerate quite well from the disturbance. In California, for example, kelp harvesters are only allowed to cut in the top 4 ft (1.4 m) of the water column, leaving the deeper parts of the forest intact. The kelp harvesting is done using a large barge-like apparatus, which can collect as much as 605 tons (550 metric tons) of kelp per day.

Kelp forests also have an extremely large indirect value to the economy, by serving as the critical habitat for many species of fish and shellfish that are harvested in the coastal fishery. The forests are also critical habitat for many species of indigenous biodiversity. This has an indirect benefit to the coastal economy, through recreational activities associated with ecotourism.

KHORANA, HAR GOBIND (1922-)

Indian-born American biochemist

Har Gobind Khorana, an organic chemist who specialized in the study of proteins and nucleic acids, shared the Nobel Prize in Physiology of Medicine with Robert W. Holley (1922–) and Marshall W. Nirenberg (1927–) in 1968 for discoveries related to the **genetic code** and its function in **protein synthesis**. In addition to developing methods for investigating the structure of the nucleic acids, Khorana introduced many of the techniques that allowed scientists to decipher the genetic code and show how **ribonucleic acid (RNA)** can specify the structure of proteins. Four years after winning the Nobel Prize, Khorana succeeded in synthesizing the first wholly artificial **gene**. In the 1980s Khorana synthesized the gene for rhodopsin, a protein involved in vision.

Har Gobind Khorana, youngest of the five children of Shri Ganput Rai Khorana and Shrimat Krishna Devi Khorana, was born in Raipur, in the Punjab region of India (now part of West Pakistan). His birth date was recorded as January 9, 1922, but the exact date of his birth is uncertain. Although his family was poor, his parents believed strongly in the importance of education. His father was a village agricultural taxation clerk in the British colonial government. Khorana attended D.A.V. High School in Multan (now West Punjab). After receiving his Bachelor of Science (1943, with honors) and Master's degree (1945, with honors) from Punjab University in Lahore, India, Khorana was awarded a Government of India Fellowship, which enabled him to study at Liverpool University, England, where he earned his Ph.D. in 1948. From 1948 to 1949, he worked as a postdoctoral fellow at the Federal Institute of Technology, Zurich, Switzerland, with Professor Vladimir Prelog, who had a major influence on his life-long approach to science.

After briefly returning to India, Khorana accepted a position in the laboratory of (Lord) Alexander Todd at Cambridge University (1950–52), where he studied proteins and nucleic acids. From 1952 to 1960, Khorana worked in the organic chemistry section of the British Columbia Research Council, Vancouver, Canada. The next year Khorana moved to the University of Wisconsin, Madison, Wisconsin, where he

served as Co-director of the Institute for Enzyme Research and Professor of **Biochemistry**. In 1964, he became the Conrad A. Elvehjem Professor of the Life Sciences. In 1970, Khorana accepted the position of Alfred P. Sloan Professor, Departments of Biology and Chemistry, at the Massachusetts Institute of Technology, Cambridge, Massachusetts. From 1974 to 1980, he was Andrew D. White Professor-at-large, Cornell University, Ithaca, New York. During his long and distinguished career, Khorana has been the author or co-author of over 500 scientific publications.

In 1953, Khorana and Todd published their only co-authored paper; it described the use of a novel phosphorylating reagent. Khorana found that this reagent was very useful in overcoming problems in the synthesis of polynucleotides. Between 1956 and 1958, Khorana and his coworkers established the fundamental techniques of nucleotide chemistry. Their goal was to develop purely chemical methods of synthesizing oligonucleotides (long chains of nucleotides). In 1961, Khorana synthesized Coenzyme A, a factor needed for the activity of certain key metabolic **enzymes**.

In 1955, Khorana learned about Severo Ochoa's discovery of the enzyme polynucleotide phosphorylase and met Arthur Kornberg, who described pioneering research on the enzymatic synthesis of **DNA**. These discoveries revolutionized nucleic acid research and made it possible to elucidate the genetic code. Khorana and his coworkers synthesized each of the 64 possible triplets (codons) by synthesizing polynucleotides of known composition. Khorana also devised the methods that led to the synthesis of large, well-defined nucleic acids.

By combining synthetic and enzymatic methods, Khorana was able to overcome many obstacles to the chemical synthesis of polyribonucleotides. Khorana's work provided unequivocal proof of codon assignments and defined some codons that had not been determined by other methods. Some triplets, which did not seem to code for any particular amino acid, were shown to serve as "punctuation marks" for beginning and ending the synthesis of polypeptide chains (long chains of amino acids). Khorana's investigations also provided direct evidence concerning other characteristics of the genetic code. For example, Khorana's work proved that three nucleotides specify an amino acid, provided proof of the direction in which the information in messenger RNA is read, demonstrated that punctuation between codons is unnecessary, and that the codons did not overlap. Moreover, construction of specific polyribonucleotides proved that an RNA intermediary is involved in translating the sequence of nucleotides in DNA into the sequence of amino acids in a protein. Summarizing the remarkable progress that had been made up to 1968 in polynucleotide synthesis and understanding the genetic code, Khorana remarked that the nature of the genetic code was fairly well established, at least for *Escherichia coli*.

Once the genetic code had been elucidated, Khorana focused on gene structure-gene function relationships and studies of DNA-protein interactions. In order to understand gene expression, Khorana turned to DNA synthesis and sequencing. Recognizing the importance of the class of ribonucleotides known as transfer RNAs (tRNAs), Khorana decided to synthesize the DNA sequence that coded for alanine tRNA. The nucleotide sequence of this tRNA had been determined in Robert Holley's laboratory. In 1970, when Khorana announced the total synthesis of the first wholly artificial gene, his achievement was honored as a major landmark in **molecular biology**. Six years later, Khorana and his associates synthesized another gene. In the 1980s, Khorana carried out studies of the chemistry and molecular biology of the gene for rhodopsin, a protein involved in vision.

In 1966, Khorana was elected to the National Academy of Sciences. His many honors and awards include the Merck Award from the Chemical Institute of Canada, the Dannie-Heinneman Prize, the American Chemical Society Award for Creative Work in Synthetic Organic Chemistry, the Lasker Foundation Award for Basic Medical Research, the Padma Vibhushan Presidential Award, the Ellis Island Medal of Honor, the National Medal of Science, and the Paul Kayser International Award of Merit in Retina Research. He holds Honorary Degrees for numerous universities, including Simon Fraser University, Vancouver, Canada; University of Liverpool, England; University of Punjab, India; University of Delhi, India; Calcutta University, India; University of Chicago; and University of British Columbia, Vancouver, Canada.

See also Genetic regulation of eukaryotic cells; Microbial genetics

KITASATO, SHIBASABURO (1852-1931)

Japanese bacteriologist

Bacteriologist Shibasaburo Kitasato made several important contributions to the understanding of human disease and how the body fights off infection. He also discovered the bacterium that causes **bubonic plague**.

Born in Kumamoto, Japan, Kitasato, completed his medical studies at the University of Tokyo in 1883. Shortly after, he traveled to Berlin to work in the laboratory of **Robert Koch**. Among his greatest accomplishments, Kitasato discovered a way of growing a pure **culture** of **tetanus** bacillus using anaerobic methods in 1889. In the following year, Kitasato and German microbiologist **Emil von Behring** reported on the discovery of tetanus and **diphtheria** antitoxin. They found that animals injected with the microbes that cause tetanus or diphtheria produced substances in their blood, called antitoxins, which neutralized the toxins produced by the microbes. Furthermore, these antitoxins could be injected into healthy animals, providing them with **immunity** to the microbes. This was a major finding in explaining the workings of the **immune system**. Kitasato went on to discover **anthrax** antitoxin as well.

In 1892, Kitasato returned to Tokyo and founded his own laboratory. Seven years later, the laboratory was taken over by the Japanese government, and Kitasato was appointed its director. When the laboratory was consolidated with the University of Tokyo, however, Kitasato resigned and founded the Kitasato Institute.

During an outbreak of the bubonic plague in Hong Kong in 1894, Kitasato was sent by the Japanese government to research the disease. He isolated the bacterium that caused the plague. (Alexandre Yersin, 1863 – 1943, independently announced the discovery of the organism at the same time). Four years later, Kitasato and his student Kigoshi Shiga were able to isolate and describe the organism that caused one form of **dysentery**.

Kitasato was named the first president of the Japanese Medical Association in 1923, and was made a baron by the Emperor in 1924. He died in Japan in 1931.

See also Antibody and antigen; Bacteria and bacterial infection; Immunity, active, passive and delayed; Immunization

KLUYVER, ALBERT JAN (1888-1956)

Dutch microbiologist, biochemist, and botanist

Albert Jan Kluyver developed the first general model of cell **metabolism** in both aerobic and anaerobic **microorganisms**, based on the transfer of hydrogen atoms. He was a major exponent of the "Delft School" of classical microbiology in the tradition of Antoni van Leeuwenhoek (1632–1723). Outside Delft, he also drew on the legacy of **Louis Pasteur** (1822–1895), **Robert Koch** (1843–1910), and Sergei Nikolayevich Winogradsky (1856–1953).

Born in Breda, the Netherlands, on June 3, 1888, Kluyver was the son of a mathematician and engineer, Jan Cornelis Kluyver, and his wife, Marie, née Honingh. In 1910, he received his bachelor's degree in chemical engineering from the Delft University of Technology, but immediately shifted his focus toward botany and **biochemistry**, winning his doctorate in 1914 with a dissertation on the determinations of biochemical sugars under the tutelage of Gijsebertus van Iterson, professor of microscopic anatomy. In 1916, on van Iterson's recommendation, the Dutch government appointed Kluyver as an agricultural and biological consultant for the Dutch East Indies colonial administration.

In 1921, again on van Iterson's recommendation, Kluyver succeeded **Martinus Willem Beijerinck** (1851–1931) as director of the microbiology laboratory at Delft, where he spent the rest of his career. He immediately acquired the most modern equipment and established high standards for both collegiality and research. The reorganized laboratory thrived. Kluyver's reputation soon attracted many excellent graduate students, such as Cornelius Bernardus van Niel (1897–1985), another chemical engineer. Van Niel received his doctorate under Kluyver with a dissertation on propionic acid **bacteria** in 1928 and was immediately offered an appointment at Stanford University.

In a landmark paper, "Eenheid en verscheidenheid in de stofwisseling der microben" [Unity and diversity in the metabolism of microorganisms] *Chemische Weekblad*, Kluyver examined the metabolic processes of oxidation and **fermentation** to conclude that, without bacteria and other microbes, all life would be impossible. Two years later he co-authored with his assistant, Hendrick Jean Louis Donker, another important paper, "Die Einheit in der Biochemie" [Unity in biochemistry] *Chemie der Zelle und Gewebe*, which asserted that all life forms are chemically interdependent because of their shared and symbiotic metabolic needs. He explained these findings further in *The Chemical Activities of Microorganisms.*

Kluyver had a knack for bringing out the best in his students. He often and fruitfully collaborated and co-published with them, maintaining professional relationships with them long after they left Delft. For example, with van Niel he co-wrote *The Microbe's Contribution to Biology.* A cheerful, friendly, popular man, he was widely and fondly eulogized when he died in Delft on May 14, 1956. Van Niel called him "The Father of Comparative Biochemistry."

See also Aerobes; Anaerobes and anaerobic infections; Azotobacter; Bacteria and bacterial infection; Bioluminescence; *Escherichia coli (E.coli)*; Microbial symbiosis; Microbial taxonomy; Microscope and microscopy; Yeast

KOCH, ROBERT (1843-1910)

German physician

Robert Koch pioneered principles and techniques in studying **bacteria** and discovered the specific agents that cause **tuberculosis**, cholera, and **anthrax**. For this he is often regarded as a founder of microbiology and **public health**, aiding legislation and changing prevailing attitudes about **hygiene** to prevent the spread of various infectious diseases. For his work on tuberculosis, he was awarded the Nobel Prize in 1905.

Robert Heinrich Hermann Koch was born in a small town near Klausthal, Hanover, Germany, to Hermann Koch, an administrator in the local mines, and Mathilde Julie Henriette Biewend, a daughter of a mine inspector. The Kochs had thirteen children, two of whom died in infancy. Robert was the third son. Both parents were industrious and ambitious. Robert's father rose in the ranks of the mining industry, becoming the overseer of all the local mines. His mother passed her love of nature on to Robert who, at an early age, collected various plants and insects.

Before starting primary school in 1848, Robert taught himself to read and write. At the top of his class during his early school years, he had to repeat his final year. Nevertheless, he graduated in 1862 with good marks in the sciences and mathematics. A university education became available to Robert when his father was once again promoted and the family's finances improved. Robert decided to study natural sciences at Göttingen University, close to his home.

After two semesters, Koch transferred his field of study to medicine. He had dreams of becoming a physician on a ship. His father had traveled widely in Europe and passed a desire for travel on to his son. Although bacteriology was not taught then at the University, Koch would later credit his interest in that field to Jacob Henle, an anatomist who had published a theory of contagion in 1840. Many ideas about contagious diseases, particularly those of chemist and microbiologist **Louis Pasteur**, who was challenging the prevailing myth of spontaneous generation, were still being debated in universities in the 1860s.

During Koch's fifth semester at medical school, Henle recruited him to participate in a research project on the structure of uterine nerves. The resulting essay won first prize. It was dedicated to his father and bore the Latin motto, *Nunquam Otiosus,*, meaning never idle. During his sixth semester, he assisted Georg Meissner at the Physiological Institute. There he studied the secretion of succinic acid in animals fed only on fat. Koch decided to experiment on himself, eating a half-pound of butter each day. After five days, however, he was so sick that he limited his study to animals. The findings of this study eventually became Koch's dissertation. In January 1866, he finished the final exams for medical school and graduated with highest distinction.

After finishing medical school, Koch held various positions; he worked as an assistant at a hospital in Hamburg, where he became familiar with cholera, and also as an assistant at a hospital for developmentally delayed children. In addition, he made several attempts to establish a private practice. In July, 1867, he married Emmy Adolfine Josephine Fraatz, a daughter of an official in his hometown. Their only child, a daughter, was born in 1868. Koch finally succeeded in establishing a practice in the small town of Rakwitz where he settled with his family.

Shortly after moving to Rakwitz, the Franco-Prussian War broke out and Koch volunteered as a field hospital physician. In 1871, the citizens of Rakwitz petitioned Koch to return to their town. He responded, leaving the army to resume his practice, but he didn't stay long. He soon took the exams to qualify for district medical officer and in August 1872 was appointed to a vacant position at Wollstein, a small town near the Polish border.

It was here that Koch's ambitions were finally able to flourish. Though he continued to see patients, Koch converted part of his office into a laboratory. He obtained a **microscope** and observed, at close range, the diseases his patients confronted him with.

One such disease was anthrax, which is spread from animals to humans through contaminated wool, by eating uncooked meat, or by breathing in airborne spores emanating from contaminated products. Koch examined under the microscope the blood of infected sheep and saw specific **microorganisms** that confirmed a thesis put forth ten years earlier by biologist C. J. Davaine that anthrax was caused by a bacillus. Koch attempted to **culture** (grow) these bacilli in cattle blood so he could observe their life cycle, including their formation into spores and their germination. Koch performed scrupulous research both in the laboratory and in animals before showing his work to Ferdinand Cohn, a botanist at the University of Breslau. Cohn was impressed with the work and replicated the findings in his own laboratory. He published Koch's paper in 1876.

In 1877, Koch published another paper that elucidated the techniques he had used to isolate *Bacillus anthracis.* He had dry-fixed bacterial cultures onto glass slides, then stained the cultures with dyes to better observe them, and photographed them through the microscope.

It was only a matter of time that Koch's research eclipsed his practice. In 1880, he accepted an appointment as a government advisor with the Imperial Department of Health in Berlin. His task was to develop methods of isolating and cultivating disease-producing bacteria and to formulate strategies for preventing their spread. In 1881 he published a report advocating the importance of pure cultures in isolating disease-causing organisms and describing in detail how to obtain them. The methods and theory espoused in this paper are still considered fundamental to the field of modern bacteriology. Four basic criteria, now known as **Koch's postulates**, are essential for an organism to be identified as pathogenic, or capable of causing disease. First, the organism must be found in the tissues of animals with the disease and not in disease-free animals. Second, the organism must be isolated from the diseased animal and grown in a pure culture outside the body, or *in vitro*. Third, the cultured organism must be able to be transferred to a healthy animal, which will subsequently show signs of infection. And fourth, the organisms must be able to be isolated from the infected animal.

While in Berlin, Koch became interested in tuberculosis, which he was convinced was infectious, and, therefore, caused by a bacterium. Several scientists had made similar claims but none had been verified. Many other scientists persisted in believing that tuberculosis was an inherited disease. In six months, Koch succeeded in isolating a bacillus from tissues of humans and animals infected with tuberculosis. In 1882, he published a paper declaring that this bacillus met his four conditions—that is, it was isolated from diseased animals, it was grown in a pure culture, it was transferred to a healthy animal who then developed the disease, and it was isolated from the animal infected by the cultured organism. When he presented his findings before the Physiological Society in Berlin on March 24, he held the audience spellbound, so logical and thorough was his delivery of this important finding. This day has come to be known as the day modern bacteriology was born.

In 1883, Koch's work on tuberculosis was interrupted by the Hygiene Exhibition in Berlin, which, as part of his duties with the health department, he helped organize. Later that year, he finally realized his dreams of travel when he was invited to head a delegation to Egypt where an outbreak of cholera had occurred. Louis Pasteur had hypothesized that cholera was caused by a microorganism; within three weeks, Koch had identified a comma-shaped organism in the intestines of people who had died of cholera. However, when testing this organism against his four postulates, he found that the disease did not spread when injected into other animals. Undeterred, Koch proceeded to India where cholera was also a growing problem. There, he succeeded in finding the same organism in the intestines of the victims of cholera, and although he was still unable to induce the disease in experimental animals, he did identify the bacillus when he examined, under the microscope, water from the ponds used for drinking water. He remained convinced that this bacillus was the cause of cholera and that the key to prevention lay in improving hygiene and sanitation.

Koch returned to Germany and from 1885–1890 was administrator and professor at Berlin University. He was highly praised for his work, though some high-ranking scientists and doctors continued to disagree with his conclusions. Koch was an adept researcher, able to support each claim with his exacting methodology. In 1890, however, Koch faltered

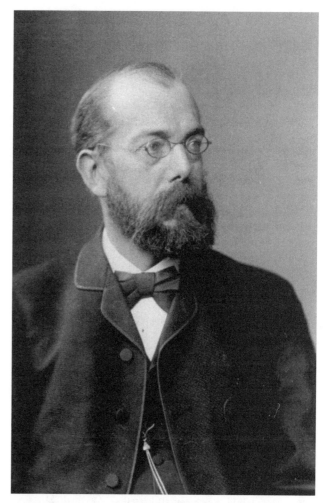

Robert Koch, whose postulates on the identification of microorganisms as the cause of a disease remain a fundamental underpinning of infectious microbiology.

from his usual perfectionism and announced at the International Medical Congress in Berlin that he had found an inoculum that could prevent tuberculosis. He called this agent tuberculin. People flocked to Berlin in hopes of a cure and Koch was persuaded to keep the exact formulation of tuberculin a secret, in order to discourage imitations. Although optimistic reports had come out of the clinical trials Koch had set up, it soon became clear from autopsies that tuberculin was causing severe **inflammation** in many patients. In January 1891, under pressure from other scientists, Koch finally published the nature of the substance, but it was an uncharacteristically vague and misleading report which came under immediate criticism from his peers.

Koch left Berlin for a time after this incident to recover from the professional setback, although the German government continued to support him throughout this time. An Institute for Infectious Diseases was established and Koch was named director. With a team of researchers, he continued his work with tuberculin, attempting to determine the ideal dose at which the agent could be the safest and most effective. The discovery that tuberculin was a valuable diagnostic tool (causing a reaction in those infected but none in those not infected), rather than a cure, helped restore Koch's reputation. In 1892, there was a cholera outbreak in Hamburg. Thousands of people died. Koch advocated strict sanitary conditions and isolation of those found to be infected with the bacillus. Germany's senior hygienist, Max von Pettenkofer, was unconvinced that the bacillus alone could cause cholera. He doubted Koch's ideas, going so far as to drink a freshly isolated culture. Several of his colleagues joined him in this demonstration. Two developed symptoms of cholera, Pettenkofer suffered from diarrhea, but no one died; Pettenkofer felt vindicated in his opposition to Koch. Nevertheless, Koch focused much of his energy on testing the water supply of Hamburg and Berlin and perfecting techniques for filtering drinking water to prevent the spread of the bacillus.

In the following years, he gave the directorship of the Institute over to one of his students so he could travel again. He went to India, New Guinea, Africa, and Italy, where he studied diseases such as the plague, **malaria**, **rabies**, and various unexplained fevers. In 1905, after returning to Berlin from Africa, he was awarded the Nobel Prize for physiology and medicine for his work on tuberculosis. Subsequently, many other honors were awarded him recognizing not only his work on tuberculosis, but his more recent research on tropical diseases, including the Prussian Order Pour le Merits in 1906 and the Robert Koch medal in 1908. The Robert Koch Medal was established to honor the greatest living physicians, and the Robert Koch Foundation, established with generous grants from the German government and from the American philanthropist, Andrew Carnegie, was founded to work toward the eradication of tuberculosis.

Meanwhile, Koch settled back into the Institute where he supervised clinical trials and production of new tuberculins. He attempted to answer, once and for all, the question of whether tuberculosis in cattle was the same disease as it was in humans. Between 1882 and 1901 he had changed his mind on this question, coming to accept that bovine tuberculosis was not a danger to humans, as he had previously thought. He presented his arguments at conferences in the United States and Britain during a time when many governments were attempting large-scale efforts to minimize the transmission of tuberculosis through limiting meat and milk.

Koch did not live to see this question answered. On April 9, 1910, three days after lecturing on tuberculosis at the Berlin Academy of Sciences, he suffered a heart attack from which he never fully recovered. He died at Baden Baden the next month at the age of 67. He was honored after death by the naming of the Institute after him. In the first paper he wrote on tuberculosis, he stated his lifelong goal, which he clearly achieved: "I have undertaken my investigations in the interests of public health and I hope the greatest benefits will accrue therefrom."

See also Bacteria and bacterial infection; History of microbiology; History of public health; Koch's postulates; Laboratory techniques in microbiology

KOCH'S POSTULATES

Koch's postulates are a series of conditions that must be met for a microorganism to be considered the cause of a disease. German microbiologist **Robert Koch** (1843–1910) proposed the postulates in 1890.

Koch originally proposed the postulates in reference to bacterial diseases. However, with some qualifications, the postulates can be applied to diseases caused by **viruses** and other infectious agents as well.

According to the original postulates, there are four conditions that must be met for an organism to be the cause of a disease. Firstly, the organism must be present in every case of the disease. If not, the organism is a secondary cause of the infection, or is coincidentally present while having no active role in the infection. Secondly, the organism must be able to be isolated from the host and grown in the artificial and controlled conditions of the laboratory. Being able to obtain the microbe in a pure form is necessary for the third postulate that stipulates that the disease must be reproduced when the isolated organism is introduced into another, healthy host. The fourth postulate stipulates that the same organism must be able to be recovered and purified from the host that was experimentally infected.

Since the proposal and general acceptance of the postulates, they have proven to have a number of limitations. For example, infections organisms such as some the bacterium *Mycobacterium leprae*, some viruses, and **prions** cannot be grown in artificial laboratory media. Additionally, the postulates are fulfilled for a human disease-causing microorganism by using test animals. While a microorganism can be isolated from a human, the subsequent use of the organism to infect a healthy person is unethical. Fulfillment of Koch's postulates requires the use of an animal that mimics the human infection as closely as is possible.

Another limitation of Koch's postulates concerns instances where a microorganism that is normally part of the normal flora of a host becomes capable of causing disease when introduced into a different environment in the host (e.g., *Staphylococcus aureus*), or when the host's **immune system** is malfunctioning (e.g., *Serratia marcescens*).

Despite these limitations, Koch's postulates have been very useful in clarifying the relationship between **microorganisms** and disease.

See also Animal models of infection; Bacteria and bacterial infection; Germ theory of disease; History of immunology; History of microbiology; History of public health; Laboratory techniques in immunology; Laboratory techniques in microbiology

KÖHLER, GEORGES (1946-1995)

German immunologist

For decades, antibodies, substances manufactured by the plasma cells to help fight disease, were produced artificially by injecting animals with foreign macromolecules, then extracted by bleeding the animals and separating the **antiserum** in their blood. The technique was arduous and far from foolproof. But the discovery of the hybridoma technique by German immunologist Georges Köhler changed revolutionize the procedure. Köhler's work made antibodies relatively easy to produce and dramatically facilitated research on many serious medical disorders such as acquired **immunodeficiency** syndrome (**AIDS**) and cancer. For his work on what would come to be known as monoclonal antibodies, Köhler shared the 1984 Nobel Prize in medicine.

Born in Munich, in what was then occupied Germany, Georges Jean Franz Köhler attended the University of Freiburg, where he obtained his Ph.D. in biology in 1974. From there he set off to Cambridge University in England, to work as a postdoctoral fellow for two years at the British Medical Research Council's laboratories. At Cambridge, Köhler worked under Dr. **César Milstein**, an Argentinean-born researcher with whom Köhler would eventually share the Nobel Prize. At the time, Milstein, who was Köhler's senior by nineteen years, was a distinguished immunologist, and he actively encouraged Köhler in his research interests. Eventually, it was while working in the Cambridge laboratory that Köhler discovered the hybridoma technique.

Dubbed by the *New York Times* as the "guided missiles of biology," antibodies are produced by human plasma cells in response to any threatening and harmful bacterium, virus, or tumor cell. The body forms a specific **antibody** against each **antigen**; and César Milstein once told the *New York Times* that the potential number of different antigens may reach "well over a million." Therefore, for researchers working to combat diseases like cancer, an understanding of how antibodies could be harnessed for a possible cure is of great interest. And although scientists knew the benefits of producing antibodies, until Köhler and Milstein published their findings, there was no known technique for maintaining the long-term **culture** of antibody-forming plasma cells.

Köhler's interest in the subject had been aroused years earlier, when he had become intrigued by the work of Dr. Michael Potterof the National Cancer Institute in Bethesda, Maryland. In 1962 Potter had induced myelomas, or plasma-cell tumors in mice, and others had discovered how to keep those tumors growing indefinitely in culture. Potter showed that plasma tumor cells were both seemingly immortal and able to create an unlimited number of identical antibodies. The only drawback was that there seemed no way to make the cells produce a certain *type* of antibody. Because of this, Köhler wanted to initiate a **cloning** experiment that would fuse plasma cells able to produce the desired antibodies with the "immortal" myeloma cells. With Milstein's blessing, Köhler began his experiment.

"For seven weeks after he had made the hybrid cells," the *New York Times* reported in October, 1984, "Dr. Köhler refrained from testing the outcome of the experiment for fear of likely disappointment. At last, around Christmas 1974, he persuaded his wife," Claudia Köhler, "to come to the windowless basement where he worked to share his anticipated disappointment after the critical test." But disappointment turned to joy when Köhler discovered his test had been a success: Astoundingly, his hybrid cells were making pure antibodies against the test antigen. The result was dubbed monoclonal antibodies. For his contribution to medical science, Köhler—who in 1977 had relocated to Switzerland to do research at the Basel Institute for Immunology—was awarded the Nobel in 1984.

The implications of Köhler's discovery were immense, and opened new avenues of basic research. In the early 1980s Köhler's discovery led scientists to identify various lymphocytes, or white blood cells. Among the kinds discovered were the T-4 lymphocytes, the cells destroyed by AIDS. Monoclonal antibodies have also improved tests for **hepatitis** B and streptococcal infections by providing guidance in selecting appropriate **antibiotics**, and they have aided in the research on thyroid disorders, lupus, rheumatoid arthritis, and inherited brain disorders. More significantly, Köhler's work has led to advances in research that can harness monoclonal antibodies into certain drugs and toxins that fight cancer, but would cause damage in their own right. Researchers are also using monoclonal antibodies to identify antigens specific to the surface of cancer cells so as to develop tests to detect the spread of cancerous cells in the body.

Despite the significance of the discovery, which has also resulted in vast amounts of research funds for many research laboratories, for Köhler and Milstein—who never patented their discovery—there was little financial remuneration. Following the award, however, he and Milstein, together with Michael Potter, were named winners of the Lasker Medical Research Award.

In 1985, Köhler moved back to his hometown of Freiburg, Germany, to assume the directorship of the Max Planck Institute for Immune Biology. He died in Freiburg in 1995.

See also Antibody-antigen, biochemical and molecular reactions; Antibody and antigen; Antibody formation and kinetics; Antibody, monoclonal; Immunity, active, passive and delayed; Immunity, cell mediated; Immunity, humoral regulation; Immunodeficiency; Immunodeficiency disease syndromes; Immunodeficiency diseases

KREBS, HANS ADOLF (1900-1981)
German biochemist

Few students complete an introductory biology course without learning about the **Krebs cycle**, an indispensable step in the process the body performs to convert food into energy. Also known as the citric acid cycle or tricarboxylic acid cycle, the Krebs cycle derives its name from one of the most influential biochemists of our time. Born in the same year as the twentieth century, Hans Adolf Krebs spent the greater part of his eighty-one years engaged in research on intermediary **metabolism**. First rising to scientific prominence for his work on the ornithine cycle of urea synthesis, Krebs shared the Nobel Prize for physiology and medicine in 1953 for his discovery of the citric acid cycle. Over the course of his career, the German-born scientist published, oversaw, or supervised a total of more than 350 scientific publications. But the story of Krebs's life is more than a tally of scientific achievements; his biography can be seen as emblematic of biochemistry's path to recognition as its own discipline.

In 1900, Alma Davidson Krebs gave birth to her second child, a boy named Hans Adolf. The Krebs family—Hans, his parents, sister Elisabeth and brother Wolfgang—lived in Hildesheim, in Hanover, Germany. There his father Georg practiced medicine, specializing in surgery and diseases of the ear, nose, and throat. Hans developed a reputation as a loner at an early age. He enjoyed swimming, boating, and bicycling, but never excelled at athletic competitions. He also studied piano diligently, remaining close to his teacher throughout his university years. At the age of fifteen, the young Krebs decided he wanted to follow in his father's footsteps and become a physician. World War I had broken out, however, and before he could begin his medical studies, he was drafted into the army upon turning eighteen in August of 1918. The following month he reported for service in a signal corps regiment in Hanover. He expected to serve for at least a year, but shortly after he started basic training, the war ended. Krebs received a discharge from the army to commence his studies as soon as possible.

Krebs chose the University of Göttingen, located near his parents' home. There, he enrolled in the basic science curriculum necessary for a student planning a medical career and studied anatomy, histology, embryology and botanical science. After a year at Göttingen, Krebs transferred to the University of Freiburg. At Freiburg, Krebs encountered two faculty members who enticed him further into the world of academic research: Franz Knoop, who lectured on physiological chemistry, and Wilhelm von Möllendorff, who worked on histological staining. Möllendorff gave Krebs his first research project, a comparative study of the staining effects of different dyes on muscle tissues. Impressed with Krebs's insight that the efficacy of the different dyes stemmed from how dispersed and dense they were rather than from their chemical properties, Möllendorff helped Krebs write and publish his first scientific paper. In 1921, Krebs switched universities again, transferring to the University of Munich, where he started clinical work under the tutelage of two renowned surgeons. In 1923, he completed his medical examinations with an overall mark of "very good," the best score possible. Inspired by his university studies, Krebs decided against joining his father's practice as he had once planned; instead, he planned to balance a clinical career in medicine with experimental work. But before he could turn his attention to research, he had one more hurdle to complete, a required clinical year, which he served at the Third Medical Clinic of the University of Berlin.

Krebs spent his free time at the Third Medical Clinic engaged in scientific investigations connected to his clinical duties. At the hospital, Krebs met Annelise Wittgenstein, a more experienced clinician. The two began investigating physical and chemical factors that played substantial roles in the distribution of substances between blood, tissue, and cerebrospinal fluid, research that they hoped might shed some light on how pharmaceuticals such as those used in the treatment of **syphilis** penetrate the nervous system. Although

Krebs published three articles on this work, later in life he belittled these early, independent efforts. His year in Berlin convinced Krebs that better knowledge of research chemistry was essential to medical practice.

Accordingly, the twenty-five-year-old Krebs enrolled in a course offered by Berlin's Charité Hospital for doctors who wanted additional training in laboratory chemistry. One year later, through a mutual acquaintance, he was offered a paid research assistantship by Otto Warburg, one of the leading biochemists of the time. Although many others who worked with Warburg called him autocratic, under his tutelage Krebs developed many habits that would stand him in good stead as his own research progressed. Six days a week work began at Warburg's laboratory at eight in the morning and concluded at six in the evening, with only a brief break for lunch. Warburg worked as hard as the students. Describing his mentor in his autobiography, *Hans Krebs: Reminiscences and Reflections,* Krebs noted that Warburg worked in his laboratory until eight days before he died from a pulmonary embolism. At the end of his career, Krebs wrote a biography of his teacher, the subtitle of which described his perception of Warburg: "cell physiologist, biochemist, and eccentric."

Krebs's first job in Warburg's laboratory entailed familiarizing himself with the tissue slice and manometric (pressure measurement) techniques the older scientist had developed. Until that time, biochemists had attempted to track chemical processes in whole organs, invariably experiencing difficulties controlling experimental conditions. Warburg's new technique, affording greater control, employed single layers of tissue suspended in solution and manometers (pressure gauges) to measure chemical reactions. In Warburg's lab, the tissue slice/manometric method was primarily used to measure rates of **respiration** and glycolysis, processes by which an organism delivers oxygen to tissue and converts carbohydrates to energy. Just as he did with all his assistants, Warburg assigned Krebs a problem related to his own research—the role of heavy metals in the oxidation of sugar. Once Krebs completed that project, he began researching the metabolism of human cancer tissue, again at Warburg's suggestion. While Warburg was jealous of his researchers' laboratory time, he was not stingy with bylines; during Krebs's four years in Warburg's lab, he amassed sixteen published papers. Warburg had no room in his lab for a scientist interested in pursuing his own research. When Krebs proposed undertaking studies of intermediary metabolism that had little relevance for Warburg's work, the supervisor suggested Krebs switch jobs.

Unfortunately for Krebs, the year was 1930. Times were hard in Germany, and research opportunities were few. He accepted a mainly clinical position at the Altona Municipal Hospital, which supported him while he searched for a more research-oriented post. Within the year, he moved back to Freiburg, where he worked as an assistant to an expert on metabolic diseases with both clinical and research duties. In the well-equipped Freiburg laboratory, Krebs began to test whether the tissue slice technique and manometry he had mastered in Warburg's lab could shed light on complex synthetic metabolic processes. Improving on the master's methods, he began using saline solutions in which the concentrations of various ions matched their concentrations within the body, a technique which eventually was adopted in almost all biochemical, physiological, and pharmacological studies.

Working with a medical student named Kurt Henseleit, Krebs systematically investigated which substances most influenced the rate at which urea—the main solid component of mammalian urine—forms in liver slices. Krebs noticed that the rate of urea synthesis increased dramatically in the presence of ornithine, an amino acid present during urine production. Inverting the reaction, he speculated that the same ornithine produced in this synthesis underwent a cycle of conversion and synthesis, eventually to yield more ornithine and urea. Scientific recognition of his work followed almost immediately, and at the end of 1932—less than a year and a half after he began his research—Krebs found himself appointed as a *Privatdozent* at the University of Freiburg. He immediately embarked on the more ambitious project of identifying the intermediate steps in the metabolic breakdown of carbohydrates and fatty acids.

Krebs was not to enjoy his new position in Germany for long. In the spring of 1933, along with many other German scientists, he found himself dismissed from his job because of Nazi purging. Although Krebs had renounced the Jewish faith twelve years earlier at the urging of his patriotic father, who believed wholeheartedly in the assimilation of all German Jews, this legal declaration proved insufficiently strong for the Nazis. In June of 1933, he sailed for England to work in the **biochemistry** lab of Sir Frederick Gowland Hopkins of the Cambridge School of Biochemistry. Supported by a fellowship from the Rockefeller Foundation, Krebs resumed his research in the British laboratory. The following year, he augmented his research duties with the position of demonstrator in biochemistry. Laboratory space in Cambridge was cramped, however, and in 1935 Krebs was lured to the post of lecturer in the University of Sheffield's Department of Pharmacology by the prospect of more lab space, a semi-permanent appointment, and a salary almost double the one Cambridge was paying him.

His Sheffield laboratory established, Krebs returned to a problem that had long preoccupied him: how the body produced the essential amino acids that play such an important role in the metabolic process. By 1936, Krebs had begun to suspect that citric acid played an essential role in the oxidative metabolism by which the carbohydrate pyruvic acid is broken down so as to release energy. Together with his first Sheffield graduate student, William Arthur Johnson, Krebs observed a process akin to that in urea formation. The two researchers showed that even a small amount of citric acid could increase the oxygen absorption rate of living tissue. Because the amount of oxygen absorbed was greater than that needed to completely oxidize the citric acid, Krebs concluded that citric acid has a catalytic effect on the process of pyruvic acid conversion. He was also able to establish that the process is cyclical, citric acid being regenerated and replenished in a subsequent step. Although Krebs spent many more years refining the understanding of intermediary metabolism, these early results provided the key to the chemistry that sustains life processes. In June of 1937, he sent a letter to *Nature* reporting these preliminary findings. Within a week, the editor notified

him that his paper could not be published without a delay. Undaunted, Krebs revised and expanded the paper and sent it to the new Dutch journal *Enzymologia,* which he knew would rapidly publicize this significant finding.

In 1938, Krebs married Margaret Fieldhouse, a teacher of domestic science in Sheffield. The couple eventually had three children. In the winter of 1939, the university named him lecturer in biochemistry and asked him to head their new department in the field. Married to an Englishwoman, Krebs became a naturalized English citizen in September, 1939, three days after World War II began.

The war affected Krebs's work minimally. He conducted experiments on vitamin deficiencies in conscientious objectors, while maintaining his own research on metabolic cycles. In 1944, the Medical Research Council asked him to head a new department of biological chemistry. Krebs refined his earlier discoveries throughout the war, particularly trying to determine how universal the Krebs cycle is among living organisms. He was ultimately able to establish that all organisms, even **microorganisms**, are sustained by the same chemical processes. These findings later prompted Krebs to speculate on the role of the metabolic cycle in **evolution**.

In 1953, Krebs received the Nobel Prize in physiology and medicine, which he shared with Fritz Lipmann, the discoverer of co-enzyme A. The following year, Oxford University offered him the Whitley professorship in biochemistry and the chair of its substantial department in that field. Once Krebs had ascertained that he could transfer his metabolic research unit to Oxford, he consented to the appointment. Throughout the next two decades, Krebs continued research into intermediary metabolism. He established how fatty acids are drawn into the metabolic cycle and studied the regulatory mechanism of intermediary metabolism. Research at the end of his life was focused on establishing that the metabolic cycle is the most efficient mechanism by which an organism can convert food to energy. When Krebs reached Oxford's mandatory retirement age of sixty-seven, he refused to end his research and made arrangements to move his research team to a laboratory established for him at the Radcliffe Hospital. Krebs died at the age of eighty-one.

See also Cell cycle and cell division; Cell membrane transport

KREBS CYCLE

The Krebs cycle is a set of biochemical reactions that occur in the mitochondria. The Krebs cycle is the final common pathway for the oxidation of food molecules such as sugars and fatty acids. It is also the source of intermediates in biosynthetic pathways, providing carbon skeletons for the synthesis of amino acids, nucleotides, and other key molecules in the cell. The Krebs cycle is also known as the citric acid cycle, and the tricarboxylic acid cycle. The Krebs cycle is a cycle because, during its course, it regenerates one of its key reactants.

To enter the Krebs cycle, a food molecule must first be broken into two- carbon fragments known as acetyl groups, which are then joined to the carrier molecule coenzyme A (the A stands for acetylation). Coenzyme A is composed of the **RNA** nucleotide adenine diphosphate, linked to a pantothenate, linked to a mercaptoethylamine unit, with a terminal S-H.Dehydration of this linkage with the OH of an acetate group produces acetyl CoA. This reaction is catalyzed by pyruvate dehydrogenase complex, a large multienzyme complex.

The acetyl CoA linkage is weak, and it is easily and irreversibly hydrolyzed when Acetyl CoA reacts with the four-carbon compound oxaloacetate. Oxaloacetate plus the acetyl group form the six-carbon citric acid, or citrate. (Citric acid contains three carboxylic acid groups, hence the alternate names for the Krebs cycle.)

Following this initiating reaction, the citric acid undergoes a series of transformations. These result in the formation of three molecules of the high-energy hydrogen carrier NADH (nicotinamide adenine dinucleotide), 1 molecule of another hydrogen carrier FADH2 (flavin adenine dinucleotide), 1 molecule of high-energy GTP (guanine triphosphate), and 2 molecules of carbon dioxide, a waste product. The oxaloacetate is regenerated, and the cycle is ready to begin again. NADH and FADH2 are used in the final stages of cellular **respiration** to generate large amounts of ATP.

As a central metabolic pathway in the cell, the rate of the Krebs cycle must be tightly controlled to prevent too much, or too little, formation of products. This regulation occurs through inhibition or activation of several of the **enzymes** involved. Most notably, the activity of pyruvate dehydrogenase is inhibited by its products, acetyl CoA and NADH, as well as by GTP. This enzyme can also be inhibited by enzymatic addition of a phosphate group, which occurs more readily when ATP levels are high. Each of these actions serves to slow down the Krebs cycle when energy levels are high in the cell. It is important to note that the Krebs cycle is also halted when the cell is low on oxygen, even though no oxygen is consumed in it. Oxygen is needed further along in cell respiration though, to regenerate NAD+ and FAD. Without these, the cycle cannot continue, and pyruvic acid is converted in the cytosol to lactic acid by the **fermentation** pathway.

The Krebs cycle is also a source for precursors for biosynthesis of a number of cell molecules. For instance, the synthetic pathway for amino acids can begin with either oxaloacetate or alpha-ketoglutarate, while the production of porphyrins, used in hemoglobin and other proteins, begins with succinyl CoA. Molecules withdrawn from the cycle for biosynthesis must be replenished. Oxaloacetate, for instance, can be formed from pyruvate, carbon dioxide, and water, with the use of one ATP molecule.

See also Mitochondria and cellular energy

L

LABORATORY TECHNIQUES IN IMMUNOLOGY

Various laboratory techniques exist that rely on the use of antibodies to visualize components of **microorganisms** or other cell types and to distinguish one cell or organism type from another.

Electrophoresis is a technique whereby the protein or carbohydrate components of microorganisms can be separated based upon their migration through a gel support under the driving influence of electricity. Depending upon the composition of the gel, separation can be based on the net charge of the components or on their size. Once the components are separated, they can be distinguished immunologically. This application is termed **immunoelectrophoresis**.

Immunoelectrophoresis relies upon the exposure of the separated components in the gel to a solution that contains an **antibody** that has been produced to one of the separated proteins. Typically, the antibody is generated by the injection of the purified protein into an animal such as a rabbit. For example, the protein that comprises the flagellar appendage of a certain **bacteria** can be purified and injected into the rabbit, so as to produce rabbit anti-flagellar protein.

Immunoelectrophoresis can be used in a clinical **immunology** laboratory in order to diagnose illness, especially those that alter the immunoglobulin composition of body fluids. Research immunology laboratories also employ immunoelectrophoresis to analyze the components of organisms, including microorganisms.

One example of an immunoelectrophoretic technique used with microorganisms is known as the Western Blot. Proteins that have been separated on a certain type of gel support can be electrically transferred to a special membrane. Application of the antibody will produce binding between the antibody and the corresponding **antigen**. Then, an antibody generated to the primary antibody (for example, goat anti-rabbit antibody) is added. The secondary antibody will bind to the primary antibody. Finally, the secondary antibody can be constructed so that a probe binds to the antibody's free end. A chemical reaction produces a color change in the probe. Thus, bound primary antibody is visualized by the development of a dark band on the support membrane containing the electrophoretically separated proteins. Various controls can be invoked to ensure that this reaction is real and not the result of an experimental anomaly.

A similar reaction can be used to detect antigen in sections of biological material. This application is known as immunohistochemistry. The sections can be examined using either an **electron microscope** or a light **microscope**. The preparation techniques differ for the two applications, but both are similar in that they ensure that the antigen is free to bind the added antibody. Preservation of the antigen binding capacity is a delicate operation, and one that requires a skilled technician. The binding is visualized as a color reaction under light microscopic illumination or as an increased electron dense area under the electron beam of the electron microscope.

The binding between antigen and antibody can be enhanced in light microscopic immunohistochemistry by the exposure of the specimen to heat. Typically a microwave is used. The heat energy changes the configuration of the antigen slightly, to ease the fit of the antigen with the antibody. However, the shape change must not be too great or the antibody will not recognize the altered antigen molecule.

Another well-establish laboratory immunological technique is known as enzyme-linked immunosorbent assay. The technique is typically shortened to **ELISA**. In the ELISA technique, antigen is added to a solid support. Antibody is flooded over the support. Where an antibody recognizes a corresponding antigen, binding of the two will occur. Next an antibody raised against the primary antibody is applied, and binding of the secondary antibody to the primary molecule occurs. Finally, a substrate is bound to a free portion of the secondary antibody, and the binding can be subsequently visualized as a color reaction. Typically, the ELISA test is

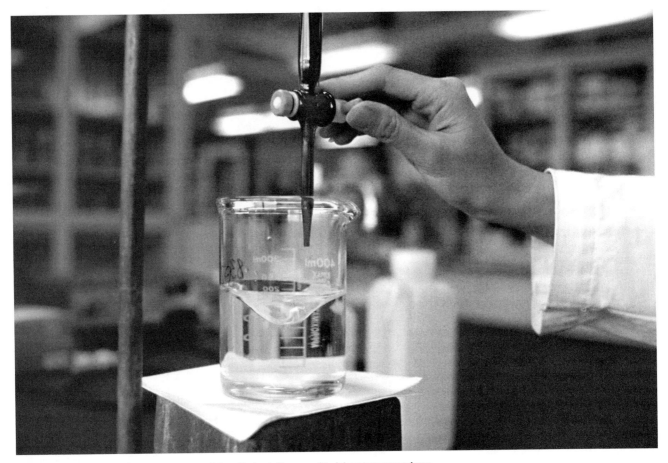

Titration burettes are used to carefully control the pH of solutions used in laboratory procedures.

done using a plastic plate containing many small wells. This allows up to 100 samples to be tested in a single experiment. ELISA can reveal the presence of antigen in fluids such as a patient's serum, for example.

The nature of the antibody can be important in laboratory immunological techniques. Antibodies such as those raised in a rabbit or a goat are described as being polyclonal in nature. That is, they do recognize a certain antigenic region. But if that region is present on different molecules, the antibody will react with all the molecules. The process of monoclonal antibody production can make antigenic identification much more specific, and has revolutionized immunological analysis.

Monoclonal antibodies are targeted against a single antigenic site. Furthermore, large amounts of the antibody can be made. This is achieved by fusing the antibody-producing cell obtained from an immunized mouse with a tumor cell. The resulting hybrid is known as a hybridoma. A particular hybridoma will mass-produce the antibody and will express the antibody on the surface of the cell. Because hybridoma cells are immortal, they grow and divide indefinitely. Hence the production of antibody can be ceaseless.

Monoclonal antibodies are very useful in a clinical immunology laboratory, as an aid to diagnose diseases and to detect the presence of foreign or abnormal components in the blood. In the research immunology laboratory, monoclonal technology enables the specific detection of an antigenic target and makes possible the development of highly specific vaccines.

One example of the utility of monoclonal antibodies in an immunology laboratory is their use in the technique of flow cytometry. This technique separates sample as individual sample molecules pass by a detector. Sample can be treated with monoclonal antibody followed by a second treatment with an antibody to the monoclonal to which is attached a molecule that will fluoresce when exposed to a certain wavelength of light. When the labeled sample passes by the detector and is illuminated (typically by laser light of the pre-determined wavelength), the labeled sample molecules will fluoresce. These can be detected and will be shunted off to a special collection receptacle. Many sorts of analyses are possible using flow cytometry, from the distinguishing of one type of bacteria from another to the level of the genetic material comprising such samples.

See also Antibody-antigen, biochemical and molecular reactions

LABORATORY TECHNIQUES IN MICROBIOLOGY

A number of techniques are routine in microbiology laboratories that enable **microorganisms** to be cultured, examined and identified.

An indispensable tool in any microbiology laboratory is the inoculating loop. The loop is a piece of wire that is looped at one end. By heating up the loop in an open flame, the loop can be sterilized before and after working with **bacteria**. Thus, **contamination** of the bacterial sample is minimized. The inoculating loop is part of what is known as aseptic (or sterile) technique.

Another staple piece of equipment is called a petri plate. A petri plate is a sterile plastic dish with a lid that is used as a receptacle for solid growth media.

In order to diagnose an infection or to conduct research using a microorganism, it is necessary to obtain the organism in a pure **culture**. The streak plate technique is useful in this regard. A sample of the bacterial population is added to one small region of the growth medium in a petri plate and spread in a back and forth motion across a sector of the plate using a sterile inoculating loop. The loop is sterilized again and used to drag a small portion of the culture across another sector of the plate. This acts to dilute the culture. Several more repeats yield individual colonies. A **colony** can be sampled and streaked onto another plate to ensure that a pure culture is obtained.

Dilutions of bacteria can be added to a petri plate and warm growth medium added to the aliquot of culture. When the medium hardens, the bacteria grow inside of the **agar**. This is known as the pour plate technique, and is often used to determine the number of bacteria in a sample. Dilution of the original culture of bacteria is often necessary to reach a countable level.

Bacterial numbers can also be determined by the number of tubes of media that support growth in a series of dilutions of the culture. The pattern of growth is used to determine what is termed the most probable number of bacteria in the original sample.

As a bacterial population increases, the medium becomes cloudier and less light is able to pass through the culture. The optical density of the culture increases. A relationship between the optical density and the number of living bacteria determined by the viable count can be established.

The growth sources for microorganisms such as bacteria can be in a liquid form or the solid agar form. The composition of a particular medium depends on the task at hand. Bacteria are often capable of growth on a wide variety of media, except for those bacteria whose nutrient or environmental requirements are extremely restricted. So-called non-selective media are useful to obtain a culture. For example, in **water quality** monitoring, a non-selective medium is used to obtain a total enumeration of the sample (called a heterotrophic plate count). When it is desirable to obtain a specific bacterial species, a selective medium can be used. Selective media support the growth of one or a few bacterial

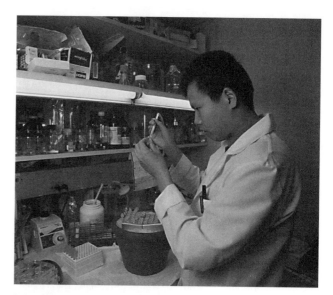

Lab technician performing medical research.

types while excluding the growth of other bacteria. For example, the growth of the bacterial genera *Salmonella* and *Shigella* are selectively encouraged by the use of *Salmonella-Shigella* agar. Many selective media exist.

Liquid cultures of bacteria can be nonspecific or can use defined media. A batch culture is essentially a stopped flask that is about one third full of the culture. The culture is shaken to encourage the diffusion of oxygen from the overlying air into the liquid. Growth occurs until the nutrients are exhausted. Liquid cultures can be kept growing indefinitely by adding fresh medium and removed spent culture at controlled rates (a chemostat) or at rates that keep the optical density of the culture constant (a turbidostat). In a chemostat, the rate at which the bacteria grow depends on the rate at which the critical nutrient is added.

Living bacteria can also be detected by direct observation using a light **microscope**, especially if the bacteria are capable of the directed movement that is termed motility. Also, living microorganisms are capable of being stained in certain distinctive ways by what are termed vital stains. Stains can also be used to highlight certain structures of bacteria, and even to distinguish certain bacteria from others. One example is the Gram's stain, which classifies bacteria into two camps, Gram positive and Gram negative. Another example is the Ziehl-Neelsen stain, which preferentially stains the cell wall of a type of bacteria called Mycobacteria.

Techniques also help detect the presence of bacteria that have become altered in their structure or genetic composition. The technique of replica plating relies on the adhesion of microbes to the support and the transfer of the microbes to a series of growth media. The technique is analogous to the making of photocopies of an original document. The various media can be tailored to detect a bacteria that can grow in the presence of a factor, such as an antibiotic, that the bacteria from the original growth culture cannot tolerate.

Various biochemical tests are utilized in a microbiology laboratory. The ability of a microbe to utilize a particular compound and the nature of the compound that is produced are important in the classification of microorganisms, and the diagnosis of infections. For example, coliform bacteria were traditionally identified by a series of biochemical reactions that formed a presumptive-confirmed-completed triad of tests. Now, media have been devised that specifically support the growth of coliform bacteria, and *Escherichia coli* in particular.

Various laboratory tests are conducted in animals to obtain an idea of the behavior of microorganisms *in vivo*. One such test is the lethal dose 50 (LD50), which measures the amount of an organism or its toxic components that will kill 50 percent of the test population. The lower the material necessary to achieve the LD50, the more potent is the disease component of organism.

See also Antibiotic resistance, tests for; Blood agar, hemolysis, and hemolytic reactions; Microscopy; Qualitative and quantitative analysis in microbiology

LACTIC ACID BACTERIA

Lactic acid **bacteria** compose a group of bacteria that degrade carbohydrate (e.g., **fermentation**) with the production of lactic acid. Examples of genera that contain lactic acid bacteria include *Streptococcus*, *Lactobacillus*, *Lactococcus*, and *Leuconostoc*.

The production of lactic acid has been used for a long time in food production (e.g., yogurt, cheese, sauerkraut, sausage,). Since the 1970s, the popularity of fermented foods such as kefir, kuniss, and tofu that were formally confined to certain ethnically oriented cuisines, has greatly increased.

Generally, lactic acid bacteria are Gram-positive bacteria that do not form spores and which are able to grow both in the presence and absence of oxygen. Another common trait of lactic acid bacteria is their inability to manufacture the many compounds that they need to survive and grow. Most of the nutrients must be present in the environment in which the bacteria reside. Their fastidious nutritional needs restrict the environments in which lactic acid bacteria exist. The mouth and intestinal tract of animals are two such environments, where the lactic acid bacterium *Enterococcus faecalis* lives. Other environments include plant leaves (*Leuconostoc*, *Lactobacillus*, and decaying organic material.

The drop in **pH** that occurs as lactic acid is produced by the bacteria is beneficial in the preservation of food. The lowered pH inhibits the growth of most other food spoilage **microorganisms**. Abundant growth of the lactic acid bacteria, and so production of lactic acid, is likewise hindered by the low pH. The low pH environment prolongs the shelf life of foods (e.g., pickles, yogurt, cheese) from **contamination** by bacteria that are common in the kitchen (e.g., *Escherichia coli,* or bacteria that are able to grow at refrigeration temperatures (e.g., *Listeria*. The drop in the oxygen level during lactic acid fermentation is also an inhibitory factor for potential food pathogens. Research is actively underway to extend the pro-

tection afforded by lactic acid bacteria to others foods, such as vegetables.

The acidity associated with lactic acid bacteria has also been useful in preventing colonization of surfaces with infectious bacteria. The best example of this is the vagina. Colonization of the vaginal epithelial cells with *Lactobacillus* successfully thwarts the subsequent colonization of the cell surface with harmful bacteria, thus reducing the incidence of chronic vaginal **yeast** infections.

Lactic acid bacteria produce antibacterial compounds that are known as bacteriocins. Bacteriocins act by punching holes through the membrane that surrounds the bacteria. Thus, bacteriocins activity is usually lethal to the bacteria. Examples of bacteriocins are nisin and leucocin. Nisin inhibits the growth of most gram-positive bacteria, particularly spore-formers (e.g., *Clostridium botulinum*. This bacteriocin has been approved for use as a food preservative in the United States since 1989. Leucocin is inhibitory to the growth of *Listeria monocytogenes*.

Lactic acid bacteria are also of economic importance in the preservation of agricultural crops. A popular method of crop preservation utilizes what is termed silage. Silage is essentially the exposure of crops (e.g., grasses, corn, alfalfa) to lactic acid bacteria. The resulting fermentation activity lowers the pH on the surface of the crop, preventing colonization of the crop by unwanted microorganisms.

See also Economic uses and benefits of microorganisms

LACTOBACILLUS

Lactobacillus is the name given to a group of Gram-negative **bacteria** that do not form spores but derive energy from the conversion of the sugar glucose into another sugar known as lactose. The name of the genus derives from the distinctive sugar use. *Lactobacillus* has a number of commercial uses, especially in aspects of dairy production, including the manufacture of yogurt. As well, *Lactobacillus* is part of the normal microbial population of the human adult vagina, where it exerts a protective effect.

Prominent examples of the genus include *Lactobacillus acidophilus*, *Lactobacillus* GG, *Bifidobacterium bifidum*, and *Bifidobacterium longum*.

A distinctive feature of the members of the genus *Lactobacillus* is the formation of lactic acid from glucose. This is the property that confers the sour taste to natural, *Lactobacillus*-containing yogurt. As well, the lactic acid lowers the **pH** of the environment that the bacteria dwell in. In the case of the vagina, this acidic change can inhibit the growth of other, harmful invading bacteria. Consistent with this, the use of suppositories containing *Lactobacillus* species has been successful in controlling recurrent bacterial vaginal infections. Similarly, use of the bacterium has been promising in the control and prevention of recurrent urinary tract infections.

Aside from the exclusion of bacteria due to the pH alteration in the vagina or urinary tract, *Lactobacillus* also adheres to cells lining the vagina and the urinary tract, and colonizes these surfaces. The luxuriant growth of these bacteria excludes other bacteria from gaining a foothold. This phenomenon is known as competitive exclusion.

Commercially, *Lactobacillus* is best known as the basis of yogurt manufacture. A mixture of *Lactobacillus bulgaricus* or *Lactobacillus acidophilus* and *Streptococcus thermophilus* produce the lactic acid that ferments milk.

Yogurt that contains live bacteria usually contains *Lactobacillus acidophilus*. There is evidence that the persistence of the bacteria in the intestinal tract for up to a week after consuming yogurt increases the number of antibody-secreting cells in the intestine. Also *Lactobacillus acidophilus* bacteria possess and enzyme called lactase that enables the bacteria are to utilize undigested starches, particularly those in milk, that would otherwise be eliminated from the body.

Yet another benefit of *Lactobacillus* is the production of beneficial compounds that are used by the body. For example, *Lactobacillus acidophilus* produces niacin, folic acid, and pyridoxine, a group of compounds that collectively are referred to as the B vitamins.

Another noteworthy strain of *Lactobacillus* is known as *Lactobacillus GG*. This strain was isolated from humans in the 1980s by Drs. Sherwood Gorbach and Barry Goldin. The initials of their last names are the basis for the GG designation. *Lactobacillus GG* has shown great promise as a nutritional supplement because the bacteria are able to survive the passage through the very acidic conditions of the stomach. They then colonize the intestinal tract. There, the bacteria produce a compound that has antibacterial activity. This may help maintain the intestinal tract free from invading bacteria.

See also Microbial flora of the stomach and gastrointestinal tract; Probiotics

LANCEFIELD, REBECCA CRAIGHILL
(1895-1981)
American bacteriologist

Rebecca Craighill Lancefield is best-known throughout the scientific world for the system she developed to classify the **bacteria** *Streptococcus*. Her colleagues called her laboratory at the Rockefeller Institute for Medical Research (now Rockefeller University) "the Scotland Yard of streptococcal mysteries." During a research career that spanned six decades, Lancefield meticulously identified over fifty types of this bacteria. She used her knowledge of this large, diverse bacterial family to learn about pathogenesis and **immunity** of its afflictions, ranging from sore throats, rheumatic fever and scarlet fever, to heart and kidney disease. The Lancefield system remains a key to the medical understanding of streptococcal diseases.

Born Rebecca Craighill on January 5, 1895, in Fort Wadsworth on Staten Island in New York, she was the third of six daughters. Her mother, Mary Montague Byram, married William Edward Craighill, a career army officer in the Army Corps of Engineers who had graduated from West Point.

Lancefield received a bachelor's degree in 1916 from Wellesley College, after changing her major from English to zoology. Two years later, she earned a master's degree from Columbia University, where she pursued bacteriology in the laboratory of Hans Zinsser. Immediately upon graduating from Columbia, she formed two lifelong partnerships. She married Donald Lancefield, who had been a classmate of hers in a genetics class. She was also hired by the Rockefeller Institute to help bacteriologists Oswald Avery and Alphonse Dochez, whose expertise on *Pneumococcus* was then being applied to a different bacterium. This was during World War I, and the project at Rockefeller was to discover whether distinct types of *Streptococci* could be isolated from soldiers in a Texas epidemic so that a serum might be produced to prevent infection. The scientists employed the same serological techniques that Avery had used to distinguish types of *Pneumococcus*. Within a year, Avery, Dochez, and Lancefield had published a major report which described four types of *Streptococcus*. This was Lancefield's first paper.

Lancefield and her husband took a short hiatus to teach in his home state at the University of Oregon, then returned to New York. Lancefield worked simultaneously on a Ph.D. at Columbia and on rheumatic fever studies at the Rockefeller Institute in the laboratory of Homer Swift, and her husband joined the Columbia University faculty in biology. Before World War I, physicians had suspected that *Streptococcus* caused rheumatic fever. But scientists, including Swift, had not been able to recover a specific organism from patients. Nor could they reproduce the disease in animals using patient cultures. Lancefield's first project with Swift, which was also her doctoral work, showed that the alpha-hemolytic class of *Streptococcus,* also called green or viridans, was not the cause of rheumatic fever.

As a result of her work with Swift, Lancefield decided that a more basic approach to rheumatic fever was needed. She began sorting out types among the disease-causing class, the beta-hemolytic **streptococci**. She used serological techniques while continuing to benefit from Avery's advice. Her major tool for classifying the bacteria was the precipitin test. This involved mixing soluble type-specific antigens, or substances used to stimulate immune responses, with antisera (types of serum containing antibodies) to give visible precipitates. Precipitates are the separations of a substance, in this case bacteria, from liquid in a solution, the serum, in order to make it possible to study the bacteria on its own.

Lancefield soon recovered two surface antigens from these streptococci. One was a polysaccharide, or carbohydrate, called the C substance. This complex sugar molecule is a major component of the cell wall in all streptococci. She could further subdivide its dissimilar compositions into groups and she designated the groups by the letters A through O. The most common species causing human disease, *Streptococcus pyogenes,* were placed in group A. Among the group A streptococci, Lancefield found another **antigen** and determined it was a protein, called M for its matt appearance in **colony** formations. Because of differences in M protein composition, Lancefield was able to subdivide group A streptococci into types. During her career, she identified over fifty types, and since her death in 1981, bacteriologists have identified thirty more.

Lancefield's classification converged with another typing system devised by Frederick Griffith in England. His typing was based on a slide agglutination method, in which the bacteria in the serum collect into clumps when an **antibody** is introduced. For five years the two scientists exchanged samples and information across the Atlantic Ocean, verifying each other's types, until Griffith's tragic death during the bombing of London in 1940. Ultimately, Lancefield's system, based on the M types, was chosen as the standard for classifying group A streptococci.

In further studies on the M protein, Lancefield revealed this antigen is responsible for the bacteria's virulence because it inhibits **phagocytosis**, thus keeping the white blood cells from engulfing the streptococci. This finding came as a surprise, because Avery had discovered that virulence in the *Pneumococcus* was due to a polysaccharide, not a protein. Lancefield went on to show the M antigen is also the one that elicits protective immune reactions.

Lancefield continued to group and type strep organisms sent from laboratories around the world. Until the end of her life her painstaking investigations helped unravel the complexity and diversity of these bacteria. Her thoroughness was a significant factor in her small but substantial bibliography of nearly sixty papers.

Once her system of classification was in place, however, Lancefield returned to her original quest to elucidate connections between the bacteria's constituents and the baffling nature of streptococcal diseases. She found that a single serotype of group A can cause a variety of streptococcal diseases. This evidence reversed a long-standing assumption that every disease must be caused by a specific microbe. Also, because the M protein is type-specific, she found that acquired immunity to one group A serotype could not protect against infections caused by others in group A.

From her laboratory at Rockefeller Hospital, Lancefield could follow patient records for very long periods. She conducted a study that determined that once immunity is acquired to a serotype, it can last up to thirty years. This particular study revealed the unusual finding that high titers, or concentrations, of antibody persist in the absence of antigen. In the case of rheumatic fever, Lancefield illustrated how someone can suffer recurrent attacks, because each one is caused by a different serotype.

In other studies, Lancefield focused on antigens. She and Gertrude Perlmann purified the M protein in the 1950s. Twenty years later she developed a more conservative test for typing it and continued characterizing other group A protein antigens designated T and R. Ten years after her official retirement, she made a vital contribution on the group B streptococci. She clarified the role of their polysaccharides in virulence and showed how protein antigens on their surface also played a protective role. During the 1970s, an increasingly high-rate of infants were born with group B **meningitis**, and her work laid the basis for the medical response to this problem.

During World War II, Lancefield had performed special duties on the Streptococcal Diseases Commission of the Armed Forces Epidemiological Board. Her task involved identifying strains and providing antisera for **epidemics** of scarlet and rheumatic fever among soldiers in military camps. After the commission dissolved, her colleagues in the "Strep Club" created the Lancefield Society in 1977, which continues to hold regular international meetings on advances in streptococcal research.

An associate member at Rockefeller when **Maclyn McCarty** took over Swift's laboratory in 1946, Lancefield became a full member and professor in 1958, and emeritus professor in 1965. While her career and achievements took place in a field dominated by men, Lewis Wannamaker in American Society for Microbiology News quotes Lancefield as being "annoyed by any special feeling about women in science." Nevertheless, most recognition for Lancefield came near her retirement. In 1961, she was the first woman elected president of the American Association of Immunologists, and in 1970, she was one of few women elected to the National Academy of Sciences. Other honors included the T. Duckett Jones Memorial Award in 1960, the American Heart Association Achievement Award in 1964, the New York Academy of Medicine Medal in 1973, and honorary degrees from Rockefeller University in 1973 and Wellesley College in 1976.

In addition to her career as a scientist, Lancefield had one daughter. Lancefield was devoted to research and preferred not to go on lecture tours or attend scientific meetings. Rockefeller's laboratories were not air-conditioned and her main diversion was leaving them during the summer and spending the entire season in Woods Hole, Massachusetts. There she enjoyed tennis and swimming with her family, which eventually included two grandsons. Official retirement did not change her lifestyle. She drove to her Rockefeller laboratory from her home in Douglaston, Long Island, every working day until she broke her hip in November 1980. She died of complications from this injury on March 3, 1981, at the age of eighty-six.

The pathogenesis of rheumatic fever still eludes scientists, and **antibiotics** have not eliminated streptococcal diseases. Yet the legacy of Lancefield's system and its fundamental links to disease remain and a **vaccine** against several group A streptococci is being developed in her former laboratory at Rockefeller University by Vincent A. Fischetti.

See also Bacteria and bacterial infection; Streptococci and streptococcal infections

LANDSTEINER, KARL (1868-1943)

American immunologist

Karl Landsteiner was one of the first scientists to study the physical processes of **immunity**. He is best known for his identification and characterization of the human blood groups, A, B, and O, but his contributions spanned many areas of **immunology**, bacteriology, and pathology over a prolific forty-year career. Landsteiner identified the agents responsible for immune reactions, examined the interaction of antigens and antibodies, and studied allergic reactions in experimental animals. He determined the viral cause of **poliomyelitis** with research that laid the foundation for the eventual development of a polio **vaccine**. He also discovered that some simple chemicals, when linked to proteins, produced an immune response. Near the end of his career in 1940, Landsteiner and immunologist Philip Levine discovered the **Rh** factor that helped save the lives of many unborn babies whose Rh factor did not match their mothers. For his work identifying the human blood groups, Landsteiner was awarded the Nobel Prize for medicine in 1930.

Karl Landsteiner was born on in Vienna, Austria. In 1885, at the age of 17, Landsteiner passed the entrance examination for medical school at the University of Vienna. He graduated from medical school at the age of 23 and immediately began advanced studies in the field of organic chemistry, working in the research laboratory of his mentor, Ernst Ludwig. In Ludwig's laboratory Landsteiner's interest in chemistry blossomed into a passion for approaching medical problems through a chemist's eye.

For the next ten years, Landsteiner worked in a number of laboratories in Europe, studying under some of the most celebrated chemists of the day: Emil Fischer, a protein chemist who subsequently won the Nobel Prize for chemistry in 1902, in Wurzburg; Eugen von Bamberger in Munich; and Arthur Hantzsch and Roland Scholl in Zurich. Landsteiner published many journal articles with these famous scientists. The knowledge he gained about organic chemistry during these formative years guided him throughout his career. The nature of antibodies began to interest him while he was serving as an assistant to **Max von Gruber** in the Department of **Hygiene** at the University of Vienna from 1896 to 1897. During this time Landsteiner published his first article on the subject of bacteriology and **serology**, the study of blood.

Landsteiner moved to Vienna's Institute of Pathology in 1897, where he was hired to perform autopsies. He continued to study immunology and the mysteries of blood on his own time. In 1900, Landsteiner wrote a paper in which he described the agglutination of blood that occurs when one person's blood is brought into contact with that of another. He suggested that the phenomenon was not due to pathology, as was the prevalent thought at the time, but was due to the unique nature of the individual's blood. In 1901, Landsteiner demonstrated that the blood serum of some people could clump the blood of others. From his observations he devised the idea of mutually incompatible blood groups. He placed blood types into three groups: A, B, and C (later referred to as O). Two of his colleagues subsequently added a fourth group, AB.

In 1907, the first successful transfusions were achieved by Dr. Reuben Ottenberg of Mt. Sinai Hospital, New York, guided by Landsteiner's work. Landsteiner's accomplishment saved many lives on the battlefields of World War I, where transfusion of compatible blood was first performed on a large scale. In 1902, Landsteiner was appointed as a full member of the Imperial Society of Physicians in Vienna. That same year he presented a lecture, together with Max Richter of the Vienna University Institute of Forensic Medicine, in which the two reported a new method of typing dried blood stains to help solve crimes in which blood stains are left at the scene.

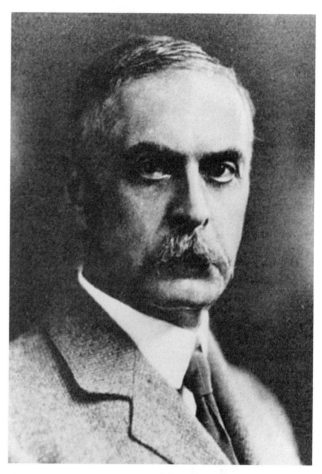

Karl Landsteiner, awarded the 1930 Nobel Prize in Medicine or Physiology for his discovery of human blood groups.

In 1908, Landsteiner took charge of the department of pathology at the Wilhelmina Hospital in Vienna. His tenure at the hospital lasted twelve years, until March of 1920. During this time, Landsteiner was at the height of his career and produced 52 papers on serological immunity, 33 on bacteriology and six on pathological anatomy. He was among the first to dissociate antigens that stimulate the production of immune responses known as antibodies, from the antibodies themselves. Landsteiner was also among the first to purify antibodies, and his purification techniques are still used today for some applications in immunology.

Landsteiner also collaborated with Ernest Finger, the head of Vienna's Clinic for Venereal Diseases and Dermatology. In 1905, Landsteiner and Finger successfully transferred the venereal disease **syphilis** from humans to apes. The result was that researchers had an animal model in which to study the disease. In 1906, Landsteiner and Viktor Mucha, a scientist from the Chemical Institute at Finger's clinic, developed the technique of dark-field microscopy to identify and study the **microorganisms** that cause syphilis.

One day in 1908, the body of a young polio victim was brought in for autopsy. Landsteiner took a portion of the boy's spinal column and injected it into the spinal canal of several species of experimental animals, including rabbits, guinea pigs, mice, and monkeys. Only the monkeys contracted the disease. Landsteiner reported the results of the experiment, conducted with Erwin Popper, an assistant at the Wilhelmina Hospital.

Scientists had accepted that polio was caused by a microorganism, but previous experiments by other researchers had failed to isolate a causative agent, which was presumed to be a bacterium. Because monkeys were hard to come by in Vienna, Landsteiner went to Paris to collaborate with a Romanian bacteriologist, Constantin Levaditi of the Pasteur Institute. Working together, the two were able to trace poliomyelitis to a virus, describe the manner of its transmission, time its incubation phase, and show how it could be neutralized in the laboratory when mixed with the serum of a convalescing patient. In 1912, Landsteiner proposed that the development of a vaccine against poliomyelitis might prove difficult but was certainly possible. The first successful polio vaccine, developed by **Jonas Salk**, wasn't administered until 1955.

Landsteiner accepted a position as chief dissector in a small Catholic hospital in The Hague, Netherlands where he performed routine laboratory tests on urine and blood from 1919 to 1922. During this time he began working on the concept of haptens, small molecular weight chemicals such as fats or sugars that determine the specificity of antigen-antibody reactions when combined with a protein carrier. He combined haptens of known structure with well-characterized proteins such as albumin, and showed that small changes in the hapten could affect **antibody** production. He developed methods to show that it is possible to sensitize animals to chemicals that cause contact dermatitis (**inflammation** of the skin) in humans, demonstrating that contact dermatitis is caused by an antigen-antibody reaction. This work launched Landsteiner into a study of the phenomenon of allergic reactions.

In 1922, Landsteiner accepted a position at the Rockefeller Institute in New York. Throughout the 1920s Landsteiner worked on the problems of immunity and allergy. He discovered new blood groups: M, N, and P, refining the work he had begun 20 years before. Soon after Landsteiner and his collaborator, Philip Levine, published the work in 1927, the types began to be used in paternity suits.

In 1929, Landsteiner became a United States citizen. He won the Nobel Prize for medicine in 1930 for identifying the human blood types. In his Nobel lecture, Landsteiner gave an account of his work on individual differences in human blood, describing the differences in blood between different species and among individuals of the same species. This theory is accepted as fact today but was at odds with prevailing thought when Landsteiner began his work. In 1936, Landsteiner summed up his life's work in what was to become a medical classic: *Die Spezifität der serologischen Reaktionen*, which was later revised and published in English, under the title *The Specificity of Serological Reactions*.

Landsteiner retired in 1939, at the age of seventy-one, but continued working in immunology. With Levine and Alexander Wiener he discovered another blood factor, labeled the Rh factor, for Rhesus monkeys, in which the factor was first discovered. The Rh factor was shown to be responsible for the infant disease, erythroblastosis fetalis that occurs when mother and fetus have incompatible blood types and the fetus is injured by the mother's antibodies. Landsteiner died in 1943, at the age of 75.

See also Antibody and antigen; Antibody-antigen, biochemical and molecular reactions; Blood agar, hemolysis, and hemolytic reactions; History of immunology; Rh and Rh incompatibility

LATENT VIRUSES AND DISEASES

Latent **viruses** are those viruses that can incorporate their genetic material into the genetic material of the infected host cell. Because the viral genetic material can then be replicated along with the host material, the virus becomes effectively "silent" with respect to detection by the host. Latent viruses usually contain the information necessary to reverse the latent state. The viral genetic material can leave the host genome to begin the manufacture of new virus particles.

The molecular process by which a virus becomes latent has been explored most fully in the **bacteriophage** designated lambda. The lysogenic process is complex and involves the interplay between several proteins that influence the **transcription** of genes that either maintain the latent state or begin the so-called lytic process, where the manufacture of new virus begins.

Bacteriophage lambda is not associated with disease. However, other viruses that can establish a latent relationship with the host are capable of causing disease. Examples of viruses include the **Herpes** Simplex Virus 1 (also dubbed HSV 1) and **retroviruses**. The latter group of viruses includes the **Human Immunodeficiency Viruses** (**HIVs**) that are the most likely cause of acquired immunodeficiency syndrome (**AIDS**).

In the case of HSV 1, the virus can become latent early in life, when many people are infected with the virus. The virus infects the mucous membranes located around the mouth. From this location the virus spreads to a region of certain nerve cells called the ganglion. It is here that the viral genetic material (**deoxyribonucleic acid**, or **DNA**) integrates into the host genetic material. The period of latency can span decades. Then, if the host is stressed such that the survival of the infected cells is in peril, the viral DNA is activated. The new virus particles migrate back to the mucous membranes of the mouth, where they erupt as "cold sores". A form of the reactivated herpes virus that is known as Herpes Zoster causes the malady of shingles. The painful sores associated with shingles can appear all over the body.

The re-emergence of HSV 1 later in life does qualify as a disease. However, it has been argued that the near universal prevalence of the latent form of the viral DNA in people worldwide qualifies HSV as being part of the normal microbial makeup of humans. Others argue that even the latent HSV state qualifies as an infection, albeit an infection that displays no symptoms and is essentially harmless to the host.

Other examples of a latent virus include the HIVs. The latent form of **HIV** is particularly insidious from the point of view of treatment, because the drugs traditionally given to treat AIDS are effective only against the actively replicating form of the virus. In the absence of detectable virus, drug therapy may be discontinued. Then, if the virus is stimulated to leave the latent state and begin another round of infection, that infection will be uncontrolled. Indeed, it has been shown that even the near continuous administration of anti-HIV drugs does not completely eliminate the pool of latent virus in the **immune system**.

A hallmark of latent viral infections is that the immune system is not stimulated to respond. Indeed, with little or no viral products or new virus produced, the immune system has no target. This complicates the development of vaccines to infections such as HSV 1 and AIDS, because the nature of the **vaccine** effect is the stimulation of the immune system.

One experimental approach that is being explored with latent viral infections is to establish whether there is some aspect of the host cell that predisposes the cells to infection with a virus capable of becoming latent. Identification of such host factors could help in the design of therapeutic strategies to target these cells against viral infection.

See also Lysogeny; Virology; Viral genetics

LEDERBERG, JOSHUA (1925-)

American geneticist

Joshua Lederberg is a Nobel Prize-winning American geneticist whose pioneering work on genetic **recombination** in **bacteria** helped propel the field of **molecular genetics** into the forefront of biological and medical research. In 1946, Lederberg, working with **Edward Lawrie Tatum**, showed that bacteria may reproduce sexually, disproving the widely held theory that bacteria were asexual. The two scientists' discovery also substantiated that bacteria possess genetic systems comparable to those of higher organisms, thus providing a new repertoire for scientists to study the genetic basis of life.

Continuing with his work in bacteria, Lederberg also discovered the phenomena of genetic **conjugation** and **transduction**, or the transfer of either the entire **complement** of **chromosomes** or chromosome fragments, respectively, from cell to cell. In his work on conjugation and transduction, Lederberg became the first scientist to manipulate genetic material, which had far-reaching implications for subsequent efforts in genetic engineering and **gene** therapy. In addition to his laboratory research, Lederberg lectured widely on the complex relationship between science and society and served as a scientific adviser on **biological warfare** to the **World Health Organization**.

Lederberg was born in Montclair, New Jersey. His family moved to New York City where he attended Stuyvesant High School. Through a program known as the American Institute Science Laboratory, Lederberg was given the opportunity to conduct original research in a laboratory after school hours and on weekends. Here he pursued his interest in biology, working in cytochemistry, or the chemistry of cells.

Lederberg was influenced early on by science-oriented writers such as Bernard Jaffe, Paul de Kruif, and H. G. Wells.

After graduating from high school in 1941, Lederberg entered Columbia University as a premedical student. He received a tuition scholarship from the Hayden Trust, which, coupled with living at home and commuting to school, made it financially possible for him to attend college. Although his undergraduate studies focused on zoology, Lederberg also received a foundation in humanistic studies under Lionel Trilling, James Gutman, and others. H. Burr Steinbach fostered Lederberg's work in zoology and helped him obtain a space in a histology lab where he could pursue his own research. This early undergraduate research included the cytophysiology of mitosis in plants and the uses of genetic analysis in cell biology. In 1942, Lederberg met Francis Ryan, whose work in the biochemical genetics of *Neurospora* (a genus of **fungi**) was Lederberg's first opportunity to see significant scientific research as it occurred. Lederberg graduated with honors in 1944 with a B.A. at the age of nineteen.

At the age of seventeen, Lederberg enlisted in the United States Navy V–12 college training program, which featured a condensed pre-med and medical curriculum to produce medical officers for the armed services during World War II. During his years as an undergraduate, he was also assigned duty to the U.S. Naval Hospital at St. Albans in Long Island. He began his medical courses at Columbia College of Physicians and Surgeons in 1944, but left after two years to study under Edward L. Tatum in the microbiology department at Yale University.

Tatum, with George W. Beadle, had made substantial contributions to biochemical genetics, including investigations proving that the **DNA** (**deoxyribonucleic acid**) of *Neurospora* played a fundamental role in many of the chemical reactions in *Neurospora* cells. Lederberg was interested in natural **selection** and helped Tatum continue his studies of *Neurospora*. Eventually, Lederberg and Tatum proceeded to embark on a more tenuous line of research, studying *Escherichia coli* (a bacterium that lives in the gastrointestinal tract) for evidence of genetic inheritance. At the international Cold Spring Harbor Symposium of 1946, Lederberg and Tatum presented their research on *E. coli* in addition to the *Neurospora* studies. An audience that included the leading molecular biologists and geneticists in the world met the scientists' announcement that they had discovered sexual or genetic recombination in the bacterium with keen interest. The prevailing theory among biologists of the time was that bacteria reproduced asexually by cells essentially splitting, creating two cells with a complete set of chromosomes (threadlike structures in the cell **nucleus** that carry genetic information). Lederberg and Tatum had found evidence that some strains of *E. coli* pass on hereditary material cell to cell. They found that a conjugation of two cells produced a cell that subsequently began dividing into offspring cells. These offspring showed that they inherited traits from each of the parent strains. Lederberg received requests for *E. coli* cultures by others who wanted to investigate his findings.

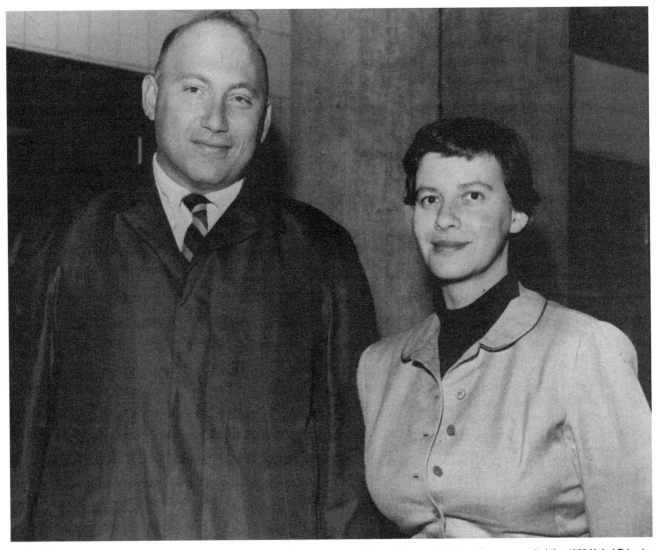

Joshua Lederberg (left) who, with his wife Esther (right), discovered the process of bacterial recombination. He was awarded the 1958 Nobel Prize in Medicine for this and other discoveries.

In 1947, while at Yale, Lederberg received an offer from the University of Wisconsin to become an assistant professor of genetics. Although only two years away from receiving his M.D. degree, Lederberg accepted the position at Wisconsin and received his Ph.D. degree from Yale in 1948. He worked at the University of Wisconsin for a decade after abandoning his medical training, although he noted his later honorary medical degrees from Tufts University and the University of Turin as being among his most valued.

Lederberg continued to make groundbreaking discoveries at Wisconsin that firmly established him as one of the most promising young intellects in the burgeoning field of genetics. By perfecting a method to isolate mutant bacteria species using ultraviolet light, Lederberg was able to prove the long-held theory that genetic **mutations** occurred spontaneously. He found he could mate two strains of bacteria, one resistant to **penicillin** and the other to streptomycin, and produce bacteria

resistant to both **antibiotics**. He also found that he could manipulate a virus's virulence.

Working with graduate student Norton Zinder, Lederberg discovered genetic transduction, which involves the transfer only of hereditary fragments of information between cells as opposed to complete chromosomal replication (conjugation). Lederberg went on to breed unique strains of **viruses**. Although these strains promised to reveal much about the nature of viruses in hopes of one day controlling them, they also posed a clear threat in terms of creating harmful biochemical substances. At the time, the practical aspect of Lederberg's work was hard to evaluate. The Nobel Prize Committee, however recognized the significance of his contributions to genetics and, in 1958, awarded him the Nobel Prize in physiology or medicine for the bacterial and viral research that provided a new line of investigations of viral diseases and cancer. Lederberg shared the prize with Beadle and Tatum.

Lederberg's work in genetics eventually proved to be one of the foundations of gene mapping, which eventually led to efforts to genetically treat disease and identify those at risk of developing certain diseases.

Known as brilliant laboratory scientist and technician, Lederberg was also concerned with the role of science in society and the far-reaching effects of scientific discoveries, particularly in genetics. In a Pan American Health Organization/World Health Organization lecture in biomedical sciences called "Health in the World Tomorrow," Lederberg acknowledged concerns of the public, and even some scientists, over the newfound ability to tamper with the **genetic code** of life. However, he was more concerned with the many ethical questions that would arise over the inevitable success of the technological advances in microbiology and genetics. Lederberg saw the biological revolution as "a philosophical one" that was to bring a "new depth of scientific understanding about the nature of life." He foresaw advancements in the treatment of cancer, organ transplants, and geriatric medicine as presenting a whole new set of ethical and social problems, such as the availability and allocation of expensive health-care resources.

Lederberg was also interested in the study of biochemical life outside of Earth and coined the term *exobiology* to refer to such studies. Along with physicist Dean B. Cowie, he expressed concern in *Science* over the possible **contamination** of biological life on other planets from microbes carried by human spacecraft. He was also a consultant to the U.S. Viking space missions to the planet Mars.

Lederberg's career included an appointment as chairman of the new genetics department at Stanford University in 1958. In 1978 he was appointed president of Rockefeller University. Working with his first wife, Esther Zimmer, a former student of Tatum's whom Lederberg married in 1946, Lederberg investigated the role of bacterial **enzymes** in sugar **metabolism**. He also discovered that penicillin's ability to kill bacteria was due to its preventing synthesis of the bacteria's cell walls. Among Lederberg's many honors were the Eli Lilly Award for outstanding work by a scientist under thirty-five years of age and the Alexander Hamilton Medal of Columbia University.

See also Escherichia coli (E. coli); Microbial genetics; Molecular biology and molecular genetics; Viral genetics

LEEUWENHOEK, ANTONI VAN (1632-1723)

Dutch microscopist

Antoni van Leeuwenhoek is best remembered as the first person to study **bacteria** and "animalcules," or one-celled organisms now known as *protozoa*. Unlike his contemporaries **Robert Hooke** and Marcello Malpighi, Leeuwenhoek did not use the more advanced compound **microscope**; instead, he strove to manufacture magnifying lenses of unsurpassed power and clarity that would allow him to study the microcosm in far greater detail than any other scientist of his time.

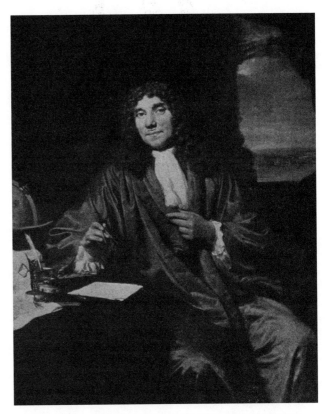

Antoni van Leeuwenhoek, the "father" of microscopy, pictured with one of his light microscopes used to observe "animalcules."

Leeuwenhoek was born on October 24, 1632, in Delft, Holland. Although his family was relatively prosperous, he received little formal education. After completing grammar school in Delft, he moved to Amsterdam to work as a draper's apprentice. In 1654, he returned to Delft to establish his own shop, and he worked as a draper for the rest of his life. In addition to his business, Leeuwenhoek was appointed to several positions within the city government, which afforded him the financial security to spend a great deal of time and money in pursuit of his hobby, lens grinding. Lenses were important tools in Leeuwenhoek's profession, as cloth merchants often used small lenses to inspect their products. His hobby soon turned to obsession, however, as he searched for more and more powerful lenses.

In 1671, Leeuwenhoek constructed his first simple microscope. It consisted of a tiny lens that he had ground by hand from a globule of glass and placed within a brass holder. To this, he had attached a series of pins designed to hold the specimen. It was the first of nearly six hundred lenses ranging from 50 to 500 times magnifications that he would grind during his lifetime. Through his microscope, Leeuwenhoek examined such substances as skin, hair, and his own blood. He studied the structure of ivory as well as the physical composition of the flea, discovering that fleas, too, harbored **parasites**.

Leeuwenhoek began writing to the British Royal Society in 1673. At first, the Society gave his letters little notice, thinking that such magnification from a single lens microscope could only be a hoax. However, in 1676, when he sent the Society the news that he had discovered tiny one-celled animals in rainwater, the interest of member scientists was piqued. Following Leeuwenhoek's specifications, they built microscopes of comparable magnitude and confirmed his findings. In 1680, the Society unanimously elected Leeuwenhoek as a member.

Until this time, Leeuwenhoek had been operating in an informational vacuum; he read only Dutch and, consequently, was unable to learn from the published works of Hooke and Malpighi (though he often gleaned what he could from the illustrations within their texts). As a member of the Society, he was finally able to interact with other scientists. In fact, the news of his discoveries spread worldwide, and he was often visited by royalty from England, Prussia, and Russia. The traffic through his laboratory was so persistent that he eventually allowed visitors by appointment only. Near the end of his life, Leeuwenhoek had reached near-legendary status and was often referred to by the local townsfolk as a magician.

Amid the attention, Leeuwenhoek remained focused upon his scientific research. Specifically, he was interested in disproving the common belief in spontaneous generation, a theory proposing that certain inanimate objects could generate life. For example, it was assumed that **mold** and maggots were created spontaneously from decaying food. Leeuwenhoek succeeded in disproving spontaneous generation in 1683, when he discovered bacteria cells. These tiny organisms were nearly beyond the resolving power of even Leeuwenhoek's remarkable equipment and would not be seen again for more than a century.

Leeuwenhoek created and improved upon new lenses for most of his long life. For the forty-three years that he was a member of the Royal Society, he wrote nearly 200 letters that described his progress. However, he never divulged the method by which he illuminated his specimens for viewing, and the nature of that illumination is still somewhat of a mystery. Upon his death on August 30, 1723, Leeuwenhoek willed twenty-six of his microscopes, a few of which survive in museums, to the British Royal Society.

See also Bacterial growth and division; Bacterial kingdoms; Bacterial membranes and cell wall; Bacterial movement; History of microbiology; Microscope and microscopy

LEGIONNAIRES' DISEASE

Legionnaires' disease is a type of **pneumonia** caused by *Legionella* **bacteria**. The bacterial species responsible for Legionnaires' disease is *L. pneumophila*. Major symptoms include fever, chills, muscle aches, and a cough that is initially nonproductive. Definitive diagnosis relies on specific laboratory tests for the bacteria, bacterial antigens, or antibodies produced by the body's **immune system**. As with other types of pneumonia, Legionnaires' disease poses the greatest threat to people who are elderly, ill, or immunocompromised.

Legionella bacteria were first identified as a cause of pneumonia in 1976, following an outbreak of pneumonia among people who had attended an American Legion convention in Philadelphia, Pennsylvania (the bacterium's name was derived from this group's name). This outbreak prompted further investigation into *Legionella* and it was discovered that earlier unexplained pneumonia outbreaks were linked to the bacteria. The earliest cases of Legionnaires' disease were shown to have occurred in 1965, but samples of the bacteria exist from 1947.

Exposure to the *Legionella* bacteria does not necessarily lead to infection. According to some studies, an estimated 5–10% of the American population show serologic evidence of exposure, the majority of whom do not develop symptoms of an infection. *Legionella* bacteria account for 2–15% of the total number of pneumonia cases requiring hospitalization in the United States.

There are at least 40 types of *Legionella* bacteria, half of which are capable of producing disease in humans. A disease that arises from infection by *Legionella* bacteria is referred to as legionellosis. The *L. pneumophila* bacterium, the root cause of Legionnaires' disease, causes 90% of legionellosis cases. The second most common cause of legionellosis is the *L. micdadei* bacterium, which produces the Philadelphia pneumonia-causing agent.

Approximately 10,000–40,000 people in the United States develop some type of Legionnaires' disease annually. The people who are the most likely to become ill are over age 50. The risk is greater for people who suffer from health conditions such as malignancy, diabetes, lung disease, or kidney disease. Other risk factors include immunosuppressive therapy and cigarette smoking. Legionnaires' disease has occurred in children, but typically, it has been confined to newborns receiving respiratory therapy, children who have had recent operations, and children who are immunosuppressed. People with **HIV** infection and **AIDS** do not seem to contract Legionnaires' disease with any greater frequency than the rest of the population, however, if contracted, the disease is likely to be more severe compared to other cases.

Cases of Legionnaires' disease that occur in conjunction with an outbreak, or epidemic, are more likely to be diagnosed quickly. Early diagnosis aids effective and successful treatment. During epidemic outbreaks, fatalities have ranged from 5% for previously healthy individuals to 24% for individuals with underlying illnesses. Sporadic cases (that is, cases unrelated to a wider outbreak) are harder to detect and treatment may be delayed pending an accurate diagnosis. The overall fatality rate for sporadic cases ranges from 10–19%. The outlook is bleaker in severe cases that require respiratory support or dialysis. In such cases, fatality may reach 67%.

Legionnaires' disease is caused by inhaling *Legionella* bacteria from the environment. Typically, the bacteria are dispersed in aerosols of contaminated water. These aerosols are produced by devices in which warm water can stagnate, such as air-conditioning cooling towers, humidifiers, shower heads, and faucets. There have also been cases linked to whirlpool spa baths and water misters in grocery store produce departments. Aspiration of contaminated water is also a potential source of infection, particularly in hospital-acquired cases of Legionnaires' disease. There is no evidence of person-to-person transmission of Legionnaires' disease.

Once the bacteria are in the lungs, cellular representatives of the body's immune system (alveolar macrophages) congregate to destroy the invaders. The typical macrophage defense is to phagocytose the invader and demolish it in a process analogous to swallowing and digesting it. However, the *Legionella* bacteria survive being phagocytosed. Instead of being destroyed within the macrophage, they grow and replicate, eventually killing the macrophage. When the macrophage dies, many new *Legionella* bacteria are released into the lungs and worsen the infection.

Legionnaires' disease develops 2–10 days after exposure to the bacteria. Early symptoms include lethargy, headaches, fever, chills, muscle aches, and a lack of appetite. Respiratory symptoms such as coughing or congestion are usually absent. As the disease progresses, a dry, hacking cough develops and may become productive after a few days. In about a third of Legionnaires' disease cases, blood is present in the sputum. Half of the people who develop Legionnaires' disease suffer shortness of breath and a third complain of breathing-related chest pain. The fever can become quite high, reaching 104°F (40°C) in many cases, and may be accompanied by a decreased heart rate.

Although the pneumonia affects the lungs, Legionnaires' disease is accompanied by symptoms that affect other areas of the body. About half the victims experience diarrhea and a quarter have nausea and vomiting and abdominal pain. In about 10% of cases, acute renal failure and scanty urine production accompany the disease. Changes in mental status, such as disorientation, confusion, and hallucinations, also occur in about a quarter of cases.

In addition to Legionnaires' disease, *L. pneumophila* legionellosis also includes a milder disease, Pontiac fever. Unlike Legionnaires' disease, Pontiac fever does not involve the lower respiratory tract. The symptoms usually appear within 36 hours of exposure and include fever, headache, muscle aches, and lethargy. Symptoms last only a few days and medical intervention is usually not necessary.

The symptoms of Legionnaires' disease are common to many types of pneumonia and diagnosis of sporadic cases can be difficult. The symptoms and chest x rays that confirm a case of pneumonia are not useful in differentiating between Legionnaires' disease and other pneumonias. If a pneumonia case involves multisystem symptoms, such as diarrhea and vomiting, and an initially dry cough, laboratory tests are done to definitively identify *L. pneumophila* as the cause of the infection.

If Legionnaires' disease is suspected, several tests are available to reveal or indicate the presence of *L. pneumophila* bacteria in the body. Since the immune system creates antibodies against infectious agents, examining the blood for these indicators is a key test. The level of **immunoglobulins**, or **antibody** molecules, in the blood reveals the presence of infection. In microscopic examination of the patient's sputum, a fluorescent stain linked to antibodies against *L. pneumophila* can uncover the presence of the bacteria. Other means of revealing

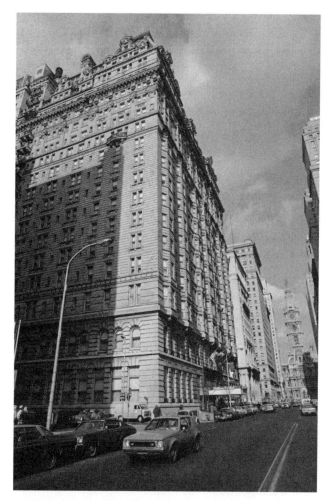

The Bellevue-Stratford Hotel in Philadelphia, where an outbreak at a Legionnaires' convention gave the disease its name.

the bacteria's presence from patient sputum samples include isolation of the organism on **culture** media or detection of the bacteria by **DNA** probe. Another test detects *L. pneumophila* antigens in the urine.

The type of antibiotic prescribed by the doctor depends on several factors including the severity of infection, potential **allergies**, and interaction with previously prescribed drugs. For example, erythromycin interacts with warfarin, a blood thinner. Several drugs, such as penicillins and cephalosporins, are normally ineffective against the infection. Although they may be deadly to the bacteria in laboratory tests, their chemical structure prevents them from being absorbed into the areas of the lung where the bacteria are present. In severe cases with complications, antibiotic therapy may be joined by respiratory support. If renal failure occurs, dialysis is required until renal function is recovered.

Appropriate medical treatment has a major impact on recovery from Legionnaires' disease. Outcome is also linked to the victim's general health and absence of complications. If the patient survives the infection, recovery from Legionnaires' disease is usually complete. Similar to other types of pneumonia, severe cases of Legionnaires' disease may cause scarring in the lung tissue as a result of the infection. Renal failure, if it occurs, is reversible and renal function returns as the patient's health improves. Occasionally, fatigue and weakness may linger for several months after the infection has been successfully treated.

Because the bacteria thrive in warm stagnant water, regularly disinfecting ductwork, pipes, and other areas that may serve as breeding areas is the best method for preventing outbreaks of Legionnaires' disease. Most outbreaks of Legionnaires' disease can be traced to specific points of exposure, such as hospitals, hotels, and other places where people gather. Sporadic cases are harder to determine and there is insufficient evidence to point to exposure in individual homes.

See also Pneumonia, bacterial and viral

LEPROSY

Leprosy, also called Hansen's disease, affects 10 –12 million people worldwide. Caused by an unusual bacterium called *Mycobacterium leprae,* leprosy primarily affects humans. Leprosy is found in tropical areas, such as Africa, South and Southeast Asia, and Central and South America. In the United States, cases of leprosy have been reported in areas of Texas, California, Louisiana, Florida, and Hawaii. Leprosy can take many forms, but the most familiar form is characterized by skin lesions and nerve damage. Although leprosy is curable with various **antibiotics**, it remains a devastating illness because of its potential to cause deformity, especially in the facial features. Fortunately, antibiotic regimens are available to treat and eventually cure leprosy.

Mycobacterium leprae is an unusual bacterium for several reasons. The bacterium divides slowly; in some tests, researchers have noted a dividing time of once every twelve days. This differs from the dividing time of most **bacteria**, which is about once every few hours. *M. leprae* cannot be grown on **culture** media, and is notoriously difficult to culture within living animals. Because of these culturing difficulties, researchers have not been able to investigate these bacteria as closely as they have other, more easily cultured, bacteria. Questions remain unanswered about *M. leprae;* for instance, researchers are still unclear about how the bacteria are transmitted from one person to another, and are not sure about the role an individual's genetic make up plays in the progression of the disease.

Because *M. leprae* almost exclusively infects humans, animal models for studying leprosy are few. Surprisingly, a few species of armadillo can also be infected with *M. leprae.* Recently, however, wild armadillos have been appearing with a naturally occurring form of leprosy. If the disease spreads in the armadillo population, researchers will not be able to use these animals for leprosy studies, since study animals must be completely free of the disease as well as the bacteria that cause it. Mice have also been used to study leprosy, but laboratory conditions, such as temperature, must be carefully controlled in order to sustain the infection in mice.

M. leprae is temperature-sensitive; it favors temperatures slightly below normal human body temperature. Because of this predilection, *M. leprae* infects superficial body tissues such as the skin, bones, and cartilage, and does not usually penetrate to deeper organs and tissues. *M. leprae* is an intracellular pathogen; it crosses host cell membranes and lives within these cells. Once inside the host cell, the bacterium reproduces. The time required by these slow-growing bacteria to reproduce themselves inside host cells can be anywhere from a few weeks to as much as 40 years. Eventually, the bacteria lyse (burst open) the host cell, and new bacteria are released that can infect other host cells.

Researchers assume that the bacteria are transmitted via the respiratory tract. *M. leprae* exists in the nasal secretions and in the material secreted by skin lesions of infected individuals. *M. leprae* has also been found in the breast milk of infected nursing mothers. *M. leprae* may be transmitted by breathing in the bacteria, through breaks in the skin, or perhaps through breast-feeding.

Leprosy exists in several different forms, although the infectious agent for all of these forms is *M. leprae*. Host factors such as genetic make up, individual **immunity**, geography, ethnicity, and socioeconomic circumstances determine which form of leprosy is contracted by a person exposed to *M. leprae*. Interestingly, most people who come in contact with the bacterium, about three-fourths, never develop leprosy, or develop only a small lesion on the trunk or extremity that heals spontaneously. Most people, then, are not susceptible to *M. leprae*, and their immune systems function effectively to neutralize the bacteria. But one-fourth of those exposed to *M. leprae* contract the disease, which may manifest itself in various ways.

Five forms of leprosy are recognized, and a person may progress from one form to another. The least serious form is tuberculoid leprosy. In this form, the skin lesions and nerve damage are minor. Tuberculoid leprosy is evidence that the body's cellular immune response—the part of the **immune system** that seeks out and destroys infected cells—is working at a high level of efficiency. Tuberculoid leprosy is easily cured with antibiotics.

If tuberculoid leprosy is not treated promptly, or if a person has a less vigorous cellular immune response to the *M. leprae* bacteria, the disease may progress to a borderline leprosy, which is characterized by more numerous skins lesions and more serious nerve damage. The most severe form of leprosy is lepromatous leprosy. In this form of leprosy, the skin lesions are numerous and cause the skin to fold, especially the skin on the face. This folding of facial skin leads to the leonine (lion-like) features typical of lepromatous leprosy. Nerve damage is extensive, and people with lepromatous leprosy may lose the feeling in their extremities, such as the fingers and toes. Contrary to popular belief, the fingers and toes of people with this form of leprosy do not spontaneously drop off. Rather, because patients cannot feel pain because of nerve damage, the extremities can become easily injured.

Lepromatous leprosy occurs in people who exhibit an efficient **antibody** response to *M. leprae* but an inefficient cellular immune response. The antibody arm of the immune system is not useful in neutralizing intracellular pathogens such as

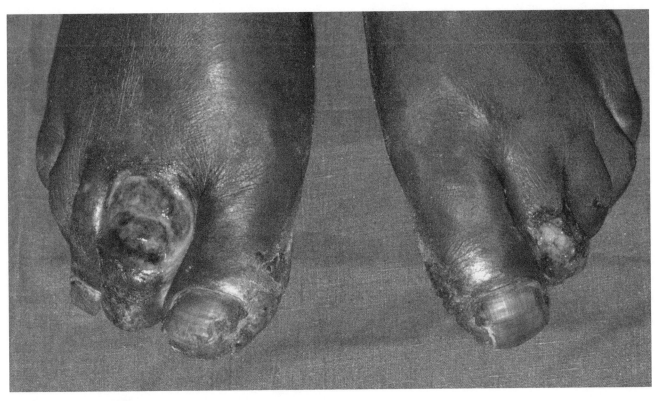

The disfiguring effect of leprosy.

M. leprae; therefore, people who initially react to invasion by M. leprae by making antibodies may be at risk for developing more severe forms of leprosy. Researchers are not sure what determines whether a person will react with a cellular response or an antibody response; current evidence suggests that the cellular immune response may be controlled by a special **gene**. If a person has this gene, he or she will probably develop the less severe tuberculoid leprosy if exposed to *M. leprae.*

Treatments for leprosy have improved considerably over the past 40 years. In fact, some experts are encouraged that the drug regimens being tested in various trials throughout the world (including the United States) may eradicate leprosy completely by the year 2010. Beginning in the 1950s, an antibiotic called dapsone was used to treat leprosy, offering the first hope of a cure for persons with the disease. Dapsone's main disadvantage was that the patient had to take the medication daily throughout his or her lifetime. In addition, the *M. leprae* in some patients underwent genetic **mutations** that rendered it resistant to the antibiotic. In the 1960s, the problem of resistance was tackled with the advent of multidrug therapy. Bacteria are less likely to become resistant to several drugs given in combination. The new multidrug treatment time was also considerably shorter-typically about four years. Currently, researchers offer a new drug combination that includes an antibiotic called oflaxicin. Oflaxicin is a powerful inhibitor of certain bacterial **enzymes** that are involved in **DNA** coiling. Without these enzymes, the *M. leprae* cannot copy the DNA properly and the bacteria die. The treatment time for this current regimen is about four weeks or less, the shortest treatment duration so far.

One risk of treatment, however, is that antigens—the proteins on the surface of *M. leprae* that initiate the host immune response—are released from the dying bacteria. In some people, when the antigens combine with antibodies to *M. leprae* in the bloodstream, a reaction called erythema nodosum leprosum may occur, resulting in new lesions and peripheral nerve damage. In the late 1990s, the drug thalidomide was approved to treat this reaction, with good results. Because thalidomide may cause severe birth defects, women of childbearing age must be carefully monitored while taking the drug.

A promising development in the treatment and management of leprosy is the preliminary success shown by two different vaccines. One **vaccine** tested in Venezuela combined a vaccine originally developed against **tuberculosis**, called Bacille Calmette-Guerin (BCG), and heat-killed *M. leprae* cultured from infected armadillos. The other vaccine uses a relative of *M. leprae* called *M. avium*. The advantage of this vaccine, currently being tested in India, is that *M. avium* is easy to culture on media and is thus cheaper than the Venezuelan vaccine. Both vaccines have performed well in their clinical trials, leading many to hope that a vaccine against leprosy might soon be available.

The **World Health Organization** announced in January, 2002, that during the previous decade, the number of active cases of leprosy worldwide had been reduced by 90%. Control of leprosy still eludes six countries, Brazil, India, Madagascar, Mozambique, Myanmar and Nepal, with approximately 700,

000 ongoing cases identified worldwide in 2002. In conjunction with the World Health Organization, these countries have committed to accelerating control efforts, including early access to current drug therapy. The worldwide reduction and control of leprosy stands as one of the major world health initiatives of modern times.

See also Bacteria and bacterial infection; Mycobacterial infections, atypical

LETHAL DOSE, LD50 · *see* LABORATORY TECHNIQUES IN MICROBIOLOGY

LICHEN PLANUS

Lichen planus is a skin rash characterized by small, flat-topped, itchy purplish raised spots on the wrists, arms, or lower legs. Although the evidence is not conclusive, many researchers assert that Lichen planus is an autoimmune disease.

Lichen planus affects approximately one to two percent of the population. Although there is no apparent correlation to race or geographic region, it is interesting to note that the majority of individuals affected are women, age 30 to 50 years. Lichen planus rashes may produce discoloration of the skin, especially in darker skinned population groups. Lichen planus lesions may develop on the genitals or in the mouth. Within a few years, most of the spots disappear, even without treatment.

Although not definitive, researchers assert Lichen planus exhibits many of the characteristics of an autoimmune disorder. Autoimmune diseases result when the **immune system** attacks the body's own cells, causing tissue destruction. Dermatologists argue that the condition may result from a viral infection that is then aggravated by stress. Lichen planus symptoms are similar to allergic reactions to arsenic, gold, and bismuth. The spots are also similar to the type produced from allergic reactions to certain chemicals used to develop film.

There is a correlation (a statistical relationship) between allergic reactions to certain medications and the appearance of a Lichen planus rash in the mouth. Oral lichen planus usually forms white lines and spots that may appear in clusters. Only a definitive biopsy can fully distinguish the rash from **yeast** infections or canker sores. Dentists find that some patients develop a Lichen planus rash following dental procedures. Other reports indicate that a Lichen planus rash may appear as an allergic-reaction like response to certain foods, candy, or chewing gum.

Because the exact cause of Lichen planus is unknown, there is no specific treatment for the rash. Treatment with various combinations of steroid creams, oral corticosteroids, and oral antihistamines appears effective at relieving discomfort caused by the rash. In more severe cases PUVA photochemotherapy, a procedure where cells are photosensitizing and then exposed to ultraviolet light and **antibiotics**.

Lichen planus may also affect the growth of nails and, if present on the scalp, may contribute to hair loss.

Lichen planus is not an infectious disease. Research also indicates that it is not, as once argued, caused by any specific dietary deficiency.

See also Autoimmunity and autoimmune diseases; Viruses and responses to viral infection; Yeast, infectious

LICHENS

Lichens are an intimate symbiosis, in which two species live together as a type of composite organism. Lichens are an obligate mutualism between a fungus mycobiont and an alga or blue-green bacterium phycobiont.

Each lichen mutualism is highly distinctive, and can be identified on the basis of its size, shape, color, and **biochemistry**. Even though lichens are not true "species" in the conventional meaning of the word, lichenologists have developed systematic and taxonomic treatments of these mutualisms.

The fungal partner in the lichen mutualism gains important benefits through access to photosynthetic products of the alga or blue-green bacterium. The phycobiont profits from the availability of a relatively moist and protected habitat, and greater access to inorganic nutrients.

The most common **fungi** in lichens are usually species of *Ascomycetes,* or a few *Basidiomycetes.* The usual algal partners are either species of green algae **Chlorophyta** or blue-green **bacteria** of the family Cyanophyceae. In general, the fungal partner cannot live without its phycobiont, but the algae is often capable of living freely in moist soil or water. The largest lichens can form a thallus up to 3 ft (1 m) long, although most lichens are smaller than a few inches or centimeters in length. Lichens can be very colorful, ranging from bright reds and oranges, to yellows and greens, and white, gray, and black hues.

Most lichens grow very slowly. Lichens in which the phycobiont is a blue-green bacterium have the ability to fix nitrogen gas into ammonia. Some lichens can commonly reach ages of many centuries, especially species living in highly stressful environments, such as alpine or arctic tundra.

Lichens can grow on diverse types of substrates. Some species grow directly on rocks, some on bare soil, and others on the bark of tree trunks and branches. Lichens often grow under exposed conditions that are frequently subjected to periods of drought, and sometimes to extremes of hot and cold. Lichen species vary greatly in their tolerance of severe environmental conditions. Lichens generally respond to environmental extremes by becoming dormant, and then quickly becoming metabolically active again when they experience more benign conditions.

Lichens are customarily divided into three growth forms, although this taxonomy is one of convenience, and is not ultimately founded on systematic relationships. Crustose lichens form a thallus that is closely appressed to the surface upon which they are growing. Foliose lichens are only joined to their substrate by a portion of their thallus, and they are somewhat leaf-like in appearance. Fruticose lichens rise above their substrate, and are much branched and bushy in appearance.

Most lichens regenerate asexually as lichen symbioses, and not by separate reproduction of their mycobiont and phycobiont. Reproduction is most commonly accomplished by small, specialized fragments of thallus known as soredia, consisting of fungal tissue enclosing a small number of algal cells. The soredia generally originate within the parent thallus, then grow out through the surface of the thallus, and detach as small bits of tissue that are dispersed by the wind or rain. If the dispersing soredium is fortunate enough to lodge in a favorable microenvironment, it develops into a new thallus, genetically identical to the parent.

Because they are capable of colonizing bare rocks and other mineral substrates, lichens are important in soil formation during some ecological successions. For example, lichens are among the first organisms to colonize sites as they are released from glacial ice. In such situations, lichens can be important in the initial stages of nitrogen accumulation and soil development during post-glacial primary succession.

Lichens are important forage for some species of animals. The best known example of this relationship involves the northern species of deer known as caribou or reindeer (*Rangifer tarandus*) and the so-called reindeer lichens (*Cladina spp.*) that are one of their most important foods, especially during winter.

Some species of lichens are very sensitive to air pollutants. Consequently, urban environments are often highly impoverished in lichen species. Some ecologists have developed schemes by which the intensity of air pollution can be reliably assayed or monitored using the biological responses of lichens in their communities. Monitoring of air quality using lichens can be based on the health and productivity of these organisms in places variously stressed by toxic pollution. Alternatively, the chemical composition of lichens may be assayed, because their tissues can effectively take up and retain sulfur and metals from the atmosphere.

Some lichens are useful as a source of natural dyes. Pigments of some of the more colorful lichens, especially the orange, red, and brown ones, can be extracted by boiling and used to dye wool and other fibers. Other chemicals extracted from lichens include litmus, which was a commonly used acid-base indicator prior to the invention of the **pH** meter.

Some of the reindeer lichens, especially *Cladina alpestris,* are shaped like miniature shrubs and trees. Consequently, these plants are sometimes collected, dried, and dyed, and are used in "landscaping" the layouts for miniature railroads and architectural models.

In addition, lichens add significantly to the aesthetics of the ecosystems in which they occur. The lovely orange and yellow colors of *Caloplaca* and *Xanthoria* lichens add much to the ambience of rocky seashores and tundras. The intricate webs of filamentous *Usnea* lichens hanging in profusion from tree branches give a mysterious aspect to humid forests. These and other, less charismatic lichens are integral components of their natural ecosystems. These lichens are intrinsically important for this reason, as well as for the relatively minor benefits that they provide to humans.

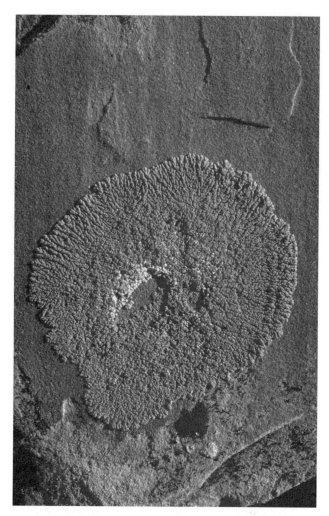

A lichen growing on a rock.

LIFE, ORIGIN OF

The origin of life has been a subject of speculation in all known cultures and indeed, all have some sort of creation idea that rationalizes how life arose. In the modern era, this question has been considered in terms of a scientific framework, meaning that it is approached in a manner subject to experimental verification as far as that is possible. Radioactive dating suggests that Earth formed at least 4.6 billion years ago. Yet, the earliest known fossils of **microorganisms**, similar to modern **bacteria**, are present in rocks that are 3.5–3.8 billion years old. The earlier prebiotic era (i.e., before life began) left no direct record, and so it cannot be determined exactly how life arose. It is possible, however, to at least demonstrate the kinds of abiotic reactions that may have led to the formation of living systems through laboratory experimentation. It is generally accepted that the development of life occupied three stages: First, chemical **evolution**, in which simple geologically occurring molecules reacted to form complex organic polymers. Second, collections of these polymers self organized to form replicating entities. At some

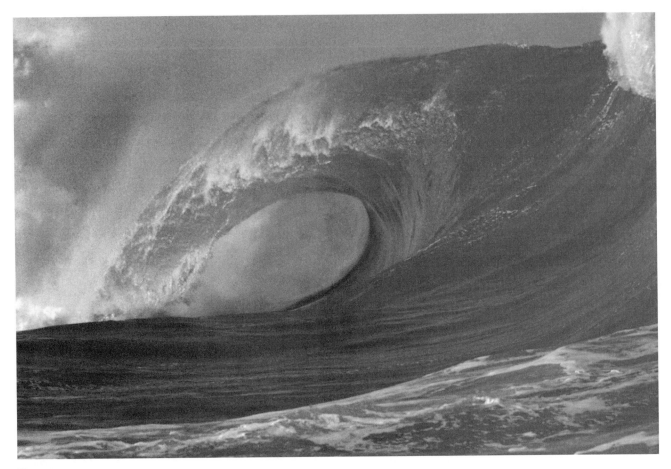

The sea.

point in this process, the transition from a lifeless collection of reacting molecules to a living system probably occurred. The third process following organization into simple living systems was biological evolution, which ultimately produced the complex web of modern life.

The underlying biochemical and genetic unity of organisms suggests that life arose only once, or if it arose more than once, the other life forms must have become rapidly extinct. All organisms are made of chemicals rich in the same kinds of carbon-containing, organic compounds. The predominance of carbon in living matter is a result of its tremendous chemical versatility compared with all the other elements. Carbon has the unique ability to form a very large number of compounds as a result of its capacity to make as many as four highly stable covalent bonds (including single, double, triple bonds) combined with its ability to form covalently linked C—C chains of unlimited length. The same 20 carbon and nitrogen containing compounds called amino acids combine to make up the enormous diversity of proteins occurring in living things. Moreover, all organisms have their genetic blueprint encoded in nucleic acids, either **DNA** or **RNA**. Nucleic acids contain the information needed to synthesize specific proteins from their amino acid components. **Enzymes**, catalytic proteins, which increase the speed of specific chemical reactions,

regulate the activity of nucleic acids and other biochemical functions essential to life, while other proteins provide the structural framework of cells. These two types of molecules, nucleic acids and proteins, are essential enough to all organisms that they, or closely related compounds, must also have been present in the first life forms.

Scientists suspect that the primordial Earth's atmosphere was very different from what it is today. The modern atmosphere with its 79% nitrogen, 20% oxygen, and trace quantities of other gases is an oxidizing atmosphere. The primordial atmosphere is generally believed not to have contained significant quantities of oxygen, having instead rather small amounts of gases such as carbon monoxide, methane, ammonia and sulphate in addition to the water, nitrogen and carbon dioxide, which it still contains today. With these combinations of gases, the atmosphere at that time would have been a reducing atmosphere providing the hydrogen atoms for the synthesis of compounds needed to create life. In the 1920s, the Soviet scientist Aleksander Oparin (1894–1980) and the British scientist J.B.S. Haldane (1892–1964) independently suggested that ultraviolet (UV) light, which today is largely absorbed by the ozone layer in the higher atmosphere, or violent lightning discharges, caused molecules of the primordial reducing atmosphere to react and form simple organic compounds (e.g., amino acids, nucleic acids and sugars). The possibility of such a process was demonstrated in 1953 by Stanley Miller and **Harold Urey**, who simulated the effects of lightning storms in a primordial atmosphere by subjecting a refluxing mixture of water, methane, ammonia and hydrogen to an electric discharge for about a week. The resulting solution contained significant amounts of water-soluble organic compounds including amino acids.

The American scientist, Norman H. Horowitz proposed several criteria for living systems, saying that they all must exhibit replication, catalysis and mutability. One of the chief features of living organisms is their ability to replicate. The primordial self-replicating systems are widely believed to have been nucleic acids, like DNA and RNA, because they could direct the synthesis of molecules complementary to themselves. One hypothesis for the evolution of self-replicating systems is that they initially consisted entirely of RNA. This idea is based on the observation that certain species of ribosomal RNA exhibit enzyme-like catalytic properties, and that all nucleic acids are prone to mutation. Thus, RNA can demonstrate the three Horowitz criteria and the primordial world may well have been an "RNA world". A cooperative relationship between RNA and protein could have arisen when these self-replicating protoribosomes evolved the ability to influence the synthesis of proteins that increased the efficiency and accuracy of RNA synthesis. All these ideas suggest that RNA was the primary substance of life and the later participation of DNA and proteins were later refinements that increased the survival potential of an already self-replicating living system. Such a primordial pond where all these reactions were evolving eventually generated compartmentalization amongst its components. How such cell boundaries formed is not known, though one plausible theory holds that membranes first arose as empty vesicles whose exteriors served as attachment sites for entities such as enzymes and **chromosomes** in ways that facilitated their function.

See also DNA (Deoxyribonucleic acid); Evolution and evolutionary mechanisms; Evolutionary origin of bacteria and viruses; Miller-Urey experiment; Ribonucleic acid (RNA)

LIGHT MICROSCOPY · *see* MICROSCOPE AND MICROSCOPY

LIPOPOLYSACCHARIDE AND ITS CONSTITUENTS

Lipopolysaccharide (LPS) is a molecule that is a constituent of the outer membrane of Gram-negative **bacteria**. The molecule can also be referred to as endotoxin. LPS can help protect the bacterium from host defenses and can contribute to illness in the host.

The LPS comprises much of the portion of the outer membrane that is oriented towards the outside of the bacterium. There are fewer phospholipid molecules in this outer

"leaflet" of the membrane than there are on the inner side of the membrane. Thus, because of the presence of lipopolysaccharide, the construction of the outer membrane is asymmetric. In contrast, the inner membrane of Gram-negative bacteria and the single membrane of Gram-positive bacteria are more symmetric, with both leaflets of the membrane comprised of much the same molecules.

A complete LPS consists of a lipid portion and a chain of sugar. The lipid region is anchored into the inner portion of the membrane by a molecule called lipid A. A core polysaccharide is also considered part of the lipid region. This core contains a compound known as 2-keto-3-deoxyoctonic acid, or KDO. The lipid A and KDO portions of LPS are common to all bacterial LPS.

The other region of LPS is the sugar chain. This portion is also known as the O-antigen. The O-antigen gets its name from the fact that it is exposed to the external environment and will be the target of **antibody formation** by the host. The hydrophilic ("water-loving") sugar side chain extends outward from the surface of the cell into the watery environment that typically surrounds many Gram-negative bacteria. There are many chemical arrangements of the sugar chain.

The manufacture of LPS is a multi-step process involving many **enzymes**. The complete LPS molecule is incorporated into the outer membrane. The biosynthetic pathway of LPS was deduced by the isolation of **mutants** defective in LPS assembly.

LPS can be detected using microscopic techniques following the binding of LPS specific **antibody**. Additionally, a biochemical test can be done. The test utilizes a compound that is obtained from the horseshoe crab.

Not all bacteria have a complete sugar chain. Depending on the bacterial species a portion of the sugar chain can be present, or sugar chain may be entirely absent. The various LPS chemistries have an affect on the appearance of the bacteria when they are grown as colonies on solid growth media. Those bacteria with the complete side chain can appear smooth and even wet, whereas those with no side chain often appear crinkly and dry. For this reason, bacteria having the complete LPS are known as smooth strains and those bacteria with no sugar side chain are designated as rough strains. Those species of bacteria that are in between, having a portion of the sugar side chain, are called semi-rough strains.

The composition of the LPS also affects the overall chemistry of the bacterial surface. Because the sugar chains protruding from the surface are hydrophilic, the bacterium tends to prefer watery environments. In contrast the lack of the side chains exposes the **hydrophobic** ("water hating") lipid portion of the LPS. The surface of such bacteria tends to be more hydrophobic. In solution, the rough bacteria tend to clump together in an effort to avoid the water. Antibacterial compounds that are hydrophobic are more likely to penetrate into rough strains than into smooth strains. In the intestinal tract of warm-blooded animals, where many Gram-negative bacteria live, the possession of a complete LPS is advantageous for the absorption of hydrophilic nutrients by the bacteria.

The LPS structure has a profound influence on the potential of infectious Gram-negative bacteria to establish an infection in humans and other animals. The sugar chains of smooth LPS can overlay the surface proteins of the outer membrane, masking the proteins from immune detection. Also, a bacterium can vary the chemistry of the O-antigen, so as to make the targeting of antibodies to the bacterial surface even more difficult. In contrast, the immune response to a rough strain, where the surface proteins are not camouflaged, is greater and more consistent.

Lipopolysaccharide is medically important to humans. When free from the bacterium, LPS is toxic. The portion of the LPS that is responsible for the toxicity is the core and lipid A portion (the endotoxin). Endotoxin can produce a fever, decrease in the number of white blood cells, and damage to blood vessels resulting in reduced blood pressure. At high enough endotoxin concentrations, shock can set in and death can occur.

See also Bacterial membranes and cell wall; Enterotoxin and exotoxin; Immunization

LIQUID MEDIA • *see* GROWTH AND GROWTH MEDIA

LISTER, JOSEPH (1827-1912)
English surgeon

Joseph Lister contributed to a fundamental revolution in surgery with the introduction of his antiseptic method. At the time Lister was practicing medicine, the mortality rate for certain injuries and surgeries was extremely high due to infection. The mortality rate dropped drastically with the use of an antiseptic method, and when used in conjunction with the anesthetics that were available at the time, surgeons dared to perform more complicated surgical procedures.

Lister was born to a well-known Quaker family at Upton, England. Lister studied medicine at University College, and received his medical degree in 1852. As a student, Lister had the opportunity to be a spectator at the first surgery performed with general anesthesia, performed by Robert Liston (1794–1847). He also studied histology under William Sharpey during which time, Lister wrote an important paper on **inflammation** where he discussed the susceptibility to disease of inflamed tissue. Lister was also interested in microscopic anatomy and physiology, perhaps because his father, Joseph Jackson Lister, was a microscopist. At one point, Lister wanted to become a surgeon and left England to study at Edinburgh University with James Syme (1799–1870), who was well known for his success with performing amputations and joint excisions. Syme, the first surgeon to adopt antisepsis and anesthesia, eventually became Lister's father-in-law.

As a surgeon, Lister was concerned with the high mortality rate of post-amputation patients and the high rate of gangrene after surgery. Applying the knowledge that **bacteria** caused disease, and drawing from Louis Pasteur's work that proved the existence of airborne **microorganisms**, Lister concluded that airborne bacteria could cause infection in surgical

wounds. Lister read about the affect of carbolic acid used on sewage bacteria in outhouses, cesspools, and stables in the nearby town of Carlisle, and developed an antiseptic system whereby he would spray carbolic acid in the operating room, and use it to sterilize the surgical instruments and his hands. In addition, he applied the acid in and around the wound, and directly on the dressings. Lister first used this method in 1865 while treating a compound fracture of a leg, an injury that often claimed about 60% of patients, and where amputation of a limb was usually the only treatment. The procedure was successful. Lister published his antiseptic method in *The Lancet,* in 1867. There was one problem: carbolic acid, especially the spray, was harmful to those who came in contact with it. However, Lister found milder **antiseptics** and later heat-sterilized the surgical instruments. At first, the medical community did not support Lister's theory, but eventually his antiseptic method gained recognition and was adopted as standard procedure for treating wounds and during surgery. Medics used Lister's antiseptic method, which proved to be effective, during the Franco-Prussian War (1870–1871). In 1877, Lister became Professor of Surgery at King's College, London.

Lister received many honors and awards. A dedicated surgeon, he treated both inflicted and surgical wounds; he experimented with various antiseptics, developed absorbable sutures, and introduced a method of draining wounds. He was the first British surgeon to be elevated to the peerage (became a member of the House of Lords), and upon his death in 1912, his remains were interred in Westminster Abbey. When he died, it was said that Lister had saved more lives than all the wars in history had claimed.

See also Bacteria and bacterial infection; History of microbiology; History of public health; Infection and resistance; Infection control

LOEFFLER, FRIEDRICH AUGUST JOHANNES (1852-1915)
German physician

Friedrich August Loeffler was a German physician who turned his career path to focus on microbiology after becoming an assistant to **Robert Koch**. Loeffler is accredited with the discovery of several **microorganisms** including *Loefflerella mallei,* the etiological agent of glanders, *Corynebacterium diphtheriae,* the infectious organism of **diphtheria**; and *Erysipelothrix rhusiopathiae,* the infectious agent that causes cholera in swine. In addition to his discoveries of **bacteria**, Loeffler determined that **foot-and-mouth disease** was due to an infectious microorganism smaller than any bacteria (a virus).

Friedrich Loeffler began his studies in medicine at the University of Würzburg but then transferred to the Army Medical School shortly before the Franco-Prussian War. In 1872, Loeffler received his medical degree and then worked as an assistant physician in Berlin at the Charté Hospital. Beginning in 1876, he worked as a **public health** officer and military surgeon in Potsdam and Hannover. This lasted until

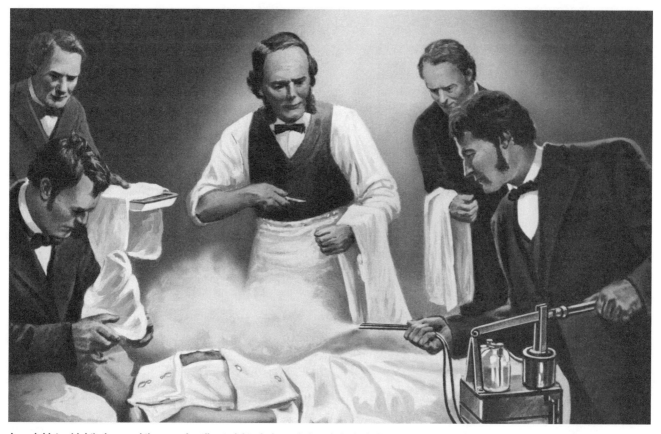

Joseph Lister (right) pioneered the use of antibacterial techniques in hospitals, including the use of disinfectant spray during operations.

1879, when he moved to Berlin and continued his work at the Kaiserliches Gesundheitsamt.

Friedrich Loeffler's transfer brought him under the supervision of Robert Koch. Loeffler and Georg Graffky began assisting Koch on his research of bacteria. Loeffler first began his bacteriological studies researching effective methods of **disinfection**. During his studies, Loeffler discovered *Loefflerella mallei,* bacteria that causes glanders, a disease seen mainly in horses. To determine the exact bacteria that causes glanders, Loeffler applied what has come to be known as **Koch's postulates**. Initially, Loeffler isolated the infectious agent from the horse and grew it in a pure **culture** of blood serum. Next, Loeffler injected the bacteria into healthy horses, which then showed symptoms of the disease. Finally, Loeffler once again isolated the bacteria from the once healthy horses. In addition to discovering *Loefflerella mallei,* Loeffler discovered the infectious agent that causes cholera in swine.

In 1884, after a long struggle to decipher the etiological agent that causes diphtheria, Loeffler isolated *Corynebacterium diphtheriae* in pure culture from the throat of humans. Problems pinpointing the exact microorganism that causes diphtheria stemmed from the fact that many different microorganisms inhabited the throats of diphtheria patients. Loeffler undertook the task of isolating pure cultures of bacteria to determine the exact etiological agent of diphtheria. Loeffler found that certain throat infections were due to streptococcal infections, which are now known to cause scarlet fever. He reasoned that the *Streptococcus* bacteria were not responsible for causing diphtheria because when injected into healthy animals, the bacteria did not produce symptoms characteristic of the disease. Additionally, the *Streptococcus* was not always abundant in diphtheria patients. The *Streptococcus* appeared to be secondary to rod shaped bacteria. When these rod shaped bacteria, called bacillus, were isolated in pure culture and injected into healthy animals, the animals exhibited the characteristic signs of human diphtheria, including the pseudomembrane in the throat of the patients that suffocate to death. Additionally, Loeffler determined that toxins produced by the infectious agent were the cause of destruction to internal organs. He reasoned that the toxins released entered the blood stream and traveled to other organs thereby poisoning them. Emile Roux and Yersin proved this theory of toxins to be correct. Loeffler made a surprising discovery when he was able to isolate the diphtheria bacillus from healthy individuals. He then determined that not all people who carry infectious microorganisms contract the disease.

Also in 1884, Loeffler began his new career as hygienic director with his first directorship position being at the First Garrison Hospital. There he was able to continue his bacteriological research in conjunction with lecturing on sanitation. Two years later, he became part of the faculty at the University of Berlin. By 1888, he had transferred to the University of Greifswald where he spent the next 25 years.

At the University of Greifswald, Loeffler studied *Salmonella typhi-murium,* the bacteriological agent that causes mouse typhoid but does not infect other animals. This research was intended to control the exuberant mouse population that was threatening to destroy the crops of Greece. Loeffler effectively killed the mice by contaminating their food sources with the bacteria.

In 1898, Friedrich Loeffler, in conjunction with Paul Frosch, determined a filterable agent proving smaller than any bacteria previously discovered caused foot-and-mouth disease. This was the first hint that **viruses** existed. At that time, Loeffler was working at the University of Greifswald as head of the department of **hygiene**. Loeffler moved his laboratory to the island of the Insel Riems in order to safely continue his research on the disease. In 1913, Loeffler's research took a back seat to his new position as director of the Robert Koch Institute in Berlin. Once World War I began, all research on the Insel Riems ceased. Loeffler worked for the army to implement proper hygiene regimens until his death in 1915.

See also Coryneform bacteria; Streptococci and streptococcal infections

LUMINESCENT BACTERIA

Luminescence is the emission of light by an object. Living organisms including certain **bacteria** are capable of luminescence (**bioluminescence**). Bacteria are the most abundant luminescent organism in nature.

Bacterial luminescence has been studied most extensively in several marine bacteria (e.g., *Vibrio harveyi, Vibrio fischeri, Photobacterium phosphoreum, Photobacterium leiognathi*), and in *Xenorhabdus luminescens,* a bacteria that lives on land. The precise molecular mechanisms of luminescence differ between these bacteria. But, the general scheme of the process is similar.

In luminescent bacteria (and other luminescent organisms as well) this general scheme involves an enzyme that is dubbed luciferase. A suite of genes dubbed lux genes code for the enzyme and other components of the luminescent system. The different bacteria are dissimilar in the sequence of their lux genes and in the enzyme reactions that produce luminescence. However, the general pattern of the reaction is the same.

A similarity between the luminescent bacteria concerns the conditions that prompt the luminescence. A key factor is the number of bacteria that are present. This is also known as the cell density (i.e., the number of bacteria per given volume of solution or given weight of sample). A low cell density (e.g., less than 100 living bacteria per milliliter) does not induce luminescence, whereas luminescence is induced at a high cell density (e.g., 10^{10} to 10^{11} living bacteria per milliliter).

The effect of cell density is particularly evident in those luminescent bacteria that live in the ocean. When living free in the ocean water, *Vibrio fischeri* is not luminescent. However, when living in a confined space such as the inside of a fish or squid, *Vibrio fischeri* is luminescent. Bacterial luminescence may have evolved as a means of enhancing the survival of the bacteria species. For example, the luminescence of *Vibrio fischeri* in a squid enables the squid to camouflage itself from undersea predators in the moonlit ocean. In return for this protection, the squid provides the bacteria with a hospitable environment.

The influence of cell density on bacterial luminescence is due to the nature of the luminescent process. The bacteria produce a chemical called homoserine lactone. At low cell densities, the chemical exits a bacterium and drifts away in the fluid that surround the cell. But at high cell densities when the bacteria are tightly packed together, the homoserine lactone stays in the immediate vicinity of the bacteria. Then, the chemical is able to stimulate the activity of the lux genes that are responsible for the luminescence. This occurs when the homoserine lactone binds to a protein in the bacterial **cytoplasm** called LuxR. The LuxR-homoserine lactone complex then binds to a region of the bacterial **DNA** that is the master control for the activity of the lux genes.

Bacterial luminescence is due to the action of the enzyme called luciferase. Luciferase catalyses the removal of an electron from two compounds. Excess energy is liberated in this process. The energy is dissipated as a luminescent blue-green light. Luminescent bacteria contain a number of genes that are found linked to each other in the bacterial genome, and which are controlled by a common regulatory region of the DNA. This arrangement of genes is called an **operon**.

The lux genes are involved in the production of luciferase, in the production and activity of the LuxR protein that detects the homoserine lactone, and in the chemicals reactions that produce the compounds on which the luciferase acts.

Bacteria utilize homoserine lactone in other cell-to-cell communications that are cell-density dependent. One example is the formation of the adherent, exopolysaccharide-enmeshed populations, known as biofilms, by the bacterium *Pseudomonas aeruginosa.* Another example is the bacterium *Agrobacterium* that produces diseases in some plants. The phenomenon has been termed **quorum sensing**.

The lux **gene** system responsible for bacterial luminescence has become an important research tool and commercial product. The incorporation of the luminescent genes into other bacteria allows the development of bacterial populations to be traced visually. Because luminescence can occur over and over again and because a bacterium's cycle of luminescence is very short (i.e., a cell is essentially blinking on and off), luminescence allows a near instantaneous (i.e., "real time") monitoring of bacterial behavior. The use of lux genes is being extended to eukaryotic cells. This development has created the potential for the use of luminescence to study eukaryotic cell density related conditions such as cancer.

See also Bacterial adaptation; Bioluminescence; Economic uses and benefits of microorganisms

LYME DISEASE

Lyme disease is an infection transmitted by the bite of ticks carrying the spiral-shaped bacterium *Borrelia burgdorferi*. The disease was named for Lyme, Connecticut, the town where it was first diagnosed in 1975, after a puzzling outbreak of arthritis. The organism was named for its discoverer, Willy Burgdorfer. The effects of this disease can be long-term and disabling unless it is recognized and treated properly with **antibiotics**.

Lyme disease is a vector-borne disease, which means it is delivered from one host to another. In this case, a tick bearing the *B. burgdorferi* organism literally inserts it into a host's bloodstream when it bites the host to feed on its blood. It is important to note that neither *B. burgdorferi* nor Lyme disease can be transmitted from one person to another.

In the United States, Lyme disease accounts for more than 90% of all reported vector-borne illnesses. It is a significant **public health** problem and continues to be diagnosed in increasing numbers. More than 99,000 cases were reported between 1982 and 1996. When the numbers for 1996 Lyme disease cases reported were tallied, there were 16,455 new cases, a record high following a drop in reported cases from 1994 (13,043 cases) to 1995 (11,700 cases). Controversy clouds the true incidence of Lyme disease because no test is definitively diagnostic for the disease, and the broad spectrum of Lyme disease's symptoms mimic those of so many other diseases. Originally, public health specialists thought Lyme disease was limited geographically in the United States to the East Coast. Now it is known that it occurs in most states, with the highest number of cases in the eastern third of the country.

The risk for acquiring Lyme disease varies, depending on what stage in its life cycle a tick has reached. A tick passes through three stages of development—larva, nymph, and adult—each of which is dependent on a live host for food. In the United States, *B. burgdorferi* is borne by ticks of several species in the genus *Ixodes,* which usually feed on the white-footed mouse and deer (and are often called deer ticks). In the summer, the larval ticks hatch from eggs laid in the ground and feed by attaching themselves to small animals and birds. At this stage, they are not a problem for humans. It is the next stage, the nymph, that causes most cases of Lyme disease. Nymphs are very active from spring through early summer, at the height of outdoor activity for most people. Because they are still quite small (less than 2 mm), they are difficult to spot, giving them ample opportunity to transmit *B. burgdorferi* while feeding. Although far more adult ticks than nymphs carry *B. burgdorferi*, the adult ticks are much larger, more easily noticed, and more likely to be removed before the 24 hours or more of continuous feeding needed to transmit *B. burgdorferi*.

Lyme disease is a collection of effects caused by *B. burgdorferi*. Once the organism gains entry to the body through a tick bite, it can move through the bloodstream quickly. Only 12 hours after entering the bloodstream, *B. burgdorferi* can be found in cerebrospinal fluid (which means it can affect the nervous system). Treating Lyme disease early and thoroughly is important because *B. burgdorferi* can hide for long periods within the body in a clinically latent state.

That ability explains why symptoms can recur in cycles and can flare up after months or years, even over decades. It is important to note, however, that not everyone exposed to *B. burgdorferi* develops the disease.

Lyme disease is usually described in terms of length of infection (time since the person was bitten by a tick infected with *B. burgdorferi*) and whether *B. burgdorferi* is localized or disseminated (spread through the body by fluids and cells carrying *B. burgdorferi*). Furthermore, when and how symptoms of Lyme disease appear can vary widely from patient to patient. People who experience recurrent bouts of symptoms over time are said to have chronic Lyme disease.

The most recognizable indicator of Lyme disease is a rash around the site of the tick bite. Often, the tick exposure has not been recognized. The eruption might be warm or itch. The rash, erythema migrans (EM), generally develops within 3–30 days and usually begins as a round, red patch that expands. Clearing may take place from the center out, leaving a bull's-eye effect; in some cases, the center gets redder instead of clearing. The rash may look like a bruise on people with dark skin. Of those who develop Lyme disease, about 50% notice the rash; about 50% notice flu-like symptoms, including fatigue, headache, chills and fever, muscle and joint pain, and lymph node swelling. However, a rash at the site can also be an allergic reaction to the tick saliva rather than an indicator of Lyme disease, particularly if the rash appears in less than three days and disappears only days later.

Weeks, months, or even years after an untreated tick bite, symptoms can appear in several forms, including fatigue, neurological problems, such as pain (unexplained and not triggered by an injury), Bell's palsy (facial paralysis, usually one-sided but may be on both sides), mimicking of the **inflammation** of brain membranes known as **meningitis** (fever, severe headache, stiff neck), and arthritis (short episodes of pain and swelling in joints). Less common effects of Lyme disease are heart abnormalities (such as irregular rhythm or cardiac block) and eye abnormalities (such as swelling of the cornea, tissue, or eye muscles and nerves).

A clear diagnosis of Lyme disease can be difficult, and relies on information the patient provides and the doctor's clinical judgment, particularly through elimination of other possible causes of the symptoms. Lyme disease may mimic other conditions, including chronic fatigue syndrome (CFS), multiple sclerosis (MS), and other diseases with many symptoms involving multiple body systems. Differential diagnosis (distinguishing Lyme disease from other diseases) is based on clinical evaluation with laboratory tests used for clarification, when necessary. A two-test approach is common to confirm the results. Because of the potential for misleading results (false-positive and false-negative), laboratory tests alone cannot establish the diagnosis.

Physicians generally know which disease-causing organisms are common in their geographic area. The most helpful piece of information is whether a tick bite or rash was noticed and whether it happened locally or while traveling. Doctors may not consider Lyme disease if it is rare locally, but will take it into account if a patient mentions vacationing in an area where the disease is commonly found.

The treatment for Lyme disease is antibiotic therapy. If a patient has strong indications of Lyme disease (symptoms and medical history), the doctor will probably begin treatment on the presumption of this disease. The American College of Physicians recommends treatment for a patient with a rash resembling EM or who has arthritis, a history of an EM-type rash, and a previous tick bite.

The physician may have to adjust the treatment regimen or change medications based on the patient's response. Treatment can be difficult because *B. burgdorferi* comes in several strains (some may react to different antibiotics than others) and may even have the ability to switch forms during the course of infection. Also, *B. burgdorferi* can shut itself up in cell niches, allowing it to elude antibiotic actions. Finally, antibiotics can kill *B. burgdorferi* only while it is active rather than dormant.

If aggressive antibiotic therapy is given early, and the patient cooperates fully and sticks to the medication schedule, recovery should be complete. Only a small percentage of Lyme disease patients fail to respond or relapse (have recurring episodes). Most long-term effects of the disease result when diagnosis and treatment is delayed or missed. Co-infection with other infectious organisms spread by ticks in the same areas as *B. burgdorferi* (babesiosis and ehrlichiosis, for instance) may be responsible for treatment failures or more severe symptoms. Lyme disease has been responsible for deaths, but that is rare.

An genetically engineered **vaccine** for Lyme disease was made available in the United States in 1999. **Immunity** requires three injections, the first two given a month apart; a third injection given a year later. Clinical trials conducted in 1997 from a large study of 10,000 adults in many locations showed strong promise of the vaccine's safety and efficacy. The **Centers for Disease Control** recommends the vaccine for those who live and work in Lyme disease endemic areas, and who have repeated and prolonged exposure to tick-infested areas (e.g., park rangers, landscape workers). The Lyme disease vaccine will not prevent other diseases spread by ticks, however, so protective measures against tick bites should still be observed. The vaccine is not recommended for travelers who will have little exposure when visiting areas where Lyme disease has occurred.

Precautions to avoid contact with ticks include moving leaves and brush away from living quarters. Most important are personal protection techniques when outdoors, such as using **repellents** containing DEET, wearing light-colored clothing to maximize ability to see ticks, tucking pant legs into socks or boot top, and checking children frequently for ticks.

LYMPHOCYTES · *see* T CELLS OR T LYMPHOCYTES

LYSOGENY

Lysogeny refers to a process whereby a virus that specifically infects a bacterium, a **bacteriophage** (which means "devourer of bacteria"), achieves the manufacture of copies of its deoxyribonucleic acid (**DNA**) genetic material by integrating the viral DNA into the DNA of the host **bacteria**. The inserted viral DNA is then replicated along with the host DNA.

The nature of lysogeny remained unresolved for many years following the discovery of the bacteriophage by Felix d'Hérelle in 1915. The sudden appearance of virus in cultures of bacteria was at first thought to be the result of viral **contamination**. The acceptance of lysogeny as a real phenomenon came almost 40 years later.

In lysogeny no new virus particles are made. Instead, the virus essentially remains dormant, while ensuring that its genetic material continues to be made. A stress to the bacterium, such as exposure of the bacterium to ultraviolet light, triggers the viral DNA to separate from the bacterial DNA. Then, new virus particles will form in what is known as the lytic cycle. The two processes of lysogeny and lysis are under a system of control first explained by the French biologist André Lwoff in the early 1950s.

Lysogeny is of benefit to the virus, allowing the genetic material to persist in the absence of a virus manufacture. Lysogeny can also be beneficial to the host bacterium. The primary benefit to bacteria occurs when the integrated viral DNA contains a **gene** that encodes a toxin. Possession of the toxin can be advantageous to those bacteria that establish an infection as part of their strategy of replication. For example, toxins encoded by bacteriophage genes are the main cause of the symptoms associated with the bacteria diseases of **tetanus**, **diphtheria**, and cholera.

The process of lysogeny has been studied most intensively in a bacteriophage that is designated as lambda. In the lambda bacteriophage, the establishment of lysogeny depends on the presence of three viral proteins. These are designated cI ("c-one"), cII, and cIII. The cI protein is manufactured first, using host molecules that interpret the information for the protein contained in the viral DNA, following the entry of the viral DNA into the host bacterium. At this point the viral DNA is not integrated into the host genome, but exists as an independent circle. CI is a so-called repressor protein that operates to occupy sequences on the viral genome that would otherwise be used to make the various viral proteins that are needed to assemble the new virus particles. By occupying these sites, cI prevents viral proteins from being produced.

At about the same time, the viral DNA becomes integrated into the host DNA and the cII and cIII proteins are manufactured. These latter proteins assist cI in the task of blocking synthesis of viral components. Accordingly, cI, cII, and cIII function to maintain the lysogenic state. The cII protein functions to make the manufacture of cI by the host's **transcription** machinery more efficient. The cIII protein helps protect the cII protein from being degraded by host **enzymes**.

Once lysogeny is established, the continued manufacture of the cI protein will maintain the integrated state of the viral DNA.

The cI protein maintains its own transcription. The binding of cI to a certain stretch of DNA promotes the recognition and use of the gene for cI to manufacture the cI protein. This is known as positive control. As well, the protein exerts a negative control of another protein (termed "cro"). In negative control, the binding of cI to a region of the DNA prevents the gene from cro from being recognized and used to manufacture the cro protein.

The "decision" to maintain lysogeny or to begin the cycle whereby new virus particles are made and the bacterium explosively releases the new particles is essentially a competition between the cI and cro proteins. This competition centers on the binding of the proteins to a stretch of DNA called the O_R operator. This stretch of DNA has three sites that the proteins can occupy. Depending on which sites are occupied by which protein, the manufacture of either the cI or the cro proteins is promoted. If more cI is made, lysogeny continues. If cro is made, the process of viral assembly (i.e., the lytic cycle) begins. The lytic cycle can be triggered by events that damage the host bacterium, including exposure to environmental stressors (e.g., ultraviolet radiation exposure).

See also Bacteriophage and bacteriophage typing; Operon; Viral genetics; Virus replication

LYSOSOME

Lysosomes are small membranous bags of digestive **enzymes** found in the **cytoplasm** of all eukaryotic cells (those with true nuclei). As the principle site of intracellular digestion, they contain a variety of enzymes capable of degrading proteins, nucleic acids, sugars, lipids, and most other ordinary cellular components. These enzymes hydrolyze (break down) their target compounds best under acidic conditions. Although lysosomes vary considerably in size even within a single cell, the normal range is usually slightly smaller than the average mitochondrion.

The membrane enclosing lysosomes appears to be similar to that of other cellular organelles, but it has several unique properties. First, hydrogen pumps in the membrane acidify the lysosomal interior to a **pH** of five, an optimal level for the activity of its internal enzymes. The membrane has docking sites on its exterior that allow both materials to be digested and the enzymes to carry out the job to be transferred into the lysosome from transport vesicles derived from the Golgi apparatus, the endoplasmic reticulum, or from endocytosis by the plasma membrane. The lysosomal membrane also has transport complexes that allow the final products of digestion such as amino acids, simple sugars, salts, and nucleic acids to be exported back into the cytoplasm, where they can be either excreted or recycled by the cell into new cellular components. Finally, by mechanisms that are not yet fully understood, the lysosomal membrane is able to avoid digestion by the enzymes it contains even though it is composed of the same compounds that those enzymes routinely destroy.

See also Cell membrane transport

180 80